SMALL ANIMAL
CLINICAL NUTRITION
III

LON D. LEWIS, DVM, PhD

MARK L. MORRIS, JR., DVM, PhD

MICHAEL S. HAND, DVM, PhD

MARK MORRIS INSTITUTE
TOPEKA, KANSAS

Dedicated To

MARK L. MORRIS, DVM

Practitioner, Pioneer, Innovator and
Father of Small Animal Clinical Nutrition

LOUISE W. MORRIS

Implementor, Organizer, Stabilizer and
Heart of these Endeavors

and

**THE VETERINARY PRACTITIONERS
OF THE WORLD**

All of Whom Made It Possible

Third Edition
Copyright 1987
Second Printing 1989
Third Printing 1990
Fourth Printing 1992
Fifth Printing 1993
Sixth Printing 1994
MARK MORRIS INSTITUTE
Box 2097
Topeka, Kansas 66601

PREFACE

In order to provide animals and their owners the most beneficial service possible, the practicing veterinarian's emphasis should be on preventive medicine first and disease treatment second. Disease prevention requires proper nutrition, immunization, dental, and parasite control programs throughout life. All, except for proper nutrition, are well covered in many veterinary texts. This text deals with nutrition, which is one of the most important factors in maximizing health, performance, and longevity, and in the management of many diseases. Proper nutrition is as important for the management of diseases, such as renal failure or heart failure, as antimicrobial drugs and vaccines are for the management of infectious diseases. However, nutritional management, like surgery and other aspects of medicine, is of benefit only if it is done properly. It is our hope this book will enhance the veterinarian's ability to use proper dietary management for both prevention and treatment of disease. The book was written for the veterinary student and practitioner, with this goal in mind.

For proper dietary management the veterinarian must know how to feed and care for an animal during all stages of life—in health and in disease. The veterinarian should have knowledge of how nutritional needs vary with each stage of an animal's life, with psychological, physical, and environmental extremes, and with disease. Causes and effects of dietary imbalances, both deficiencies and toxicities, must be known so that the resulting maladies can be diagnosed, treated, and prevented. For proper dietary management, the veterinarian must be familiar with the foods available or those that are commonly fed. This book is intended to provide such information in an organized fashion:

First—Nutrients: their characteristics, functions, use, optimal amounts in the diet, and effects of excesses and deficiencies.

Second—Pet foods: types, forms, determining nutrient content, evaluating quality, factors affecting palatability, and the concepts on which pet foods are marketed.

Third—Methods of feeding and care for maintaining optimal health and longevity, and maximizing performance during reproduction, growth, maintenance, physical exertion, and environmental and psychological stress, including orphans, and healthy or sick neonates.

Fourth—Dietary energy deficiencies and excesses: anorexia, inanition, and critical care nutrition, including fluid and electrolyte therapy, appetite stimulation, force feeding, orogastric, nasogastric, pharyngostomy, gastrostomy, and enterostomy tube feeding, and intravenous feeding. Obesity: incidence, diagnosis, effects, causes, stages, types, treatment, and prevention, including psychology, exercise, caloric restriction, starvation, drugs, and surgery.

Finally—Dietary management of diseases: gastrointestinal, pancreatic, hepatic, renal, cardiac, neuromuscular, and skeletal diseases, and urolithiasis, including causes, pathophysiology, clinical signs, diagnosis, treatment, and dietary management. Although diet may or may not play a role in causing or predisposing to these diseases, diet is important in their proper management.

Many other aspects of medicine, in addition to diet, are necessary for proper clinical management of these diseases. This book covers both dietary and medical management, since both must be used to provide the best possible results. This combination, along with the factors necessary for diagnosis, is what makes this a **clinical** nutrition text, rather than a nutrition text, of which there are many. Clinical nutrition is neither nutrition nor medicine alone—but both together. In nutrition texts the discussion revolves primarily around nutrients because they are the main interest of the intended readers—nutritionists. In a clinical nutrition text, the discussion should revolve around disease prevention and management, because these are the main concerns of the intended readers—future and current veterinary practitioners. We hope that readers will continue to inform us as to additional topics and improvements that will make the book more useful to them and ultimately their clients and patients.

The book concludes with an index for the dietary management of approximately 40 common clinical conditions; a list of specialized diets categorized according to their nutritional characteristics (including diets high or low in a specific nutrient, and hypoallergenic, meat free, soy free, lactose free, gluten free, and additive free diets); a description and nutrient contents of dietary foods, both prepared and homemade (along with recipes); and the nutrient contents of human foods occasionally fed to dogs and cats.

This book is intended as a reference to which the busy practitioner can refer and quickly find methods for optimal feeding and care for healthy or diseased dogs and cats. To further this goal, the Summary of Management Recommendations can be utilized for rapidly determining how to manage a given disease. A more detailed description, and

the reasons for the recommended management practices are provided in the body of the chapter. Although the major aspects needed for the proper total management of the diseases covered are discussed, emphasis is placed on medicine, particularly dietary management. The reader is referred to surgery and pharmacology texts for a more complete discussion of these aspects of therapy. In addition, only clinical nutrition for the dog and cat is covered.

For nutrition of other species, the reader is referred to other sources, such as: "Feeding and Care of the Horse" (Lea and Febiger, 1982); "Zoo and Wild Animal Medicine" (W. B. Saunders, 1986), which includes amphibians, reptiles, bats, birds, ratites, raptors, nonhuman primates, rabbits, rodents, invertebrates, and many other zoo and wild animals; several NRC booklets from the Printing and Publishing Office, Washington, D.C., on amphibians, poultry, wild birds, coturnix, fish, guinea pigs, hamsters, gerbils, mice, voles, rats, mink, foxes, nonhuman primates, and rabbits; "Diseases of Caged and Aviary Birds" (Lea and Febiger, 1982); "Ferrets" (Barron's, 1985); "Captive Turtles" (AMS Publishing, 1982); and numerous texts that cover clinical nutrition for food animals.

We are grateful to, and wish to acknowledge, the many people who contributed to this book. In the past several years, veterinary students in the United States and Canada have made many helpful suggestions, which have been incorporated in this third edition. We owe special thanks to our colleagues, James N. Ross, Jr. and Francis A. Kallfelz, for providing chapters on Heart Failure, and Skeletal and Neuromuscular Diseases; to Charles A. Buffington and Aunna C. Lippert for their help with sections dealing with critical care nutrition; to Stanley M. Teeter, who contributed substantially with assistance in organization of data; and to George G. Doering and his colleagues at Theracon, Inc. for generation of research results.

Several persons contributed in other ways. Our thanks go to: Betty Cleland, who provided the impetus to use word processing by placing the second edition on computer disc; Ray Ottinger, who converted our writings to reasonable English grammar; and John Ives, and his cohorts at H. M. Ives & Sons who patiently worked with us and were responsible for layout and printing. We owe a special debt to Karen Smith, who typed relentlessly and to Mary Raines who proofed draft after draft and somehow managed to find order in the chaos of revised manuscripts and references, always knowing where something was that we were sure was lost.

Finally, we are forever grateful for Nancy, Bette, Ruth and our families who sacrificed all those nights and weekends so that this book could be a reality. We appreciate your patience and support.

Lon D. Lewis   Mark L. Morris, Jr.   Michael S. Hand

AUTHORS

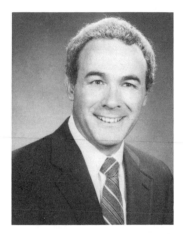

Lon D. Lewis, DVM, PhD

Dr. Lon D. Lewis received a B.S. in chemical engineering from the University of Wyoming and a D.V.M. from Colorado State University. After several years of operating his own veterinary practice he returned to Colorado State University, where he received a Ph.D. in physiology. Two years of research and study were conducted at the Universities of Lund, Sweden and Texas Medical Schools. For eight years he was Professor of Clinical Nutrition in the Veterinary Teaching Hospital at Colorado State University before joining the clinical nutrition research group, Mark Morris Associates. He is the author of over a hundred scientific papers, numerous chapters in several veterinary textbooks and the book "Feeding and Care of the Horse." He has conducted research on canine obesity, intestinal absorption, cerebral energy metabolism, hypoglycemia, hypoxia and equine nutrition, but is best known for his research on the role of diet in the etiology and clinical management of feline urolithiasis and nutrient, fluid and electrolyte needs in diarrhea, for which he has developed several widely used products. He has consulted with veterinarians and animal owners throughout the world in providing nutritionally sound feeding programs for animals under a wide variety of situations. He teaches clinical nutrition at several veterinary schools, is an adjunct professor at two, and lectures widely at both domestic and international veterinary meetings. He received the American Feed Manufacturers' nutritional research award in 1980, and the Norden distinguished teaching award in 1982.

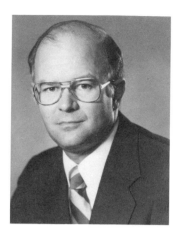

Mark L. Morris, Jr., DVM, PhD

Dr. Mark L. Morris, Jr. was reared in the small animal hospital built by his father, and by cleaning cages and feeding sick dogs and cats became aware at an early age of the importance of diet in the management of clinical diseases. He received his D.V.M. degree from Cornell University, and M.S. and Ph. D. degrees from the University of Wisconsin in veterinary pathology and biochemistry, in which he described the lesions associated with taurine deficiency in the cat and magnesium deficiency in the dog. He is an adjunct professor at Cornell University, heads the clinical nutrition research group, Mark Morris Associates and serves as Research Vice President of the Morris Animal Foundation, the leading independent sponsor of companion animal research. He has authored numerous publications on dietary management of disease, and lectured widely, both domestically and internationally, to veterinary students, practicing veterinarians and companion animal owners. The dietary foods his organization develops are found throughout the world, and have been used for over 40 years by veterinarians to manage and prevent a wide variety of diseases of dogs and cats. His research on the dietary needs of military working dogs led to the development of the medicated food used by U.S. Armed Forces to properly nourish guard dogs and, at the same time, prevent heartworms and intestinal parasites. His revolutionary approach to zoo nutrition has led to the widespread use of prepared diets in feeding exotic animals in captivity, which has led to the conservation of several endangered species. In addition to his own research endeavors, he heads a private research laboratory which provides testing services for the pet food industry. He is one of the few veterinarians in the world that has an intimate knowledge and understanding of the pet food industry, but is not employed by a pet food company.

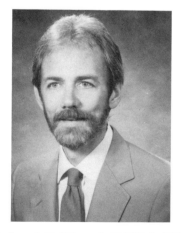

Michael S, Hand, DVM, PhD

Dr. Michael S. Hand received his D.V.M. from Colorado State University. He spent 10 years in a mixed practice. During this time he served as an instructor in the state college animal health technician program, was a member of the public school board, and was a recipient of the Outstanding Young Men of America award. He returned to Colorado State University where he received a Ph.D. in physiology and the C.S.U. Teaching Award. After 3 years as Associate Professor of Clinical Nutrition at the School of Veterinary Medicine at North Carolina State University, he joined the clinical nutrition research group, Mark Morris Associates. He has conducted research on sepsis, diabetes mellitus, the effects of alcohol on the response to trauma, and critical care nutrition. He is adjunct professor at two veterinary colleges. He has lectured at numerous state and national meetings and has consulted on nutritional problems with veterinarians and animal owners in the United States and abroad. He has authored over 25 scientific papers and 10 veterinary textbook chapters.

Small Animal Clinical Nutrition

CONTENTS

CHAPTER 1

Nutrients

CONTENTS

INTRODUCTION

Proper diet is among the more important considerations in health maintenance and is essential in the management of many diseases. To feed correctly or to properly advise on feeding, a knowledge of dietary nutrients and their availability is important. This chapter presents a discussion of nutrients and their use. Chapters two through four deal with the types of foods available and feeding management programs for maintaining optimal health. Subsequent chapters cover nutritional causes and management of disease.

A nutrient is any food constituent that helps support life. Nutrients accomplish this by performing a number of functions, including:

1. Acting as structural components of the body
2. Enhancing or being involved in chemical reactions that occur in the body (metabolism)
3. Transporting of substances into, throughout, or out of the body
4. Regulating temperature
5. Affecting food palatability and, therefore, consumption
6. Supplying energy

Nutrients are divided into six basic classes:
1. Water
2. Carbohydrates
3. Proteins
4. Fats
5. Minerals
6. Vitamins

Some nutrients fulfill a number of functions. For example, water and several minerals are needed for all of the functions listed, except supplying energy. Carbohydrates, fats, and proteins may all be used for energy but they are structural components as well. In contrast, vitamins are involved primarily in metabolic functions.

Although all nutrients are necessary for health, their absolute requirements vary. Following are the nutrients listed in the order of the amount needed.

1. Water—At rest in a comfortable environmental temperature, two to three parts of water are required per part of dietary dry matter.
2. Energy-yielding nutrients (carbohydrates, fats and proteins)—Approximately 50-80% of dry matter intake is used for energy.

3. Protein—Amount needed varies inversely with the digestibility and essential amino acid content (quality) of the protein. In nonprescription commercial pet foods, crude protein ranges from 20-50% of the diet dry matter.
4. Minerals—Total mineral requirements comprise about 2-3% of the diet dry matter.
5. Vitamins—Vitamin requirements are met at levels constituting 0.2-0.3% of the diet dry matter.

The order of nutrient precedence, or importance for body function, relates directly to the amount of that nutrient needed in the diet. Nutritional adequacy of the diet should always be evaluated in the order listed above.

WATER

Water is the most important nutrient. An animal can survive after losing almost all of its glycogen and storage fat and half of its protein, but a 10% loss of total body water causes serious illness; a 15% loss results in death.

Animals have two basic sources of water: metabolic and ingested. Metabolic water results when oxygen combines with hydrogen ions cleaved from carbohydrates, proteins or fats when they are used for energy. Approximately 10-16g of water are generated for each 100 kcal of energy utilized. Ingested water is that acquired by drinking or eating. Because the water contents of pet foods vary, pet foods are categorized accordingly into dry (6-10% water), soft-moist (23-40% water) or canned (68-78% water) forms. When the amount of water consumed in food increases, the amount the animal drinks decreases. Thus, total water intake is independent of the diet's water content.

The total amount of water consumed, if the water is readily available and palatable, is more than the amount required for maintenance. **The water requirement of the dog or cat, expressed in ml/day, is roughly equivalent to the energy requirement in kcal/day.** This relationship exists because, in the healthy animal, changes in water requirement are due primarily to water loss from urinary excretion of metabolic wastes and thermoregulatory activity. Both of these factors are directly affected by energy utilization. The amount of water consumed by mature, healthy, nonreproducing dogs and cats at a comfortable environmental temperature is about 2.5 times the amount of dry matter consumed in food. Water consumption increases with:

1. Habit
2. Increased salt or electrolyte intake
3. Anything that increases body water loss, such as increased thermoregulatory activity associated with physical exertion, increased ambient temperature, pyrexia, lactation, diarrhea, hemorrhage, or polyuria.

For practical feeding purposes, water of good quality should **always** be available. An exception is during persistent vomiting. In case of persistent vomiting, a period of approximately 24 hours with nothing consumed orally is recommended. Inadequate water intake reduces food intake, thereby adversely affecting production (physical activity, reproduction, lactation, or growth). Decreased water intake may result from reduced availability, improper temperature (too warm or too cold) or poor quality.

The amount of **total dissolved solids (TDS)** provides a useful overall index to the quality of drinking water. Total dissolved solids is the concentration of all constituents dissolved in water and is the most reliable parameter by which water can be evaluated.[58] Water containing less than 5000 parts per million (ppm or mg/liter) TDS is generally considered acceptable, whereas more than 7000 ppm is considered unsuitable for livestock or poultry.[58] Dogs and cats are usually allowed access to tap water. Water suitable for human consumption is also suitable for dogs and cats. Besides TDS, excessive amounts of some specific contaminates may make the water unsuitable for consumption, either because of a direct effect on the body after consumption or, indirectly, by decreasing the palatability of water and therefore, consumption.

The term "salinity" as applied to fresh water is often used synonymously with TDS. However, these terms are not synonymous with hardness. The **hardness** of water indicates its tendency to precipitate soap or to form a scale on heated surfaces. Highly saline water may contain small amounts of the cations responsible for hardness. Hardness is often expressed as the sum of calcium and magnesium reported in equivalent amounts of calcium carbonate. Other cations, such as strontium, iron, aluminum, zinc, and manganese, also contribute to water hardness. Cations such as sodium and potassium do not contribute. Hard water, containing high amounts of magnesium, has been implicated as a cause of urinary calculi. However, the amount of magnesium consumed in drinking water is insignificant compared to the amount consumed in the diet. The magnesium content of food is measured in parts per hundred (%) whereas that of water is measured in parts per million (a 10,000-fold difference).

ENERGY

The nutrients that provide energy are carbohydrates, fats, and proteins (Figure 1). Excepting water, dietary energy is the most critical item to be considered in nutrition.

All living things are solar-powered. As described by the first law of thermodynamics, energy can be changed from one form to another but is neither created nor destroyed. The energy in sunlight is captured by plants and, via photosynthesis, is stored as energy nutrients (carbohydrates, proteins, and fats) in the plants. Animals eat plants or other animals that have eaten plants. The energy nutrients in plants are digested, absorbed and transported to individual body cells. In these cells, chemical reactions transfer the energy stored in the nutrients to high energy phosphate compounds (e.g. adenosine triphosphate [ATP]) and heat. Cells can use the energy derived from these compounds for pumping ions, for molecular synthesis and/or to activate contractile proteins. The sum of these three processes (and heat production) essentially describes total energy expenditure by an animal.

Energy has no measurable dimension or mass, but it can be converted to heat, which can be measured. Thus, the energy available in food can be determined by the complete combustion or burning of a sample of the food (i.e. oxidizing the nutrients) in a bomb calorimeter and measuring the heat produced. The heat produced, called "the heat of combustion," represents the gross energy content of the food. The amount of heat required to raise the temperature of 1ml of water from 14.5-15.5°C is defined as 1 calorie. One kilocalorie (kcalorie, kcal

FIGURE 1

ENERGY-SUPPLYING NUTRIENTS
CHEMICAL COMPOSITION AND END PRODUCTS OF METABOLISM

Nutrient	Chemical Composition	End Products When Used for Energy
Protein	H_2N–CH–CO ———————— [NH–CH–CO] ———————— NH–CH–COOH | | | Alpha Carbon → R_1 R n R_2 N-Terminal Amino Acid Peptide Bond Many Amino Acids Peptide Bond Carboxyl Amino Acid R = different chemical groups and thus different amino acids.	Carbon dioxide (CO_2) Water (H_2O) Ammonia (NH_3) which is converted to urea (H_2N–CO–NH_2) in the liver and excreted by the kidney.

Carbohydrate	HCO
	  |
	(HCOH)$_{1-4}$
	  |
	H_2COH
	
	Monosaccharides, e.g. glucose (dextrose), fructose, and galactose 2 Monosaccharides = 1 Disaccharide. e.g., glucose + glucose = maltose
	glucose + fructose = sucrose (table sugar)
	glucose + galactose = lactose (milk sugar).
	
	Many Monosaccharides = Polysaccharides, e.g. starch, glycogen, and fiber are many glucose molecules connected by alpha bonds or for fiber, beta bonds.
		Carbon dioxide (CO_2)
		
		Water (H_2O)

Fat	H_2CO———— (CH)———— COOH
	  | 16–20
	HCO———— (CH)———— COOH
	  | 16–20
	H_2CO———— (CH)———— COOH
	           16–20
	Glycerol 3 Fatty acids
	Triglyceride
		Carbon dioxide (CO_2)
		
		Water (H_2O)

or Calorie) is equal to 1000 calories. In nutrition, use of the word calorie always refers to the term kilocalorie. Occasionally the terms megacalorie, therm or joule are used. One megacalorie and 1 therm equal 1000 kcal, and 1 kilocalorie equals 4186 joules.

As shown in Figure 2, an animal cannot use all of the gross energy in food. Some is lost in the feces, urine, and the combustible gases produced during fermentation. Only the remaining energy, called "net energy," is available for maintenance and production (work, growth, gestation, lactation). The net energy is used first for maintenance. If additional energy is available, production can occur.

After an animal's initial adjustment to the palatability of the diet, the average amount of food consumed will be the amount necessary to meet the animal's energy requirement. Thus, to ensure intake of the proper amount of non-energy nutrients, they

FIGURE 2

PARTITION OF ENERGY IN NUTRITION

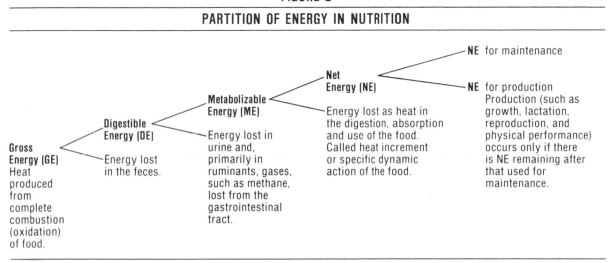

FIGURE 3

EFFECT OF CALORIC DENSITY OF THE DIET ON THE AMOUNT CONSUMED

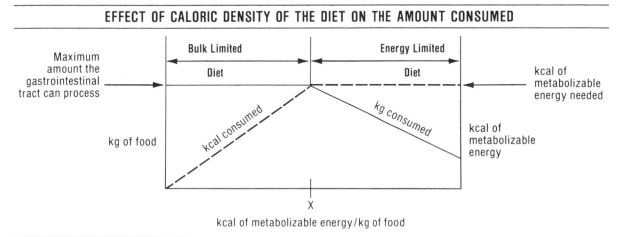

With a diet containing less than X kcal/kg the animal eats the maximum amount its gastrointestinal tract will hold but is unable to meet its energy requirement. Thus, the amount of food eaten is bulk-limited. As the energy content of the diet increases up to point X, the animal continues to eat the same amount of food but gets more energy. With a diet containing more than X kcal/kg, the animal eats until its energy requirement is met and quits. Thus, less food is eaten the higher its energy content, i.e., food intake is energy-limited. Some animals may eat more than their energy requirement, particularly if the diet is especially palatable, which will result in obesity.

should be balanced relative to the energy density of the diet. Thus, when the amount of the diet consumed meets the animal's energy needs, the requirements for non-energy nutrients are automatically met. However, if the energy density of the diet is inadequate, gastrointestinal capacity will limit diet intake before the animal's energy requirement is satisfied. In this instance, the diet is said to be "bulk limited" since, as illustrated in Figure 3, the amount of diet consumed is limited by the bulk or amount of the diet the gastrointestinal tract can process.

If the non-energy nutrients are balanced relative to the energy density of a bulk-limited diet, deficiencies of all nutrients will occur. This happens most commonly during growth and lactation when a poor-quality, low-energy commercial pet food, or a food formulated for maintenance, is fed. In an attempt to meet its energy requirement, the animal consumes large quantities of the food. As a result, puppies and kittens consuming these diets have distended abdomens and exhibit slow growth and underdevelopment of musculoskeletal tissue. Lactating females lose weight and produce inadequate amounts of milk, resulting in poor growth, or even death, of neonates. Certain diets intended to correct or prevent obesity are designed to be bulk-limited for energy nutrients, but not for non-energy nutrients.

When the energy density of a diet is high enough that an animal can consume a sufficient amount of the diet to meet its energy needs, the main factor determining the amount of diet consumed is the diet's energy density (Fig 3). This type of diet is said to be "energy-limiting." Increasing the energy density of a previously balanced diet by supplementing it with large amounts of fat and/or carbohydrate can result in deficiencies of non-energy nutrients. This occurs because the animal usually stops eating after its energy requirement has been met.

Feeding the amount needed to meet the animal's energy requirement provides the proper amount of all nutrients needed if the diet is correctly balanced. The amount to feed can be determined by dividing the animal's energy requirement by the energy density of the food.

DETERMINATION OF THE ENERGY REQUIREMENT

Basal energy expenditure is the amount of energy used following sleep, 12-18 hours after food consumption, and during thermoneutral conditions.[42]

It is also referred to as the **basal metabolic rate** (basal energy requirement [BER]). **Resting metabolic rate** (resting energy requirement [RER]) differs from BER because it includes energy expended for recovery from physical activity. Depending on the level of activity and the time between cessation of activity and determination of metabolic rate, RER may range from almost the same as BER to as much as 25% higher.[41] **Maintenance energy requirement (MER)** is the amount of energy used by a moderately active adult animal in a thermoneutral environment. It includes energy expended for obtaining and using food in amounts necessary to maintain body weight, but would not support additional physical activity or production such as growth, gestation or lactation.[54] The MER for the dog is approximately twice BER,[56] whereas MER for the cat is about 1.4 times BER[36] (65 to 70 kcal metabolizable energy/kg/day for inactive domestic cats[55]). The lower MER value for cats may be because they are generally more quiet and reserved than dogs. Cats have been reported to spend as much as 15-16 hours per day sleeping.[60] It is most practical to determine BER first, and then estimate MER from BER.

Most of the energy used by the body is given off as heat. The main avenue of heat loss under basal conditions is via radiation and convection from the body surface.[4] Therefore, the energy expended is directly related to body surface area. Basal energy requirement is approximately 1000 kcal per square meter of body surface area.[41] The smaller the animal, the greater the body surface area per unit of body weight.[40] Thus, the smaller the animal, the greater its rate of heat loss and BER per unit of body weight. This discrepancy in surface area per unit of weight can vary widely among breeds of dogs. A dog weighing 2.5 kg has 300% more surface area per kilogram than a dog weighing 50 kg.[59]

Determination of surface area requires the use of a weight to surface area conversion table[59] or the use of rather unwieldy formulas using body weight and length measurements.[40] However, body surface area is directly related to kilograms of body weight to the 0.75 power ($Wt_{kg}^{0.75}$) which is referred to as "metabolic body size."[40] This value can be determined by cubing the number and then taking its square root twice. Basal metabolic rate is approximately 70 metabolizable kcal/day kg metabolic body size, i.e. $70(Wt_{kg})^{0.75}$ Data indicate that although this formula provides a reasonable interspecies estimate for BER, it is less accurate within species in which large variability in body size occurs, such as the dog. Also, fractional exponents are awkward to use.

A linear equation has been derived that appears to be more accurate and is simpler to use. **For dogs and cats weighing more than 2 kg, BER (metabolizable kcal/day) = 30Wt$_{kg}$ +70.** The equation is derived from a linear formula for determining canine MER, where canine MER (metabolizable kcal/day) = 62.2 Wt$_{kg}$ + 144.4.[57] Since canine BER is one-half MER, BER = 31.1 Wt$_{kg}$ + 72.2; or simplified, canine BER = 30Wt$_{kg}$ + 70. When this equation is applied to the average sized domestic cat (2.7 to 5kg), a mean of 50 kcal/kg/day is obtained for BER, as compared to 52.2 kcal/kg/day derived by indirect calorimetry.[17] Because there is little variation in the body weight of mature domestic cats, feline BER may simply be assumed to equal 50 metabolizable kcal/kg/day.

Energy requirements of sick or injured patients are a function of BER since these animals are usually resting indoors in a thermoneutral environment (in a cage). Excluding the metabolic burden of disease, these animals have an energy expenditure near basal. However, surgery, trauma, sepsis, or burn impose varying degrees of hypermetabolism[28,39] and appropriate increases in BER (discussed in Chapter 5). In contrast, energy requirements for weight control or various physiologic states, such as growth, gestation, lactation, stress, and different levels of physical activity, are more closely related to maintenance energy needs and, therefore, are factored from MER (Table 1).

TABLE 1

WATER AND METABOLIZABLE ENERGY REQUIREMENTS

Daily Maintenance Requirement*		Factors To Be Applied To Maintenance Energy Requirement (MER)* To Obtain Daily Energy Requirement For:
Dog Body Weight	Water (ml)** Energy (kcal)**	
(lb)	(per lb)	Work—1 hour light work (hunting) = 1.1 × MER+
6	50	1 full day light work = 1.4–1.5 × MER
12	40	1 full day heavy work (sled dog) = 2–4 × MER
20	35	Inactivity = 0.8 × MER (dog)
50 or more	30	Gestation—first 6 weeks = 1 × MER
(kg)	(per kg)	last 3 weeks = 1.1–1.3 × MER
3	110	Peak Lactation—3–6 weeks = [1 + 0.25 (number in litter)] × MER
6	85	= 2–4 × MER
10	75	Growth —Birth to 3 mo. = 2 × MER
25 or more	65	3 mo. to 6 mo. = 1.6 × MER
		6 mo. to 12 mo. = 1.2 × MER
Cat		3 mo. to 9 mo. (giant dog breeds) = 1.6 × MER
6–12 lb inactive = 30/lb		9 mo. to 24 mo. (giant dog breeds) = 1.2 × MER
active = 40/lb		Cold—wind-chill factor of 8.5°C (47°F) = 1.25 × MER
2.5–5.5 kg inactive = 65–70/kg		subfreezing wind-chill factor = 1.75 × MER[10]
active = 85/kg		Heat—tropical climates = up to 2.5 × MER
		++Disease = BER* × appropriate disease factor

*Maintenance energy requirement (MER) includes basal energy requirement (BER) plus energy expended for obtaining and utilizing food in order to maintain body weight in a thermoneutral environment. Determine the caloric requirement for MER from tabulated data above or calculate:

Dogs over 2 kg—MER (metabolizable kcal/day) = 2 (30 wt$_{kg}$ + 70).
Cats over 2 kg—MER (metabolizable kcal/day) = 1.4 (30 wt$_{kg}$ + 70).
                                    or
All dogs—MER (metabolizable kcal/day) = 2 [70 (wt$_{kg}^{0.75}$)].
All cats—MER (metabolizable kcal/day) = 1.4 [70 (wt$_{kg}^{0.75}$)].

Multiply MER by the appropriate factor to obtain the approximate daily energy requirement for a given situation (see Table 5, p. 1–9).

Interpolate between these values to get the approximate amount needed for a dog of any size. These values should be used only as an approximation of the needs. Many factors, such as environmental conditions, activity, stage of life and temperament, alter the amount needed. There is also much individual variation. Good-quality water should always be readily available. For long-term feeding adjust the amount fed to **maintain optimal body weight and condition, i.e., so the ribs cannot be seen but are easily felt with no appreciable subcutaneous or abdominal fat evident, and so that most breeds have some indentation behind the rib cage when viewed from above. This may require substantially more or less food than the amount calculated.

+Based on running at 8 km (5 mi) for 1 hr on a 6% incline.

++See Table 3, page 5–12 or Figure 6, page 5–13.

DETERMINATION OF
FOOD ENERGY DENSITY

The caloric density of a food must be known in order to determine the amount of that food an animal must consume to meet its energy requirement. The average caloric densities of popular, private label and generic brands of pet foods are listed in Table 2. Products referred to as premium brand foods were not included in these averages because their energy content is usually higher (a description of brand categories is given on page 2-15). Some manufacturers specify the energy content of their products. The Association of American Feed Control Officials (AAFCO), an association of state officials responsible for regulating commercially prepared animal foods, has designated that if the energy content of a pet food is reported, it will be as metabolizable energy. However, it is not required that the energy content of a pet food be stated, and usually this information is not made available. Even if the energy content is specified, it may not be in units of metabolizable energy.

Any energy unit may be used to determine the amount to feed, as long as the animal's energy requirement is stated in the same unit. However, if no energy terms are provided (e.g. gross, digestible, metabolizable, or net), the product information should not be used. If the animal's energy requirement is established as metabolizable energy, and the caloric density of the food is reported as digestible energy, the metabolizable energy content can be estimated. If the food contains 10% protein (dry matter basis), or less, multiply the digestible energy value by 0.97. If the food contains 50% protein or more (dry matter basis), multiply the digestible energy value by 0.88. For foods that contain intermediate amounts of protein, interpolate accordingly. The higher the protein content of the diet, the greater the difference between its digestible and metabolizable energy content. This is due to energy lost in the urine as urea (Figure 2, page 1-7). Loss of energy due to the production of combustible gases is negligible in dogs and cats.

If the caloric density of a food is not known, it can be calculated using the following formula: caloric density = energy provided by each nutrient × the amount of that nutrient in the food. The gross calories generated when proteins, fats or carbohydrates are completely oxidized are 5.65, 9.4 and 4.15 kcal/g, respectively. However, only the portion of these energy nutrients that is digested, absorbed and retained, is available for metabolism. When protein is used for energy, the constituent amino acids are deaminated, and the ammonia is combined with carbon dioxide in the liver to form

TABLE 2

ESTIMATED ENERGY CONTENT OF PET FOODS*

Type and Form of Food	Metabolizable Energy Content (kcal/unit as fed)
Dog Food:	
Dry	350/8 oz measuring cup**
Soft-moist	425/6 oz package
	275/8 oz measuring cup**
Canned	500/14–15 oz can
	250/6–6.5 oz can
Cat Food:	
Dry	300/8 oz measuring cup**
Soft-moist	110/1.5 oz package
	250/8 oz measuring cup**
Canned	400/14–15 oz can
	180/6–6.5 oz can
	85/3 oz can

*Estimates made from averages of laboratory analyses of 120 commercial pet foods including generic, private label, and popular brands sold in grocery stores. Premium-brand foods were excluded. Note that considerable variability may exist between products.

**An 8 oz (volume) measuring cup holds 3–3.5 oz by weight (85 to 100g) of most dry foods or 3.5–5 oz by weight (100 to 150g) of most soft-moist foods.

urea (H_2N-CO-NH_2), which is excreted in the urine. Urea contains 5.4 kcal of gross energy/g. This decreases the energy available from protein from 5.65 kcal/g to 4.4 kcal/g.[25] As shown in Table 3, when urinary energy losses are factored out, the metabolizable energy provided by each energy nutrient is the gross energy available from that nutrient multiplied by the digestibility of the nutrient. Often the digestibility of these nutrients is not known and estimates of digestibility must be made. When the digestibility of protein is 91%, and the digestibility of fat and soluble carbohydrate is 96%, these nutrients provide the commonly used values of 4, 9 and 4 metabolizable kcal/g, respectively. These are referred to as the Atwater factors and are accurate for human subjects consuming specified diets.[25] However, the digestibility of energy nutrients is less in average-quality pet foods consumed by dogs and cats. This results in factors lower than those of Atwater (see Table 3). The appropriate digestibility factor must be multiplied by the amount of the energy nutrient in the food to determine the amount of metabolizable energy supplied by that nutrient. The sum of these products gives the energy density of the food. This is demonstrated by the example shown in Table 4. The only accurate way to determine the nutrient content of a food is by laboratory analysis. Some manufacturers provide

TABLE 3

ENERGY AVAILABLE FROM PROTEIN, FAT AND SOLUBLE CARBOHYDRATE

Species	Metabolizable Energy (kcal/g)		
	Crude Protein	Crude Fat	Soluble Carbohydrate (NFE)
All*	4.4 × digestibility*	9.4 × digestibility*	4.15 × digestibility*
Dogs[38,56]**	3.5	8.7	3.5
Cats[37]**+	3.9	7.7	3.0
Humans[25]**	4	9	4

*The most accurate value to use when the digestibility of the nutrient is known.

**Available to human subjects consuming specified diets and to dogs and cats consuming average quality commercial dog and cat foods, respectively. This includes dry, soft-moist and canned forms of pet foods. More energy is provided by nutrients from better quality pet foods and less from poorer quality pet foods.

+The most accurate estimate of metabolizable energy available to the cat from average quality dry cat foods is:[37] Kcal/100g food (as fed) = 0.84 [(% protein × 4.4) + (% fat × 9.4) + (% soluble carbohydrate × 4.15)] − 60.

analytical information, or food samples can be analyzed by commercial laboratories. If an analysis of a given food is not available, the guaranteed analysis, required by law on all pet food labels, may be used. **However, the guaranteed analysis is not the same as the actual analysis of a food.** The guaranteed analysis simply indicates that the diet contains at least, or not more than, the amounts stated. In addition, the label guarantee sometimes is not even met. If the guaranteed analysis on the label is used for calculating energy density, multiply the resulting energy density by 1.2 for canned pet foods and 1.1 for soft-moist or dry pet foods. These factors were established from comparisons between

TABLE 4

EXAMPLE CALCULATION OF CALORIC DENSITY OF A PET FOOD

Analysis			Metabolizable Energy		
Nutrient	%	×	(kcal/g of nutrient)*	=	kcal/100 g of diet
Protein	22	×	3.5	=	77.0
Fat	9	×	8.7	=	78.3
Fiber**	3	×	0	=	0
Moisture	10	×	0	=	0
Ash**	5	×	0	=	0
Soluble Carbohydrate (NFE)***	51	×	3.5	=	178.5
				Total	333.8+

% protein calories = 77 ÷ 333.8 = 23%

3.338 kcal/g × amount of food/measuring cup = kcal/measuring cup++

*From Table 3.

**If not available these may be estimated as 3% fiber and 9% ash in dry foods, 1% fiber and 6% ash in soft-moist foods, and 1% fiber and 2.5% ash in canned foods.

***Percent NFE (nitrogen free extract or soluble carbohydrate) usually is not stated but can be calculated by subtracting the percent protein, fat, fiber, moisture, and ash from 100 (see Figure 2, page 2-6).

+If the nutrient percentages were obtained from the label guarantee, multiply the diet caloric density by 1.2 for canned pet foods and 1.1 for soft-moist and dry pet foods. In this example, 333.8 × 1.1 = 367 kcal/100g of dry diet.

++An 8 oz (volume) measuring cup holds 3 to 3.5 oz by weight (85 to 100g) of most dry pet foods or 3.5 to 5 oz by weight (100 to 150g) of most soft-moist pet foods. It is more accurate to use the average weight of three individual measuring cups of food in determining kcal/cup.

TABLE 5

EXAMPLE CALCULATIONS OF AMOUNT OF FOOD TO FEED

Animal	Wt (lb)		Energy Needs*				Total Daily Energy Need (kcal/animal/day)		Energy Density of Food**		Amount of Food Needed Daily
			Maintenance Energy (MER) (kcal/lb/day)	Situation	Increased Need (Factor)						
Cat	7	×	30	Maintenance	1	=	210	÷	300 kcal/cup	=	0.7 cup
Kitten (4 mo)	4	×	38***	Growth	1.6	=	243	÷	180 kcal/6 oz can	=	1⅓ can
Dog	13	×	40	Active	1.1	=	570	÷	500 kcal/14 oz can	=	1.1 can
Dog	50	×	30	Peak Lactation (6 puppies)	2.5	=	3750	÷	350 kcal/cup	=	10.7 cups
Puppy (4 mo)	20	×	35	Growth	1.6	=	1120	÷	475 kcal/can	=	2.35 cans

*Obtain from Table 1, page 1-6.
**Obtain from Table 3, page 1-8 or Table 4, page 1-8.
***Calculated from Table 1, page 1-6.

caloric densities derived from label guarantees and laboratory analyses of 120 different pet foods. These factors improve the accuracy of an energy density calculated from a guaranteed analysis, because pet foods usually contain more protein and fat, and less water, fiber, and ash than are listed on the label. The ingredients are listed this way to ensure the product meets its label guarantee.

ESTIMATION OF FOOD DOSAGE

Four steps are involved in calculating estimated food dosage:

1. Calculate basal metabolic rate (BER) as required for hospitalized patients (page 1-5 or Figure 6, page 5-13) and maintenance energy requirement (MER) for all others (page 1-5 or Table 1, page 1-6).

2. Multiply BER or MER by the appropriate factor to determine the estimated energy requirement (Table 3, page 5-12 or Table 1, page 1-6, respectively).

3. Select the food to be fed and determine its energy density Tables 10, 11, 12 & 13, Chapter 5, for hospitalized patients or Table 2, page 1-7 or Table 4, page 1-8 for normal dogs and cats).

4. Divide the estimated energy requirement by the energy density of the food to obtain daily food dosage.

Sample calculations of estimated amounts to feed are given in Table 5.

Although food dosages can be estimated, the efficiency of food utilization varies among individuals due to differences in psychologic temperament, level of physical activity, body condition, insulative characteristics of the hair coat, and differences in external environment.[56,57] Even when environmental conditions and physical activity are similar, individual variability exists. Several different studies have provided data on the amount of dietary energy consumed by mature, nonreproducing dogs and cats kept in cages or runs under similar environmental conditions and maintaining body weight. As shown in Figure 4, with the average energy consumed set at 100%, in 95% of 120 dogs it varied from 65% to 135% (range 43-152%); in 95% of 76 cats it varied from 61% to 139% (range 50-146%). Thus, the amount of food needed by both dogs and cats for maintenance, even under similar environmental conditions and when kept in cages or runs, varies three-fold. Even when the extremes are excluded (the top and bottom 2.5%) the amount needed varies more than two-fold.

Therefore, **a calculated food dosage should only be considered an estimate or starting point, or an amount to feed for a short time (few days).** Start with the estimate. Then adjust the amount fed to produce optimal body condition. Optimal condition is when the ribs cannot be seen but can readily be felt. Rapidly growing puppies may normally appear somewhat thin. Overweight cats tend to accumulate excess subcutaneous and abdominal fat which is especially visible along the underline (Chapter 6).

FIGURE 4

VARIATION IN ENERGY REQUIREMENT FOR BODY WEIGHT MAINTENANCE IN DOGS AND CATS*

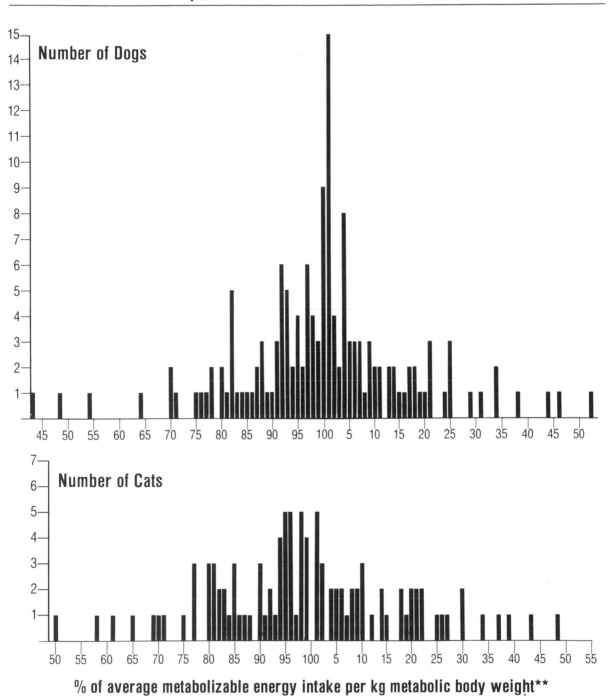

% of average metabolizable energy intake per kg metabolic body weight**

*Data were collected from 120 dogs and 76 cats kept under similar conditions and fed the amount of a variety of commercial pet foods necessary to maintain their body weight.

**For explanation of metabolizable energy see Figure 2, page 1–4. For explanation of metabolic body weight (size) see page 1-5.

ENERGY IMBALANCES

Chronic excessive energy intake by the growing pup can increase the risk of development of metabolic bone disease (Chapters 3 and 12) and/or may predispose to obesity throughout life (Chapters 3 and 6). Excessive energy intake by the mature dog or cat can cause obesity (Chapter 6). Inadequate energy intake is usually accompanied by insufficient intake of non-energy nutrients. Inadequate energy intake most commonly occurs during lactation or other period of high-energy need (Chapters 3 and 4). It is common in hospitalized pets and may compromise recovery from disease or injury if not treated (Chapter 5).

CARBOHYDRATES

Dietary carbohydrates provide energy and affect gastrointestinal function. Some question exists regarding the need of dogs and cats for dietary carbohydrate. From a practical sense, the answer to this question is of little importance because there are carbohydrates in most food ingredients used in commercially prepared dog and cat foods.

Carbohydrates are often classified into either of two groups, based on their solubility (digestibility) characteristics. Monosaccharides are considered soluble because they require no digestion. They are the only carbohydrates that can be absorbed and, therefore, used by the animal. Monosaccharides can have either alpha or beta configuration. Carbohydrates consisting of alpha monosaccharide units link together through alpha bonds (e.g. starch) and are very different in physical structure from those comprised of beta monosaccharide units, which link together through beta bonds (e.g. cellulose). Carbohydrates consisting of alpha monosaccharide units are readily digested by endogenous enzymes (digestive enzymes actually produced by the animal) and are called **"soluble carbohydrates."**

The carbohydrates comprised of beta monosaccharide units resist the action of endogenous digestive enzymes and are called **"insoluble carbohydrates."** However, microbes that inhabit specialized areas of the gastrointestinal tract secrete enzymes (cellulases) that digest insoluble carbohydrates; then they ferment the constituent monosaccharides to carbon dioxide, combustible gases, and volatile fatty acids.

Volatile fatty acids are a significant source of energy for herbivorous animals. However, microbial digestive/fermentative capacity is severely limited in non-herbivores, such as the dog and cat, because they have no rumen and only a relatively small, simple, large intestine. Thus, dietary insol-uble carbohydrates provide no significant amount of energy to the dog and cat. In fact, they reduce the energy density of a diet by displacing soluble carbohydrate, protein, or fat.

Therefore, diets high in insoluble carbohydrates are inappropriate for dogs and cats that have high energy requirements (growth, late gestation, lactation, stress, work). However, the dietary energy restriction imposed by high levels of insoluble carbohydrate is appropriate in diets designed for weight reduction or weight control. Soluble carbohydrates are also referred to as nitrogen-free extract (NFE) due to a commonly used analytical method by which it is determined in a food as described in Figure 2, page 2-6.

The alpha bond in all carbohydrates, excepting disaccharides, is cleaved by the digestive enzyme amylase. This enzyme is secreted by the pancreas and, in some species, in small amounts by the salivary gland. The final alpha bond connecting the two monosaccharides making up a disaccharide is cleaved by a disaccharidase, such as maltase, isomaltase, sucrase or lactase. These enzymes are not secreted. Instead, they are an integral part of the intestinal epithelial cell brush border.

If the brush border is lost, as with enteritis, or there is a lack of these enzymes, the animal cannot use the disaccharides. In these circumstances, the disaccharides remain in the intestinal lumen, where they may be used by bacteria. This action leads to intestinal bacterial overgrowth and an increase in the osmolality of luminal fluid . The result is an osmotic gradient for fluid flow into the gut that can cause diarrhea. For this reason, an animal may be unable to tolerate carbohydrates other than monosaccharides for several days after enteritis. It is also why excessive consumption of milk, which is high in lactose, may cause diarrhea. The occurrence of diarrhea does not necessarily mean that milk cannot be fed, but that the amount fed should be reduced. (See page 7-42.)

Soluble carbohydrates supply relatively inexpensive calories and comprise a moderately high percentage of most pet foods other than those composed entirely of meat, fish, or organ tissues. Because of the calories they provide, dietary carbohydrates play an important role in sparing dietary protein. In this way dietary protein can be used to meet the animal's amino acid requirements rather than its energy needs. Carbohydrates exceeding the amount needed to meet the animal's energy requirements are stored in the body as glycogen or fat, for later use. Thus, obesity is the only effect of excess usable carbohydrate intake. In general, the absence of dietary carbohydrate will not affect blood glucose

levels or cause an energy deficiency; this is because the body can use protein and the glycerol portion of fat for glucose production, and fat and protein for energy.

Digestibility of glucose, sucrose, lactose, dextrin, and starch mixed with animal tissue in a properly cooked diet may be as high as 94%.[61] However, the digestibility of soluble carbohydrates in average quality commercial dog foods is about 85%[57] and in average cat foods is about 73%.[37] Although cats and dogs can digest some of the starch in uncooked cereal grains, digestibility is increased by heating such as occurs during the processing of pet foods.[8,47]

Insoluble carbohydrates, referred to collectively as **"dietary fiber,"** include cellulose, hemicellulose, pectin, gum, mucilage, and lignin (a noncarbohydrate constituent). Lignin is a structural component of plants that is resistant to the digestive enzymes produced by higher animals, and to anaerobic microbial digestion as well. Certain aerobic microbes can digest lignin and are responsible for its degradation such as in the rotting of wood.

The different fractions of dietary fiber vary widely in their physical and chemical properties. The effect of fiber in regulating bowel function has led to its use in many clinical settings. The addition of fiber to the diet has successfully alleviated both diarrhea and constipation in hospitalized human patients.[16,23,29,30,62-64] Fiber, particularly cellulose and hemicellulose, alters intestinal function by increasing stool bulk.[12,18,19,34,62] This seems to be due to the water-holding capacity of fiber, the osmotic effect of volatile fatty acids produced by bacterial fermentation of fiber, and/or alteration of colonic bacteria, which may account for up to 75% of fecal wet weight.[18] Regardless of the mechanism(s), the increase in stool bulk causes rectal distention and stimulation of the defecation reflex. The result is a larger, softer stool that is more easily passed.[21]

Components of dietary fiber have also been shown to alter lipid and glucose metabolism. Pectin and guar gum can inhibit lipid absorption, increase excretion of cholesterol and bile acids, and decrease blood lipids;[32,34,62,65] whereas cellulose has little or no effect on serum cholesterol.[32,34,62] Glucose and insulin kinetics can be altered with dietary fiber. The effect of fiber to lower blood insulin and glucose values may be due to a reduced rate of glucose absorption, slower gastric emptying and/or altered secretion of gastrointestinal peptides.[5] There are also indications that fiber increases peripheral sensitivity to insulin, perhaps by increasing the number of insulin receptors.[6] Guar gums and pectins were shown to be most beneficial in this regard.[31]

Fiber has been shown to decrease the absorption of nutrients other than glucose and lipids. Total energy and protein absorption are less when high levels of dietary fiber are consumed.[20,34,62] Effects of fiber on mineral absorption vary.[35] Guar gum and pectin decrease absorption of some minerals, whereas cellulose has little effect on mineral absorption. Thus, if the mineral content of a diet is marginally low, increasing guar or pectin intake without an appropriate mineral increase may lead to a mineral deficiency.[35]

If a diet contains too much fiber, the dog or cat may be unable to consume enough to meet its energy needs. The inability of dogs and cats to digest fiber is used to advantage in formulating reducing diets for these species. Much emphasis has been placed on the value of adding fiber to the diet of humans for preventing intestinal cancer and other abnormalities. Similar benefits would not be expected from diets for dogs and cats because most pet foods already contain two to four times the fiber content of typical human diets.

PROTEIN

As shown in Figure 1 (page 1-3), proteins consist of many amino acids attached to each other by peptide bonds. Body proteins function as components of enzymes, hormones, a variety of body secretions, and structural and protective tissues. These proteins are in a constant state of flux, i.e. degradation and synthesis. Even though the constituent amino acids are reused, the recycling process is not 100% efficient. Also, some amino acids are used for energy and some proteins are lost from the body. In the case of growing or gestating animals, additional body tissue (which contains protein) is being produced. Since animals cannot synthesize amino acids *de novo*, as can plants, they require en exogenous protein source (dietary) or there will be a loss of body function and/or an inability to produce new tissue.

There are 22 different alpha amino acids. All animals need all of them. However, all animals can synthesize 12 of these amino acids in sufficient quantity to meet their needs. Therefore, it is not essential that these amino acids be included in the diet. Therefore, they are called "dispensable" or "non-essential" amino acids. The remaining amino acids cannot be synthesized in sufficient quantity and must be absorbed from the intestinal tract. In herbivores, many of these amino acids are produced by microbes in the rumen or large intestine. In non-herbivores such as the dog and cat, gastrointestinal production is minimal. Therefore, these amino acids are essential in the diet and are called

TABLE 6

MINIMAL AMINO ACID REQUIREMENTS FOR GROWTH

Amino Acid	mg/kcal of Metabolizable Energy	
	Kitten[61]*	Puppy
Arginine	2.5	1.4[26]
Histidine	0.6	0.5[15]
Isoleucine	1.1	1.0[53]
Leucine	< 2.6**	< 1.6[53]**
Lysine	1.7	1.5
Methionine or	0.8 or	1.2 or
Methionine + Cystine	1.6	1.5[9]
Phenylalanine or	1.1 or	1.3[51]
Phenylalanine + Tyrosine	2.2	----
Taurine	0.1	0
Threonine	1.5	1.2[15]
Tryptophan	0.25	0.4[15]
Valine	< 1.3**	< 1.0[53]**

*The essential amino acid nitrogen/nonessential amino acid nitrogen ratio in the kitten's diet should be equal to or greater than 0.70.[7]

**< indicates that less than this amount is needed.

indispensable or **essential amino acids.** The essential amino acids and the amounts required by dogs and cats for growth are shown in Table 6. Non-essential amino acids in the diet are beneficial because they have a sparing effect on the essential amino acids present. If an inadequate amount of non-essential amino acids is absorbed, or produced from breakdown of normal body protein, non-essential amino acids are produced from dietary essential amino acids.

The amino acid arginine was thought to be essential for dogs only during growth.[56] However, results of recent studies have shown that it is also an essential amino acid for adult dogs[14] and cats.[61] Arginine is a component of the urea cycle. In case of arginine deficiency, conversion of ammonia to urea is suppressed, resulting in an increased blood ammonia concentration, which can reach toxic levels. Clinical signs, which occur within hours after the animal has consumed an arginine-deficient diet, include hypersalivation, hyperesthesia, emesis, muscular tremors, ataxia, tetanic spasms, and, in some cases, coma and death.[57,61] This is of little practical significance because most protein sources contain adequate arginine. Cataracts caused by an arginine deficiency have occurred in dog and wolf pups being raised on commercially available canine milk replacers.[74]

Taurine is an essential amino acid for cats (but not dogs). Taurine (H_2N-CH_2-CH_2-SO_3H) differs from other amino acids in that it is a beta amino acid.* It contains a sulfonic rather than a carboxylic group and thus cannot form a peptide bond. It is present in bile as taurocholic acid and in high concentrations in the retina and olfactory bulb.[61] In dogs, sufficient taurine synthesis occurs from the sulfur-containing amino acids methionine and cystine.[61] However, cats, unlike many other placental mammals, exclusively conjugate cholic acid with taurine and are unable to alternate between taurine and glycine conjugations in producing bile.[61]

Therefore, the cat has a continual dietary requirement for taurine to replace fecal losses which occur because of less than 100% recovery by the enterohepatic circulation. As the fiber content in the cat's diet increases, fecal taurine losses increase. This necessitates a corresponding elevation of taurine in the diet. The taurine requirement of cats is also increased with decreasing intake of other sulfur-containing amino acids. Based on the amount of fiber and sulfur-containing amino acids in most cat

TABLE 7

TAURINE CONTENT OF FOODS (mg/kg, as fed)*

Food	Uncooked		Cooked or Processed**	
	Mean	Range	Mean	Range
Mammalian				
Muscle	444	150–690	203	96–390
Liver	181	110–270	113	68–184
Kidney	232	128–440	146	81–290
Avian				
Muscle	337	300–380	229	140–310
Poultry by-product meal	—	—	969	962–975
Cod	314	233–396	294	260–328
Tuna*				
Canned (water)	—	—	681	329–1004
Canned (oil)	—	—	572	440–588
Oysters	698	390–1238	264	217–308
Clams	2400	1450–3700	1017	587–1700
Egg (dried)*	—	—	57	—
Milk	151	104–200	—	—
Soybean meal* (solvent extracted)	—	—	trace	—

*Values were adapted from reference 55 except for asterisked items which were analyzed.

**Baked unless otherwise stated. Generally boiling reduces the taurine content of foods by approximately 50% of baked values, unless the cooking fluid remains with the food.

*Amino or NH_2 group is attached to the second (beta) carbon atom.

foods, a level of 500 mg of taurine/kg of diet dry matter has been recommended.[61]

Dietary taurine deficiency has also been shown to suppress reproductive performance in queens.[66] Surviving kittens from taurine-depleted mothers exhibited a number of neurologic abnormalities. Milk from these taurine-deficient queens had only 10% of the taurine content of milk from queens whose diet was supplemented with taurine.

Inadequate taurine intake by cats produces central retinal degeneration that can cause irreversible blindness. The most common cause is the feeding of dog food to cats. Compared to cat foods, most dog foods contain lesser amounts of protein and, therefore, sulfur-containing amino acids. In addition, most dog foods contain more ingredients from plant sources and fewer from animal sources than do cat foods. Plants are devoid of taurine, whereas fish and animal tissue are high in taurine content (Table 7).

However, the presence of central retinal degeneration does not necessarily indicate that the cat's diet is deficient in taurine. Retinal degeneration can be familial.[2] Cats have developed retinal degeneration and hypotaurinemia after long-term consumption of diets containing more than adequate taurine (greater than 1000 mg/kg). Acquired or inherited defects in taurine metabolism in such cats is certainly possible.

The quality of a protein varies directly with the number and amount of essential amino acids it contains. There are many ways to measure or estimate protein quality. The method most commonly used is **biologic value.** The biologic value is the percentage of a nutrient absorbed and retained; i.e. not excreted in the urine or feces and, therefore, presumably used by the body. The biologic value of a protein has meaning only if there is sufficient intake of non-protein calories to meet the animal's

FIGURE 5
FOOD ACCEPTABILITY, DIGESTIBILITY, UTILIZATION AND BIOLOGIC VALUE

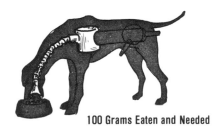

100 Grams Eaten and Needed

100% ACCEPTABLE

Acceptability of a food is the relationship between the quantity needed to meet caloric needs and the quantity eaten.

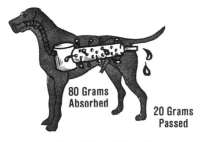

80 Grams Absorbed

20 Grams Passed

80% DIGESTIBLE

Digestibility is the relationship between the quantity of a food or nutrient eaten and the quantity absorbed.

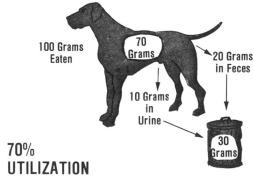

100 Grams Eaten

70 Grams

20 Grams in Feces

10 Grams in Urine

30 Grams

70% UTILIZATION

Utilization is the relationship between the quantity of a food or nutrient eaten and the quantity retained, i.e. not excreted. This is the best overall indication of nutrient quality.

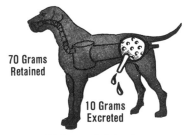

70 Grams Retained

10 Grams Excreted

70 Grams Retained ÷
80 Grams Absorbed =

87% BIOLOGIC VALUE

Biologic Value is the relationship between the quantity of a nutrient absorbed and the quantity utilized, i.e. retained. An accurate determination requires the subtraction of endogenous from total excretion. It is most commonly used in regard to protein.

needs, and the animal is in a steady state (not gaining or losing weight). The method for determining digestibility and biologic value of a food or nutrient is shown in Figure 5.

Protein digestibility in dog foods of average quality is approximately 80%[38,57] but may be as high as 90% in certain diets.[45] Protein digestibility in cat foods of average quality is approximately 74%.[37] Digestibility is less for poor-quality protein and poor-quality diets. The heat used in producing a diet increases the digestibility of carbohydrates, but excessive heat can have the opposite effect on protein digestibility.

Cereal proteins, which are a common component in commercially prepared diets, are low in certain amino acids, notably lysine, methionine, leucine and tryptophan. Most commercial pet foods contain a mixture of animal tissues, soybean meal, and cereal grains. **Methionine** is the most limiting amino acid in these mixtures with arginine, threonine, and leucine being second, third and fourth most limiting.[61] The biologic value of the protein in some pet food ingredients is shown in Table 8.

The higher the biologic value of a protein, the less the amount of that protein needed in a diet to meet all of an animal's essential amino acid requirements. For example, if a puppy needs 1% arginine in a particular diet and arginine makes up 5% of the protein in that diet, then (1% ÷ 5% = 20%) 20% of that protein is needed in that particular diet to supply the puppy's arginine requirement. If the protein in that diet has an optimal amino acid

content, 20% of it in the diet would provide just enough, but little excess, of all other essential amino acids. No single protein meets these requirements. For example, a diet containing 17.1% egg protein would just meet the puppy's arginine requirement for growth.[26,45] However, this amount of egg protein in the diet provides 3.2 times the needed valine,[45,53] 2.5 times the needed lysine,[45,52] and 1.6 to 1.9 times the required amount of all the other essential amino acids.[15,45] (see Table 6, page 1-13). An excess of some of these amino acids may be just as detrimental as a deficiency. For example, a 1.7-fold excess of lysine[52] and a 1.5-fold excess of threonine,[15] in a purified amino acid diet, slowed the growth of puppies. Thus, comparing the essential amino acid content of a protein in a diet or food, to the essential amino acid content of another protein, does not give a good indication of protein quality.

There is a better way to determine protein quality: Compare the amino acid content of a protein to the amount of each amino acid the animal needs to perform the particular function for which the diet is intended. The amount of amino acids needed varies with different body functions. For example, the dog needs 1.12% arginine for growth[26] but only 0.28% for maintenance. Thus, the quality of a protein in a diet intended for growth should be compared to the amount of essential amino acids needed for growth; and the quality of a protein in a diet intended for maintenance should be compared to the amount of essential amino acids needed for maintenance.

However, even when the amount of amino acids a protein contains is compared to the amount of amino acids needed, the value obtained may still be relatively meaningless because amino acid requirements differ with the amount of many other substances in the diet. For example, dietary arginine,[26] lysine,[52] and threonine[15] requirements become greater as amounts of dietary protein increase. The amounts of all amino acids needed in the diet increase with increasing energy density of the diet and may vary with the fiber and fat contents, independent of its energy density. Differences also exist in the availability of amino acids from different protein sources.

In addition, if the amount of protein (amino acids) in the diet substantially exceeds all of the animal's amino acid requirements, protein quality has little importance except where the protein provides an excess of amino acids that could be detrimental. Results of studies in rats have suggested that protein quality may be determined by measuring the percent nitrogen excreted in the urine

TABLE 8

PROTEIN BIOLOGIC VALUE OF COMMON PET FOOD INGREDIENTS

Food	Biologic Value
Egg	100
Fish Meal	92
Milk	92
Liver	79
Beef	78
Casein	78
Casein + Methionine	100
Soybean Meal	67
Meat and Bone Meal	50 (variable)
Whole Wheat	48
Whole Corn	45
Gelatin	0*

*Does not contain any of the essential amino acid tryptophan.

TABLE 9

MINIMAL PROTEIN REQUIREMENTS[61]

Animal	Ideal Protein*		In Non-Dietary Pet Foods**	
	% in Diet	% of Gross Energy	% in Diet	% of Metaboliz-able Energy
Kitten	16[7]	22	30	25
Adult Cat	8[11]	9	25–30	20–25
Puppy	11	12	29	29
Adult Dog	4	4	18	18

*An ideal protein is one that is 100% digestible and has a biologic value (BV) of 100%. The amount of protein needed in a diet increases with decreasing protein digestibility and BV, and with increasing caloric density of the diet. The values listed are based on a diet caloric density of 4 kcal of metabolizable energy/g.

The minimum % protein needed in the diet as fed = minimum % ideal protein needed ÷ [(% protein digestibility ÷ 100) × (% BV ÷ 100) × (4 ÷ kcal per gram of diet, as fed)]. For example, for the adult dog, the amount of protein needed from meat, that is 90% digestible and has a BV of 78%, in a canned diet providing 1.25 kcal/g as fed, is: 4 ÷ (90/100 × 78/100 × 4/1.25) = 1.8% in the diet as fed. If the diet contained 75% moisture, 1.8 ÷ (1 − 0.75) = 7.2% meat protein needed in the diet on a dry-matter basis. The protein content of many meat-type canned dog foods exceeds 50% of the diet dry-matter, which is seven times the dog's requirement.

**Based on a diet providing 4 kcal of metabolizable energy/g. For diets with different caloric contents, multiply the % protein in the diet by the quotient of (the caloric density of the diet divided by 4). For example, a diet providing 5 kcal/g for kittens should contain 30% × (5/4) = 37.5% protein.

after oral administration of alanine.[13] The only totally effective method of evaluating the amino acid or other nutrient content of a diet is to feed that diet and evaluate the results.

The amounts of protein needed by cats and dogs are shown in Table 9. Cats need much more protein than do dogs, yet they do not require substantially more of any amino acid (see Table 6, page 1-13). Cats have a high protein requirement because they always use a given amount of protein for energy. In most animals, including dogs, hepatic transaminases adapt to the amount of protein consumed. This allows the animal to conserve nitrogen on a low-protein diet and excrete nitrogen on a high-protein diet. Cats do not have this metabolic flexibility. The transaminases, urea cycle and gluconeogenic enzymes of the cat are fixed at relatively high levels of activity.[61] However, this is not a disadvantage because the cat's natural diet is composed of animal tissue consistently high in protein. Thus it appears that during evolution, the cat as well as other members of the suborder feloidea (genets and hyenas) and some canoidea (weasels) remained carnivorous, whereas other members of the sub-order canoidea became omnivorous (dogs, raccoons, and bears) or even herbivorous (pandas).[61]

PROTEIN IMBALANCES

The use of protein and consumption of calories are closely related. Regardless of caloric intake, if more protein is consumed than the animal needs,

the excess protein (amino acids) will be deaminated and the keto acid portions used for energy. If energy is not needed, the amino acids can be converted to glycogen or fat and stored for future use. The ammonia removed from the protein is converted by the liver to urea and other nitrogenous wastes which are normally excreted primarily by the kidneys.

Chronic excessive protein intake by a dog (and perhaps a cat) can result in renal glomerulosclerosis and a disproportionate increase in renal aging (page 8-10). In addition, there appear to be no detriments to health associated with preventing excess protein intake. Thus, it seems prudent to avoid chronic excessive protein intake, because doing so may slow renal deterioration, contributing to longevity. In addition, excessive protein intake in an animal with a sufficient decrease in renal function results in the accumulation of nitrogenous waste products in the body (page 8-18). Accumulation of these compounds is responsible for most of the clinical signs that occur with renal failure. Thus, the ideal diet should provide the required amount of all amino acids while avoiding excessive intake of protein.

If dietary sources of soluble carbohydrate or fat are inadequate, the animal will use dietary protein for energy. Body protein catabolism occurs when total energy intake is inadequate. Therefore, caloric needs must be met before protein needs can be satisfied. This concept is particularly important when nutritional support for anorectic patients is considered.

Inadequate protein intake is detrimental. The most obvious manifestations of protein deficiency are reduced growth in young animals and weight loss and reduced performance or production (such as reduced milk production during lactation) in adult animals. Growth and shedding of hair are slowed, resulting in a rough, coarse, unkempt appearance. The plasma albumin concentration and albumin/globulin ratio are decreased, which lowers the plasma oncotic pressure. Sufficient depression of plasma oncotic pressure can cause edema or ascites. In case of a protein deficiency, food intake may be decreased. The result is insufficient energy intake, which contributes to the clinical signs. However, if food intake is not decreased so that energy intake remains adequate, protein deficiency may lead to increased deposition of fat in the liver.[3] Hepatic fibrosis or cirrhosis may also occur. Plasma alkaline phosphatase activity increases as a result of these hepatic changes.

Protein deficiencies are caused by:
1. Inadequate food intake
2. Poor quality or poorly digestible dietary protein
3. Bulky low-energy diets which cause the marginal protein present to be converted to energy
4. Insufficient total protein in the diet
5. Inability to digest or absorb sufficient protein
6. Excessive protein losses from the body, e.g. from burns or protein-losing enteropathy or nephropathy

Insufficient total protein intake often occurs in kennels or catteries whose owners attempt to economize by feeding low-cost, poor-quality commercial pet foods, or such foods as corn bread, biscuits, oatmeal, boiled potatoes, or other foods high in carbohydrate content. Such foods may constitute up to 90% of these animals' diet. Inexpensive proteins of low biologic value such as gelatin and collagen, or those contained in low-quality meat and bone meal and cereal wastes, are often present in poor-quality pet foods.

Inadequate protein intake and amino acid deficiencies may occur in cats because they have been fed dog foods or a single food item. Although dog foods may be quite adequate for dogs, they may be inadequate for cats because of the cat's relatively high protein requirement and requirement for taurine.

FATS

Fats are referred to as oils, lipids, and ether extract. They are required dietarily as follows:

1. For the absorption of the fat soluble vitamins A, D, E, and K
2. To enhance palatability so the animal will eat the food
3. As a source of essential (unsaturated) fatty acids

If a diet contains adequate carbohydrate and protein, fats are not needed as a source of energy. However, fats are an excellent source of dietary energy. In most diets, increasing the fat content results in an increase in the caloric density. On a weight basis, fats yield approximately 2.25 times more energy than either soluble carbohydrates or proteins. Also, since fats tend to be more digestible, dietary fats may provide 2.5 times as much energy as dietary soluble carbohydrates or proteins. The digestibility of fat in average commercial dog foods is approximately 90%.[57] In a recent study the digestibility of fat in average commercial cat foods was found to be somewhat less, at 74%.[38] However, this study employed a more rigorous fecal fat extraction process which would provide a lower calculated digestibility than methods used previously.[38] The digestibility of fat in a diet can also be influenced by the ingredient source, as demonstrated in another study where fat digestibility in a commercial cat food was greater than 91%.[48] Dogs as well as cats can readily use most fats or oils of either animal or plant origin. However, a few hydrogenated fats, including hydrogenated coconut oil, are poorly digested. **Hepatic lipidosis** developed in cats fed this form of fat. This was thought to result from a specific deleterious effect of the **medium-chain triglycerides** in coconut oil.[50]

The type and amount of fat in the diet also affects its palatability. Up to a relatively high level, fats generally enhance palatability of a diet for both dogs and cats. In one study cats preferred diets containing bleached tallow over the same diets containing chicken or butter fat. The amount of fat in the diet also affected its palatability.[33] Diets containing 25% yellow grease were preferred over those containing either 10% or 50%; those containing 40% bleached tallow were preferred over those with 12% or 25%. The effect of fat content (type and amount) on the palatability of a diet may result either from the flavor of the fat or from the consistency (mouth feel) it imparts to the diet.

From 25-50% of the daily energy requirement of dogs or cats can be supplied by fat. Although from 5-20% fat in the diet dry matter is generally recommended, the percentage of fat has been increased to 40% for dogs[56] and 64% for cats[55] with no observable negative results, including steatorrhea or pancreatitis. Large amounts of dietary fat are

advantageous during periods of high caloric need such as growth, lactation or physical exertion. However, if the amount of dietary fat exceeds the animal's ability to assimilate it, steatorrhea occurs. The **acute** ingestion of very high levels of fat (e.g. meat trimmings) has been related to bouts of **acute pancreatitis,** particularly in overweight dogs. Possibly as a result of this association, **chronic** excessive fat consumption has also been thought to be involved in the development of acute pancreatitis. However, clinical data do not support this hypothesis unless dietary fat levels greatly exceed the amounts in commercial pet foods. Most commercial dog foods contain from 7-25% fat (Table 9, page 2-22). A diet composed of 77% fat (dry-matter basis) caused acute pancreatitis in dogs.[49] However, 16 racing sled dogs fed double maintenance amounts of a 66% fat diet for nine weeks developed no clinical signs of pancreatitis nor an elevation of serum amylase activity.[44] Acute pancreatitis, induced by injecting bile and trypsin into the pancreatic duct, developed more readily in dogs fed a diet that contained 40% fat, than in dogs fed a 10% fat diet.[27] However, no increased risk of pancreatitis was associated with dogs eating canned diets containing 20-30% fat.[46] In another study no differences were noted in serum amylase activity in dogs that had consumed diets containing 17, 25, or 37% fat, over a six month period.[43] See page 7-17 for a discussion of acute pancreatitis.

Inadequate dietary fat may lead to a fatty acid deficiency and/or an energy deficiency resulting in poor growth, poor physical performance, lowered reproductive performance, and weight loss. As shown in Figure 1 (page 1-3), triglyceride, the chief dietary fat, consists of 1 glycerol molecule and 3 fatty acid molecules. The specific fatty acids present determine the fat's physical and nutritional characteristics. Lipids containing a high percentage of either short-chain or unsaturated fatty acids are liquid at room temperature; they are called "oils." Those with a low percentage of unsaturated fatty acids or that contain longer chain fatty acids are solid at room temperature; they are referred to as "fats." Most plant oils contain 30-60% unsaturated fatty acids, excepting palm, olive, and coconut oils, all of which contain less than 10% (Table 10).

Linoleic acid is an essential fatty acid required by all animals. It is the main unsaturated fatty acid in most vegetable oils and makes up 15-25% of poultry and pork fat but less than 5% of beef tallow, fish oil, and butter fat (Table 10). In addition to linoleic acid, at least 0.17% (dry-matter basis) of the unsaturated fatty acid, arachidonic acid, is also required in the diet of cats. Arachidonic acid is synthesized from linoleic acid by animals other than domestic cats and possibly lions.[61] Arachidonic acid is a constituent of animal fats and is not present in plant products of any type (Table 10). Linoleic acid is converted to linolenic acid by both cats and dogs. Therefore, neither specie requires linolenic acid in the diet. Essential fatty acids should constitute at least 1% of the diet dry matter or 2% of caloric intake.

FATTY ACID DEFICIENCY

Essential fatty acids are necessary as constituents of cell membranes, for the synthesis of prostaglandins and related compounds, and in controlling epidermal loss of water. An essential fatty acid deficiency may result in impaired reproductive efficiency. If pregnancy does occur, there may be neonatal abnormalities and death. Also a deficiency of essential fatty acids can impair wound healing, cause a dry lusterless coat and scaly skin, and change the lipid film on the skin, which may predispose to skin infection or pyoderma. If deficiency persists, alopecia, edema, and exudation from localized areas of the skin (moist dermatitis) may ensue. Lesions of moist dermatitis are most common in the external ear canals and between the toes. However, they may develop anywhere on the body, resulting in what are referred to as **"hot spots."** Emaciation may result from severe persistent essential fatty acid deficiency. Essential fatty acid deficiency occurs most commonly in dogs receiving low-fat dry dog foods containing beef tallow, or dry foods that have been stored too long, particularly under warm, humid conditions.

Unsaturated fatty acids, including the essential fatty acids, contain double bonds that become oxidized (rancid) if sufficient antioxidants are not present. The oxidation process is hastened by increased temperature and humidity. Unsaturated

TABLE 10

FATTY ACID COMPOSITION AND FATTY ACID CONTENT OF COMMON FATS AND OILS[57,68]

Fat/Oil	Unsaturated Fatty Acids (%)	Linoleic Acid (%)	Arachidonic Acid (%)
Pork Fat (lard)	64.1	18.3	0.3- 1.0
Poultry Fat	60.9	22.3	0.5- 1.0
Tallow	52.4	4.3	0.0- 0.2
Fish Oil	60.0	2.7	20.0-25.0
Corn Oil	87.7	55.4	—
Coconut Oil	9.7	1.1	—
Linseed Oil	91.8	13.9	—
Safflower Oil	89.5	72.7	—
Butter Fat	35.8	2.5	—

fatty acids that become oxidized lose their nutritional value.

In suspected cases of fatty-acid deficiency, addition of one teaspoonful of soy or corn oil per 8 oz measuring cup of dry food will correct the problem. If a specific arachidonic acid deficiency is suspected in a cat, the diet should be supplemented with such sources of animal fats as poultry fat or lard (Table 10). However, most pathologic changes associated with essential fatty-acid deficiency in cats can be prevented by feeding fats containing linoleic acid.[50] If a clinical response to supplementation is not observed within three weeks, other causes of pathologic change should be considered.

Excessive dietary unsaturated fat in conjunction with inadequate antioxidants may result in **pansteatitis.** Accumulation of reactive peroxides (end products of rancidification) in adipose tissue results in a yellow, brown, or orange discoloration of body fat. The discoloration is the basis for a common name for the condition, **"yellow fat disease."** Affected animals are anorectic, depressed, febrile, and lethargic. They move stiffly and generally show obvious signs of cutaneous pain upon handling, as a result of inflamed subcutaneous fat. Nodular subcutaneous fat or fibrous deposits are palpable. Occasionally, an ascitic fluid low in protein may develop. These signs may resemble feline infectious peritonitis. However, with feline infectious peritonitis, the ascitic fluid is high in protein. Cats with pansteatitis usually have a history of fish, particularly red-meat tuna, comprising a major part of their diet. Treatment involves correction of diet and oral administration of 30 mg/day of vitamin E (alpha tocopherol) until clinical signs disappear.[17a] Initially, corticosteroids are helpful as supportive therapy.

MINERALS

Although important for a variety of functions, minerals constitute only a small fraction of the body weight. That fraction reflects the quantity needed in the diet. On a weight basis the body consists of 63% hydrogen, 25.5% oxygen, 9.5% carbon, and 1.4% nitrogen. Collectively, minerals make up less than 0.7% of the body, most of which is comprised of the macrominerals calcium, phosphorus, potassium, sodium and magnesium. Macrominerals are minerals for which the dietary requirements are best expressed as a percent (parts per hundred). Trace or microminerals are those for which dietary requirements are best expressed as parts per million (ppm or mg/kg). Microminerals include iron, zinc, copper, manganese, iodine, and selenium.

The macrominerals maintain the following:
1. Acid-base balance
2. Osmotic pressures needed for maintaining body fluid balance
3. Transmembrane potentials needed for a variety of general cellular functions, nerve conduction, and muscle contraction
4. Structural integrity

Most of the microminerals are needed as components of metalloenzymes. These enzymes are involved in controlling enormous numbers of diverse biochemical reactions. Iodine is a necessary constituent of thyroid hormone, iron of hemoglobin and myoglobin, and cobalt of vitamin B_{12}.

Dietarily, minerals should be regarded as a group rather than individually. As the intake of a mineral increases above an animal's requirement, the amount absorbed and/or excreted in urine and/or feces also increases. The excess amount absorbed may be harmful. The unabsorbed amount can bind other minerals, preventing their absorption and possibly resulting in a deficiency or imbalance of these other minerals. If the intake of the other minerals is increased to compensate for this binding, decreased absorption of still other minerals may occur, leading to a deficiency of these other minerals.

It is the balanced amount of all minerals in the diet that is important. **Indiscriminate supplementation with one or even several minerals is likely to be more harmful than beneficial, and is the main cause of mineral imbalances in dogs and cats.** The recommended amount of minerals in the diet and major causes and symptoms of mineral deficiencies and excesses are listed in Table 11.

Some minerals, such as calcium or phosphorus, are major constituents of bone that provide its compressional strength. However, these minerals also have biochemical functions in a variety of tissues. Dietary imbalances of these minerals often manifest clinically as bone disease because the skeleton releases its mineral stores to subserve the more critical biochemical functions. If the mineral imbalance persists, integrity of the skeleton may be compromised to the point of failure. Bone abnormalities from mineral imbalances most often occur during the growth period and respond slowly to treatment. Clinical improvement will often not become apparent until the animal's growth rate slows as the animal nears maturity. The only diagnosis that frequently can be made in animals exhibiting skeletal problems is that dietary intake is incorrect or that growth rate is too rapid for optimal bone development. (See page 3-14.)

TABLE 11

MINERAL REQUIREMENTS AND EFFECTS OF DEFICIENCY AND EXCESS

| Mineral | Requirement (Dog and Cat) | | Deficiency | Excess |
	Units	In Diet*		
Calcium	%	0.5**– 0.9	Occurs when meat or organ tissue comprise majority of diet. **Initially:** lameness, stiffness, reluctance to move, constipation, enlarged metaphyses, splayed toes, carpal and tarsal hyperextension. When **chronic:** spontaneous fractures, limb deviations, anorexia, dehydration, loose teeth. When **acute:** tetany.	Most common cause is oversupplementation. May cause phosphorus, zinc, iron and copper deficiencies. Slows growth, decreases thyroid function and may predispose to bloat.
Phosphorus	%	0.2**– 0.6	Generally due to excessive calcium supplementation. Causes depraved appetite and same signs as a calcium deficiency.	From oversupplementation or high P diets. Major effect is to cause Ca deficiency. If Ca is increased enough to offset excess P, it results in excess Ca. Excess P promotes renal damage.
Potassium	%	0.4	Due to excess losses from diarrhea or diuretics, or inadequate intake because of anorexia. Causes anorexia, weakness, lethargy and decreased muscle tone, which may cause head drooping, ataxia and ascending paralysis.	Does not occur unless there is oliguria. Causes hyperkalemia, same signs as a deficiency, cardiotoxicity and death.
Sodium	%	0.1– 0.5†	Polyuria, salt hunger, pica, wt. loss, fatigue, agalactia, and slow growth.††	**Acute:** Occurs only if there is inadequate nonsaline, good quality water available. Causes thirst, pruritus, constipation, anorexia, seizures and death.†† **Chronic:** High amounts in many pet foods may induce hypertension resulting in increased heart and renal diseases.
Magnesium	%	0.05– 0.10†	Retarded growth, spreading of toes and hyperextension of carpus and tarsus, hyperirritability, convulsions, soft tissue calcification, enlargement of the metaphysis of long bones.††	Acute excess intake causes diarrhea because of poor absorption.†† Chronic intake of high amounts present in many cat foods contributes to urolithiasis and cystitis.
Iron	mg/kg	60	May occur if fed milk exclusively for an extended period or secondary to blood loss. Causes microcytic-hypochromic anemia, anisocytosis and poikilocytosis of erythrocytes.	Anorexia, wt. loss, hypoalbuminemia, hemochromatosis.†† Death following excess administration to young, particularly if they are vitamin E or selenium deficient.††
Zinc	mg/kg	50	Anorexia, wt. loss, slow growth, emesis, generalized thinning of hair coat, scaly dermatitis, parakeratosis, hair depigmentation, decreased testicular development and wound healing, depression, and peripheral lymphadenopathy.	Causes a calcium and/or copper deficiency.††
Copper	mg/kg	7	May be caused by excess zinc, iron or molybdenum. Slow growth, bone lesions similar to calcium deficiency, pica[8] and liver copper less than 20 μg/g wet wt.[61] Reported that anemia, hair depigmentation and diarrhea don't occur in cats as they do in other species.[22]	Occurs in Bedlington Terriers due to inability to mobilize hepatic copper, resulting in signs of liver disease.
Manganese	mg/kg	5	Impaired reproduction, abortion, enlarged joints, stiffness, reluctance to move, short, thick and brittle bones.††	Partial albinism, impaired fertility.††
Iodine	mg/kg	1.5	Hypothyroidism, goiter, alopecia, fetal resorption, cretinism, myxedema, lethargy, drowsiness, timidity. At necropsy, feline thyroid wt. > 12 mg/100 g body wt.	Same as a deficiency.††
Selenium	mg/kg	0.1	"White muscle disease," skeletal and cardiac myopathy.	Based on data in other species: Nervousness, anorexia, vomiting, weakness, ataxia, dyspnea and death due to pulmonary edema within hours to days.††

*Based on a diet providing 4.0 kcal metabolizable energy/g. For diets with a different caloric density multiply the amount given times the quotient of (kcal/g of that diet ÷ 4).

**Ca should equal or exceed P and twice these amounts are recommended during growth and lactation.

†The greater amount is recommended during lactation.

††This mineral imbalance is rare in dogs and cats.

When a mineral imbalance is present, determining the specific mineral involved is difficult because the same clinical signs and similar lesions often characterize several mineral deficiencies or excesses. In these cases, analysis of the diet, with or without blood profiling, can be helpful in establishing a diagnosis (see chapters 2 and 12). Regardless of whether or not a definitive diagnosis can be made, the best approach in most cases is to feed a diet known to contain the proper amount and balance of minerals for normal growth. This is better than attempting to correct the amount of any one or several suspect minerals by using a mineral supplement, thereby risking intensifying the imbalances or causing additional mineral imbalances.

VITAMINS

Vitamins are regulatory molecules that function as enzymes, enzyme precursors, or coenzymes. Their chemical structure and function are widely diverse. Vitamins are not used as an energy source or for structural purposes; their primary function is to promote and regulate a wide variety of physiologic processes.

Vitamins are divided into two groups, based on their solubility rather than their function. However, as shown in Table 12, their solubility does relate to the mechanisms by which they are absorbed, stored, and excreted. There are some functional similarities within the two groups, particularly the water-soluble B-complex vitamins. Many of the B-complex vitamins assist in regulating energy metabolism and participate in so many biochemical reactions that individual vitamin deficiencies produce similar clinical signs, often making specific diagnosis difficult. Generally, deficiencies of these energy regulating vitamins will manifest earliest in tissues composed of rapidly dividing cells. Common clinical signs of deficiencies of these vitamins include dermatitis, glossitis, cheilitis, enteritis, and a variety of neuropathies (depression, confusion, and motor incoordination).

Vitamins are often incorrectly administered therapeutically in lieu of an accurate diagnosis. This is a frequent practice in cases of reduced food intake. Because of the emphasis on vitamin supplementation, hypervitaminosis is more common clinically than are vitamin deficiencies. Cases of true dietary vitamin deficiency are rare, primarily because vitamins are available in natural sources and prepared pet foods are fortified with vitamins.

Processing and storage of foods decreases their active vitamin content. The least stable are vitamins B_1 (thiamin), folic acid, A, E, and K. However, these vitamin losses are readily determined and manufacturers of quality pet foods anticipate and compensate for them by adding vitamins to their products.[11] **Routine vitamin supplementation of a quality prepared pet food with vitamins incurs additional expense, is usually unnecessary, and may induce toxicity depending on the vitamin and the dosage.** Vitamin supplementation is justified during periods when loss of water soluble vitamins (B-complex and C) from the body is increased, as occurs with polyuria or diarrhea or the ingestion of antibiotics or antivitamins. Antivitamins are substances that prevent vitamin utilization. These include thiaminase, avidin, folic acid antagonists, and dicoumarol.

Avidin is a protein that binds biotin, preventing its absorption. Avidin is present in raw egg white. Because egg yolks are high in biotin content they negate the effect of avidin if ingested simultaneously with raw egg whites. Also, cooking the egg white destroys the antivitamin effect of avidin. **Dicoumarol** or its derivatives (warfarin, pindone and diphacinone) are the active ingredients in some rodenticides (D-Con, Prolin, etc.) They inhibit hepatic synthesis of vitamin K-dependent clotting factors, thus prolonging blood coagulation time. Diphenylhydantoin (Dilantin, Primidone), methotrexate, and aminopterin interfere with folic acid metabolism. Their administration to dogs has, in rare instances, been associated with megaloblastic anemia induced by folic acid deficiency.[67] **Thiaminase** is an enzyme in the viscera of certain raw fish (smelt, bullhead, herring, catfish, carp, and others). It destroys thiamin (vitamin B_1). Because cats, mink, and foxes require more thiamin than other animals, and are occasionally fed raw fish, they are the species most commonly affected. Excessive heating while processing, or prolonged storage, particularly at high temperatures and humidity, may also result in a thiamin deficient diet. The main signs of vitamin deficiencies and toxicities, and vitamin requirements are given in Table 13.

TABLE 12

CHARACTERISTICS AND FUNCTIONS OF VITAMINS

	Vitamins A, D, E and K	Vitamins B and C (ascorbic acid)
Absorbed and Excreted with	Fats	Water
Required in diet of healthy animals	Yes, although minimal for K since it is produced by intestinal bacteria.	No, or minimal amounts needed because B vitamins are produced by bacteria in the intestinal tract, which decreases dietary need. The B-vitamin niacin is also produced, although quite inefficiently, from the amino acid tryptophan by all animals except cats. Vitamin C is produced from glucose in the liver in adequate quantities to meet the needs of all animals except primates, guinea pigs, fruit bats, red vented bulbul birds, coho salmon, and rainbow trout.
Major dietary sources	Liver, fats and oils, egg yolks and cereal grain germ.	Liver, yeast, egg yolks and whole cereal grain, and for vitamin C fresh fruits and vegetables.
Form in foods	All but vitamin E occur as inactive pro-vitamins in non-animal source foods. Cats, in contrast to other animals, are unable to convert the inactive pro-vitamin, beta-carotene, to vitamin A. The cat, therefore, must consume preformed vitamin A, which is present only in animal tissues.	Occur as the active form in all foods.
Body storage	Yes, except K.	No, except B_{12} of which a 3–5 year supply is stored in the liver.
Deficiencies occur when	Body storage is depleted.	Water excretion increases, or intake or synthesis in body decreases (e.g., oral antibiotics at high levels for prolonged periods).
Functions Deficiencies are manifested by alterations in these functions.	A = vision, hearing, tract lining, skin and bone (controls cell differentiation and regulates rate of mitosis). D = bone, teeth and, calcium and phosphorus absorption and utilization. E = antioxidant, muscle, fat and reproduction. K = blood clotting.	B's = appetite and metabolism. C = wound healing and capillary fragility, i.e., anti-hemorrhage, anti-scurvy.
Toxicities	Excesses can't be excreted so toxicities of A and D occur. 4 times the vitamin D requirement increases plasma cholesterol and 10 times causes calcium deposition in soft tissue. 50–100 times the vitamin A requirement is necessary to cause toxicity. Excess carotene intake won't cause vitamin A toxicity.	Excesses excreted so toxicities usually don't occur.

TABLE 13

VITAMIN REQUIREMENTS AND SIGNS OF DEFICIENCY AND TOXICITY

Vitamin	mg (or for A&D IU)/kg			Major Signs of a	
	Dogs[56]		Cats[55]		
	Body Wt.*/day	Diet**	Diet**	Deficiency†	Toxicity
A (3.3 IU = 1 mg retinol)	110	5000	5000	Reproductive failure, retinal degeneration, tearing, papilledema, keratomalacia, night blindness, photophobia, conjunctivitis, poor coat, weakness of hind legs, increased susceptibility to infectious diseases. Plasma vitamin A less than 10 μg retinol or 45 IU/dl.	Anorexia, wt. loss, bone decalcification, hyperesthesia, plasma vitamin A above 600 μg retinol or 1800 IU/dl (normal is 40–100 μg/dl).
D (40 IU = 1 μg)	11	500	500	Rickets in young, osteomalacia in adults, lordosis, chest deformity and poor eruption of permanent teeth.	Anorexia, wt. loss, nausea, fatigue, soft tissue calcification, hypercalcemia, diarrhea, dehydration, death.
E (alpha-tocopherol)	1.1 50 50 Up to 3-fold increase with increased unsaturated fat intake.			Reproductive failure with weak or dead feti. Muscular dystrophy, pansteatitis, progressive retinal atrophy, intestinal lipofuscinosis (brown gut disease), impaired immunity.	Anorexia. None others recorded.
K	Not required except during antibacterial therapy or chronic ileal or colonic disease.			Increased clotting time and hemorrhage.	None recorded, but high levels probably dangerous.
C	Not required for normal dogs and cats.			Retarded healing, increased susceptibility to disease, hemorrhage, anemia, rickets.	Generally considered non-toxic.
Thiamin (B$_1$)	0.02	1	5	Anorexia, vomiting, weight loss, dehydration, paralysis, prostration, abnormal reflexes, ataxia, convulsions, cardiac disorders, ventral flexion of neck, called "Chastek Paralysis," mydriasis.	Non-toxic.
Riboflavin (B$_2$)	0.1	2.2	4	Dry scaly skin, erythema, posterior muscular weakness, anemia, sudden death, cheilosis, glossitis, pannus, reduced fertility, fatty liver, testicular hypoplasia.	Non-toxic.
Niacin	0.25	11	40	"Black tongue," hemorrhagic diarrhea, anemia, reddening and ulceration of mucous membranes of mouth and tongue, death. In cats only signs may be diarrhea, emaciation and death.	Dilation of blood vessels, itching, burning of skin.
Pyridoxine (B$_6$)	0.02	1	4	Microcytic hypochromic anemia, high serum iron, atherosclerosis, convulsions.	None recorded.
Pantothenic Acid	0.22	10	5	Anorexia, hypoglycemia, hypochloremia, BUN increase, gastritis, enteritis, convulsions, fatty liver, coma and death.	None recorded.
Folic Acid (Pteroyl-glutamic Acid)	0.004	0.18	0.8	Due to blood loss, or prolonged malabsorption, or sulfonamide administration. Hypoplasia of bone marrow, macrocytic anemia, glossitis.	Non-toxic.
Biotin	0.002	0.1	0.07	Scaly dermatitis, alopecia, anorexia, dried saliva around mouth and secretions around eyes, weakness, diarrhea, progressive spasticity and posterior paralysis.	Non-toxic.
Cobalamin (B$_{12}$)	0.0005	0.02	0.02	Doesn't occur clinically, experimentally causes a macrocytic anemia.	Non-toxic.
Choline††	26	1200	2000	Fatty liver, hypoalbuminemia, and increased alkaline phosphatase, prothrombin time, hemoglobin and hematocrit.	Persistent diarrhea caused by 10 g/day or greater.

*Twice these amounts are recommended during growth and lactation.

**Based on a diet providing 4.0 kcal metabolizable energy/g. For diets with a different caloric density, multiply the amount given times the quotient of (kcal/g of that diet ÷ 4).

†All result in retarded growth or weight loss and most in anorexia.

††Although routinely listed as a vitamin it is not and is not needed for metabolism. It is needed as a structural component of fat and nervous tissue.

REFERENCES

1. Adams CR: Stability of vitamins in processed dog food. Petfood Industry pp 20-21 (Jan-Feb 1981).

2. Aquirre GD: Retinal degeneration associated with the feeding of dog food to cats. J Amer Vet Med Assoc 172:791-796 (1978).

3. Allison JB: Calories and protein nutrition. Ann NY Acad Sci 69(5):1009-1018 (1958).

4. Anderson BE: Temperature regulation and environmental physiology. In Dukes Physiology of Domestic Animals, ed MJ Swenson, Publisher Cornell University Press, Ithaca p 721 (1984).

5. Anderson JW: Dietary fiber and diabetes. In Dietary Fiber in Health and Disease, eds GV Vahouny and D Kritchevsky, Publisher Plenum Press, New York pp 151-167 (1982).

6. Anderson JW: Physiological and metabolic effects of dietary fiber. Federation Proc 44:2902-2906 (1985).

7. Anderson PA, Baker DH, Sherry PA, Corbin JE: Nitrogen requirement of the kitten.Amer J Vet Res 41:1646-1649 (1980).

8. Bernard R, Smith SE, Maynard LA: The digestion of cereals by minks and foxes with special reference to starch and crude fiber. Cornell Vet XXXII, 29-36 (1942).

9. Blaza SE,Burger IH, Holme DW, Kendall PT: Sulfur-containing amino acid requirements of growing dogs. J Nutr 112:2033-2042 (1982).

10. Blaza SE: Energy requirements of dogs in cold conditions. Canine Pract 9:10-15 (1982).

11. Burger IH, Blaza SE, Kendall PT, Smith PM: The protein requirement of adult cats for maintenance. Feline Pract 14:8-14 (1984).

12. Burkitt DP, Painter N: Gastrointestinal transit times; stool weights and consistency; intraluminal pressures. In Refined Carbohydrate Foods and Disease:Some Implications of Dietary Fibre, eds DP Burkitt and HC Trowell, Publisher Academic Press, London (1975).

13. Burnette MA, Babcock MJ: Oral amino acid load test of protein nutrition:effect of protein quantity and quality in the rat. J Nutr 108:465-474 (1978).

14. Burns RA, Milner JA, Corbin JE: Arginine:An indispensable amino acid for mature dogs. J Nutr 111:1020-1024 (1981).

15. Burns RA, Milner JA: Threonine, tryptophan and histidine requirements of immature beagle dogs. J Nutr 112:447-452 (1982).

16. Burrows CF, Kronfeld DS, Banta CA, Meritt AM: Effects of fiber on digestibility and transit time in dogs. J Nutr 112:1726-1732 (1982).

17. Carpenter TM: The effects of sugars on the respiratory exchange of cats. J Nutr 28:315-323 (1944).

17a. Collins DR: Nutrition, In Feline Medicine, ed Pratt PW, Publisher, American Veterinary Publications, Santa Barbara, pp. 15-29 (1983).

18. Cummings JH, Stephan AM: The role of dietary fibre in the human colon. Can Med Assoc J 123:1109-1114 (1980).

19. Cummings JH: Consequences of the metabolism of fibre in the human large intestine. In Dietary Fibre in Health and Disease, eds GV Vahouny and D Kritchevsky, Publisher Plenum Press, New York pp 9-22 (1982).

20. Cummings JH: Nutritional implications of dietary fiber. Amer J Clin Nutr 31:521-529(1978).

21. Davenport HW: Physiology of the Digestive Tract, Publisher Year Book Medical Publishers Inc, Chicago (1977).

22. Doong G, Keen CL, Rogers Q, et al: Selected features of copper metabolism in the cat. J. Nutr 113:1963-1971 (1983).

23. Frank HA, Green LC: Successful use of a bulk laxative to control the diarrhea of tube feeding. Scand J Plast Reconstr Surg 13:193-194 (1979).

24. Glaze MB, Blanchard GL: Nutritional cataracts in a Samoyed litter. J Amer Anim Hosp Assoc 19:951-954 (1983).

25. Goranzon H, Forsum E, Thilen M: Calculation and determination of metabolizable energy in mixed diets to humans. Amer J Clin Nutr 38:954-963 (1983).

26. Ha YH, Milner JA, Corbin JF: Arginine requirements in immature dogs. J Nutr 108:203-210 (1978).

27. Haig BTH: Experimental pancreatitis intensified by a high fat diet. Surg Gynecol Obstet 131:914-918 (1970).

28. Hand MS, Crane SW, Buffington CA: Surgical nutrition. In manual of Small Animal Surgical Therapeutics, eds CW Betts and SW Crane. Publisher Churchill Livingstone, New York pp 91-115 (1986).

29. Hull C, Greco RS, Brooks DL: Alleviation of constipation in the elderly by dietary fiber supplementation. J Am Geriatr Soc 28:410-414 (1980).

30. Iseminger M, Hardy P: Bran works! Geriatr Nurs Nov/Dec: 402:404 (1982).

31. Jankins DJA, Leeds AR, Gassull MA, Cochet B, Alberti KGM A: Decrease in post prandial insulin and glucose concentration by guar and pectin. Ann Int Med 86:20-23 (1977).

32. Jenkins DJA, Reynolds D, Leeds AR, et al: Hypocholesterolemic action of dietary fiber unrelated to fecal bulking effect. Am J Clin Nutr 32:2430-2435 (1979).

33. Kane E, Morris JG, Rogers QR: Acceptability and digestibility by adult cats of diets made with various sources and levels of fat. J Anim Sci 53:1516-1523 (1981).

34. Kelsay JL: A review of research on effects of fiber intake on man. Am J Clin Nutr 31:142-159 (1978).

35. Kelsay JL: Effects of fiber on mineral and vitamin bioavailability. In Dietary Fiber in Health and Disease, eds GV Vahouny and D Kritchevsky, Publisher Plenum Press, New York, pp 91-103 (1982).

36. Kendall PT, Blaza SE, Smith PM: Comparative digestible energy requirements of adult beagles and domestic cats for body weight maintenance J Nutr 113:1946-1955 (1983).

37. Kendall PT, Burger IH, Smith PM: Methods of estimation of the metabolizable energy content of cat foods. Feline Prac 15:38-44 (1985).

38. Kendall PT, Holme DW, Smith PM: Methods of prediction of the digestible energy content of dog foods from gross energy value, proximate analysis and digestive nutrient content. J Sci Food & Agric 33:823-831 (1982).

39. Kinny JM: Energy metabolism. In Surgical Nutrition, ed JE Fischer, Publisher Little, Brown and Company, Boston, pp 97-126 (1983).

40. Kleiber M: Body size and metabolic rate. In the Fire of Life, Publisher Robert E Krieger Publishing Co, Huntington, pp 179-222 (1975).

41. Kleiber M: Energetic efficiency for animal production. In the Fire of Life. Publisher, Robert E. Krieger Publishing Co., Huntington, pp 297-332 (1975).

42. Kleiber M: Food as fuel. In the Fire of Life. Publisher, Robert E. Krieger Publishing Co., Huntington, pp 257-258 (1975).

43. Kronfeld DS, Hammell EP, Ramburg CF Jr, Dunlap HL Jr: Hematological and metabolic responses to training in racing sled dogs fed diets containing medium, low, or zero carbohydrate. Am J Clin Nutr 30:419 (1977).

44. Kronfeld DS: Diet and the performance of racing sled dogs. J Am Vet Med Assoc 162:470-473 (1973).

45. Kronfeld DS: Protein quality and amino acid profiles of commercial dog foods. J Amer Anim Hosp Assoc 18:679-683 (1982).

46. Kronfeld DS: Some nutritional problems in dogs. In Canine Nutrition, ed DS Kronfeld, Publisher University of Pennsylvania School of Veterinary Medicine, p 26 (1972).

47. Lee PC, Lebenthal E: Digestibility of modified starches, Amer J Clin Nutr 39:665-666 (1984).

48. Lewis LD, Boulay JP, Chow FHC: Fat excretion and assimilation by the cat. Feline Pract(1)9:46-49 (1979).

49. Lindsay S, Entenmann C, Chaikoff IL: Pancreatitis accompanying hepatic disease in dogs fed a high fat, low protein diet. Arch Pathol 45:635 (1948).

50. MacDonald ML, Anderson BG, Rogers QR, Buffington CA, Morris JG: Essential fatty acid requirements of cats:pathology of essential fatty acid deficiency. Am J Vet Res 45:1310-1317 (1984).

51. Milner, JA: Assessment of essentiality of methionine, threonine, tryptophan, histidine and isoleucine in immature dogs. J Nutr 109:1351-1357 (1979).

52. Milner JA: Lysine requirements of the immature dog. J Nutr 111:40-45 (1981).

53. Milner JA, Burns RA: Leucine, isoleucine and valine requirements of immature beagle dogs. Proc Pet Food Institute Annual Meeting, pp 53-63 (Sept 1982).

54. Morrison FB: Maintaining farm animals. In Feeds and Feeding. Publisher The Morrison Publishing Co., Ithaca. pp 149-167 (1957).

55. Nutrient Requirements of Cats. National Academy of Sciences, Washington DC, pp 1-49 (1978).

56. Nutrient Requirements of Dogs, National Academy of Sciences, Washington DC, pp 1-71 (1974).

57. Nutrient Requirements of Dogs. National Academy of Sciences, Washington DC, pp 1-79 (1985).

58. Nutrients and Toxic Substances in Water for Livestock and Poultry. Washington DC, National Academy of Sciences, pp 1-93 (1974).

59. Owen LN: Cancer Chemotherapy and immunotherapy. In Textbook of Veterinary Internal Medicine, ed SJ Ettinger, Publisher W.B. Saunders Co., pp 368-392 (1983).

60. Prescott CW: Feeding the cat. The University of Sydney Postgraduate Committee in Veterinary Science. Refresher Course on Cats. Sydney, N.S.W., Australia. Proceedings No. 53, pp 53:603-53:638 (1981).

61. Rogers QR, Morris JG: Protein and amino acid nutrition of the cat. Amer Anim Hosp Assoc Proc pp 333-336 (1983).

62. Royal College of Physicians of London, a Report:Medical aspects of dietary fiber. Publisher, Pitman Medical Ltd. (1980).

63. Smalley JR, Klish WJ, Campbell MA, Brown MR: Use of psyllium in the management of chronic non-specific diarrhea of childhood. J Pediatr Gastroenterol Nutr 1:361-363 (1982).

64. Spiller GA, Amen RJ: Dietary fiber in human nutrition. Crit Rev Food Sci Nutr, Nov:39-70 (1975).

65. Story JA: The role of dietary fiber in lipid metabolism. Adv Lipid Res 18:229-246 (1981).

66. Sturman JA, Gargano AD, Messing JM, Imaki H: Feline maternal taurine deficiency:effect on mother and offspring. J Nutr 116:655-667 (1986).

67. Switzer JW: Anemia. In Current Vet Therapy IV, Small Animal Pract, Ed R W Kirk, WB Saunders Co, Philadelphia (1971).

68. Watt BK, Merrill AL: Composition of Foods. Agricultural Handbook No. 8. Agricultural Research Service. United States Dept. Agriculture. U.S. Government Printing Office, Washington D.C. p. 124 (1975).

CHAPTER 2

Pet Foods

CONTENTS

INTRODUCTION

The majority of people who take their pets to the veterinarian ask about feeding. The veterinarian receives more questions on feeding, or nutrition, than on any other topic. One of the most common questions asked is, "What and how do I feed my pet?" The question may be phrased any number of ways: "How many times per day should I feed? Should I feed free-choice? Do I need to supplement? What brand do you recommend? Is brand X alright to feed? Are table scraps OK?"

The basis of modern food animal medicine is herd health management where feeding is recognized as an important component. However, proper advice on feeding is also an important part of the overall health management of small animal patients. This includes preventive as well as therapeutic nutrition.

To provide proper feeding advice, the veterinarian must have knowledge of the foods available, how to use them, and what nutrients they contain. Nutrients are described in Chapter 1. This chapter describes the foods available to feed dogs and cats. Chapters 3 and 4 describe how to use these foods to best nourish the normal dog and cat for maximum health and longevity. To perform these functions properly:

1. A diet must contain the proper amount and balance of all nutrients.
2. The ingredients in the diet must be such that the animal is able to digest, absorb, and utilize these nutrients.
3. The diet must be palatable enough so that an animal will consume an amount sufficient to meet its nutrient requirements.

FOOD PALATABILITY AND ACCEPTABILITY

Implementing veterinary recommendations on proper feeding of pets often requires the owner to change the pet's diet. Some pets readily accept dietary change; others do not. To change the diet of those that do not readily accept a new diet, or to induce an anorectic animal to eat, an understanding of factors that affect the palatability and acceptability of food is helpful.

Palatability is a measure of how well an animal likes a food. **Acceptability** is an indication of whether the amount of a food eaten will be enough to meet the animal's caloric requirement. A balanced diet needs only to be palatable enough to assure acceptability and, therefore, adequate nutrient intake. Although palatability receives considerable marketing attention, palatability above a level of acceptability will not improve a diet's performance. In fact, highly palatable diets are often precluded from free-choice feeding because they can result in excess nutrient intake and obesity. A variety of factors affect both the palatability and acceptability of a diet.

PALATABILITY

Factors affecting the palatability of a diet include:
1. Odor
2. Temperature
3. Texture or mouth feel
4. The amount of certain nutrients or foods in the diet
5. Habit

These factors may be interrelated. For example, water or fat content affects both the odor and texture of a diet. Knowledge of the effect of these various factors on food palatability provides for more logical and successful management of anorectic patients, or diet changes required in treating many diseases.

Odor is an important palatability factor for both dogs and cats. The dog's sense of smell is legendary and well documented. Olfaction has been shown to have an important influence on canine food preferences.[10] Cats also use their sense of smell in food selection, often sniffing carefully at food before eating it. Cats also exhibit definite preferences for certain odors in foods.[21] If the nasal passages are blocked, as often occurs with feline upper respiratory disease, olfaction and food acceptance may be improved by reestablishing patency using intranasal instillation of 5% saline drops. Warming food, particularly wet food, volatilizes odors and may improve palatability.

The temperature of food also appears to have a direct effect on palatability. In healthy cats, warming a canned food from 0°C to 40°C changed preference from approximately 4% to 80%, respectively, compared to the same food at 20°C; whereas, continued warming to 50°C reduced preference to 25% (Figure 1).[21] Dogs exhibit similar a preference for food temperature.[22] Therefore, warming food to no more than body temperature, may help entice an anorectic or reluctant dog or cat to eat.

Texture or mouth feel affects food palatability for both dogs and cats.[21] Cats tend to be individualistic and like either a canned or a dry food, generally preferring the one to which they are accustomed. Most cats do not like sticky foods. Dogs uniformly tend to prefer canned over dry foods, primarily because of the higher water con-

FIGURE 1

INFLUENCE OF FOOD TEMPERATURE ON FOOD PREFERENCE* IN THE CAT[21]

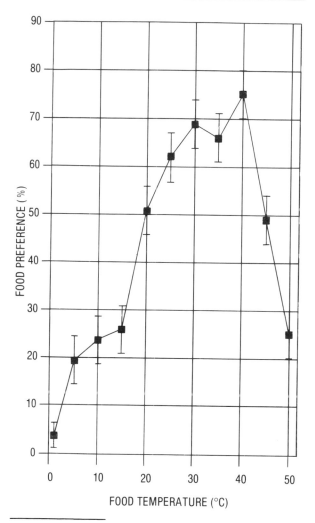

*Mean (±SEM) food preference demonstrated by 23 cats fed canned food at various temperatures as compared to same food at 20°C.

with an acid pH (3.5-5) over neutral or alkaline foods. As a result, acids are a common ingredient in commercial cat foods, especially dry and soft-moist forms. In addition, to increase their palatability, many dry cat foods have a coating of acid, digest, and/or fat sprayed on the exterior after they have been dried.

Digest is probably the most important factor discovered in recent years for enhancing the palatability of dry food for cats and, to a lesser degree, dogs. Digest is produced by controlled enzymatic degradation of a variety of animal tissues. The animal tissues most commonly used are ground poultry viscera, fish, liver, and beef lungs. Proteolytic enzymes, present in or added to the tissues, partially digest the protein. Degradation is stopped by the addition of acid (usually phosphoric), which creates a pH unfavorable for enzymatic action. The resulting liquid material, called digest, is sprayed on the exterior of dry foods at the 3-5% level. Digest may also be dried and dusted on a dry food following application of fat. Different digests are often used to justify a different flavor designation for pet foods that contain basically the same ingredients.

Many animals prefer the diet to which they are accustomed. If they are accustomed to variety, it is relatively easy to change their diet. However, if they are always fed a single ingredient, or flavor, or form of diet, they may develop a marked fixed preference for that diet. The diet then becomes a "habit." This makes it difficult to change the animal's diet regardless of the new diet's average palatability. Feeding a ration-type, rather than a gourmet-type pet food may prevent this "addiction." This is because ration-type pet foods contain a number of different food items, whereas gourmet pet foods contain a limited number of food items. When an animal has a fixed food preference, its diet may have to be changed gradually. Begin by feeding the old food mixed with a small amount of the new. When the animal accepts this mixture, over a period of several days, gradually reduce the amount of old food and increase the amount of new. However, many pets do not require a gradual change. In fact, some will initially eat more of a new diet than they ate of their previous diet. In one study, started at the time of weaning, kittens were fed exclusively one of three different types of palatable canned cat foods.[12] At 22 weeks of age the cats were allowed a choice of two diets; one being the food they were eating previously and the other, a canned cat food of equal palatability. Almost all the cats initially preferred the new food. This preference diminished with time, resulting in equal consumption of both foods.

tent of canned foods. Adding water to a dry food increases its palatability for most dogs,[22] but most cats do not like a dry food that has been wetted. The shape of dry food pellets, i.e. nuggets, stars, etc., has little effect on palatability, provided that the product does not irritate the oral cavity. However, many cats develop a preference for certain shapes of dry foods, which is one reason manufacturers produce specifically-shaped products.

Up to a certain level, increasing the protein and fat content will improve the palatability of a diet for most dogs and cats. Cats also tend to prefer foods

ACCEPTABILITY

Acceptability of the diet is affected by palatability, but is also influenced by two other factors:

1. Nutritional need. This is called "true appetite."
2. Previous experience; that is, a learned appetite, or aversion if the food is avoided.

In contrast to popular belief, animals seek out and consume only three nutrients in accordance with body need. These are water, sodium, and those nutrients providing energy. If these three nutrients are readily available, and diets providing them are sufficiently palatable, animals may consume more of all of these nutrients than they require. However, if animals are physically capable and are not anorectic, they will not consume less of these three nutrients than they need. This does not apply to other nutrients. With the exception of sodium, the amounts of all other minerals, as well as vitamins, are ingested according to taste preference, or palatability, rather than the amount needed.

Many diseases, both nutritional and non-nutritional, may cause a change in taste perception or preference.[18,19] When this occurs as a result of a nutritional deficiency, and the animal happens to eat more of a food or substance containing that nutrient, the situation is often cited as evidence that the animal somehow perceives it needs more of that nutrient and, therefore, has a true appetite for it. However, if the animal's taste perception has changed, it may eat more of certain foods, if they are available, or less of others. The particular food for which the animal is showing a preference may contain more or less of the nutrient that is deficient. If it contains more, it is easy to reach the incorrect conclusion that the animal has a true appetite for that nutrient.

Studies conducted in several species have proven that animals do not consume amino acids, fatty acids, fiber, vitamins, or minerals (with the exception of sodium) according to their needs.[6,20] When animals are allowed to select and consume specific nutrients, free-choice, there is much individual variation. Some animals ingest the correct amount, others an excess, and others little or none. Consumption is not related to requirements. Thus, **the only way to ensure that each animal receives the proper amount of each nutrient is to feed a food containing the proper balance of nutrients with respect to the caloric density of the diet.** When the animal consumes enough food to meet its caloric requirement, it will automatically obtain the proper amount of all other nutrients.

DETERMINATION OF FOOD ACCEPTABILITY AND PALATABILITY

Food acceptability is determined by a 1-pan test and palatability by a 2-pan test. In the 1-pan test, access to a single food is provided, and the amount of food consumed is measured. Sometimes the eagerness with which it is eaten is observed, or the time it takes to eat the food is measured. This is the procedure used by animal owners in feeding their pets. Scientists, however, routinely use the 2-pan test to determine palatability. In this test, excessive amounts of two foods are offered at the same time to a number of animals for several days. The amount of each food consumed daily by each animal is measured. Examples of the results of three actual 2-pan palatability tests are shown in Table 1.

Even when a majority of animals find one diet much more palatable than another, some animals prefer the less palatable diet; just as the majority of people may not prefer liver, some people consider it quite palatable. Thus, **it is normal for some animals to prefer one diet over another, even though the average palatability of that diet for the entire population is low.**

FOOD NUTRIENT CONTENT

DETERMINING FOOD NUTRIENT CONTENT

Foods are nutrient packages containing different nutrients in different amounts and availability. In order to determine if a food provides the nutrients needed, or if the total diet provides the proper amount of nutrients, the nutrient levels in a food must be known. There are three ways to accomplish this:

1. Obtain a laboratory analysis (proximate analysis) of the food. This is the most accurate method.
2. From the label on a prepared food
3. Calculate the nutrient content of the diet from the average nutrient contents of its ingredients. The average nutrient content of human foods fed to dogs and cats are listed in Appendix Table 4.

The most common method of determining the nutrient content of a food is the **proximate analysis** which provides the percent moisture, protein, fat, ash, and fiber, and allows calculation of the soluble carbohydrate or nitrogen-free extract (NFE). The determination is conducted as shown in Figure 2. Many commercial laboratories conduct proximate analyses of foods.

TABLE 1

TWO-PAN PALATABILITY TEST

% of Total Food Intake	Example 1 Number Eating*		Example 2 Number Eating*		Example 3 Number Eating*	
	Diet A	Diet B	Diet C	Diet D	Diet E	Diet F
40–60	46		5		5	
60–90	5	3	10	8	44	2
90–100	4	2	20	17	7	2
Total preferring	9	5	30	25	51	4
Consumption Ratio**	1.35:1		1.20:1		5.27:1	
Statistical Significance	No		No		p<0.001	
Conclusions†	No difference		No difference		E preferred	

*Indicates the number of animals whose percent of total food intake of each diet was within the range, i.e. Example 1, 46 animals ate fairly equal amounts (40–60%) of each diet; whereas 60% or more of total food intake for 9 animals was diet A, and for 5 was diet B.

**Ratio of the total amount of each diet consumed by all animals throughout the test.

†Although most animals did not care whether they ate diet A or B, some did have a preference. This effect is even greater with diets C and D. Although there is no significant difference in the total number that preferred diet C or D, or the total amount of each diet consumed by all of the animals, 30 preferred C while 25 preferred D. Even with two diets, such as E and F, which one is greatly preferred over the other by the majority of animals, some animals still preferred the diet which had lower palatability (F).

FIGURE 2

PROXIMATE ANALYSIS OF FOODS

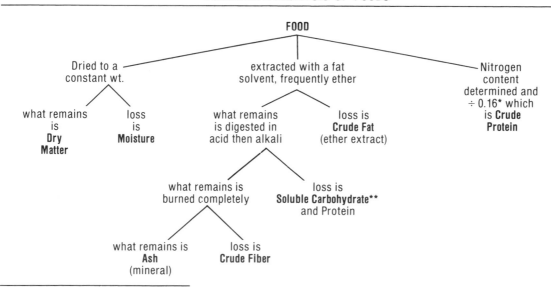

*Proteins contain 16 ± 2% nitrogen. Crude protein = nitrogen × 6.25, or nitrogen ÷ 0.16. Protein determined by this method will be erroneously high if the food contains non-protein nitrogen such as urea or ammonia.

**Frequently called nitrogen free extract or NFE. It is determined as the difference between 100% and the amount of everything else in the food, i.e. 100% − % moisture − % crude protein − % crude fat − % crude fiber − % ash. Any errors in these analyses also will appear in the NFE value.

The use of the **guaranteed analysis** listed on the label of prepared foods is much less accurate than the proximate analysis because the quantities listed in the guaranteed analysis are minimums or maximums only. Label values are **not** the nutrient content of the food. They are a guarantee by the manufacturer that the food contains not more or less than the stated amount. Label guarantees are useful only to provide a general idea of the nutrient content and classification of the food; they are of little or no value in comparing specific nutrient levels between foods. In many instances, label guarantees are more confusing than helpful because of the erroneous assumption that they represent the actual nutrient contents of the food. Two foods with the same label guarantee may contain nutrient levels that vary by more than 100%, yet both meet their label guarantees as shown in Table 2.

METHODS OF EXPRESSING FOOD NUTRIENT CONTENT

Regardless of how the nutrient content of a food is obtained, the basis on which these values are expressed must be understood. The nutrient content of a food is generally expressed by one of the following methods:

1. "As is," "as fed" or "as purchased" basis
2. Dry-matter basis
3. Calorie basis

Failure to understand the differences in these methods is a common reason for errors made in feeding, in statements about pet foods types and in comparisons between brands of pet foods. For example, 100 g of a diet contains 10 g of protein and 75 g of water. If the water is removed, the remaining 25 g of dry matter still contains 10 g of protein. Thus, the diet contains 10 g of protein/100 g diet as is (or as fed) and, therefore, contains 10% protein on an as fed basis; whereas on a dry-matter basis the diet contains 10 g of protein/25 g of dry matter and, therefore, 40% on a dry-matter basis.

Because the water content of pet foods can vary from less than 5% to more than 80% (more than 95% to less than 20% dry matter, respectively), there can be almost a five-fold difference in the nutrient content in the same diet depending on how it is expressed, or a five-fold difference in the dry matter content of a nutrient in two diets that have the same amount of that nutrient reported on the label. Therefore, the only way that the nutrient content between different diets can be compared, or that the nutrient content of a diet can be compared to an animal's requirements, is if all are expressed on an identical moisture or calorie basis. Because the moisture contents of diets differ, the best way to ensure that the nutrient contents of diets are compared on an identical moisture basis, is to determine the amount of nutrients in the diet dry matter.

In comparing foods, even greater accuracy can be achieved by comparing nutrients on a calorie basis because most animals eat to meet their energy requirement. Thus, the amount of food consumed, and therefore the amount of nutrients consumed, depends on the calorie content of the food. For example:

Diet A provides 300 kcal and 4 g protein/100 g of food, whereas diet B provides 600 kcal and 4 g protein/100 g of food.

Assume the energy requirement of an animal is 600 kcal/day.

When fed diet A the animal would need 600 Kcal/day ÷ 300 kcal/100 g of food, or 200 g of food.

When fed diet B the animal would need 600 kcal/day ÷ 600 kcal/100 g of food, or 100 g of food.

The amount of protein provided daily by diet A would be 200 g of food × 4 g protein/100 g of food or 8 g protein.

TABLE 2

VARIABILITY IN NUTRIENT CONTENT OF PET FOODS
(Guaranteed vs Actual Analysis)

Food	Guaranteed Analysis		Actual Analysis					
	Water %	Calcium %	Water %	Calcium %		Dry Matter Fraction		Calcium % in Dry Matter
A	78 max.	0.4 min.	70.0	0.40	÷	0.30	=	1.33
B	78 max.	0.4 min.	78.0	0.60	÷	0.22	=	2.73
Difference	None		50%					105%

The amount of protein provided daily by diet B would be

100 g of food × 4 g protein/100 g of food or 4 g protein.

Therefore, although both diets A and B contained the same amount of protein on a dry-matter basis (4%), the higher energy density of diet B results in less of it being eaten to meet the animal's energy requirement and, accordingly, less protein being consumed.

If the caloric content on a dry-matter basis differs between diets, the only accurate way to compare the amount of nutrients in these diets (or to an animal's requirements) is: 1) to convert to an isocaloric basis (as is done in all tables or nutrient requirements in this book) or 2) to express it as the amount of nutrient per kcal of metabolizable energy. However, the amount of nutrients in the diet dry matter is used more often for two reasons: 1) an accurate estimate of the metabolizable energy content of the food usually is not available, and 2) the caloric content in the dry matter of pet foods does not vary as much as the moisture content. Most pet foods of average quality provide 3.5-4.0 kcal of metabolizable energy/g of dry matter. However, in specific-purpose diets, ranging from those intended for weight reduction to those for stress or physical exertion, energy density can vary more than 100%, and obviously should be considered. **To determine the amount of nutrient per kcal of metabolizable energy, divide the nutrient content by the energy density of the food.** For example, to determine the amount of magnesium on a calorie basis in a cat food containing 0.16% magnesium and 4 kcal/g as fed:

$$\frac{0.16 \text{ g Mg}/100 \text{ g diet as fed}}{400/\text{kcal}/100 \text{ g diet as fed}} =$$

$$\frac{0.16 \text{ g Mg}}{400 \text{ kcal}} = \frac{160 \text{ mg Mg}}{400 \text{ kcal}} =$$

$$\frac{0.4 \text{ mg Mg}}{\text{kcal}} = 40 \text{ mg Mg}/100 \text{ kcal}$$

Occasionally it is desirable to express the amount of fat, soluble carbohydrate, or protein in a diet on the basis of the relative amount of energy supplied by each. This may be done as shown for protein in Table 3 (page 1-8).

Nutrient values obtained from a laboratory analysis or listed by a food manufacturer are generally on an "as is" or "as fed" basis unless stated otherwise. To convert an amount of nutrient from an as-fed to a dry-matter basis, divide the amount of the nutrient, as fed, by the fraction of dry matter. For example (also, see Table 2):

10% protein as fed ÷ 0.25 dry-matter fraction as fed = 40% protein (dry-matter basis)

Two errors are commonly made in making this conversion: 1) using the moisture content rather than the dry matter content, and 2) multiplying rather than dividing.

DIET— FORMULATION AND EVALUATION

Most pet owners use a commercially prepared diet for feeding their dogs and cats. Different types of diets may be used for different purposes. However, in some instances it may be necessary to formulate a diet to meet nutrient requirements for a specific condition. The same procedure is used to determine the amount of any nutrient provided by a mixture of two or more foods. The procedure can also be used to determine how much of a food or supplement containing a specific nutrient is needed to meet the animal's requirements, or to provide a specific amount of that nutrient.

To formulate or evaluate a diet, three things must be known:

1. The nutrient content of the foods in the diet (determined as shown in Figure 2, page 2-5).
2. The amount of the nutrient of concern needed by the animal (the animal's requirements)
3. The procedures used to formulate or evaluate the diet

The nutrient requirements for the normal healthy dog and cat are given in Chapter 1, Tables 1, 6, 9, 11 and 13; those for sick animals are given in subsequent chapters on nutritional management of various diseases. The following examples illustrate how to determine the quantity of each food needed to meet the animal's requirement, or the amount of each nutrient provided by a combination of foods.

Example 1:

A mature non-reproducing dog is being fed 0.5 lb/day of beef fat and 10 cups (2 lb) of dry dog food. What is the protein content of this diet? The guaranteed analysis on the food container indicates that it contains a minimum of 22% protein. The fat being added does not provide any protein. The protein content of the ration can be calculated as shown in Table 3.

TABLE 3

DIET CALCULATION — EXAMPLE 1

Food	Amount Fed (lb)		Total Intake		Fraction in Diet		Protein (%) in Feed		Protein (%) in Diet	kcal/g in Food		kcal/g in Diet
Beef Fat	0.5	÷	2.5	=	0.2	×	0	=	0	7.36	=	1.47
Dry Food	2.0	÷	2.5	=	0.8	×	22	=	17.6	4	=	3.20
Total	2.5				1.0				17.6			4.67

Thus, there is 17.6% protein in this diet which provides 4.67 kcal/g. This would be equivalent to 15.1% protein in a diet providing 4 kcal/g [17.6% × (4 ÷ 4.67)].

As given in Table 9, page 1-16, a diet providing 4 kcal/g should contain at least 18% protein. Thus, to determine if this diet meets the dog's protein requirement, the percent protein in this diet must be corrected to a diet containing 4 kcal/g. The caloric density of the fat is 7.36 kcal/g (Appendix Table 4) and the caloric density of the dry food can be determined as shown in Table 4, page 1-8. For this example, 4 kcal/g was used. Using these values, as shown in Table 3, the caloric content of the fat supplemented diet can be determined and the percent protein corrected to a caloric density of 4 kcal/g. The result is 15.1%, compared to 18% needed.

Example 2:

How much calcium carbonate containing 33% calcium must be added to an all-meat diet to increase its calcium content from 0.01% to 0.3% (1% of the dry matter)? This can be determined in a number of ways. The easiest way is called the **Pearson square.** As shown in Table 4, the percent of the specific nutrient required is placed in the center of the square—in this example 0.3%. The percentage of that nutrient in the food or diet (in this case meat) is placed at the upper left corner—in this example 0.01%. The percent of that nutrient in

TABLE 4

DIET CALCULATION — EXAMPLE 2

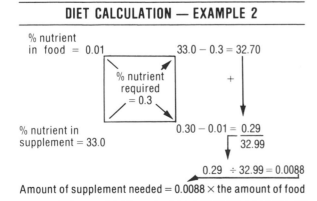

% nutrient in food = 0.01

33.0 − 0.3 = 32.70

% nutrient required = 0.3

% nutrient in supplement = 33.0

+

0.30 − 0.01 = 0.29

32.99

0.29 ÷ 32.99 = 0.0088

Amount of supplement needed = 0.0088 × the amount of food

the other food, diet, or supplement (in this case calcium carbonate) is placed at the lower left corner—in this example 33%. Next, the number in the middle is subtracted from the number at the lower left corner, and the answer is placed at the upper right corner—in this example 33 - 0.3 = 32.70. Then the number at the upper left corner is subtracted from the number in the middle, and the answer is placed at the lower right corner—in this sample 0.3 - 0.01 = 0.29. Add the two numbers at the right corners—in this example 32.70 + 0.29 = 32.99. Then divide the number at the lower right corner by this sum—in this case 0.29 ÷ 32.99 = 0.0088. This value multiplied by 100 is the percent calcium carbonate containing 33% calcium required for addition to the meat diet to increase its calcium content from 0.01% to 0.3%. Thus, for each 1 lb (454 g) of meat, 0.0088 × 454 or 4 g (approximately 1 level teaspoonful) of calcium carbonate is needed.

Example 3:

A dog is consuming 1 kg/day of dry food. The guaranteed analysis on the label indicates that the food contains a minimum of 21% protein. Because of a protein-losing enteropathy estimated at 20-25 g/day, an increase in the protein content of the diet is desired. To accomplish this objective, 500 g (1.25 cans) of a meat-type dog food is fed. Its guaranteed analysis indicates that it contains at least 14% protein. It is calculated or known that the dry food provides 3000 kcal/kg and the canned food 1200 kcal/kg. As shown in Table 5, when 0.5 kg of canned food is consumed:

1. Dry food intake is reduced from 1 to 0.8 kg in order to maintain the same caloric intake.
2. Protein intake is increased by 28 g/day which replaces the estimated protein loss.

If this increase in protein intake was not sufficient, the amount of canned food fed could be increased. As shown, feeding the canned food in place of the dry food at the same caloric level increases protein intake by 140 g/day.

TABLE 5

DIET CALCULATION — EXAMPLE 3

Food Fed	kg/day Fed		kcal/kg in				Protein in Food (%)		Food Eaten (g/day)		Protein Eaten (g/day)
			Food		Diet						
Previous Diet:											
Dry	1	×	3000	=	3000		21	×	1000	=	210
New Diet:											
Dry	0.8	×	3000	=	2400		21	×	800	=	168
Can	0.5	×	1200	=	600		14	×	500	=	70
			Total		3000						238
			Change		0						+ 28
Canned Diet:											
Can	2.5	×	1200	=	3000		14	×	2500	=	350
			Change		0						+140

OPTIMAL DIETARY NUTRIENT CONTENT

Inadequate intake of any nutrient or the excess intake of a number of nutrients can be harmful. For example, the effects of an inadequate intake of nutrients such as protein, calcium, and phosphorus occur quite rapidly and are easily demonstrated. A protein deficiency impairs growth, reproduction, physical performance, health, and resistance to infectious diseases. A deficiency in either calcium or phosphorus, or both, results in skeletal disease, especially in growing animals. Providing more calcium, phosphorus, or protein than necessary to meet the animal's requirements will prevent a deficiency of these nutrients. However, if the amount consumed greatly exceeds the animal's requirements, other problems may arise. These excesses may induce dietary imbalances, some of which can result in clinical signs identical to those occurring when intake of that nutrient is inadequate.

Nutritional deficiencies are rare when a good quality pet food constitutes most of the diet for the healthy dog or cat. Nutritional excesses are more common and are caused by an excess amount of certain nutrients in commercial pet foods, and/or inappropriate dietary supplementation by the owner. These two factors occur for three major reasons:

1. Failure to appreciate that the excessive intake of some nutrients is just as harmful as a deficiency.
2. Regulations used to substantiate claims of nutritional adequacy require that commercial pet foods only meet or exceed established minimums.
3. Many manufacturers ensure that their products, regardless of the purpose for which the diet is intended, contain even more of all the nutrients than the National Research Council recommends for growth and lactation, the periods of greatest nutritional need.

A committee of nutritionists is periodically formed by the National Academy of Sciences to make recommendations on the minimum amount of the various nutrients required by different species of animals. These recommendations have been based on the minimum amount of most nutrients needed when that nutrient is provided by an ingredient from which it is poorly utilized. Then a margin of safety is added. These recommendations are widely published as the National Research Council Nutrient Requirements for that particular species of animal, including one for the dog[15] and one for the cat.[13] The National Research Council recommendations are the guidelines used by most pet food manufacturers in formulating their products. However, for most nutrients these recommendations are stated as minimums only. Unfortunately, neither maximum nor optimum recommendations are made.

The most recent edition of the National Research Council Nutrient Requirements of Dogs was released in 1985.[15] In this edition, minimum nutrient requirements are listed as **available** nutrients. Because availability of nutrients in most pet food ingredients is not known, the new publication cannot be used as a comparison standard to substantiate nutritional adequacy of a diet. As an alternative, the Pet Food Institute, the trade association of the pet food industry, has commissioned feeding studies to determine minimum diet standards based on availability of nutrients in commonly used ingredients. In the interim, the Association of

American Feed Control Officials (AAFCO) has extended the use of the 1974 edition of the Nutrient Requirements of Dogs[14] until these studies are completed and new standards are developed.

Many manufacturers produce pet foods that contain a far greater amount of most nutrients than are recommended by the National Research Council for growth and lactation. This is done for the following reasons:

1. So that the manufacturer can advertise that the product exceeds National Research Council recommendations. Many consumers assume that this means that the product has a "government stamp of approval."

2. To protect against the development of nutritional deficiencies, regardless of the activity or function of the animal to which the food is fed. A diet that just meets the needs for the inactive mature or older dog would be deficient for growth, reproduction, or increased physical activity and would result in noticeably poor performance during these periods. This would be damaging to a company's reputation and might even result in litigation. In contrast, the amount of excess nutrients, such as protein, calcium, phosphorus, and sodium, provided to the mature inactive dog being fed a diet adequate for growth, reproduction, or extensive physical activity, takes months or years to cause any detrimental effects. Such effects are frequently not recognized as having dietary causes.

   Thus, from the manufacturer's point of view, it is safest to formulate a food that contains adequate nutrients for all feeding situations rather than one for specific feeding situations. However, this does not mean that many companies do not market multiple foods. Many companies produce as many products as possible. Often the nutritional differences in these products are minimal. By using different names, different flavors, and featuring different ingredients, a large number of products can be developed and marketed, which takes up more shelf space in the supermarket, resulting in increased sales. Gourmet canned cat foods are an illustration of this type of product.

3. To protect against a deficiency due to variability in the nutrient content and nutrient availability in the ingredients used to make their foods.

4. Because many inexpensive pet food ingredients contain high levels of certain nutrients. For example, meat and bone meal, poultry meal, and fish meal contain large amounts of ground bone (ash) and as a result are high in calcium, phosphorus, and magnesium. These ingredients are available with lower levels of these nutrients, but they are more expensive and currently there is little incentive to use them.

5. Many people believe that "more is better." This is one reason that some pet owners (particularly dog owners) give nutritional supplements. Because of this misconception, if pet food "X" contains more of certain nutrients than pet food "Y," it is often concluded that "X" is better than "Y."

These are the major reasons that many commercial pet foods contain certain nutrients in quantities that, if consumed over a prolonged period, can predispose to, or promote, progression of a variety of diseases.

Excess protein, phosphorus, or sodium intake induces renal hyperperfusion and hypertension which in turn can cause and promote the progression of renal damage (Chapter 8). Diets restricted in these nutrients can help prevent renal failure and are important in managing animals with this disease which, after cancer, is the leading non-accidental cause of death of dogs.

The sodium (salt) content of most commercial pet foods is much greater than needed to meet the requirement of either dogs or cats. Too much sodium intake may induce hypertension, which in turn is a major risk factor for the development of congestive heart disease. Numerous organ systems can be adversely affected by congestive heart disease, thereby reducing longevity (page 8-11). In addition, excessive sodium intake is harmful for animals with pre-existing renal or heart disease, both of which are common in older dogs and cats. Reducing sodium intake decreases or prevents hypertension and its associated detrimental effects.

In addition to protein, phosphorus, and sodium, excess calcium and magnesium can also be harmful. Too much calcium impairs absorption of several minerals, including zinc, iron, iodine, and phosphorus (for effects of this see Table 11, page 1-20). Chronic excessive calcium ingestion, even below that necessary to interfere with the absorption of other minerals, can retard growth rate and possibly predispose to bloat (page 3-16). Excessive magnesium intake and a high urine pH are prerequisites for the production of urinary crystals and calculi associated with cystitis, urethritis, and/or urethral obstruction in the cat. This condition, referred to as the "feline urologic syndrome" (FUS) or lower urinary tract disease, is described in Chapter 9.

Because of these effects, emphasis should be focused on feeding diets that contain only as much protein, calcium, phosphorus, sodium, and magnesium as necessary to meet the requirements of the

animal being fed. A diet higher in all of these nutrients, as well as energy, should be fed during growth, reproduction, and lactation. A diet high in caloric density should be fed for physical performance or to any animal in which maintaining optimal body weight is a problem. The mature inactive dog or cat should be fed a diet containing lower levels of all of these nutrients than the diet fed to growing puppies, kittens, or reproducing females. For animals past middle age, a diet even lower in protein, calcium, phosphorus, and sodium should be fed because older animals have less ability to tolerate nutrient excesses. For disease, diets modified for that specific condition (as described in detail in other chapters) should be fed, These include:

1. Low-sodium diets for hypertension, heart disease, ascites, or edema from any cause
2. Diets low in protein, phosphorus, and sodium for kidney or hepatic disease
3. Highly digestible diets for bloat, liver disease, pancreatic disease, most cases of diarrhea of small intestinal origin, as well as underweight animals
4. Diets that result in acid urine and are restricted in protein, calcium, phosphorus, and magnesium for dogs with struvite urolithiasis, and diets that are magnesium restricted and result in acid urine for cats with struvite urolithiasis
5. Diets restricted in urate precursors (DNA and RNA) and cystine (protein) that maintain an alkaline urine for dogs and cats with ammonium urate or cystine uroliths
6. Diets restricted in calcium, oxalate and sodium for dogs and cats with calcium oxalate uroliths
7. Diets high in fiber for diabetes mellitus, colitis, and constipation
8. Diets high in fiber and low in caloric density for the overweight dog or cat
9. Hypoallergenic diets for pets with food-induced allergies
10. Highly palatable diets, with increased nutrient density for the malnourished, anemic, and/or anorectic dog or cat

Emphasis in pet nutrition must be switched from the minimum amounts of nutrients needed to prevent deficiency diseases, to the optimal amounts of nutrients necessary for health, longevity and performance. This concept is further emphasized by reviewing the definitions of two common nutritional terms, i.e. **malnutrition** and **balanced diet.** Malnutrition is defined as abnormal nutrition. The definition includes overnutrition as well as undernutrition. A balanced diet is defined as one that provides the proper (optimal) amounts of all the required nutrients. Diets that are nutrient excessive and/or deficient are not balanced. Optimal dietary nutrient levels may vary with environmental changes, as well as changes in the animal's health, activity, function, and stage of life. As stated by Shakespeare in *The Merchant of Venice:*

"They are sick that surfeit with too much, as they that starve with nothing."

SUPPLEMENTATION

The harm resulting from nutrient excesses may be caused or worsened by adding to prepared diets supplements that provide additional energy, protein, calcium, phosphorus, trace minerals, or vitamins. Supplements are often given to dogs and cats by well-intentioned pet owners who believe the practice is beneficial to the pet. Unfortunately this belief is often based on promotional literature or uncontrolled studies or observations.

Nutritional supplements should not be given unless they are needed for managing a specific condition. None are needed for routine feeding if a good-quality prepared pet food makes up all, or most of, the animal's diet. A poor quality diet is unlikely to be improved by supplementation. The problem with a poor quality diet is not simply one of a specific nutrient deficiency which can be corrected by addition of a supplement. Inferior diets more often contain mineral excesses and imbalances, as well as poorly digestible energy and protein. If a diet produces poor results, it is much easier, safer, more effective, and usually less expensive, simply to switch to a diet that contains the proper amounts of available nutrients for the condition for which the diet is being fed. Then it should be fed without supplementation. Supplementing a good diet will not improve its nutrient balance and may result in nutrient excesses as well as secondary deficiencies. Therefore, routine diet supplementation is **not** recommended. However, if an owner is determined to supplement a pet's diet, the veterinarian should help them select a supplement, and determine a dosage that has the least probability of unbalancing the diet.

Human Food and Other Dietary Supplements

Since certain foods for human beings are often fed (or considered for feeding) as supplements to a commercially prepared pet food, it is helpful to know something about the more commonly used

human foods. **None of the following items should make up more than 25%, and preferably not more than 10%, of a normal dog's or cat's dry-matter intake if the animal is being fed a prepared pet food as the basic diet:**

1. **Meat**—As shown in Table 6, meat is inadequate in calcium, phosphorus, sodium, iron, copper, iodine, vitamins A, D and E, and provides excess protein. Thus, even if a calcium supplement is given, meat is still deficient in these other minerals and vitamins. Meat should not be fed raw because of the danger of transmitting parasites. In addition, most dogs and cats prefer cooked meat.

TABLE 6

COMPARISON OF THE NUTRIENT CONTENT OF MEAT TO THE NUTRIENT REQUIREMENT OF DOGS

Nutrient	Needed by 20 lb Dog Daily for Maintenance	Provided by Raw Beef (355g)	
		Amount	% of Requirement
Calories	700	700	100
Protein (g)	15–20	90	450–600
Calcium (mg)	1000	40	4
Phosphorus (mg)	880	700	80
Ca/P Ratio	1 to 2:1	1:17	——
Sodium (mg)	530	230	40
Potassium (mg)	710	1250	175
Iron (mg)	11	10	90
Copper (mg)	1.5	0.3	20
Magnesium (mg)	55	77	140
Iodine (mg)	0.3	0.03	10
Vitamin A (IU)	1000	70	7
Vitamin D (IU)	100	50	50
Vitamin E (IU)	10	2	20

2. **Fish** is a good source of protein but has many of the same deficiencies and excesses as meat (Table 6). The bones should be removed to prevent choking. If the whole fish is cooked and finely ground, it is not deficient in calcium or phosphorus. In fact, it contains too much of these minerals. Fish should be cooked to avoid parasite transmission and to destroy thiaminase, an enzyme in certain fish (particularly carp and herring) that destroys thiamin and may cause thiamin deficiency (see page 12-13). Ingestion of raw salmon or trout infected with *Neorickettsia helminthoeca* or *Neorickettsia elokominica* causes an acute systemic disease called salmon poisoning.[4,8] Severe depression, fever, generalized enlargement of lymph nodes, oculonasal discharge, hematemesis, and diarrhea, with 90% mortality in untreated cases, occur 5-12 days after inges-

tion of the organism. Diagnosis is confirmed by finding light brown, 45 x 90 μm trematode eggs in fecal smears or by sugar flotation (1.27 specific gravity), or rickettsiae in lymph node cells.[8] Treatment with oxytetracycline, fluids, and supportive therapy is effective.[4] Cooking the fish prevents the disease.

3. **Fats and oils** can be used to increase the energy density of a diet during periods of high energy need. However, there are limitations on how much fat or oil to add to a prepared food. Oversupplementation with either fats or oils increases the caloric density of a diet so that energy needs are met with less food. This situation could lead to a nutrient deficiency (see Example 1, page 2-7). One tablespoon of lard, bacon drippings, or vegetable oil added to each pound of canned food, or to each 8 oz measuring cup of dry food, is the maximum amount recommended. Vegetable oils may be used to improve the coat, particularly for dogs or cats fed an inferior quality dry food, a dry food that has been stored too long, or a food containing unstabilized fat. Adding one teaspoon of oil per 8 oz measuring cup of dry food will supply sufficient linoleic acid to improve the coat if any effect is to be realized. Vegetable oils are superior to animal fats for this purpose because they contain 5-10 times the amount of linoleic acid (see Table 10, page 1-18). Avoid giving hydrogenated coconut oil to cats, as it may cause hepatic lipidosis.

4. **Eggs** are among the best sources of protein available, but should be fed cooked. Raw egg white contains avidin, which destroys the vitamin biotin. However, this is of no concern if egg yolks are also being fed because the effect of avidin is offset by the high biotin content of egg yolk. Egg yolks contain 33% fat (65% of their dry matter) and 4% linoleic acid. Improvement in coat is often seen when eggs are added to the diet of dogs or cats eating low-fat dry foods. Credit for this response is frequently given to the protein in the egg, but it is usually the fat or linoleic acid in the yolk that produces the response. Whole egg contains more calcium than does meat, but similar amounts of phosphorus. Ground eggshells are composed of calcium carbonate and are a good source of calcium (see Appendix Table 4).

5. **Milk** is an excellent source of calcium, phosphorus, protein, and many vitamins. Due to the high lactose content of cow's milk (see Table 4, page 3-18), excessive intake may cause diarrhea in some dogs and cats. Cow's milk is a common cause of diarrhea in puppies (see page 7-42).

6. **Cheese** and **cottage cheese** are excellent sources of protein and fat for dogs and cats and are quite palatable for both. Unlike milk, cottage cheese is not a good source of calcium as it contains a 1:2 ratio of calcium to phosphorus (see Appendix Table 4).

7. **Liver** contains high biologic-value protein, fat, carbohydrate, trace minerals, and vitamins. It is deficient in calcium as it contains only 0.01%. The calcium/phosphorus ratio of liver is about 1:35. It is most nutritious when fed raw and is particularly helpful for the sick, weak or anemic dog or cat. Feeding diets composed exclusively of liver will rapidly cause a calcium deficiency and may create a vitamin A toxicity, depending on the source of the liver and its level of stored vitamin A. Diets high in liver content can cause diarrhea in some dogs and cats. There is no evidence to support the argument that liver should not be fed because it functions as an excretory organ and contains "toxic products."

8. **Vegetables,** when properly balanced in the diet with protein and mineral-supplying ingredients, are good foods for dogs. Vegetables are high in moisture (80-95%). On a dry matter basis they are high in carbohydrates (60-80%) and fiber (7-10%), and low in protein (8-14%), fat (1-4%), calcium (0.25-0.5%), and phosphorus (0.25%) (see Appendix Table 4). Occasionally vegetarians desire to impose their own food preferences on their pet. Prepared diets free of animal tissue are available and can be made at home (see Meat Free Diets, Appendix Table 1). However, it is difficult to develop a balanced diet for dogs (and impossible for cats) that is free of products from animal sources.

Other items occasionally fed to or consumed by pets are:

1. **Vitamin and mineral supplements**—Normal dogs and cats being fed a good quality pet food as 90% or more of their diet **do not need vitamin and mineral supplements.** Medical problems resulting from oversupplementation are much more common than deficiencies when prepared diets are fed. This is particularly true of the fat-soluble vitamins A and D. Vitamin-mineral supplements should be given routinely if homemade diets are being fed, or in specific medical situations where food intake is reduced, or losses or needs are increased. See Table 11, page 1-20 and Table 13, page 1-23, for mineral and vitamin requirements for the dog and cat.

2. **Bones**—Dogs enjoy chewing on bones, and chewing bones helps prevent build-up of tartar on their teeth. However, small bones, and those that splinter, may lodge in the mouth or gastrointestinal tract. Giving large "knuckle bones" that do not readily splinter is better but may result in broken teeth.

3. **Table scraps** should not be used as the primary diet of a dog or cat. The only exception is **fat trimmings** from meat, if the trimmings are added to dry food in amounts **not exceeding 10% of the diet by weight.** Feeding large amounts of fat trimmings at one meal may induce diarrhea and has been associated with episodes of acute pancreatitis in susceptible dogs (see pages 1-18 and 7-17).

4. **Chocolate and candy** are highly palatable for many dogs and some cats. The problem with feeding pets these high-calorie foods is that the pet may not then eat enough prepared food to be properly nourished. The animal may also become obese and may develop dental caries. In addition, chocolate contains theobromine which is toxic to dogs and cats. Milk chocolate contains about 1.5 mg of theobromine per gram. Unsweetened baking chocolate contains almost 16 mg/g. An animal ingesting unsweetened chocolate is at a far greater risk of experiencing toxic effects.[9] The LD_{50} for theobromine in dogs is reported to be between 240 and 500 mg/kg body weight. However, the death of a dog after ingestion of as little as 114 mg/kg has been reported.[15] To reach a potentially lethal dose of 100 mg/kg, a dog weighing 10 kg would have to ingest 63 g (2.2 oz) of unsweetened chocolate, or about 670 g (23.5 oz or 1.5 lb) of milk chocolate.

Since theobromine has been used as a diuretic in dogs at 20 mg/kg body weight, ingestion of small amounts of chocolate would be expected to produce diuresis, but no other clinical signs.[9]

Clinical signs in dogs with theobromine toxicosis include: 1) vomiting, 2) depression and lethargy, 3) diuresis, 4) muscular tremors, 5) diarrhea, and 6) death.[9] Dogs seem to clear theobromine from the body more slowly than do people.[1]

5. **Onions and garlic** will not control worms or fleas, but will make the pet's breath unpleasant. These foods do not increase diet palatability unless the pet has been fed table food by a family that commonly uses large amounts of garlic and onions in their diet. Consumption of a sufficient amount (an amount equal to more than 0.5% of body weight) of onions causes the formation of Heinz bodies in erythrocytes,

and results in hemolytic anemia, fever, darkened urine, and death. The toxic principle is n-propyldisulphide, an alkaloid.

6. **Grass**—Why dogs and cats eat grass is not known. It has been hypothesized as being due to its fiber content. Some animals may like the taste of grass. Green grass is high in moisture. Animals may vomit after consuming grass.

7. **Vitamin C** requirements increase with stress. It is possible that some dogs or cats may not produce adequate vitamin C when stressed. However, there are no published controlled studies indicating that vitamin C is beneficial for stressed dogs or cats. Even though human beings require vitamin C dietarily, several good controlled studies in people show **no** improvement in physical performance as a result of vitamin C supplementation.[23] However, if vitamin C is given, a dose of 25-100 mg of sodium or potassium ascorbate (daily per dog) has been recommended for stressed dogs and is not harmful. Larger dosages are not recommended.

8. **Brewer's yeast** is high in vitamin B_1 (thiamin). Ingestion of brewer's yeast allegedly helps control fleas and mosquitos in dogs, cats, and people. Controlled studies refute these allegations. In one study, weekly flea counts on flea-inoculated dogs were the same in dogs that were not given brewer's yeast, dogs fed active brewer's yeast, and dogs fed inactive brewer's yeast at 14 g/day for five weeks.[2] In another study, neither flea counts nor the percent of fleas biting were different between flea-inoculated dogs fed 100 mg of thiamin twice daily for two weeks and in those given a placebo.[7]

9. **Bee pollen** ingestion is occasionally alleged to provide many benefits, all of them doubtful and none of them demonstrated in controlled studies. Although nutrient content of bee pollen varies, it generally contains 50-60% soluble carbohydrate, 10-40% protein, 5-20% fiber, 3-6% moisture, 1% fat, and 2-3% ash consisting primarily of potassium (0.4-0.5%) and phosphorus (0.3-0.4%), with smaller amounts of calcium, sodium and magnesium.[3] The protein generally has a biologic value of 50-70% and is only 50-60% digestible.[3]

10. **"Health foods"**—People that believe in "health foods" for themselves sometimes want to feed them to their pets. These people are generally unaware of two important facts:

    a. The nutritional differences between typical human diets and prepared pet foods. Pet foods contain more fiber and calcium and usually are more nutritionally balanced than human diets.

    b. The nutritional needs of the dog and cat differ from those of people. The dog and cat have greater protein needs, different vitamin needs, etc. Many "health foods" are supposedly better than other food items because they have more fiber and less sugar (sucrose), or are free of additives. See page 2-21 for a discussion of additives in pet foods and Table 1, Appendix 1, for additive-free pet foods. Although sugar is commonly present in human foods, it is rarely included in prepared pet foods because of its cost. Additional fiber may be beneficial in human diets, but is not of benefit in the diet of dogs or cats unless they are overweight, constipated, or have diabetes or colitis.

11. **Chelated minerals** are metallic ions combined with, or formed into, cyclical structures. Minerals of nutritional concern most often chelated are iron, cobalt, copper, and zinc. The compounds frequently used for chelation are amino acids, inorganic or organic acids, ketones, acetone, dihydroxy compounds, disulfides or, the one most often used, ethylenediamine tetracetic acid (EDTA). Naturally occurring chelated mineral compounds include chlorophyl, hemoglobin, vitamin B_{12}, and cytochromes. Chelation shields the mineral from external influences and thereby affects intestinal absorption of these minerals and also affects interference that other minerals may have on the absorption of these minerals. For example, calcium binds zinc, decreasing its absorption. However, chelated zinc is protected from binding by calcium. If the compound to which the mineral is chelated is more readily absorbed than the mineral, chelation will increase the mineral's rate of absorption. This is beneficial if the animal needs more of that mineral. If more is not needed, it may be harmful. However, if the compound to which the mineral is chelated is less readily absorbed than the mineral itself, chelation will reduce the absorption of the mineral.

Chelated minerals are occasionally promoted as being superior to nonchelated minerals. This may or may not be true depending on: 1) the mineral and compound to which it is chelated, 2) the animal's need for that mineral, and 3) other minerals in the diet. **If** chelation increases that mineral's absorption, **if** more of that mineral is needed by the animal, and **if** there are excesses of other minerals or other substances in that diet that interfere with the mineral's

absorption, chelation is beneficial. If any of these three factors is untrue, chelation is of no benefit and may be harmful. It is better to ensure that a diet contains the proper amounts of all nutrients, including minerals, than to try to compensate for improper dietary amounts by adding, or including in the diet, chelated minerals which may or may not be of benefit.

TYPES OF PET FOODS

There are two major types of pet foods: 1) homemade and, 2) commercially produced. Most pet owners prefer the convenience, lower feeding costs, better performance, and fewer problems associated with feeding commercially produced foods. One study indicated that 92% of dog and cat owners in the United States feed their pets commercially prepared foods as the main part of the diet.[5] However, some pet owners prefer to prepare their pet's food themselves. Recipes for this purpose are given in Appendix Table 3. If a homemade diet is used, it should be prepared from recipes that produce a nutritionally complete and adequate diet. Feeding single food items, or diets consisting of an indiscriminate mixture of human foods, often results in dietary induced disease.

When homemade diets are fed, frequently one food that the owner perceives the animal likes best, or that is least expensive, is fed to the exclusion of other foods. The result is a nutritionally unbalanced diet. The animal may develop a marked preference for this food. After this occurs, getting the animal to accept a balanced diet becomes difficult. Owners may feed diets that are nutritionally adequate for people but are not adequate for dogs or cats. Even though a well-balanced diet for a dog or cat can be prepared from human foods by following a carefully developed recipe, many homemade diets are unbalanced and result in nutritional disease. Homemade diets and indiscriminate supplementation (sometimes on the advice of a veterinarian) are two of the more common causes of nutritional imbalances in dogs and cats.

A number of different types of commercially produced pet foods are available. These include:

1. Generic
2. Private label
3. Those marketed in grocery and feed stores called "popular brands"
4. Those marketed in pet stores or veterinary clinics, called "premium brands"

There are certainly individual company and product exceptions, but in general the quality of the product increases from generic to premium brands.

However, in a recent analysis of 55 cat foods, there was no difference in the nutritional quality or nutritional imbalances, such as an inverse calcium/phosphorus ratio and excess magnesium, between generic, private label, regionally marketed, and nationally marketed popular brands (Table 5, page 9-10). Also, in the generic, private label, and popular brands, nutritional quality varied widely between different products produced by the same company. These findings suggest that **the common practice of recommending "any good national brand" does not necessarily increase the likelihood of obtaining a better quality pet food.**

Generic products are those which carry no brand name. They are usually produced and marketed locally or regionally to reduce transportation costs. Generic pet foods consist of the least expensive ingredients available in that area. Manufacturers of these products may or may not have:

1. Formulated the product to meet the animal's needs
2. Considered the potential detrimental effects of nutrient excesses or toxic substances that may be present
3. Considered the availability and variability of the nutrients in the ingredients used
4. Fed the product to animals for a sufficient length of time to demonstrate palatability, prove nutritional adequacy, and assure that no ingredients are present that might cause toxicity
5. Provided adequate product quality control

Generic and private label brands are the least expensive and poorest quality types of commercially produced pet foods.

Private label brand foods are usually marketed by grocery chains under their house brand. These pet foods are produced by pet food manufacturers (often the same ones that produce generic brands) on a least-cost bid basis according to the specifications of the marketing company. Because the incentive for the manufacturer is to produce the least expensive product possible, in order to obtain the order, there is little concern for nutritional content and consistency of the product. The manufacturer knows that next month his competition may get the order. Therefore, as with generic products, private label brands are highly unlikely to provide optimal nutrition for pets. Private label products can be identified by referring to the label which will state "Distributed by_____ ," or "Manufactured **for** _____ ," instead of "Manufactured **by**_____." Unless a veterinarian or animal owner has experience or knowledge about the nutritional adequacy of a particular private label or generic food, it is better to avoid using or recom-

mending these products because performance usually parallels cost.

The main differences between pet foods marketed nationally in grocery or feed stores (popular brands) and those sold exclusively in pet stores or veterinary clinics (premium brands) are:

1. The variability and quality of ingredients used
2. The emphasis on palatability versus optimal nutrition

Most popular pet foods are variable formula diets. The ingredients used vary, depending on availability and cost. In contrast, many premium brand pet foods are produced from fixed formulas, i.e. the ingredients are not varied depending on their cost.

The quality of the ingredients also causes variations in the nutrient content of pet foods. Some ingredients such as salt, dicalcium phosphate, corn oil, etc., are uniform. On the other hand, whole ground fish, poultry by-product meal, meat and bone meal, cereals, etc., vary widely from one source to another. Unless carefully controlled, these ingredients introduce nutrient variables into the food which may have adverse effects on the quality of the food. For example, one batch of a food made using only whole ground fish might be nutritionally balanced, whereas another batch made with fish waste from a filleting plant could be unbalanced.

The primary concerns of many people buying popular brands of pet foods are cost and palatability. If a diet is inexpensive, readily consumed, and does not cause loose stools or any other immediately noticeable detrimental effect, pet owners will buy it. When nutrition is considered, the perception of many pet owners is that more is better; i.e. more protein, more calcium, more phosphorus, etc. Popular brands of pet food are produced to meet these perceptions, and their advertising is frequently geared to support and enhance them.

Premium brands of pet foods emphasize **optimal** nutrition for health maintenance, longevity, and performance, rather than palatability and prevention of readily recognized nutritional deficiencies or excesses. Ingredients that do not contain too much of certain nutrients are used and not varied depending on their cost. As a result, these foods are more expensive per unit of weight. However, because they are frequently higher in nutrient density and availability, less food is needed, which partially offsets the higher cost per unit of weight. In order for pet owners to justify paying the additional cost for the premium quality pet foods, they must understand these differences. Also, some manufacturers of premium foods offer special-purpose diets with distinct nutrient differences. These may be diets for growth and lactation, diets for maintenance of active or inactive pets, and diets for various forms of stress, i.e. emotional, physical, or environmental. The proper use of these diets requires that the purchaser receive specific instructions. For these reasons, premium brands and specific purpose diets are marketed through pet stores or veterinary clinics rather than grocery stores. Knowledgeable pet professionals and veterinarians can educate their clients and explain the differences; whereas it is virtually impossible to accurately communicate these differences through media advertising, which is the primary method used to sell the popular grocery store brands.

ASSESSING PET FOOD QUALITY

Considering the assets and liabilities of: 1) entirely homemade diets, 2) a specific food, foods, or supplement(s), or 3) commercially prepared diets (generic, private label, popular, and premium brands), the overall best option is the latter. A **good quality** commercial pet food, designed for the purpose for which it is being fed, and fed as the animal's sole diet, is most likely to maintain optimum health. The problem becomes one of identifying a good quality product. A number of factors are useful in this regard, including the product label, physical examination of the food, feeding trials, and cost.

PET FOOD LABELS

Pet food labels carry potentially useful information. However, to properly interpret the information, as well as appreciate the limitations of that information, some understanding of the regulations governing the labeling of pet foods is required. The items required on all pet food labels are:[14]

1. The product name
2. The net weight
3. The guaranteed analysis containing at least the minimum amounts of crude protein and fat and the maximum amounts of moisture and crude fiber. Additional guarantees are optional, but must be located in the guaranteed analysis panel to prevent their use in a promotional manner.
4. A list of ingredients in descending order of predominance by weight
5. The name and address of the manufacturer, packer, or distributor
6. The words "Dog Food" or "Cat Food"
7. A statement of the nutritional adequacy or purpose of the product

Guaranteed Analysis

The Guaranteed Analysis **does not guarantee that the product contains the amounts listed;** it only guarantees the tolerances the manufacturer claims the product meets. For example, if the label claims that a product contains a minimum of 10% protein, it could have 15% protein without being in violation. As shown in Table 2 (page 2-6), two foods with the same guaranteed analysis may contain nutrient levels that vary by more than 100%, yet both meet their label guarantees. However, the guaranteed analysis can be useful. Foods that are not at least as digestible and do not contain at least as much fat as given in Table 7, have such a low caloric density that excessive amounts will have to be consumed to meet the animal's energy requirements. Therefore, they should not be used unless dietary energy restriction is desired, such as with obesity treatment or prevention.

While a maximum ash guarantee is not required, many pet food manufacturers include one on the labels of their foods. Cat foods not containing an ash guarantee on the label should not be recommended as the absence of one suggests the manufacturer is trying to disguise the ash content of the product. Also, cat foods containing more than 6% ash in their dry matter are not recommended for adult maintenance. A high ash content, particularly in dry or soft-moist foods, generally indicates a high magnesium content (Fig. 3, page 9-13). Excessive magnesium intake and a urine pH which is consistently above 6.4 are risk factors for feline urolithiasis (FUS) (Chapter 9). A low ash content does not ensure that the food is low in magnesium, but it is the best indication available if the magnesium content of the food is not known. The ash content of **canned** cat foods correlates poorly with the food's magnesium content.

Subtle differences in moisture content of canned products can result in significant differences in dry matter content and therefore the economics of using a given diet. For example, a canned diet containing

TABLE 7

FACTORS USEFUL IN SUGGESTING PET FOOD QUALITY[a]

Animal	Function	Moisture (%)[c]	Food Dry Matter (%)[b]			
			Digestibility[d]	Ash	Fat	Protein[e]
Dog	Maintenance	≤ 75[f]	> 75[g]	—	> 8[g]	15-25
Dog	Growth and Reproduction	≤ 75	> 80	—	≥ 17	> 29
Dog	Physical Exertion	≤ 75	≥ 82	—	> 23	> 25
Cat	Maintenance	≤ 75	> 75[g]	≤ 5[h]	> 10[g]	> 25
Cat	Growth and Reproduction	≤ 75	> 80	≤ 7[h]	≥ 17	> 35

[a]The following factors should also be considered:
1) The name and address of the manufacturer should be given on the label. Do not use or recommend if the label says "Manufactured for _____" or "Distributed by _____."
2) It should indicate on the label that the diet is adequate for the purpose for which it is intended. Evidence based on feeding trials is much better than analysis of nutrient levels, e.g. statements such as "Guaranteed to meet or exceed all NRC recommendations."
3) The results of a physical examination of the food, as described in the text.
4) An animal source protein should be one of the first two ingredients in a canned food, and the first three in a dry food. Dog foods fed long-term should contain at least one cereal grain in the list.
5) The lowest priced product is usually the poorest quality.

[b]To determine the amount of a nutrient in the dry matter for the food being considered, divide the values given in the Guaranteed Analysis, or preferably the actual analysis, by the dry matter content of the food, which is 1 − (% moisture in the food ÷ 100). For example, if the Guaranteed Analysis indicates that the food contains 5% protein and 75% moisture, it would contain 5% ÷ (1 − 75/100) or 5% ÷ 0.25, which equals 20% protein in the food dry matter. This value may then be compared to the values given in this table to determine if the food contains the amount of nutrients recommended.

[c]More than 75% moisture is not detrimental but may be uneconomical.

[d]Percent digestibility equals [(food dry matter consumed − stool dry matter weight) ÷ (food dry matter consumed)] × 100.

[e]Based on the quality and digestibility of the protein present in average quality commercial pet foods. Lower or higher amounts are needed in a variety of disease conditions.

[f]≤ indicates less than or equal to, ≥ indicates more than or equal to.

[g]Lower values are beneficial if excess weight is a problem.

[h]Ash as an indicator of magnesium content correlates only for dry or soft-moist foods (page 9-11).

70% moisture contains over 36% more nutrients than one containing 78% moisture:

$$[(100-70) - (100-78)] \div (100 - 78) =$$
$$(30 - 22) \div 22 = 36\%$$

List of Ingredients

The list of ingredients may be helpful, although it has some shortcomings that limit its usefulness in evaluating pet foods. The ingredients are supposed to be listed in descending order of predominance by weight. However, this is an unenforceable regulation as it is generally impossible to determine the presence or absence of a specific ingredient, or the amount of each ingredient present, by examining or analyzing the finished product. A manufacturer thus faces the option of either providing competitors with proprietary information regarding formulation of their product or not complying with a law that is essentially unenforceable. Also, it is possible to list the ingredients in a product containing 10% beef, 10% soybean meal, 0.5% horsemeat, and 0.5% liver, as beef, soybean meal, horsemeat, and liver. This makes it appear that the product is predominantly animal tissue (AT), when it is actually 76% soybean meal (SBM) on a dry matter (DM) basis:

$$10\% \text{ SBM} \times 90\% \text{ DM} = 9\% \text{ SBM DM}$$

$$10.0 + 0.5 + 0.5 \text{ or } 11\% \text{ AT} \times 25\% \text{ DM} =$$
$$2.75\% \text{ AT DM}$$

$$9\% \text{ SBM DM} \div$$
$$(9\% \text{ SBM DM} + 2.75\% \text{ AT DM}) = 76.6\%$$

Therefore, 76.6% of the total dry matter of these four ingredients is soybean meal, yet it is listed as the second most abundant ingredient in the diet.

This basic principle is commonly used in canned meat-type dog foods where textured vegetable protein (TVP - soy flour) comprises a major portion of the dry matter in the product, but is listed well down in the list of ingredients because it is added in dry form; whereas the ingredients listed first are added in wet form. If the added water used to bring the dry TVP up to the moisture content of the finished food were included, soy flour would be the predominant ingredient and would be required to be listed first on the label.

Another example of a misleading list of ingredients from an actual commercial dog food label is: "Poultry By-Product Meal, Fish Meal, Kibbled Yellow Corn, Kibbled Wheat, Soybean Oil, Ground Wheat, Ground Corn, Peanut Oil, Flaked Corn, Flaked Wheat, Meat and Bone Meal, Corn Germ Meal, Lard, Wheat Bran, Sodium Chloride," etc. This list of ingredients gives the impression that poultry by-product meal and fish meal are the major ingredients. However, six of the first 10 ingredients listed are different forms of corn and wheat, i.e. kibbled, ground, and flaked. When these different cereal forms are grouped together, the product is composed primarily of corn and wheat with smaller amounts of poultry and fish meals.

Another serious limitation of the ingredient list is that general terms such as "meat by-products" and "cereal grain products" are impossible to evaluate. The actual ingredients termed meat by-products may be liver, kidney, and lungs, or udder, guts, and connective tissue. Cereal grain products may be whole grain cereals, or may be by-products derived from cereal milling such as wheat middlings, oat hulls or bran. There are considerable differences in nutritive value among various meat and cereal by-products.

The list of ingredients on the label will be of even less value in evaluating pet food products if the Collective Terms Petition becomes law. This petition would allow ingredients to be grouped in classes. The class name, such as processed animal protein products, cereal grains, plant protein products, etc., would be listed on the label. Products with ingredients listed in this manner are impossible to evaluate and should not be recommended unless the veterinarian has specific knowledge of the food's nutritional adequacy.

A few generalities about the list of ingredients may be helpful as they may give an indication of nutritional content and quality. An animal protein source should be one of the first two ingredients in a canned dog food and one of the first three in a dry dog food. Canned dog foods fed long-term as the main diet should contain at least one cereal grain in the list (page 2-24). Canned pet foods should contain at least one source of calcium. This may be a calcium salt such as calcium carbonate or an animal protein source that contains bone, such as chicken parts, poultry by-product meal, or fish meal. Listing different forms of the same ingredient separately (e.g. ground, kibbled, and flaked corn) suggests a purposeful misrepresentation of the product's ingredient contents.

Statement of Nutritional Adequacy or Purpose of the Product

Since January 1, 1984, regulations have required that the label of all pet foods (except those clearly identified as a snack or treat or those intended for use by or under the supervision or direction of a veterinarian), contain a statement indicating that the product, when fed as the sole diet without any other food or supplement of any type, meets or exceeds the requirements or is nutritionally ade-

quate for one or more of the following: gestation, lactation, growth, maintenance, or all stages of the life cycle. The statement may limit the claim of nutritional adequacy to maintenance, include maintenance and growth but exclude reproduction (gestation and lactation), or be an unqualified claim for all stages of the life cycle which is referred to as complete and balanced for all dogs or all cats.[4] Use of products with limited claims, i.e. nutritionally adequate for maintenance, should be limited to that stage of the life cycle and not fed to pets in more demanding stages such as growth or reproduction. Unfortunately, in contrast to what is commonly believed, **none of the claims need to be proven by feeding trials and, therefore, the claim does not insure nutritional adequacy or quality.** The claim can be made if the food meets **either** of the following alternatives:

1. Passes feeding tests conducted according to protocols approved by the Association of American Feed Control Officials (AAFCO)[16]
2. Contains at least the minimum amount of each nutrient as recommended by the National Research Council (NRC)[13,14]

Because it is less expensive and faster, many manufacturers use the analysis of nutrient content alternative, rather than feeding tests, to substantiate this nutritional claim for their foods. However, there are several liabilities to this method. It gives no indication of:

1. Nutrient excesses which may be just as harmful as a deficiency
2. Presence of toxic substances which, if fed over a long or even short period of time, may be harmful
3. Acceptability, i.e. whether the animal will eat sufficient quantities to meet its energy need
4. Nutrient availability (digestibility)

The presence of nutrients in a diet does not mean they can be absorbed and utilized. A diet composed of shoe leather, motor oil, vitamins, and minerals will analyze to meet National Research Council nutrient recommendations for dogs or cats, but obviously would not be a good diet for a dog or cat. Thus, the claim "balanced, complete, adequate, or guaranteed to meet or exceed all National Research Council nutrient recommendations" has little meaning. However, if the "complete and balanced" claim is substantiated by successful feeding tests according to established protocols, it is useful in evaluating the product for nutritional adequacy. A letter to the manufacturer asking which method was used to substantiate the label claim should provide the necessary information.

PHYSICAL EXAMINATION OF THE FOOD

Physical examination of a pet food can provide useful information in assessing quality. For canned foods, a swelled can indicates bacterial fermentation and its contents should not be fed. A partially collapsed can may merely be dented or indicate rapid cooling following sterilization (panelling), neither of which affect food quality. Open one end of the can and check for putrid, rancid, or sour odors. A darkened depression on the surface of the product is not contamination. The depression is the result of an air pocket called the "head space." It aids in creating a vacuum during the canning process, which reduces oxidation of vitamins and other nutrients and extends the shelf life of the product. The darkened color is caused by partial oxidation of the carbohydrates in the food. Next, empty the contents onto a plate. Lacquer on the inside of the can protects the food from the can. If the can is not lacquered, the food will have a metallic smell which usually indicates a poor-quality product. Generic and private label canned pet foods are usually packaged in unlacquered cans.

Cut lengthwise through the food (ration type loaf) or spread a portion on the plate (meat-type or stew products) and attempt to identify the ingredients. A good-quality canned ration-type food should have a heterogeneous or non-uniform textured appearance containing whole cereal grains and small chunks of animal tissue, with no evidence of undesirable ingredients (hair, feathers, cereal hulls, etc.) or foreign material (sand, wire, paper). A good meat-type food should contain pieces of striated muscle. Large blood vessels, ligaments, tendons, or other connective tissue indicate the presence of meat by-products. Examine these carefully as many meat-type canned foods contain a considerable quantity of textured vegetable protein (TVP), an extruded soybean product containing food coloring, that looks like pieces of meat or liver. Black particles in the food may be charcoal used to "decharacterize" the ingredients so that they cannot be used for human consumption. This does not mean that the food is not suitable for dogs or cats.

To evaluate dry foods, check the container for evidence of fat soaking through to the outside ("grease out"). Dry foods in bags or boxes with evidence of grease out are highly susceptible to vermin infestation. Next, take a sample of food from the top and bottom of the bag or box and observe it on a sheet of paper. A great number of tiny food particles or "fines" in a dry product is generally indicative of a low-quality product. Mold

can often be detected by odor (musty, stale smell) and by sight (white, blue, green, or black dusty coating on food).

When physically examining soft-moist foods, check the packaging (wrapper or bag) carefully for any sign of leakage. Soft-moist foods can easily become dry or contaminated if a small break occurs in the package. A desirable soft-moist product should be free of any unusual odors or colors. It should have a soft, slightly spongy, and "lubricated" feel but should not feel wet. Break the soft-moist particle, and examine it for the presence of cereal by-products. Low-quality soft-moist products contain considerable quantities of hulls, bran, or cereal wastes.

FEEDING TRIALS

Even though the label and physical examinations provide a great deal of valuable information about a pet food, these factors do not indicate the true nutritional value. The only way to be certain of the palatability, the protein and fat quality, and the vitamin and trace mineral adequacy, is to feed the diet to the animal for which it is intended.

There are three ways to obtain results of feeding trials:
1. From the manufacturer
2. From animal owners
3. From your own testing

If it is not stated that feeding trials have proved a diet to be nutritionally adequate for its intended purpose, write to the manufacturer and request this information. If the name and address of the manufacturer are not given on the label, or if this information is requested and not received, eliminate the product from consideration.

Veterinarians can obtain the results of feeding trials by routinely reviewing the dietary histories of all animals they examine. Adequate weight and physical condition, a shiny, well kept coat, good reproductive performance (particularly maintaining weight during lactation, even when nursing a large litter), good growth, and normal stools all indicate animals being fed a good-quality diet. If a diet history is taken on each animal, veterinarians can quickly form qualified opinions on the pet foods available in their practice area.

An easily conducted feeding trial that will provide useful information is to correlate the weight of the food consumed with the weight of feces produced. With the exception of a low energy, high fiber reducing diet, a large stool volume indicates poor digestibility and a poor-quality food. The test can be conducted as follows:

Determine how much to feed from Tables 1, 2 and 5, in Chapter 1. Feed exactly the same amount for six days, keeping the animal's daily activity as uniform as possible. Give no further consideration to foods that cause loose stools for the last four days of the test. During the last four days, collect all stools. Either weigh the stools daily or combine them in an air-tight plastic bag, and keep them frozen or refrigerated to limit evaporation of moisture. Either way, at the end of the test, determine the total weight of stool produced. Divide the stool weight by the weight of the food eaten during the last four days. The resultant fraction indicates total diet digestibility.

The food is acceptable if its digestibility is at least 75%. This is indicated when the weight of the stool is less than 25% of the weight of a canned-food intake, 70% of a soft-moist food intake, or 90% of a dry-food intake. These values take into consideration the average dry-matter contents of the foods and well formed stools. The actual digestibility of the food dry matter can be determined by obtaining the dry matter of both the food and stools (by drying at 105°C to constant weight) and using these values instead. However, this is less practical and generally unnecessary as the digestibility obtained without the stool and food dry matter is usually sufficiently accurate for screening pet foods.

Another rapid feeding trial is to confirm that the food will supply enough energy to maintain an adult animal's weight. Offer the diet free-choice for three weeks and record weight changes. A food should not be used if it cannot at least maintain optimal weight in an adult animal.

One of the most reliable and practical tests of the nutritional adequacy of a food for growth and reproduction is its ability to support growth and to allow the mother that is nursing a large litter to maintain optimal body weight. To test for adequacy for growth, a litter of weaned puppies or kittens is offered the food free-choice. Their growth (weight) is compared to a standard growth curve for their breed or a similar breed (page 3-11 or 4-5). Any food that fails to support a growth rate comparable to the standard, or that does not prevent the development of pathologic conditions, should be considered inadequate.

In feeding trials, any food being evaluated should be given without supplementation. This is the only way a food can be judged solely on its own merit.

COST

Accurate cost determinations require comparisons of the actual expense of feeding different foods to an animal, rather than simply comparing

TABLE 8

COMPARING THE COST OF PET FOODS

Diet	Net Weight	Moisture Content (%)	Metab. Energy (kcal)	Cost (cents)			
				Per Pkg.	as fed*	dry matter**	per 100 kcalories†
A	6.5 oz.	78	200/can	39	6.0/oz.	27.3/oz.	19.5
B	15 oz.	72	550/can	99	6.6/oz.	23.6/oz.	18.0
C	25 lb.	12	1350/lb.	900	36/lb.	40.9/lb.	2.7
D	25 lb.	8	2200/lb.	1500	60/lb.	65.2/lb.	2.7

*(¢/pkg.) ÷ (pkg. size).

**(¢/oz or lb as fed) ÷ (1—% moisture content/100).

†(¢/oz or lb as fed) ÷ kcal/oz or lb as fed. This is the most accurate value to use in comparing the cost of feeding different foods.

Conclusions: Diet B is a more economical canned diet than diet A. Although diet D costs 67% more per pound than diet C, because of the higher caloric density of diet D, less of it would need to be fed; as a result there is no difference between the cost of feeding diets C or D, as indicated by the cost per 100 kcalories. For either the canned or the dry diets, if the cost/oz or lb as purchased were used it would result in an incorrect conclusion. If the digestible or metabolizable calorie content of the food is not known, the cost/unit of dry matter is the best value to use for comparative purposes. However, as shown in this example, this value would have led to the incorrect conclusion that diet C was more economical than diet D.

pet food prices per unit weight. Another good way is to compare cost per kilocalorie of metabolizable energy, since 70-90% of the food consumed is used to meet energy needs. Units of metabolizable energy take into account food digestibility not indicated by comparison of price per unit weight. Examples of how to compare the costs of pet foods are given in Table 8. Obviously the cost should not be the only criterion in determining which food to use or recommend. The least expensive foods per unit of weight should be eliminated from consideration. Because the costs of manufacturing and marketing are similar, the lowest priced foods simply cannot contain quality ingredients. Ingredients constitute the chief expense in manufacturing a pet food. This is in contrast to products such as carbonated beverages, for which the major cost is packaging. Pet foods are a good example of "you get what you pay for."

RECOMMENDING PET FOODS

To recommend means to counsel or advise. The implication is that the advice proceeds from specific knowledge of the subject. Veterinarians routinely form qualified opinions about biologics and pharmaceuticals and make decisions or recommendations accordingly. The quality of the food an animal eats (every day of its life) is at least as important as the brand of vaccine used in an immunization program, or the specific antibiotic used to treat a clinical condition for a 3-5 day period. However, the veterinarian who simply advises the feeding of "any good commercial pet

food," without knowledgeably specifying which ones are "good," is failing to provide an important service to the pet owner. This type of "recommendation" forces the client to make the definitive decision based on promotional factors rather than scientific knowledge. Even though the number of commercial pet foods on the market is overwhelming (several thousand), the veterinarian needs in-depth knowledge of only a few good quality products to be able to make responsible recommendations. After screening pet foods by label, physical examination, feeding trials, and cost, veterinarians should be able to identify several good-quality commercially prepared diets sold in their practice areas. Once this has been accomplished, the foods should be recommended by brand name. A summary of factors useful in determining the quality of pet foods is given in Table 7 (page 2-17).

ADDITIVES

Some pet food additives do not provide direct nourishment to the animal, but they can be very beneficial to the quality of the product at the time of consumption. Additives are included in pet foods to enhance quality and prevent deterioration after processing. Some additives are included to enhance the appearance of a product. Whether or not such additives are beneficial to the animal is debatable. If the owner will not buy a food because it lacks the color perceived to indicate quality or a certain flavor, the pet obviously has no opportunity to benefit from eating the food. The additives com-

monly used in pet foods are emulsifiers or surface-active agents, colors, antioxidants, antimicrobial agents, and flavors.

Emulsifiers (which keep water and fat from separating) and colors contribute to the physical appearance of pet foods. Antioxidants (which prevent fat from oxidizing or becoming rancid), and antimicrobial agents, such as mold inhibitors, prevent spoilage. Flavors are used to assure acceptability by the pet or to justify marketing a product of a certain flavor. Most of the additives used in pet foods are also used in foods for people. Some additives such as sucrose, salt and propylene glycol have nutritive value in addition to their function as preservatives.

Pet owners often ask veterinarians about the safety of food additives and if these additives are detrimental to the health of pets. Additives used in both human and pet foods have been extensively investigated. Most are designated by the Food and Drug Administration as "generally regarded as safe." If findings suggest even a remote possibility of detrimental effects associated with the use of a particular additive, that additive is eliminated from use in both human and pet foods.

Concern over the use of these substances in pet foods is understandable but should be kept in logical perspective. Additives are expensive and therefore are incorporated into pet foods only when necessary, and at the minimum level needed to perform the desired function. Even salt, fat soluble vitamins, calcium, and proteins—all of which are important dietary nutrients—are detrimental to health, and even potentially lethal, if consumed in excessive amounts. Like additives, they are beneficial in proper amounts.

A number of additive-free pet foods are available to pet owners that are particularly concerned about additives (see Appendix Table 1). However, marketing of foods on the basis that they contain no additives or are "all natural," is a marketing gimmick only designed to increase sales (see page 2-27). An additive-free food is not necessarily any better, or worse, than foods containing additives. The factors described previously, summarized in Table 7 (page 2-17), are the best determinants of pet food quality.

Sometimes pet owners inquire about the presence of steroid-growth promotants in ingredients from poultry sources in pet foods. The poultry industry relies primarily on nutrition, genetics, and management to improve growth performance in birds. Steroids have not been used for many years.

TABLE 9

NUTRIENT CONTENT OF COMMERCIAL PET FOODS

Form of Food	Water (%)	Metab. Energy (kcal/oz as fed)	In Food Dry Matter (%)					
			Digestibility	Protein	Fat	Ca	P	Sodium
Dog Foods:								
Dry	6–10[b]	95[a]	75	22–31	7–13	1–3	1–2	0.3–0.8
Soft-Moist	23–38	85[a]	90	25–33	9–15	1–3	1–2	0.3–1.0
Canned Ration[c]	68–78	33	85	30–40	10–25	1–3	1–2	0.8–1.2
Canned Gourmet[d]	70–78	37	85	45–60	16–37	1–3	1–2	0.8–0.9
Cat Foods:								
Dry	6–10	100[a] (97–106)	80	34 (30–40)	12 (9–15)	1.6 (1.1–2.1)	1.1 (0.9–1.4)	0.6 (0.3–0.9)
Soft-Moist	30–40	75[a] (60–90)	90	36 (33–39)	16.5 (12–23)	2.4 (1.4–4.1)	2.2 (1.7–3.2)	0.85 (0.6–1.5)
Canned Ration[c]	70–78	29 (23–41)	85	41 (31–56)	14 (3–30)	2.0 (1.0–4.3)	1.4 (0.8–2.6)	0.6 (0.2–0.9)
Canned Gourmet[d]	72–78	35 (29–46)	90	53 (39–78)	27 (11–40)	1.5 (0.2–3.5)	1.5 (0.7–4.0)	0.9 (0.4–4.2)

[a] An 8 oz. (by volume) measuring cup holds 3–3.5 oz. (by wt.) of most dry foods or 3.5–5 oz. (by wt.) of most soft-moist foods.

[b] Average and/or (range) for those available in grocery stores.

[c] Multiple ingredient type food. These are generally in 13 oz. or larger cans.

[d] Foods consisting exclusively, or primarily, of a single ingredient. These cat foods are in 3 to 6.5 oz. cans.

FORMS OF COMMERCIAL PET FOODS

At the present time three major forms of commercially produced pet foods are available. They are:

1. Dry (6-10% moisture)
2. Soft-moist (23-40% moisture)
3. Canned (68-78% moisture)

Mixtures of dry and soft-moist in the same package are also available. The different types of commercially prepared foods are available in all of these different forms. Dry foods are by far the most popular for both dogs and cats, and their popularity is increasing. In 1985, on an energy basis for dog foods, 81% sold was in dry form, 11% in canned, 4% in soft-moist form, and 4% as snack foods. For cat foods, 63% sold was in dry form, 26% in canned, and 11% in soft-moist form.[17] In recent years total sales of cat foods have increased almost twice as fast as dog foods. This reflects the growing popularity of cats. The nutrient content of the three different forms of commercial pet foods is given in Table 9. **The quality of a food is in no way related to its form.** Good quality and poor quality products are available in all three forms. Each form has its individual advantages and disadvantages.

DRY FOODS

Dry pet foods may be produced as kibbles, meals, or expanded particles. Kibbled food is baked on a sheet, then broken into small pieces called kibbles. The only national brand of kibbles is the dog food Ken-L ration Biskit (Quaker Oats). A meal-type food is one in which prepared dry ingredients are simply mixed together. Meal-type dog foods were common before 1960, but they have been replaced by expanded products. There are currently no nationally marketed meal-type foods (Gaines Meal is an expanded dog food).

Expanded pet foods are cooked in an extruder and forced through a die, which results in expansion. During extrusion the product reaches temperatures approaching 150°C, which cooks (dextrinizes) the carbohydrates in the cereals, increasing their digestibility. This temperature also flash-sterilizes the product, eliminating pathogenic organisms in the ingredients. Obviously the product loses sterility during the subsequent drying, fat-coating, and packaging stages of the manufacturing process. Many soft-moist foods are produced by extrusion-cooking for a shorter time at lower temperature. Soft-moist and regular dry rations are similar except for differences in the firmness, moisture content, and preservation systems used. After extrusion and drying, fat is sprayed on the exterior of expanded dry pet foods. At this time, digest is also sprayed on most cat foods and some dog foods to increase their palatability. This process of spraying substances on the exterior of the product is called enrobing. Most currently marketed dry pet foods are of the expanded type.

The major advantages of dry foods are:

1. They are less expensive to feed.
2. They may be fed free-choice.
3. Their abrasive effect reduces (not prevents) accumulation of dental tartar, which promotes healthier gums and teeth.

The cost of feeding a dry food is approximately one-half to one-third that of feeding a canned or soft-moist food of equal quality. The accumulation of dental tartar predisposes to gingivitis, halitosis, periodontal disease, pyorrhea, and eventual loss of teeth. These advantages are the reason dry foods are the most popular form of commercial pet food and are especially preferred for large dogs.

Dry pet foods do have some disadvantages. They are less palatable than soft-moist or canned forms for most dogs and cats. However, some cats prefer the dry form after they have become accustomed to it. Moistening a dry food will often increase its palatability for dogs,[22] but usually not for cats. If water is added to dry food, it should be just enough to moisten the food (1 cup of water/4-5 cups of dry food), but not enough to make the food mushy. Moistening a dry food negates its beneficial effect on teeth and gums. If left in a feeding bowl too long, a wetted dry food may become moldy and sour.

Another disadvantage of dry foods is that only dry ingredients can be used in their formulation. Harsh drying can reduce the nutrient content and digestibility of some ingredients. Fresh animal tissues cannot be used in dry foods. This restricts the ingredients available for use in dry foods. Because of the processing and packaging used to produce most dry foods, the amount of fat that can be included in the product is restricted. This limits the caloric density of dry foods. During lactation or physical exertion the animal may be unable to consume enough of some dry foods (particularly poor-quality products) to meet its energy needs. Dry foods also tend to have lower digestibility than soft-moist or canned foods, as well as a shorter shelf life.

Of the three forms, dry pet foods tend to be the lowest in essential fatty acid content because of the small amount and type of fat (beef tallow) frequently used in their manufacture. Due to their contact with the oxygen in the air, the fatty acids may

become oxidized (rancid) during storage, destroying their nutritional value. As temperature and humidity increase, oxidation occurs more rapidly. As a general rule, dry foods should be fed within six months of manufacture. However, because the purchaser cannot tell when most commercial foods were produced, they should be bought from an active outlet and in an amount no greater than a 1-2 month supply.

Most dry pet foods tend to be lower in digestibility and fat content and higher in fiber. For this reason their consumption may increase excretion of water in the feces and decrease excretion of water in the urine. This increases urine mineral concentration, which increases the risk of urolithiasis in both dogs and cats. The incidence of feline urolithiasis is greater in cats fed primarily or exclusively dry foods, as compared to those rarely fed dry foods (page 9-12). However, some premium brand dry foods are as high, or higher, in caloric density, digestibility, fat, and essential fatty acids, as canned or soft-moist foods. Thus, **it is the quality of the individual pet food, not its form or water content, that is important.**

Most dry dog foods contain 8-20% fat and provide 300-400 metabolizable kcal/8 oz volume measuring cup. As fat content increases, the caloric content of the food also increases. Dry dog foods containing 25% or more fat provide 600 kcal/cup, whereas some containing 5-6% fat, that are also high in fiber, provide less than 200 kcal/cup.

CANNED FOODS

Canned pet foods are usually more palatable and digestible than dry foods but are more expensive per unit weight of dry matter. Approximately 75% of the content of a canned pet food is water, as compared to an average of only 9% water in dry foods and 35% in soft-moist foods.

An advantage of the canned form is that either dry or wet ingredients can be used in formulation. Many canned foods are composed of a mixture of cereals and animal tissues. These products usually contain more fat and, thus, provide more calories per pound of dry matter than most dry foods. This makes them desirable when energy needs are high. Canned foods are cooked in the can at a temperature approaching 120°C to achieve sterility. A certain amount of nutrient destruction takes place during the processing of all three forms of pet food. This is not a problem in good-quality products, since the quantity destroyed is easily determined and the formulation adjusted accordingly. Losses incurred in processing may not be considered in poor-quality

foods because of the expense of research required to determine the losses.

There are two types of canned pet foods for both dogs and cats:
1. Ration type
2. Gourmet or meat type

The ration-type foods are composed of a variety of different ingredients, including animal tissues, soy products, and cereals. They are less expensive, good nutritionally, and help prevent development of fixed food preferences.

The gourmet products may appear to contain a substantial amount of skeletal muscle (meat) but actually contain a variety of animal by-products and textured vegetable protein (TVP), which is composed of extruded soy flour mixed with red or brown coloring to make it resemble chunks of meat or liver. Unless one is familiar with the appearance of textured vegetable protein chunks, they are easily mistaken for meat or liver chunks (which is the manufacturer's objective).

The high protein content of gourmet-type canned foods requires the animal to use protein as a major energy source. Extensive protein catabolism results in renal hyperperfusion, which has been shown to cause renal damage (see page 8-10). Therefore, these foods are not recommended for long-term feeding. However, because of their elevated protein and fat content and high palatability, the gourmet foods are excellent to feed when food intake is suppressed because of anorexia from any cause (except renal failure), and when protein requirements are increased, as for wound healing and protein-losing nephropathy or enteropathy. Cat foods, particularly the canned gourmet types, are extremely palatable and, therefore, are a good diet for inducing voluntary food consumption in either anorectic dogs or cats (Chapter 5).

Gourmet cat foods are sold in 3, 6, or 6.5 oz cans, whereas ration type cat foods are sold in 12-22 oz cans. The gourmet cat foods are composed primarily of animal tissues such as shrimp, chicken, tuna, kidney, liver, poultry and animal by-products, and numerous combinations. Because these foods are highly palatable, cats often develop marked fixed preferences for one variety if it is fed exclusively for a sufficient period of time. In contrast, most good-quality ration-type cat foods contain several different ingredients; this reduces the probability of a cat becoming "addicted" to a specific ingredient. Some of the gourmet cat foods, even the nationally available brands produced by reputable companies, are not nutritionally complete. For example, one contained less than 0.2% calcium and more than 0.6% phosphorus on a dry-matter basis

(Table 5, page 9-10). Thus, it was deficient in calcium and contained a calcium/phosphorus ratio of less than 1:3. If fed for a sufficient length of time, this food would cause nutritional secondary hyperparathyroidism, and bone demineralization.

SOFT-MOIST FOODS

Soft-moist foods require no refrigeration, have a fairly long shelf life, and may be fed free-choice. Most soft-moist foods are quite palatable and, when purchased as individual portions or pouches, cost about the same as canned foods. Soft-moist foods are marketed in individual bags or patties or in 10 and 25 lb bags, which lowers their cost per feeding.

Of the three forms of commercial dog foods, soft-moist foods often have the highest energy digestibility (but not necessarily the highest energy density). This is because of the high digestibility of the carbohydrate portion, which is composed of corn syrup and polyhydric alcohols (propylene glycol) used to provide antibacterial and antifungal stability of the foods and retention of moisture. When first marketed, soft-moist foods contained sugar (sucrose), which was subsequently replaced by corn syrup.

Many soft-moist foods, especially cat foods, contain acids. Phosphoric, hydrochloric, or malic acids are most commonly used in soft-moist cat foods. Acidification aids in the manufacture of soft-moist foods and lowers the pH to retard bacterial growth and spoilage. Sugars, corn syrup, and salts elevate the soluble solids in the product and actually bind water so it is unavailable to bacteria and fungi. Propylene glycol is hygroscopic and binds moisture in the product to keep the food pliable and prevent drying. A major advantage of the soft-moist form is that more ingredients, including fresh animal tissues, can be used in formulation. However, to minimize cost, and make the soft-moist foods more cost competitive, they often contain ingredients similar to those used in dry products.

MARKETING CONCEPTS

A marketing concept is the basis on which a product is advertised and sold, i.e. why a purchaser should buy that brand rather than a competing brand. When evaluating pet foods and pet food advertising, and for answering pet owners' questions, veterinarians should be knowledgeable about the basic concepts used in pet food marketing because many companies take advantage, and perpetuate the public's nutritional ignorance. Average pet owners know little about their animal's nutritional needs and thus can be quite susceptible to skillfully presented advertising claims, whether or not the claims are valid. Occasionally there is evidence to show that a claim is invalid or in some instances is actually detrimental. Pet foods are marketed under nine basic concepts:

1. Specific purpose foods
2. "All-purpose" foods
3. Low price
4. "People-food" concept
5. Flavor varieties
6. Presence of a food item
7. Absence of a food item
8. Nutrient content
9. Product name

There may be a multitude of modifications and combinations of these basic concepts. Many marketing organizations use several concepts so that if one does not appeal to a particular pet owner, perhaps another will.

The **specific-purpose food** concept is based on the fact that animals have different nutritional requirements for growth, maintenance, reproduction, physical exertion, old age, and with numerous diseases. Examples of products marketed on the basis of this concept are Science Diets, Prescription Diets, Iams, many puppy foods (Purina Puppy Chow, Wayne Puppy O's, etc.), Cycle products, and Fit & Trim. This is a well proven and valid concept based on scientific evidence.

Even though a product may be marketed on this concept, it may or may not satisfy the concept. For example, when a popular brand of pet food was introduced as a food for the overweight dog, it was 15% less in caloric density than other foods of the same form and was advertised as such. However, the reduced caloric density of the food resulted in a less palatable product than competitive brands. Since most people who buy pet foods at a grocery store make their selection based on palatability and price, rather than the nutritional performance of the product, less palatability resulted in poor sales. As a result a "new and improved" version became available. In the "new and improved" product the fiber content was reduced and the fat content was increased to improve palatability. However, these changes also increased the caloric density so that the new product was only 3% lower in energy density than average dog foods of the same type. The advertising and positioning of the product as a food for overweight dogs was continued although the product no longer satisfies the concept under which it is marketed.

Successful marketing of a product based on the "specific purpose" concept, indicates that the pur-

chaser or retailer has some familiarity with proper nutrition. This often requires that the person selling the product be able to explain the proper use of the product to the consumer. This is why most products that actually adhere to this concept are sold through pet stores, breeders, and veterinary clinics, where the concept can be adequately explained. Sale of products through grocery stores is limited in this regard as grocery markets must rely on time-constrained media advertising to educate clients to the proper use of the product.

"All-purpose" food products are based on the premise that one product satisfies all nutritional needs in all situations. The owner feeds, and the pet eats, more or less of the food according to the pet's caloric needs; in the process, the pet gets more or less of all other nutrients. Many products are based on the "all-purpose" concept. Examples include Gaines Meal, Friskies, Purina Dog Chow, Jim Dandy, Iams Chunks, Ken-L ration, Gaines Burgers and most generic and private label brands. Extensive research has repeatedly shown that this concept is not valid for all feeding situations. However, if the products are properly formulated, they will provide **average** performance in most healthy dogs and cats. Controlled studies are often needed to demonstrate that health, longevity, or performance are adversely affected when all-purpose products are fed, as compared to feeding a diet that specifically meets the animal's nutritional needs. Because all-purpose products can be fed to all pets and no one need explain their proper use, they can be sold in grocery stores. Most foods sold in grocery stores combine the "all-purpose" concept with one or more of the following concepts.

Low price is a major criterion used by consumers to determine which product to buy. Obviously low price is a good concept to apply to marketing pet foods. Although it is a valid concept, it bears three major liabilities. First, to produce a less expensive food, ingredients that are cheaper, of poorer quality, and more variable must be used. Second, when prices of pet foods are compared, the actual cost of feeding the animal should be considered rather than simply basing a purchase on the cost per unit of food. The lowest priced foods routinely contain the least dry matter digestibility, fat content and, therefore, the lowest caloric density. As a result (Table 8, page 2-21), feeding a higher priced, better quality food may actually cost less. The third major liability of the low-price concept is that most low-priced products are produced by companies that have little or no research capability. Thus, many of their products are not test-fed to dogs or cats to assure nutritional adequacy before marketing. The main method used to support nutrition claims is that

the product meets the National Research Council recommendations, which has many short-comings (as described on page 2-9). Examples of products whose marketing is based on the low-price concept are Strongheart, Vets, Pooch, Jazz, Sturdy, Bolo, and Kozy Kitten, as well as many private label and generic brands.

The **people-food** concept suggests that animals like and need the same foods that people eat. To quickly dispel this concept, one need only observe a dog eagerly eating feces, vomitus, garbage, and many other items equally repulsive to people. This is a gimmick concept designed to attract the purchaser (people) rather than the consumer (pet). Dogs and cats do not need or necessarily desire "people food." This does not mean that an excellent diet cannot be produced using foods intended for human consumption, or that pet foods that promote this concept are either good or bad, but simply that the concept is not scientifically valid. Gravy, stew, meat, and textured vegetable protein made to look like chunks of meat are used. Examples of products using this concept are Recipe, Gravy Train, Ken-L ration Stew, Chuck Wagon, Gaines-Burgers, Alpo Beef Chunks Dinner, Kal Kan Beef Burgers, Chicken Dinner, and Meat Stew.

Flavor variety is a gimmick concept based on the idea that pets like a variety of the same flavors people do. In reality, many dogs and cats prefer what they are accustomed to. In the wild, their natural diets are somewhat monotonous. This is further emphasized by the common problem encountered with many dogs and cats when their diets must be changed. There are two reasons that this concept is used. First, it appeals to many pet owners because people like specific flavors and different flavors, and they assume their pets do too. Second, and more important to the manufacturer, it greatly increases the number of products a company can market, which is very beneficial for sales. Results of many studies have shown that a company's sales relate directly to the amount of grocery-store shelf space their products occupy. More flavors means more products, more shelf space, and increased sales. Often the different products are identical except for a small amount of flavoring, which the pet may or may not care about. The guaranteed analysis and list of ingredients on the labels of these products are identical except for the item used to justify the separate flavored product. Examples of products using this concept are Happy Cat, Catviar, and Tender Vittles soft-moist cat foods and many dry and canned cat foods available in grocery stores (liver, tuna, chicken, beef, fish, seafood, etc., and multiple combinations of these).

The **presence of a particular food item** is

another gimmick concept. The food item most often promoted for dogs is meat and for cats is fish. This concept is based on the belief that dogs need meat and that cats prefer fish. Dogs do not need meat nor, in the wild, do they necessarily prefer it. Usually the first part of a carcass consumed by wild dogs is the internal organs and gastrointestinal contents. Wild cats do not prefer or eat primarily fish. If they did, they might develop pansteatitis, thiamin deficiency, and other nutritional diseases. Fish are not even available to most cats in the wild. Fish are used as a protein source in foods for domestic cats because large quantities of trash fish are available at a low price. In order to use this source of animal protein profitably, pet food companies using fish in their cat foods designed a media campaign to convince the cat owning public that fish was a good food for cats. It has been very successful. The problem with fish in cat food is that, in addition to protein, whole ground fish contains quantities of minerals far exceeding the cat's needs. Thus, when the cat eats the food, it must excrete the excess minerals; this increases the risk that the feline urologic syndrome will occur or recur (Chapter 9). Examples of products using this concept are Alpo Beef Chunks, Kal Kan Horsemeat, and 9-Lives, Friskies Buffet, and Purina 100 cat foods. Other examples of featured ingredients are lecithin, wheat germ meal, and a whole list of "health food" items. No controlled research exists to support the benefit of adding these items to foods for dogs and cats.

The **absence of a food item** concept promotes the fear that certain ingredients are harmful. Whether or not this concept is valid is not essential for it to succeed in improving pet food sales. If the manufacturer can convince the purchaser that an ingredient is harmful and that the manufacturer's product contains none of that ingredient, it sells the product; the purchaser has been given a reason to buy that product rather than a competitive one.

An example of this concept is the all-natural, no-preservative, no-additive foods. This is a false concept. Preservatives are added to pet foods at considerable expense to make a product that is more stable or nutritious when the animal consumes it. If there is any evidence that an additive or preservative is harmful in any way, its use is prohibited. Many natural ingredients, such as salt, are much more harmful than most preservatives and additives used in pet foods.

Another example of marketing based on the "absence of a food item" concept is products advertised as being soy-free, such as Iams or Solid Gold. This concept is based on the mistaken idea that consumption of soy products by dogs may cause or predispose to bloat (acute gastric dilata-

tion and volvulus, as discussed on page 7-23). This problem is a major concern of many dog owners. There are no controlled studies that support this contention. In fact, what little evidence exists refutes it. However, products still adhere to the concept and perpetuate the misconception.

A third example of the "absence of a food item" concept is no corn, only wheat, as in Nutro Pet Foods, or the reverse: no wheat, only corn, as in Iams Pet Foods. Both corn and wheat in pet foods can be well utilized, are excellent sources of energy, and are certainly not harmful.[13,14]

The **nutrient content** concept is based on the premise that either more or less of a nutrient is beneficial. An example is Purina Hi-Pro dog food. Protein is the featured nutrient, and the product is promoted for active and stressed dogs, which supposedly need more protein (see Chapter 3, page 3-26). However, during increased physical activity or stress, the primary need is not for protein, but for more dietary energy, which is best provided by fat. This has been well demonstrated in dogs (see page 3-26). But, to the nutritionally naive public, fat has the negative connotation of obesity, cholesterol, and heart disease. In contrast, protein has the positive connotation of strong muscles, athletic ability, and prowess. The animal's increased need for dietary energy results in more food and, as a result, more protein being consumed. Thus, a higher percentage of protein in the diet is not needed even though the animal may need more protein. However, specific-purpose diets designed to be fed for stress have a greater energy density and, therefore, usually have a higher percentage of protein in the diet, but they may not necessarily be higher in protein on a calorie basis (see page 2-6). Also, diets high in protein content have even been promoted to enhance renal function because they increase renal perfusion. Recent studies demonstrate that this is harmful rather than beneficial (Chapter 8).

Another version of the nutrient content concept is low-ash, or low-magnesium, cat foods. Examples are Prescription Diet Feline c/d and Science Diet Feline Maintenance. Extensive data document that excessive magnesium intake and a urine pH above 6.4 significantly increase the incidence of the feline urologic syndrome (Chapter 9). A diet's ash content may or may not correlate to its magnesium content and, therefore, its potential for inducing the feline urologic syndrome. Correlation is good in dry and soft-moist cat foods, but there is no correlation between ash and magnesium contents of canned cat foods. Thus, low ash may or may not be a valid concept, whereas the concept of low magnesium is valid.

The nutrient content concept is also the basis for diets used by veterinarians to manage various disease conditions in dogs and cats. Foods such as Prescription Diets k/d and u/d are low in protein, phosphorus, and salt for renal failure; h/d is low in sodium for heart disease, hypertension, edema, or ascites; s/d is severely restricted in struvite calculi-forming constituents so as to allow dissolution of these uroliths; and r/d is low in calories for managing and controlling obesity.

Product name is also a marketing concept. This concept may be used as a sales gimmick, when names are used that are amusing, easy to remember, or that sound authoritative. Examples are Snoopy Dog Food, Happy Cat, Eukanuba, Bow Wow, Meow Mix, Strongheart, Vets, and Dr. Ballard's. However, product names can also be used to identify the intended application of the diet, thus reinforcing its proper use. Examples include Puppy Chow, Senior, Feline Maintenance, h/d (heart diet), r/d (reducing diet), etc.

When evaluating pet foods, their advertising and claims, and in answering questions and advising pet owners on the use of pet foods, consider the following:

1. Is the concept of the product scientifically valid?
2. Does the concept of the product actually relate to the purpose of the product?
3. Does the product adhere to the concept or just promote it as a sales gimmick?

Whether the product is based on a valid or invalid concept, and whether the product adheres to it or not, does not mean that the product is necessarily either good or bad. It does, however, make it possible to evaluate the claims made for the product, sort scientific fact from promotional gimmickry, and form an opinion of the company marketing the product.

REFERENCES

1. Animal Health Newsletter, College of Veterinary Medicine, Cornell University. Ithaca, NY Vol 1 No 8, Oct 1983.

2. Baker NF, Farver TB: Failure of brewer's yeast as a repellent to fleas on dogs. J Amer Vet Med Assoc 183:212-214 (1983).

3. Bell RR, Thornber EJ, Sheet JLL, et al: Compensation and protein quality of honeybee-collected pollen. J Nutr 113:2479-2484 (1983).

4. Booth AJ, Stogdale L, Grigor JA: Salmon poisoning disease in dogs on southern Vancouver Island. Can Vet J 25:2-6 (1984).

5. Doyle Dane Bernback International: DDB study documents belief in animal rights. Pet Food Industry March/April:20-22 (1984).

6. Goorich RD, Pamp DE, Meiske JC: Free choice minerals. Proc Minnesota Nutrition Conf Sept 1977 pp 171-177.

7. Halliwell REW: Ineffectiveness of thiamine (Vitamin B_1) as a flea-repellent in dogs. J Amer Anim Hosp Assoc 18:423-426 (1982).

8. Hibler SC, Hoskins JE, Greene CE: Rickettsial infections in dogs. Part III. Salmon Disease complex and hemobartonellosis. Comp Cont Ed 8:251-256 (1986).

9. Hooser S: Chocolate poisoning in dogs. Topics 1984, Vol 9, #4, University of Illinois.

10. Houpt KA, Hintz HA Shepherd P: The role of olfaction in canine food preferences. Chemical Senses and Flavour 3:281-290 (1978).

11. MacDonald ML, Anderson BG, Rogers QR, et al: Essential fatty acid requirements of cats: pathology of essential fatty acid deficiency. Amer J Vet Res 45:1310-1317 (1984).

12. Mugford R: The Chemical Senses and Nutrition. Academic Press, New York, NY (1977).

13. Nutrient Requirements of Cats. National Academy of Sciences, Washington DC pp 1-49 (1978).

14. Nutrient Requirements of Dogs. National Academy of Sciences, Washington DC pp 1-71 (1974).

15. Nutrient Requirements of Dogs. National Academy of Sciences, Washington DC pp 1-79 (1985).

16. Official Publication Association of American Feed Control Officials, Inc (1983).

17. Sadler M: Pet food sales hit $5.1 billion. Pet Food Industry 27:6-10 (1985).

18. Schiffman SS: Taste and smell in disease. New England J Med 308:1275-1279 (1983).

19. Schiffman SS: Taste and smell in disease. New England J Med 308:1337-1343 (1983).

20. Schryver HF, Hintz HF: Recent developments in equine nutrition. Anim Nutr and Health 4:6-10 (1975).

21. Sohail MA: The ingestive behavior of the domestic cat—a review. Nutritional Abstracts and Reviews—Series B, 53:177-186 (1983).

22. Waterhouse HN, Fritsch CW: Dog food palatability tests and sources of potential bias. Lab Animal Care 17:93-102 (1967).

23. Williams MH: Vitamins supplementation and physical performance. In Nutrient Utilization During Exercise. Editor EL Fox. Ross Laboratories, Columbus, Ohio pp 26-30 (1983).

Chapter 3

Dogs—Feeding and Care

CONTENTS

INTRODUCTION

For optimal health, and maximal longevity and productivity, the dog must be properly fed, and cared for, throughout its life. Proper feeding requires a basic understanding of nutrients (Chapter 1), a knowledge of available foods (Chapter 2), and the application of appropriate feeding management programs for the various phases of the life cycle (as discussed in this chapter). Subsequent chapters include the dietary management of diseases, to assist in returning the dog to optimal health.

Nutritional requirements, recommended feeding management programs, and general care may differ substantially during various stages of life and for different functions and situations including maintenance, pregnancy, lactation, pre- and post-weaning, orphaned animals, inactivity, old age, physical exertion, psychologic stress, and environmental extremes. The type of food and method of feeding to meet the nutritional needs, and thus maintain optimal health, during each of these situations, are described in this chapter. This chapter also includes recommendations regarding aspects of canine care not directly related to feeding but which are important for maintaining optimal pet health.

METHODS OF FEEDING

There are three methods of feeding:
1. Free-choice, *ad libitum*, or self-feeding
2. Time-restricted meal-feeding
3. Food-restricted meal-feeding

Free-choice feeding is that situation in which more food than the animal will consume is always available, and therefore the animal can eat as much as it wants, whenever it chooses. With time-restricted meal-feeding, the animal is given more food than it will consume within a specified period of time, generally 5-30 minutes. With food-restricted meal-feeding the animal is given a specific, but lesser, amount of food than it would eat if the amount fed were not restricted. Both types of meal-feeding are repeated at a specific frequency such as one or more times a day. Some people combine feeding methods, such as free-choice feeding a dry or soft-moist food and meal-feeding a canned food or other food(s) such as meat, table scraps, etc.

Each feeding method has advantages and disadvantages. A major advantage of free-choice feeding is that it takes the least amount of work, thought and knowledge. All that is necessary is to assure that reasonably fresh food is always available. Free-choice feeding has other advantages as well:

1. It has a quieting effect in a kennel.
2. It discourages coprophagy.
3. When dogs are group-fed, the less aggressive animal has a better chance of getting its share.

Free-choice feeding does, however, have some disadvantages. If a dog becomes anorectic it may not be noticed for several days, especially if two or more dogs are fed together. In contrast, if food is always available, some dogs (and cats) overeat and become obese. Obese-prone animals should be meal-fed a high-fiber low-calorie diet, in whatever amount is necessary to maintain optimal body weight. A high-fiber low-calorie diet maintains a greater degree of gastrointestinal fullness but provides fewer calories. Gastrointestinal fullness is an important satiety factor (see page 6-12). To assist in preventing obesity, some foods intended for free-choice feeding are marginally bulk-limited; that is, they are designed so that gastric fullness occurs before the animal has ingested too many calories, but not before it has consumed enough food to meet its energy needs. The individual feeding habits of dogs fed free-choice can vary greatly. Some eat small meals several times a day, whereas others eat a large meal once daily, or even less frequently.

During periods of increased caloric need, such as growth, lactation, stress, or extensive physical exertion, a food providing less than 1500 kcal of metabolizable energy/lb of dry matter is generally bulk-limited. Diets of even higher energy density are bulk-limited for some situations of physical and/or psychologic stress. When this happens, the dog cannot consume enough food to meet its energy requirement. The result is an energy deficit with an associated impairment of performance and/or weight loss. In contrast, if a food high in energy content and palatability (as is typical of puppy foods) is fed free-choice during growth, some puppies will overeat and develop obesity. The occurrence of obesity during growth can predispose to obesity throughout life (see page 6-31). In puppies of larger breeds, overeating may predispose to the development of skeletal disease (see page 3-14). Although many puppies can be fed free-choice without these problems developing, it is safer **not** to use free-choice feeding until the puppy has attained most (90%) of its anticipated mature weight. Instead, the use of time-restricted meal-feeding is recommended (as discussed on page 3-15).

When starting a dog on free-choice feeding, first feed the usual amount of the food being meal-fed. After this has been consumed and the dog's appetite has been somewhat satisfied, set out the

food to be fed free-choice. This procedure helps prevent engorgement by a dog unaccustomed to free-choice feeding. Although most dogs unaccustomed to free-choice feeding will overeat initially, they generally stop doing so within a few days, once they learn that food is always available. During this transition period, avoid taking the food away from the animal at any time. Each time it is taken away it increases the difficulty in getting that animal on a free-choice feeding regimen. However, some dogs will continually overeat if food is always available and, therefore, cannot be fed free-choice; instead, they must be meal-fed.

There are both advantages and disadvantages of frequent food consumption that result from frequent meal- and free-choice feeding. Feeding small meals frequently throughout the day results in a greater loss of energy as a result of meal induced heat production (see page 6-16), and generally results in greater total food intake than does less frequent feeding. However, frequent feeding of small meals is beneficial for animals with dysfunctions in the ability to ingest, digest, absorb, or utilize nutrients, such as, gastrointestinal or hepatic dysfunctions, pancreatic exocrine insufficiency, diabetes mellitus, and any cause of hypoglycemia, debilitation, suboptimal body weight, anorexia, or increased dietary needs. These animals may have some degree of malassimilation or an inability to regulate blood glucose. Continued input of small amounts of food is less likely to overburden a compromised digestive system or a poorly operating blood glucose homeostatic mechanism (see Chapters 6 and 7). Frequent feeding is also desirable in normal animals that require a high food intake. Toy breed puppies under 6 months of age, some dogs engaged in heavy work (high levels of physical activity), dogs experiencing ambient temperature extremes, and lactating bitches should be fed at least three times per day to assure that their nutritional needs are met. These animals may require 1.5 to 4 times as much food per unit of body weight than most normal adult dogs (see Table 1, page 1-6). A lower feeding frequency could limit total food intake in these situations. More frequent feeding during periods of variable appetite suppression, such as occurs with psychologic stress or high ambient temperatures, helps ensure adequate food intake. Feeding at least twice daily is recommended for growing dogs other than toy breeds, the bitch during the last month of gestation, for moderate work (physical activity), and for many small dogs (less than 5 kg) because of their increased caloric needs per unit of body weight (see page 1-5).

Dogs in these categories may be unable to consume enough food at one feeding per day to meet their needs. Even if they could eat enough in one meal to meet all their requirements, some dogs fed only at night may be restless and beg for food all day or, if fed in the morning, may beg at the dinner table or whine during the night. Feeding both morning and evening minimizes these problems. Most clinically normal adult dogs that are not lactating, working, or stressed will have a sufficient appetite, and the physical capacity, to consume all the food needed daily in a single 10-minute period. Although many of these dogs are fed once daily with no noticeable detrimental effects, more frequent feeding is preferred. Once a day feeding predisposes to alterations that allow acute gastric dilatation and volvulus (bloat) to occur[78] (see page 7-23). In contrast, frequent feeding has the disadvantage in that it results in more continuous renal hyperperfusion, which, if sufficient, could result in a more rapid progression of renal dysfunction (see page 8-12). Feeding twice daily appears to be a good compromise to assist in minimizing both of these effects.

Avoid between-meal snacks and table scraps. The excessive feeding of these foods may result in an inadequate or unbalanced diet, obesity, and the development of a finicky eater or food begger. If occasional scraps are fed, avoid sweets, rich gravies, and smaller bones. Poultry bones, chopped bones, or other small bones may lodge in the dog's mouth or gastrointestinal tract. Although they do help clean the teeth, chewing large bones may result in broken teeth. Table scraps or any single food item should not constitute more than 25% of the dog's ration, and preferably not more than 10% (see pages 2-11 to 2-15).

AMOUNT TO FEED

The amount of food needed to meet the average dog's nutrient requirements can be determined by dividing the animal's caloric needs by the caloric density of the diet (Table 5, page 1-9). Using this calculation, the amounts of the various forms (dry, soft-moist, canned) of average-quality commercial dog food needed for **maintenance,** have been determined and are listed in Table 1. These estimates, or those stated by the manufacturer of a particular product, are helpful as an **initial** indication of the approximate amount of food to feed healthy dogs. Considerable variability normally exists between individual dogs in the amount of food they need (see Figure 4, page 1-10). Ultimately, the proper amount of food to feed a dog is whatever amount is necessary to maintain optimal body weight and condition.

TABLE 1

AMOUNT OF AVERAGE QUALITY DOG FOOD NEEDED DAILY BY THE MATURE DOG FOR MAINTENANCE*

Body Weight		Dry	Soft-Moist		Canned
(lb)	(kg)	(cup)**	(6 oz package)	(cup)**	(15 oz can)
4.4	2	0.75	0.50	1	0.5
11	5	1.25	1	1.5	1
22	10	2.0	1.75	2.75	1.5
33	15	3.0	2.5	3.75	2.0
44	20	3.75	3.25	4.75	2.75
66	30	5.5	4.5	7.0	4.0
88	40	7.25	6.0	9.25	5.0
110	50	9.0	7.5	11.5	6.25
154	70	12.5	10.25	15.75	8.75
220	100	17.5	14.5	22.25	12.25

*The amount needed by any individual dog may vary as much as 50% above or below the amounts given (see Figure 4, page 1-10). See Table 1, page 1-6 for modifications for conditions other than maintenance.

**8 oz. cup (volume) which holds 3-3.5 oz. by weight (85-100g) of average quality dry dog food and provides approximately 350 kcal/cup, or which holds 3.5-5 oz. by weight (100-150g) of average quality soft-moist dog food and provides approximately 275 kcal/cup. These amounts must be adjusted if food of higher or lower caloric density is fed. For example, most dry dog foods contain 8-20% fat and provide 325-400 kcal/cup, being higher the more fat in the diet. However, some dry diets contain over 20% fat and provide as much as 600 kcal/cup; while others, containing 5-6% fat, and a high fiber content, provide less than 200 kcal/cup.

Optimal body weight and condition are when the ribs are not easily seen but are readily felt, without noticing appreciable subcutaneous fat. Generally, individuals of most breeds should have an hour-glass shape when viewed from above, which means that there should be some indentation behind the rib cage. Light fleshiness over the hips and a trim abdomen also indicate good body condition.

The animal should be weighed weekly during the time when the quantity to feed is being established, then its weight should be monitored monthly. Changes of more than 5-10% from the previously established optimal weight should be accompanied by a change in the amount of food fed. Changes in amount fed should be in about 10% increments.

The amount of food needed to maintain optimal body weight and condition is affected by numerous factors including:

1. Individual variation
2. Environmental temperature, humidity, air movement, and stress
3. Physical activity with or without human inducement
4. Stage of life
5. Health status

Even dogs with the same genetic background, general activity, and environment may vary as much as 50% above or below the amount of food needed to maintain the average dog's optimal weight (see Figure 4, page 1-10). Moderate work requires about 40% more food; hard work requires even more. Sedate dogs require approximately 20% less food than normal active dogs. Dogs on the average decrease their food intake about 1-1.5% for each 1°C rise in the environmental temperature above 25°C (77°F) and increase their food intake about 3.5% for each 1°C decrease in wind-chill factor below 8°C (56°F).[4,15]

Simple mathematical factors have been determined for the different stages of the life cycle, and for various conditions (see Table 1, page 1-6). These factors can be applied to the amount of food needed for maintenance (Table 1) to determine an estimated amount to feed for these different situations. Additional information for determining "food dosage" is provided in Chapter 1 (pages 1-5 to 1-9).

Before determining the amount to feed, **the proper diet** must be selected for the dog's specific stage of life or situation (Table 2).

FEEDING AND CARE FOR MAINTENANCE

The recommended nutrient content for good-quality maintenance-type diets are listed in Table 2. For normal adult dogs weighing less than 50 lb

(23 kg), feed a good-quality maintenance-type canned, soft-moist, or dry food. Normal adult dogs weighing more than 50 lb should be fed primarily, or exclusively, a good-quality maintenance-type **dry** dog food. A dry food substantially reduces the cost of feeding, may help maintain healthier teeth and gums, and in larger breeds can aid in preventing obesity. Most dry foods contain less fat and thus have a lower caloric density, which is more appropriate for maintenance of larger dogs because they have a lower caloric need per unit of body weight than do smaller dogs (see page 1-5). If canned or soft-moist food is fed to larger dogs, the quantity should be limited to prevent obesity.

For inactive, obese-prone adult dogs feed a maintenance-type diet that is moderately restricted in energy density and increased in fiber to prevent the development of obesity (Table 15, page 6-26). In some breeds and/or in some situations it may be advisable to institute this type of diet shortly after the dog reaches its optimal adult weight. Obesity prevention is an important goal in maintenance feeding.

Some adult dogs may require a food higher in caloric density than regular maintenance-type dog foods, particularly adult dogs that are active, hyperactive, or stressed (physically, psychologically, or environmentally). In such cases a stress/performance-type diet should be fed (Table 2).

Do not feed a diet intended for growth or lactation during maintenance. These foods usually are higher in caloric density than those intended for maintenance, but also contain higher amounts of protein and a number of minerals, including calcium and phosphorus. The excessive amount of these nutrients provided by a growth/lactation-type food is not harmful during maintenance when fed for short periods. However, these foods may be harmful if fed indefinitely. The greater energy content of these diets makes them inappropriate for the inactive adult dog because of the risk of obesity. The continued use of these diets after growth, in combination with a sedentary lifestyle, may explain the early onset of obesity in many dogs (see Table 2, page 6-3). In addition to energy, the excessive intake of protein, calcium, and phosphorus causes, predisposes to, or promotes the progression of several diseases (see page 2-10). The excesses provided by feeding the non-growing non-lactating dog throughout its life, foods with nutrient levels adequate for growth and lactation, may accelerate renal aging, thereby being an important risk factor for renal failure (see page 8-10). Only the many types of cancer exceed renal failure as the leading non-accidental cause of death among dogs.

Feeding a variety of different foods is unnecessary. Dogs do not require, and most do not prefer, a variety of foods. Dogs can be maintained on

TABLE 2

DIET CHARACTERISTICS RECOMMENDED FOR DOG FOODS

Situation	Minimum Metabolizable Energy Density (kcal/g)[a]	Digestibility (%)[b]	Nutrients in Diet Dry Matter[a] (%)					
			Protein	Fat	Fiber	Calcium[c]	Phosphorus[c]	Sodium
Maintenance	3.5[d]	> 75[e]	15–25	> 8	< 5[d]	0.5–0.9	0.4–0.8	0.2–0.5
Growth Gestation Lactation	3.9	> 80	> 29	≥ 17	< 5	1.0–1.8	0.8–1.6	0.3–0.7
Old Age	3.75[d]	> 80	14–21	> 10	< 4[d]	0.5–0.8	0.4–0.7	0.2–0.4
Stress: Environmental Psychological Physical	4.2	≥ 82	> 25	> 23	≤ 4	0.8–1.5	0.6–1.2	0.3–0.6

[a]Dry matter basis. To determine the amount of the nutrient in the dry matter, divide the values (preferably obtained by laboratory analysis—if unavailable use guaranteed analysis) by the dry matter content of the food which is 1 − (% moisture in the food ÷ 100). The nutrient percentages given apply to a diet with the specific dry matter energy density listed. For diets of greater energy density, adjust the nutrient percentages accordingly (see Table 3, page 2-8).

[b]% digestibility = [(food dry weight necessary for maintaining body weight − stool dry weight) ÷ (food dry weight necessary for maintaining body weight)] × 100.

[c]The amount of calcium should be greater than the amount of phosphorus.

[d]Obese-prone dogs should be fed a diet lower in energy density and higher in fiber than listed here (see Table 15, page 6-26).

[e]> indicates greater than; < indicates less than; ≥ indicates greater than or equal to; ≤ indicates less than or equal to.

a constant diet of a complete and balanced pre-pared dog food and fresh water. If the dog's diet is changed, the change should be accomplished gradually over several days to prevent diarrhea or vomiting, which may occur if the change is abrupt. Digestive upsets may also occur when a different batch of the same dog food is fed, since the ingredients in different batches of the same food may differ. Fixed-formula diets are the excep-tion (see page 2-16).

FEEDING AND CARE DURING REPRODUCTION

NUTRITIONAL PROBLEMS

Malnourishment of the bitch, both before and during gestation, may be an important contribu-tory factor in the 20-30% mortality of neonatal pups.[20] The demands of gestation and lactation drastically alter the bitch's nutritional require-ments. Reproduction draws upon nutrients deposited in the body before and during pregnancy. Females fed improperly balanced diets of low digestibility prior to estrus will not have sufficient stores of amino acids, minerals, vitamins, or energy. Rations of poor quality, such as those with a low digesti-bility, are often the underlying cause of low conception rates, fetal abnormalities, and mam-mary gland changes which affect the quantity of milk produced, and probably the quantity and quality of colostrum. Clinical signs resulting from feeding such foods to the bitch are:

1. An "out of condition" appearance, which often goes unnoticed until the pups are born. A loss of fat stores, muscular atrophy, and dehydra-tion are noted on clinical examination. An actual loss of body weight will be recorded after adjustment of the tissue fluids following whelping.

2. Uncontrollable diarrhea during lactation. In an attempt to consume adequate nutrients to meet her needs, the bitch increases her food intake. The low utilizable caloric content of a poor-quality diet prevents her from deriving sufficient energy, and the excessive food intake further reduces the overall digestibility of the diet, resulting in diarrhea.

3. The "fading puppy" syndrome. The pups may or may not appear normal at birth. At varying lengths of time after whelping an examination of a pup may reveal any one or more of the following:
   a. Excessive crying
   b. That the stomach is not well-filled
   c. Failure to gain weight
   d. Hypothermia
   The bitch may ignore or disown these pups.

4. Lactation problems such as agalactia or hypo-galactia. These conditions in the bitch will impair the growth of the pups. Also in certain cases of bacterial mastitis, "acid milk" may be produced, which may cause death of the pup-pies if the milk is ingested.

5. Anemia is commonly observed in both the bitch and pups and is one of the most helpful diagnostic indices.

When nutritionally-related gestation/lactation problems are diagnosed, they may be associated with one or more of the following feeding prac-tices:

1. **Feeding insufficient digestible nutrients to the bitch.** The most common cause occurs when the amount of food is not increased during the latter stages of gestation and during lactation.

2. **Feeding an imbalanced diet.** Deficiencies may occur under this type feeding regimen, even when feeding for maintenance. However, during lactation, nutrient deficiencies are much more obvious because of greater needs.

3. **Feeding maintenance diets.** This is one of the most frequent causes of poor reproductive performance. Maintenance diets of marginal nutritive value are commonly fed to bitches during reproduction. Although the diet is suffi-cient to meet body demands for maintenance, feeding maintenance-type diets during gestation induces nutrient depletion, and feeding them during lactation induces nutrient deficiency.

To prevent these problems, specific management practices are recommended at each stage of gesta-tion and lactation.

PRE-BREEDING FEEDING AND CARE

Prior to breeding, the bitch should be:

1. Given a thorough physical examination

2. Checked and treated as necessary for internal and external parasites

3. Vaccinated for all diseases that are potential problems in that geographic area to ensure that she has optimal immunity to pass to the pup-pies

4. Weighed, and if necessary, alter the amount or type of food being fed so that the bitch is at optimal body weight when she is bred. If a bitch is noticeably over- or underweight, she may have difficulty conceiving, problems suc-

cessfully carrying all puppies to term, dystocia, and/or after whelping may be unable to produce adequate colostrum or milk.

Before the bitch is bred, her hematocrit should be greater than 37%, her hemoglobin concentration above 10 g/dl, and her plasma protein above 5 g/dl. Values below these amounts indicate a poor nutritional state or the presence of disease. Either of these problems should be corrected prior to breeding. Ideally, all bitches used for breeding should be tested for brucellosis and bred only to stud dogs that have recently tested negative for this disease. If the bitch has previously had breeding or reproductive problems such as bacterial infections, before or during gestation, bacterial cultures and sensitivities should be conducted early in estrus so that appropriate antibiotics can be administered before breeding.

PREGNANT BITCH FEEDING AND CARE

A growth/lactation-type diet (Table 2, page 3-5) may be fed throughout pregnancy, but is particularly important during the last 3-4 weeks of gestation and throughout lactation. It is also important that the diet is of good quality (see page 2-16 for assessing the quality of pet foods). Do not supplement (meat, milk, calcium, phosphorus, or vitamins) or feed anything other than a good-quality diet meeting the specifications listed in Table 2 (page 3-5). Calcium or vitamin D supplementation may cause soft-tissue calcification and physical anomalies in the puppies and does not help prevent eclampsia (see page 12-11). Gestating bitches also require soluble carbohydrate in their diet.[53] Feeding carbohydrate-free diets, such as diets containing meat as the only energy source, causes hypoglycemia in late gestation and results in fewer live births.[53]

Nutritional deprivation during pregnancy can compromise immunologic competence of offspring. There is evidence that severe malnutrition during pregnancy can adversely affect immunocompetence not only from that pregnancy, but also in those offsprings' subsequent young, even though they are adequately fed. Evidently the reticulo-endothelial system is highly vulnerable to nutritional and metabolic derangement during its period of formation and development.[66]

Most dogs will decrease their food consumption during the fourth week of pregnancy; although in some bitches this decrease occurs during the third, and in others the fifth week of pregnancy. In our colony of Beagles, this decrease is an accurate indication of pregnancy (see Figure 1).

Less than 30% of fetal growth occurs during the first 5-6 weeks of gestation. As a result, there is little or no change in the bitch's body weight or nutritional need during this period (Figure 1). However, fetal size rapidly increases during the last 3-4 weeks of gestation. As a result the body weight of the bitch should increase 15-25% by the time of whelping (Figure 1). For the bitch at optimal body weight at breeding, the same amount of food needed for maintenance should be fed during the first 5-6 weeks of gestation. After that the amount fed should be gradually increased so that the bitch is receiving 15-25% more food by the time of whelping. During this period, feeding should be twice-a-day or free-choice. During the last 10 days of gestation, a pregnant bitch carrying a large litter may have such an enlarged abdomen that she may not eat all the food she needs in only two meals per day. In these cases, meal-feed at more frequent intervals or feed free-choice.

MANAGEMENT AT PARTURITION

Several days before whelping, the bitch may present a sagging appearance. Her mammary glands enlarge and become pink and her food intake decreases. Milk may appear in the breasts from 4-5 days to just before, parturition. The bitch begins nesting about 24 hours before whelping. Food will be refused about 12 hours prior to parturition and the bitch's rectal temperature may drop at least 1°C, often to 37°C (98°F), 12-8 hours before she gives birth.

A sturdy whelping box of suitable size should be provided. It should be large enough to house the growing puppies until they are weaned. Depending on its location, the box may need sides high enough to exclude drafts and be raised off the floor to keep it from becoming cold and damp. A railing around the inside which is about three inches tall and three inches from the sides (vary as needed based on size of puppies) will help to protect puppies from being crushed between the bitch and the sides of the box. At least one side of the box should be low enough to permit the bitch to readily enter and leave as desired. A nervous bitch may feel more secure if the box is covered.

Indoor-outdoor carpeting makes excellent bedding for the whelping box. Two pieces should be available so that one can be cleaned and dried while the other is in use. Newspapers are slippery and provide insufficient traction for puppies learning to walk. Heavy towels, mattress pads, and scatter rugs give good traction and are suitable bedding

FIGURE 1

BODY WEIGHT AND FOOD INTAKE DURING GESTATION AND LACTATION IN THE BITCH

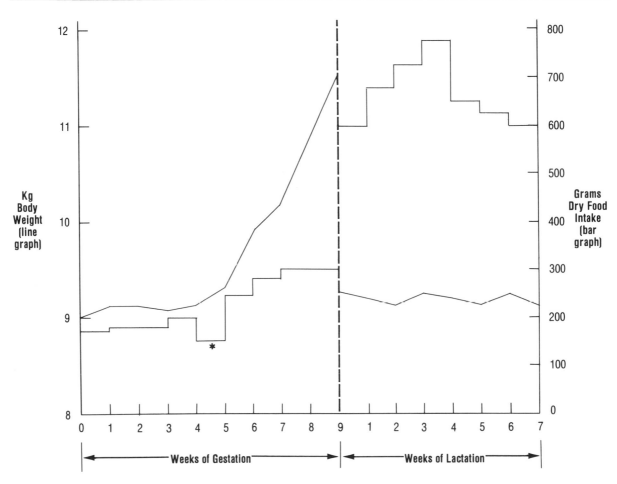

*Transient decrease in food intake at approximately the fourth week after conception is indicative of pregnancy.

if they are disposable or washable. Disposable baby diapers are excellent for toy-breed puppies. The bedding should not be so flimsy that the bitch can easily scratch it up under her and possibly smother a puppy in the folds. Small puppies should never be put in deep loose bedding that might interfere with breathing.

During whelping, an afterbirth should be passed following the birth of each puppy. The bitch normally removes the membranes from the puppy, bites off the umbilical cord, eats the afterbirth, and licks the puppy dry. If the bitch does not remove the sac within the first couple of minutes, the person in attendance should quickly intervene or the puppy will smother. However, it is better not to interfere unless a puppy is in danger. Some

bitches resent outside assistance and will not care for the puppies if too much help is given. With excessive interference some bitches become nervous and thus may be too exuberant or persistent when licking the puppies to dry and stimulate them. This can result in skin abrasions unless the puppies are protected.

Make certain that the bitch has expelled all of the afterbirths. A retained afterbirth usually results in uterine infection and systemic toxicity, which may be fatal if not promptly treated. A dark red or reddish-brown discharge after whelping usually means all afterbirths have been expelled. A bright red discharge may indicate hemorrhage. A discharge any other color, and particularly a brown or greenish-colored discharge, which generally ap-

pears 48-72 hours after whelping, indicates a retained afterbirth, a retained puppy, or a uterine infection. These problems are also suggested by a lethargic attitude in the bitch and a poor appetite for the first few days after whelping.

The whelping box and general environment should be kept scrupulously clean. This reduces parasite infestations and the possibility of bacterial and viral infections. Outside visitors should be discouraged and handling should be restricted until the pups are 2-3 weeks old. The puppies should be left alone to eat and sleep. Kennel-raised puppies should be isolated from the kennel population until they are given their first vaccinations.

FEEDING DURING LACTATION

A readily accessible source of good-quality water is of utmost importance in the proper feeding of lactating bitches. Throughout lactation, feed the bitch enough food to maintain optimal body weight. If at optimal weight at whelping, a bitch with an average-to-large litter generally requires the following amounts of food during lactation:

1. First week—1.5 times the amount needed for maintenance
2. Second week—twice as much as maintenance
3. Third week to weaning—triple that needed for maintenance

However, the amount of food required depends on the size of the litter. During peak lactation (third through sixth week of lactation), 100 kcal of metabolizable energy/lb of litter/day is needed in addition to the energy required for maintenance. This can be provided by feeding 25% more food for each puppy than the bitch needed for maintenance (see Table 1, page 1-6). For example, if prior to pregnancy the bitch ate 3 cups of dry food per day and maintained optimal body weight and now, during peak lactation, she is nursing 8 pups, she needs 3 cups/day for maintenance plus (8 pups × 25%/pup) × (3 cups/day) for lactation, for a total of 9 cups/day. However, during lactation it is usually best to feed free-choice and to encourage the bitch to eat as much as possible. Free-choice feeding also ensures that food is available for the puppies and encourages them to consume solid food at an early age. If meal-feeding is used, feed the bitch and puppies all they will eat at least three times daily.

A major problem during lactation is to provide a sufficient amount of energy to the bitch so that she will produce enough milk to meet the needs of the nursing puppies. For example:[29] a Labrador bitch weighing 28 kg with a litter of 8 puppies whose total weight is 12 kg at 4 weeks of age. At this stage the pups' daily energy requirement is about 200 kcal/kg, which they obtain primarily or exclusively from the bitch's milk. Therefore the bitch has to produce 2400 kcal/day in the form of milk. Bitch's milk contains about 1260 kcal/L, so 2400 kcal ÷ 1260 kcal/L = 1.9 L of milk is required (almost 1/2 gallon). This assumes that all of the energy of the milk is available to the pups at 100% efficiency. If lactation in the bitch is assumed to be 75% efficient, to produce 2400 kcal as milk she must obtain (2400 ÷ 0.75 =) 3200 kcal from her food. In addition she will need 1820 kcal for her own maintenance needs (Table 1, page 1-6) for a total of 5020 kcal which is 2.75 times her maintenance requirement.

The energy requirement not only depends upon the number of pups in the litter, but also on the breed (size), and temperament of the bitch. Small bitches have a higher energy requirement per pound of body weight than larger bitches (page 1-5), and nervousness or emotional stress also increases energy expenditure. The feeding of a **good-quality** growth/lactation-type cat food often works well for small bitches during lactation since many of these cat foods have higher nutrient and energy contents than dog foods.

Throughout lactation, be sure to feed a good-quality growth/lactation-type diet (Table 2, page 3-5). Lactation is the phase of the life cycle when the quality of the food is particularly important. Lactation presents one of the most severe tests of a diet's nutritional adequacy. The bitch must eat, digest, absorb, and use very large amounts of nutrients to produce sufficient milk to support the rapid growth and development of several puppies. Many commercial dog foods do not have sufficient nutrient density to meet the needs of a bitch nursing a large litter of pups. Although the requirements for all nutrients are increased, energy is usually most limiting. A lactating bitch fed free-choice should be able to maintain her body weight. If she is thin at weaning and has been fed free-choice throughout lactation, the diet fed does not contain adequate utilizable calories. In such cases, it is best to switch to a diet with a higher caloric density. A less desirable alternative is to add 1 tablespoon (15ml) of fat/cup of dry food. The type of fat (animal or vegetable) is not important, as the increased need is for calories rather than essential fatty acids. Grease, lard, tallow, or vegetable oil are all satisfactory. Adding this amount of fat increases the caloric density

of the diet about 30%. Increasing the caloric density above this recommendation may decrease food intake sufficiently to result in deficiencies of nutrients other than energy. Therefore, more fat than recommended should not be added. It is safer to switch to a higher-quality diet.

Occasionally, an attentive or inexperienced bitch will be reluctant to leave her puppies for the first 24 to 48 hours after whelping. Bitch's should be monitored for this type of behavior postpartum and be offered food and water if necessary.

Some even-mannered bitches with several puppies may become antagonistic or disgruntled during lactation. This change of attitude often begins about the second or third week. Giving 250-500 mg of vitamin C daily reportedly alleviates this condition.[51] While there is no physiologic basis for this recommendation, it may be helpful and short-term supplementation with vitamin C at this dosage would not be harmful.

Before and during weaning, restricting the food intake of the bitch may prevent excessive distention of the mammary glands and the associated discomfort following weaning. This is particularly helpful for bitches that are lactating heavily, such as those with large litters. This can be accomplished by separating the bitch from the litter during the day, withholding food from her, and allowing the puppies access to food. Reunite the bitch and pups that night and remove all food. Wean the pups the next day and begin to gradually increase the amount fed the bitch so that by several days after weaning she is receiving the amount needed for her **maintenance.**

PUPPY FEEDING AND CARE

NEONATAL CARE

As is the case with all newborn animals, it is important that pups receive adequate amounts of good-quality colostrum shortly after birth. Every effort should be made to see that pups nurse from the bitch soon after birth so that transfer of passive immunity from colostrum is maximized. The pup receives about 90% of its passive immunity from colostrum and the remainder transplacentally.[20] Early ingestion of adequate amounts of colostrum also appears to be important to the puppy because initial fluid intake contributes significantly to immediate postnatal circulatory volume. Lack of intake could cause circulatory failure. The fading-puppy complex (see page 3-20) is sometimes considered to have two separate causes: infectious and non-infectious (which in-

cludes cardio-pulmonary failure).[20] Therefore, early ingestion of adequate amounts of colostrum would help prevent both major causes of the fading-puppy complex. Holding the pup up to a nipple soon after whelping helps ensure adequate ingestion of colostrum.

During the first few weeks of life, the puppy should just eat and sleep. Much of this is activated sleep, during which the puppy twitches and jerks. This activity is important for normal muscle development. The puppy should nurse vigorously and compete with littermates for a nipple. At birth their eyes and ears are sealed shut. The eyes open between 10 and 16 days, and the ears begin to function between 15 and 17 days. The respiratory rate is 8-18 breaths/minute for the first 24 hours of life, then 15-35 per minute until 5 weeks of age. The heart rate accelerates from 120-150 beats/minute for the first day of life to 220/minute through 5 weeks of age. These rates are much faster than the adult whose average respiratory rate is 10-30/minute and average heart rate is 80-140/minute.

The puppy's body temperature is 34.5 - 36°C (94-97°F) for the first two weeks of life. They have no shivering reflex for the first 6 days and, therefore, depend on an external heat source, such as the mother, to sustain normal body temperature. In addition, pups often pile up, which decreases their total exposed body surface area and effectively reduces heat loss from the litter (see page 1-5). The puppy's body temperature drops rapidly with an environmental temperature of less than about 30°C (86°F). Mild hypothermia is not of necessity lethal, and it may be that this level of hypothermia, or an inability to produce heat, was an advantageous response for pups in the wild. A lack of response to cooling would result in no increase in energy demands. This would result in prolonged survival while the mother was away seeking food.[20] However, moderate or severe hypothermia can seriously affect survival. Moderate hypothermia is characterized by a pup which becomes progressively more lethargic and exhibits diminished reflex activity. Attempts may be made to suckle but milk is not ingested. Heart rate is slowed and the rectal temperature decreases to 15-20°C (60-70°F). With severe hypothermia there is no perceptible respiration, only occasional gasps. Heart rate is slowed and reflexes are extremely sluggish. The rectal temperature is between 10-15°C (50-60°F). The pup does not feed and eventually dies. However, even pups in deep hypothermia can be resuscitated by slow re-warming at 30°C (85°F).[20]

Hypothermia inhibits feeding and thus chances of survival. In addition, hypothermia is one of the factors inducing the cardiopulmonary syndrome of the fading-puppy complex. Hypothermia may also enhance invasion by certain pathogens (e.g. herpes virus), thereby inducing the infectious component of the fading-puppy complex[20] (see page 3-20). A bitch's rejection of a puppy may be caused in part by its cold body temperature. The rejection further deprives the puppy of a source of heat—that of its mother's and littermates' bodies.

At 6 days of age, puppies can shiver and begin to be self-sustaining. From the second to the fourth weeks of life, their body temperature rises to 36-37°C (97-99°F) and after the fourth week is near adult body temperature. By 18 days of age, puppies begin walking, which helps stimulate and maintain a higher body temperature. For puppies with the bitch and littermates, the environmental temperature should be 21°C (70°F) for at least the first few weeks.[20] If the puppy is separated from the bitch and littermates, the environmental temperature should be maintained as described for orphans (page 3-19).

Neonatal puppies have little subcutaneous fat. Their energy source is almost entirely glycogen, which is rapidly depleted after birth and not restored until after several days of nursing. If the puppy does not receive adequate nourishment, it soon becomes dehydrated, cold, weak, and debilitated; its survival is doubtful. To prevent these problems, puppies should be kept in a warm environment, weighed daily, and supplementary feeding instituted (see Tables 3 and 5, pages 3-18 and 3-19) if weight gain is not normal.

One of the more beneficial management practices is to weigh the pups, daily for the first two weeks and then every three days until the pups are 1 month old. Periodic weight checks should be made thereafter, using a gram scale. This scale is one of the best investments a breeder can make. A steady weight gain and normal stools are the best indications of good health and the adequacy of the puppy's diet. As shown in Figure 2, compared to the human infant, the pup's capacity for rate of growth is phenomenal. They should gain weight the first day of life and continue to gain daily. The birth weight usually doubles within 7-10 days and increases 6-10 times by weaning at 6 weeks of age. A more precise guide is that **puppies should gain 1-2 g/day/lb (2-4 g/day/kg) of anticipated** adult weight. For example, if the anticipated weight of the adult dog is 40 lbs, the dog as a pup should

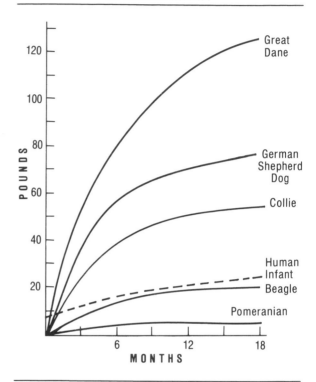

FIGURE 2

GROWTH RATE OF DOGS AS COMPARED TO HUMAN INFANT

gain 40-80 g (1.5 to 2.5 oz) per day during the first 5 months of life. Weighing should be done often to ensure that the growth rate is adequate. If it is not, supplemental feeding should be instituted, or a better quality diet should be fed. Most dogs reach 50% of their mature weight by 4 months of age. This rapid rate of growth continues until the pup is 6-9 months of age. Adult weight is approached at approximately 1 year of age. The growth rate of giant breeds (e.g. Great Danes) does not slow until about 18 months of age. Mature weight of giant breeds is not reached until the dogs are almost 2 years of age (Figure 2).

While nursing, the pups should be observed occasionally to be sure they all get a chance to nurse. If one is crowded out, it should be assisted in reaching a nipple. It is essential that the puppies receive adequate amounts of the bitch's milk. If the bitch is healthy and well-nourished, whelping is uneventful and no post-whelping problems arise. Nutritional management of the litter will be handled completely by the mother for the first three weeks. If puppies cry constantly or do not achieve the weight gain described, they are probably not receiving enough milk.

PUPPY CARE
WHEN MILK IS INADEQUATE

If the bitch is not giving enough milk, as indicated by the puppies not gaining enough weight, the following procedures should be instituted:

1. Give the bitch a physical examination and eliminate as a cause and/or treat any disease condition present.

2. Ensure that the bitch is receiving an adequate amount of a good-quality growth/lactation-type diet (Table 2, page 3-5). If a dry diet is being fed, adding water may increase intake.[76] Do not use milk, and add only enough water to moisten the food (1 cup water/4-5 cups food), not enough to make it mushy. Adding 1 tablespoon of fat or oil/cup of dry food may also be beneficial. Do **not** add more than this amount of fat.

If these procedures do not adequately increase milk production, supplemental food must be fed to the pups, as described in raising orphans (page 3-18).

FEEDING PUPPIES
FOR AND FOLLOWING WEANING

Weaning

Feeding in preparation for weaning should start when the puppies are 3 weeks old. However, if necessary, puppies may be started as soon as their eyes are open. If given the opportunity, most puppies will start eating the food being fed to the bitch when they are about 4 weeks old. This should be encouraged. A thick gruel can be made by mixing the diet with water and is helpful in starting the pups on solid food. The gruel may be smeared on their lips, or the pups may even be placed in a shallow pan of the gruel. They will lick it off their lips or feet and thus start eating it. Gradually decrease the water in the gruel until it is omitted. When making the gruel, add just enough water to make the food mushy, not sloppy. Do not use milk. The lactose content of cow's milk (whole, condensed, or skimmed) is higher than that of bitch's milk (Table 4, page 3-18) and may cause diarrhea and dehydration. Some bitches will wean puppies as early as 4 weeks, although 6-7 weeks is more desirable. By this time, they must be able to eat enough solid food to meet their needs.

Weaning and separation from littermates before 4-6 weeks of age may result in behavioral problems (see page 3-20). However, puppies older than 10 weeks of age that have had little or no human contact can make equally undesirable pets. Such dogs may be timid or may resist human domination, making them difficult to train and possibly aggressive and dangerous.[31] To minimize the development of behavioral problems, weaning should not be attempted until the puppies are 6 weeks old. In addition, close human contact should be encouraged when the puppies are 4-10 weeks of age.

Diets for Growth

The food fed the weaned pup should be one specifically formulated for this purpose, i.e. a good quality growth/lactation diet (Table 2, page 3-5). Under no circumstances should the calcium content of the diet dry matter exceed 1.8%, or phosphorus exceed 1.6%, nor should supplemental calcium or phosphorus be given. Excessive calcium and phosphorus can be harmful (see page 3-16). However, neither meeting the specifications listed in Table 2 (page 3-5), nor meeting the National Research Council's nutrient requirements for dogs,[53] will assure that the food will support optimal growth. Quantitative content of nutrients in the diet does not provide information concerning palatability, nutrient availability, or protein quality. Thus, in addition to the recommended nutrient levels, ensure that the food has been shown to be nutritionally adequate for growth by successful feeding tests (see page 2-16 for indications of pet food quality). Feed only the selected food. Supplementation with meat, table scraps, or other items can create either a finicky eater or nutritional imbalances, or both.

Feeding a soft, easily digested food is particularly important for pups weaned before 6 weeks of age. If dry foods are fed to weaning pups, water should be added. This not only softens the food, but also frequently increases the dry matter consumption by increasing palatability.[76]

The owner should be cautioned to be certain that the pup has sufficient food during its growth phase. Puppies require less total food if a high-quality diet is fed. Inferior diets are less digestible; therefore, they require that the puppy consume more diet in order to obtain the necessary amount of available nutrients.

As total food consumption increases, digestibility decreases and is a factor that should be considered when a food is chosen for the pup. If poor-quality foods with low digestibility are selected, the resulting high intake will only further reduce the digestibility of the food. Owners should be guided by the performance of the diet rather than by how much the pup eats.

A problem often develops clinically when pups (particularly of large breeds) are fed low caloric-density foods such as maintenance-type diets, poor quality foods, or inexpensive dry foods, in an effort to save money. In these instances, because of the low caloric density, the pup cannot possibly consume sufficient quantities of digestible nutrients to meet the requirements for optimal growth. As a result of being fed these diets, puppies may have a "pot-bellied" appearance with slower growth, inferior muscle and skeletal development, and decreased resistance to infectious diseases. Feeding the proper amount of a good-quality food will prevent the development of these problems.

Well-nourished, vigorous pups have a greater resistance to disease and to the devitalizing effects of intestinal parasitism than do malnourished pups. A deficiency of certain amino acids, vitamins, and energy, can markedly reduce several aspects of an animal's immune response as well as other natural host defenses.[2] Dietary protein deficiency has been associated with skeletal disease. An increased incidence of hip dysplasia was observed in growing dogs fed diets containing 20% protein.[58] (At least 29% is recommended.)

Studies have been conducted to determine the amount of dietary protein, carbohydrate, and fat needed for optimal growth. In one study, nine diets, with energy derived from carbohydrate ranging from 0-62% and energy from protein ranging from 20-48%, were fed to dogs for 8 months, starting when they were 2 months old.[59] The dogs readily consumed each of the diets. Regardless of the diet, all dogs had a similar positive nitrogen balance and weight gain. Consumption of carbohydrate-free diets did not influence postprandial concentrations of plasma glucose or insulin. Plasma cholesterol concentrations were increased in dogs consuming diets high in fat and cholesterol, but plasma triglyceride content was not influenced by diet composition. Consumption of high-protein (46-48% of energy) diets increased plasma urea nitrogen content to about 30 mg/dl but had minimal influence on plasma amino acid concentrations. At the end of the study, dogs fed the high-carbohydrate (62% of energy) diet had less body fat but an equal muscle mass as compared with dogs fed low-carbohydrate (20-42% of energy) diets containing a similar quantity of protein.

In another study, no difference in hip dysplasia was detected in growing dogs fed four different diets despite a 32% overall incidence of hip dysplasia. The diets ranged from 0-62% carbohydrate, 13-76% fat, and 24-48% protein as a percent of metabolizable energy.[73] On the basis of these studies, it appears that as long as the amino acid and fatty acid contents of the diet meet the requirements for growth, and the diet is acceptable, the proportion of energy supplied by carbohydrate, fat, and protein is not an important consideration for the growing dog.

Feeding Procedures for Growth

The goal in feeding weaned puppies should be to attain the average growth for that breed (Figure 2, page 3-11). From the standpoints of health and longevity, the optimal growth rate is probably the average growth rate for that breed. Overfeeding for maximal weight gain should be avoided. Slight underfeeding is preferable to overfeeding. Studies have shown that the growth of puppies can be slowed through underfeeding without inducing deleterious effects. However, if underfeeding is severe, mature size will be stunted. Underfeeding has been shown to increase the life span of other species and probably has the same effect in dogs. Restriction of caloric intake in amounts that do not retard growth has been shown to increase longevity of rats.[61] Limiting food intake from weaning up to 10 months of age is reported to be the most effective means of increasing longevity. The protein content of the diet is not a factor. Only the total quantity of food consumed appears to be important.[62] In contrast to mild underfeeding, overfeeding during growth predisposes to obesity and, in larger breeds, to skeletal problems.

Excessive dietary energy intake during growth can result in obesity in puppies of many breeds. As discussed in Chapter 6, the development of **obesity during growth** is due to increases in both **size and numbers of fat cells.** Growing animals are in an anabolic phase and, therefore, body cell numbers are more easily increased during growth. **Obesity in the adult is due** primarily **to an increase in fat cell size,** rather than numbers. Weight reduction, regardless of age, decreases the size of fat cells but not their number. (Once established, the number of fat cells is difficult to decrease.) Thus, excess fat deposition during growth increases total fat cell numbers and thus predisposes to obesity throughout life. Obesity is associated with several serious medical problems in adult dogs which limit their activity, productivity, longevity, and enjoyment of life (page 6-7). When the detrimental effects of obesity in the adult are considered, the "cute," fat "roly-poly" puppy is probably the one with a higher risk for health problems throughout its life.

Several breeds of dogs are predisposed to obesity (see page 6-3). Owners of all puppies, but particularly owners of obese-prone breeds, should be counselled to feed carefully to avoid obesity during growth. This would include recommending meal-feeding rather than feeding free-choice. This point is emphasized by a study in which Beagle and Labrador Retriever puppies were fed free-choice, or were meal-fed 80% of the amount consumed by those fed free-choice.[39] At 1 year of age, puppies of both breeds fed free-choice were 22-25% heavier. The Beagles fed free-choice were more obese than the Labradors fed free-choice. However, the increased weight in both breeds fed free-choice was the result of increased body fat. There was no difference in body length, height, bone size, or muscle mass. The conclusions were that free-choice feeding, even of only moderately palatable dry dog foods, can produce a marked degree of obesity in Labrador and Beagle puppies.[39] This study demonstrates that overfeeding during growth (versus controlled feeding) increases the risk of obesity but does not increase mature size or improve musculoskeletal development. In fact, overfeeding puppies may directly predispose to skeletal disease.

Overfeeding during growth may not cause obesity in large breed puppies, but does accelerate growth rate, which predisposes to development of a number of serious skeletal problems. [26,27,38,56] These include hip dysplasia, osteochondritis dissecans, dropped hocks, splayed feet, angular limb deformities, elbow subluxations, wobbler syndrome, and lameness. However, care must be taken in assessing skeletal development of puppies. Nearly all puppies, particularly larger breeds, normally show some dropping of the hocks and enlarged joints during rapid growth. A moderate degree of broadening of the metaphyseal regions of the long bones is a physiologic event during growth and accompanies longitudinal growth of the bone. During periods of rapid growth, especially in large breeds, metaphyseal enlargening is sometimes so pronounced that it is difficult to distinguish from pathologic processes including rickets.[27] Physiologic broadening of the metaphysis will regress, and at maturity no signs of impaired skeletal development will remain. Giving additional minerals or vitamins including calcium, vitamin D, or both, does not alter physiologic broadening of the metaphysis.[27] However, physiologic, as well as pathologic, bone alterations can be decreased by decreasing food intake and, thus, slowing growth rate.

Overfeeding, particularly of a good-quality highly digestible food containing the proper amount of all nutrients to permit maximum growth rate, can result in skeletal problems. The larger faster-growing puppy is more predisposed to skeletal problems due to overfeeding. Puppies on a high calorie intake after weaning have been shown to develop hip dysplasia more frequently, earlier, and more severely, than littermates fed less of the same diet.[27] Free-choice feeding of Great Danes resulted in more osteochondrosis than resulted in littermates fed one-third less of the same diet.[26] This study and the Beagle/Labrador study[39] discussed earlier demonstrate that **controlled intake of food during growth allows good development with no reduction in mature body size, but decreases the risk of obesity and skeletal problems, observed in free-choice fed dogs.**

During peak growth, puppies consume an amount of food dry matter equal to from 5.5-7% of their body weight daily when fed a palatable diet free-choice. This is apparently all the gastrointestinal tract of the puppy can process. With an increase in energy density of the diet, more calories are consumed. As caloric intake increases, growth rate and/or the amount of fat deposited increases, with an attendant increase in the risk of skeletal problems and obesity, respectively. There are two ways to prevent excessive growth rate and excessive fat deposition: 1) restrict the amount fed or 2) feed a diet that will not allow maximum growth rate or fat deposition to occur, regardless of how much is consumed. There are several types of diets that will not permit maximum growth rate and/or fat deposition. However, these diets cause problems. Following is a description of these diets and the problems they can cause:

1. A diet with inadequate metabolizable calories, such as even an average-quality maintenance-type diet. The puppy's gastrointestinal tract cannot process enough of this type of diet to provide the energy needed for maximum growth, or excess fat deposition and, as a result, growth rate and fat deposition are reduced. In an attempt to take in more dietary energy, the puppy eats continually and its gastrointestinal tract is almost always full, which, in conjunction with the puppy's normally high level of physical activity, may result in development of gastrohepatic ligament laxity. This may predispose the pup to acute gastric dilatation-volvulus (bloat) later in life (see page 7-23).

2. A diet containing excessive amounts of minerals. Certain dietary mineral excesses can decrease the absorption of other minerals and, as a re-

sult, may cause a secondary mineral deficiency. This type of diet not only slows growth, it may also result in dermatologic problems, testicular degeneration, impaired immunity, hypothyroidism, and skeletal problems.[24,25,36,37,48] Also, this type of diet may predispose the mature dog to bloat (see page 7-23).

3. A diet containing inadequate amounts of essential amino acids. This may be the result of either inadequate protein quantity, digestibility, or quality. Such a diet not only slows growth, it decreases immunity, causes a poor coat, impairs wound healing, and decreases muscle development.[2,53]

Because of: 1) the problems caused by feeding puppies a diet that will not support maximum growth rate no matter how much is consumed, and 2) the problems that may occur when a diet that does support maximum growth rate is fed free-choice, **puppies should be fed diets that are adequate to support maximum growth rate, but these diets should not be fed free-choice to growing dogs until they have attained 80-90% of their anticipated adult weight.** For most dogs this occurs at 9 months of age, and in giant breeds, such as Great Danes, at 18 months of age (see Figure 2, page 3-8). Instead of feeding free-choice, **twice daily time-limited meal-feeding is recommended for most breeds. Feed toy breeds three times daily until 6 months of age, after which and for all other breeds, feed twice daily until 12 months of age (12 to 18 months for giant breeds). At each feeding, allow the puppy approximately 20 minutes to eat all it wants.** The daily metabolizable energy intake recommended for the growing puppy is approximately twice the maintenance energy requirement (MER) up to 3 months of age, then decreases incrementally to the MER as they approach mature body size, as listed in Table 1, page 1-6.[53]

Supplementation During Growth

Growing pups should be fed **only** a high-quality balanced growth/lactation-type dog food (Table 2, page 3-5), and water. Supplementation with vitamins, minerals, or protein is not necessary and, in many instances, is harmful. High-quality growth/lactation-type foods are nutritionally balanced and therefore have the proper amount (not too much or too little) of all nutrients including protein, minerals, and vitamins to meet the needs for growth. Additional protein, vitamins or minerals can upset the balance of nutrients in the food.

If the owner or veterinarian previously has observed clinical signs of nutritional imbalance in dogs consuming a particular brand of food, the proper action is to change to a better-quality nutritionally-adequate diet, rather than attempt to supplement an unbalanced diet (see page 2-11). However, if the food has been proved by well-controlled feeding studies to be nutritionally adequate for growth, the proper action is to limit the amount consumed. Overfeeding a balanced diet results in nutrient excesses. The prophylactic use of vitamin/mineral supplements in conjunction with a good-quality balanced dog food is unnecessary and can be harmful. Supplements are often given in the hope of decreasing or preventing skeletal problems during growth, in lieu of more appropriate management.

Skeletal problems may be caused by, or predisposed to, not only by excessive energy intake, but also by feeding an unbalanced diet containing inadequate protein, or an excess or deficiency of calcium, phosphorus, and vitamins A or D. Feeding diets containing protein levels higher than the growing dog's requirement does not decrease the incidence of skeletal problems, such as hip dysplasia, below that observed when the diet contains adequate protein.[73]

A popular misconception is that most canine skeletal disease is related to inadequate dietary calcium or vitamin D intake. However, supplementing with calcium, vitamin D or both, above the dog's requirements, has not been shown to alleviate or prevent skeletal problems.[27] There have been numerous studies conducted on calcium and phosphorus requirements for dogs, under a variety of different regimens and diets, and in different breeds. No difference between breeds has been demonstrated. For all breeds and all physiologic situations, the optimal calcium/phosphorus ratio is in the range of 1.1-1.4 parts calcium to 1 part phosphorus.[53] The ratio of dietary calcium to phosphorus is important, but means little unless the absolute amounts of these minerals are considered first (see page 3-16). The National Research Council (NRC) recommends at least 1.1% calcium and 0.9% phosphorus in the diet dry matter for the dog.[53] These amounts are about 30% higher than studies suggest are needed even during growth and are adequate even in a primarily cereal-base diet.[53] Calcium and phosphorus are not as available from plant source food ingredients as they are from animal tissue, or calcium- and phosphorus-containing salts, or bone meal. Thus, the amounts recommended by the NRC are more than adequate for all breeds during growth and, in addition, provide a fairly

substantial safety margin. Many dog foods contain from 20-120% more calcium and 10-60% more phosphorus than the amounts recommended by the NRC.[42] Thus, if growing dogs are fed good-quality dog food as most of their diet, supplemental calcium and/or phosphorus should not be given, regardless of breed. Under these circumstances, calcium and phosphorus supplementation is of no benefit and may be harmful.

Excessive dietary calcium causes hypercalcemia, hypophosphatemia, and hypercalcitoninism, which retards bone resorption, cartilage maturation, bone maturation, and bone remodeling, as well as causing disturbances in endochondral ossification in both articular and physeal growth plate cartilage. These skeletal changes result in osteochondrosis, retained cartilage cones, radius curvus syndrome, wobblers syndrome, and reduced growth rate and mature size.[25] In one study using Great Dane puppies, these detrimental effects were observed when dietary calcium was supplemented to 3.3% (dry matter basis).[25] Most popular selling brands of commercial dog foods contain 1.2-2.5% calcium, and some contain more than 3% calcium. Adding as little as 2-3 teaspoonsful of calcium carbonate daily to most commercial diets can raise total dietary calcium to levels that are harmful to growing puppies. Hypertrophic osteodystrophy, hip dysplasia, wobblers syndrome, eosinophilic panosteitis, osteochondritis dissecans, and failure of conversion of woven bone to lamellar bone result from the combined action of excessive dietary calcium, protein, and energy.[45]

Vitamin C deficiency has been postulated as a cause of canine skeletal diseases, and therefore supplementing with vitamin C has been proposed to be helpful in preventing bone and joint problems in dogs. However, controlled studies have shown that vitamin C supplementation has no beneficial effect. In contrast, large doses may aggravate osteodystrophy.[36]

Excessive dietary calcium decreases phosphorus, iron, zinc, and copper absorption and may cause a deficiency of these minerals.[24,36] Zinc deficiency resulting from excessive calcium intake is not uncommon in dogs, particularly puppies. The cause is usually excessive calcium supplementation or a poor-quality commercial pet food that has a high calcium content and is marginal in zinc. The skin of **affected dogs** is crusty and scaled. Some zinc deficient dogs exhibit depigmentation of hair.[47] Affected puppies, are frequently smaller than normal because of decreased food intake, which commonly occurs with zinc deficiency. Zinc deficiency induced testicular degeneration, and as a result impaired reproductive ability, has been

shown to occur at zinc levels that are adequate for normal growth.[37] Other effects of zinc deficiency include delayed healing, poor protein utilization, nervous system dysfunctions, impaired immunity, and skeletal abnormalities (Table 11, page 1-20).

Excessive dietary calcium may slow or prevent growth, even at levels that do not cause other signs. During one study, puppies gained 4.9 lb and their body length increased by 4.8 inches when the calcium content of the diet was 2.3%.[48] In contrast, littermates fed the same diet with the calcium content increased to 4.3% (which would only be 1.5 teaspoonfuls of calcium carbonate per puppy daily) lost 0.3 lb, and their body length increased only 1.2 inches. These marked differences occurred even though the calcium/phosphorus ratio of both diets was 1.1:1.

The prolonged ingestion of excess calcium, as well as excess food intake, may predispose to acute gastric dilatation and volvulus (bloat). This disease is of major concern to owners of large, deep-chested breeds of dogs in which the condition most often occurs. A dog may be predisposed to bloat not only because of the deep-chest conformation, but also because these dogs are often free-choice fed diets that are low in energy content (see page 3-14) and are commonly supplemented with calcium, particularly during growth, pregnancy, and lactation. Although prolonged excessive dietary calcium intake has not been proven to predispose to bloat, the physiologic effects of calcium suggest it is a likely factor.

Calcium ingestion stimulates gastrin secretion, and excessive calcium intake over a prolonged period results in chronically increased gastrin secretion.[74] Gastrin increases the tone of the gastroespohageal and pyloric sphincters while simultaneously decreasing contractions of most of the rest of the stomach. Continued gastrin stimulation also causes hyperplasia of the gastric mucosa at the pylorus.[74] Hyperplasia and hypertrophy of the gastric mucosa are routinely present in dogs with bloat. Gastric mucosal hyperplasia and increased sphincter tone may interfere with gastric emptying and gas eructation and, in conjunction with a gastrin-induced decrease in gastric contractions, may lead to a pendulous atonic stomach which is susceptible to bloat. Pentagastrin administration during pregnancy caused hypertrophy of the muscular layers of the stomach and fibrosis of the submucosa in the bitch and puppies.[12] Thus, excessive calcium intake during pregnancy may predispose the puppies to bloat later in life. This predisposition would be greater if the puppies also ingest excessive calcium during growth and

continue to do so as adults (see page 7-23 for a complete discussion of bloat).

In summary, **ideally puppies should be meal-fed the proper amount** (see page 3-15) **of a good-quality dog food designed for growth** (see Table 2, page 3-5) **and should not be supplemented with anything.**

CARE FOLLOWING WEANING

Besides nutrition, other factors that are important for optimal health and physical development of the puppy include adequate exercise and proper vaccination and parasite control. The psychologic development and training of the puppy are also quite important. When the newly weaned pup is first taken from its mother and littermates and exposed to a new home, it should be a quiet get-acquainted time. The pup should not be handled excessively. If there are other dogs in the household, it is better if they are not present for the first 4-8 hours after the puppy is brought into the home. This gives the puppy an opportunity to begin acclimating to the environment without social pressure from another dog. Also, the resident dogs are less likely to exhibit territorial defense reactions after an absence from the premises.

Animal behaviorists recommend that when dogs are introduced to each other, they should be supervised with minimal intervention. If the dogs are to live peacefully in close proximity, a dominant-subordinate relationship must be established. This relationship evolves through their interaction, which may appear harsh or excessive. However, human intervention could reduce the chances that the order of dominance, and therefore social stability, will be achieved.

Usually the resident dog begins asserting itself by aggressively dominating the puppy. The resident dog usually does this by grabbing the pup by the muzzle, or scruf of the neck, and pushing the pup to the floor. Growling, piloerection, and lip curling may precede this activity. The resident dog may then briefly stand over the pup while signaling with direct eye contact. This is normal secondary socialization behavior and should be allowed to proceed without interference.

All dogs should be fed at the same time, but in separate locations. Neither dog should be allowed access to the other's food bowl until the bowl is empty. Social tension may arise over such objects as toys or bones. As during introduction, intervention by the owner in these instances should be kept to a minimum. During these encounters, the resident dog may inflict pain. Although the pup may howl and whine when challenged, it must learn just how far it can go. If the owner overreacts to the pup's vocalization by disciplining the resident dog, comforting the puppy, or both, establishment of a stable social order may be impaired.

Once the social order stabilizes, the dominant animal's status should be reinforced by greeting it first, putting its feeding bowl down first, putting its leash on before the other dog's, allowing it into the car, house, or any other location before the other, petting it first, and playing with it first, and as often as the other dog(s).

When the pup is first brought home, put a box lined with newspapers and padded with some soft material (rags, etc.) in a warm quiet spot. For the first night or two, a warm water bottle and a ticking clock placed with the puppy may allow other inhabitants of the household to get more sleep.

The most important principles to consider when house-training a puppy are: 1) confinement, 2) a regular schedule, 3) simple but not lavish praise, and 4) no punishment. One method that works well for a dog that is 6-8 weeks of age, and often even for a mature dog, is when the dog cannot be watched, place it in a box, cage, or crate from which it cannot escape. The crate should only be large enough to allow the dog to lie down with legs extended. Dogs will not urinate or defecate in their sleeping area. Therefore, the puppy (or dog) will whine or bark to be let out when it needs to relieve itself. The animal should then be carried to the desired area and praised for eliminating. The puppy should be watched at all times when not in the crate and should be taken to the area for elimination when showing any suspicious activity such as circling, sniffing, or squatting.

Always use the same area (inside or outside) for elimination so that the dog will learn that this is the proper place to relieve itself. Dogs develop a preference for a surface of one type or texture for elimination, to the exclusion of all others. Thus, the surface of the preferred elimination area should always be the same and ideally would differ from the surface texture of other areas. Newspapers are good indoors, and grass, asphalt or concrete are good outdoors. Any time the puppy lies down to sleep, it should be put in the crate. Thus, it need not be watched until it awakens and whines. Puppies typically eliminate within 15-30 minutes after awakening, after eating, and before bedding down at night. The puppy should be taken to the elimination area at these times, and as close as possible to the same time each day. Improvement is usually seen within 1 week, and complete housetraining attained within 2-4 weeks.

Additional benefits of this method of house-training are that if the dog needs to be hospitalized or shipped, it will feel more comfortable in a cage or crate than a dog that has not been confined. Also, the puppy cannot be destructive at times when the family is sleeping or away from the house. The disadvantage of this method is that if the dog is not removed from the crate when it needs to eliminate, accidents will occur and, as a result, the dog learns to disregard its natural tendency not to soil its bedding area. Because of this problem, some pet owners, rather than using a crate, prefer to confine the puppy to a small room with a clearly defined bedding area, but a limited amount of space in which accidents can occur.

ORPHAN FEEDING AND CARE

FEEDING

Commercially prepared formulas (Table 3) are preferred for feeding orphaned puppies or kittens, although the homemade formulas given in Table 3 may be used. As shown in Table 4, on a caloric basis, the lactose content of cow's milk is nearly 3 times that of bitch's milk and is about the same as in queen's milk. Puppies or kittens that are overfed milk can develop diarrhea due to lactose intolerance (see page 7-42). This is more likely to occur in puppies than kittens when they are fed cow's milk, due to its higher lactose content.

TABLE 3

FORMULAS* FOR FEEDING ORPHANED PUPPIES AND KITTENS

For Puppies:

1. Esbilac (Borden) and Unilac (Upjohn).
2. Evaporated milk (not skimmed) diluted to contain 20% total solids (3 parts milk to 1 part water). If diarrhea develops, use one of the other formulas given.
3. 2 parts canned puppy food blended with 1 part water.**
4. Blend 1 cup whole milk, 1 tsp. salad oil, 1 drop multiple infant vitamins.

For Kittens:

1. KMR (Borden).
2. Blend 0.5 cup whole milk, 1 egg yolk, 1 drop multiple infant vitamins.

---

*All provide 1 kcal of metabolizable energy per ml. For amount to feed, use Table 5, page 3-19. Wean to solid food as soon as possible, starting at 3 weeks of age.

**Blend 1 minute and strain through a kitchen strainer.

Also, on a calorie basis, cow's milk contains 15% less protein than bitch's milk (54 vs 64 mg/kcal), and one-third less protein than queen's milk (84 mg/kcal). As shown in Table 4, goat's milk offers no advantage over cow's milk for feeding kittens or puppies.

The recommended amounts to feed orphans are listed in Table 5. These amounts provide a food intake of about 10-15% of body weight/day

---

TABLE 4

NUTRIENT CONTENT OF MILK[3,20]

| Nutrient | % Nutrient as Fed (% Nutrient in Dry Matter)* | | | | |
	Bitch's Milk	Cow's Milk	Evaporated** Milk + Water	Queen's Milk	Goat's Milk
Moisture	77.2 (0)	87.6 (0)	80 (0)	81.5 (0)	87 (0)
Dry Matter	22.8 (100)	12.4 (100)	20 (100)	18.5 (100)	13 (100)
Protein	8.1 (35.5)	3.3 (26.6)	5.32 (26.6)	8.1 (43.8)	3.3 (25.4)
Fat	9.8 (43.0)	3.8 (30.6)	6.12 (30.6)	5.1 (27.6)	4.5 (34.6)
Lactose	3.5 (15.4)	4.7 (37.9)	7.58 (37.9)	6.9 (37.3)	4.0 (30.8)
Calcium	0.28 (1.23)	0.12 (0.97)	0.19 (0.97)	0.035 (0.19)	0.13 (1.0)
Phosphorus	0.22 (0.96)	0.10 (0.77)	0.15 (0.77)	0.07 (0.38)	0.11 (0.85)
Metabolizable Energy (ME), kcal/100g***	126	61	98	97	65
Lactose, mg/kcal ME***	28	77	77	71	62

*% nutrient in the dry matter = % nutrient in the diet (as fed) divided by the dry matter fraction of the diet.

**Evaporated milk (not skimmed) diluted to 20% solids by mixing 3 parts milk with 1 part water.

***Metabolizable energy (ME) content (as fed) was estimated using nutrient energy densities of 3.5 kcal/g for protein and lactose and 8.7 kcal/g for fat (see Table 3, page 1-8).

TABLE 5

ORPHAN-FORMULA DOSAGE FOR PUPPIES[55] AND KITTENS

Age (weeks)	Dosage* (ml/100g body weight/day)
1	13
2	17
3**	20
4	22

*Divide and feed four times daily.

**Make available and encourage the consumption of solid food (see page 3-12).

TABLE 6

BIRTH WEIGHTS AND GROWTH RATES FOR NORMAL PUPPIES AND KITTENS*

Puppies	Birth Weight (g)
Pomeranian	120
Miniature Schnauzer	180
Beagle	280
Cocker Spaniel	280
German Shepherd Dog	400
Great Dane	450–550
Kittens	90–110

*Puppies should gain 1–2 g/day/lb (2–4 g/day/kg) of anticipated adult weight for the first 5 months of life.

Kittens should gain 50–100 g/week.

at birth; this gradually increases to 20-25%. Orphans should be fed four times daily. After feeding, the abdomen should be enlarged but not over-distended. The degree of abdominal distention is sometimes used as a guide to the amount to feed. It is better to underfeed for the first several days, then gradually increase to the recommended amounts over the next few days. Enough food should be fed to satisfy the orphan's appetite. During the first several weeks of life, normal puppies and kittens do little other than eat and sleep. If they cry excessively, they may be hungry or cold, or both. The normal birth weights and growth rates for kittens and for several breeds of puppies are listed in Table 6.

When feeding orphans, always warm the formula, and keep all feeding equipment scrupulously clean. Spoon- and dropper-feedings are slow and tedious and are more likely to result in aspiration pneumonia and death. It is much better to use a nipple bottle or to tube-feed. If using nipple bottles, those made especially for feeding orphans (Borden's) are preferred, although toy baby bottles or premature infant bottles may be used. The hole in the nipple should be such that when the bottle is inverted, milk oozes out slowly. If necessary, it can be enlarged with a hot needle. When feeding, squeeze a drop of milk onto the tip of the nipple. Then, insert it into the pup's or kitten's mouth. Never squeeze milk out of the bottle while the nipple is in the mouth; doing so may result in aspiration pneumonia and death.

Most find tube-feeding is the easiest, cleanest, fastest, and safest way to feed orphans. A number 8-10 French infant feeding tube (available from many hospitals, pharmacies, or pediatricians), or a soft, male urethral catheter can be used. Once weekly, mark the tube at a point 75% of the distance from the orphan's nose to its last rib.

This is the length necessary to reach the caudal esophagus. If more is inserted, the tube may double over in the stomach and, when withdrawn, could damage the esophagus. Attach the tube to a syringe, aspirate the amount of formula needed, and expel any aspirated air. Moisten the tube lightly to lubricate it. Position the orphan horizontally, open its mouth slightly, and holding the head in a natural position (not over-extended), gently pass the tube to the mark. If resistance is felt before reaching the mark, the tube is probably in the trachea. Once the tube is positioned in the stomach, slowly administer the formula over a 2-minute period, to allow the stomach to dilate. If resistance is felt, stop injecting the formula; the stomach may be full. When these precautions are followed, regurgitation rarely occurs. If the orphan does regurgitate, withdraw the tube and feed no more formula until the next scheduled feeding. For the first few weeks of life, after each feeding, burp the animal (just like a human infant), and swab the genital area with warm, moistened cotton (to simulate licking by the mother) to stimulate defecation and urination.

HOUSING FOR ORPHANS

The newborn pup or kitten is poikilothermic for the first week of life, and does not gain full control over body temperature regulation until nearly 1 month of age. From birth to 4 weeks of age body temperature can vary 1-5°C below that of an adult, depending on the ambient temperature and the degree of association with the mother and littermates. If young are separated from the mother and littermates, the ambient temperature should be kept near 30°C (86°F) for the first week

of life, 27°C (80°F) for the second and third weeks, and 24°C (75°F) for the fourth and fifth weeks. The immune response of 3-10 day old puppies separated from the body warmth of other animals is greatly depressed at ambient temperatures below 30°C.[64] However, ambient temperatures of 37-39°C, and above, cause dry mucous membranes and increase heart and respiratory rates.

Adequate housing for orphans can be made from readily available household items. A cardboard box containing a thermostatically-controlled electric heating pad covered with a waterproof material, and then covered with old towels or a blanket, works nicely. One-half of the heating pad should be placed against one side of the box and the rest on the bottom, leaving part of the bottom of the box uncovered. This allows the animal to get close to the heat if it is cold, and to get away if it is too warm. Heating lamps and heating pads that the animal cannot avoid can be harmful and are not recommended. Additional bedding such as old blankets or rags (not newspapers), should be provided.

BEHAVIORAL ASPECTS OF ORPHANS

Some puppies and kittens, raised as orphans, do not make good pets. The artificial upbringing and lack of contact with their mother and littermates may result in significant psychologic problems. These animals are often afraid of others of their species or, less frequently, are aggressive toward them. They may be physically defective, less than robust, and refuse to mate. Dogs raised as orphans often become excessively human-oriented and the males may direct their sexual attention toward people. Overdependence on people can lead to separation anxiety when the dog is left alone. This sometimes results in destructive behavior or other undesirable habits such as incessant barking, whining, and even self-mutilation. These problems not only occur in orphans, but in any dog or cat separated from its mother and littermates at too young an age (before 4-6 weeks).[31] However, not all orphans or dogs or cats weaned early develop these problems. The degree to which problems occur appears to be related to the age at which the animals were orphaned or isolated from their own species. The orphaned puppy or kitten has less chance of becoming a satisfactory pet as the age at which it is isolated decreases.

Kittens raised without contact with a queen or other kittens may develop behavioral abnormalities.[41] Normal exploratory behavior is inhibited. These kittens may be markedly passive to physi-

cal restraint, have magnified responses to auditory stimuli, show self-aggression, and lack appropriate social responses to other animals. The development of abnormal behavior patterns can be reduced to a considerable extent by allowing contact with littermates and/or a foster mother.[41] Peer contact greatly compensates for maternal deprivation. Therefore, allowing an orphaned kitten to associate with its littermates is more important than finding a foster mother.

The first choice in raising orphaned pups or kittens is to transfer them to another mother who has young of a similar age. If this is not possible, the second choice is to hand-raise the orphans, leaving the litter as intact as possible. Every attempt should be made to allow maximum interaction with littermates, or other young, for at least the first 4-6 weeks of life. If another animal, even of a different species, will act as a foster mother, encourage it. Even though she cannot feed the orphans, her warmth and mothering are helpful. The most undesirable arrangement is to raise the orphans alone without contact with other animals or people.

SICK PUPPY OR KITTEN FEEDING AND CARE

Of all puppies whelped alive, 28% die within the first week of life, and another 10% die during the second week.[33] Mortality in neonatal kittens is similar to that in dogs, ranging from approximately 10%-40%.[32] Crushing by the mother, exposure, and starvation are major causes of neonatal deaths. Crushing most often results from confined, crowded housing or an inexperienced, temperamental, or obese bitch. Another common cause of neonatal death is the "fading-puppy" or "fading-kitty" syndrome, which is characterized by neonates that are apparently normal at birth, and that may even go through motions of suckling, but die within a few days. The syndrome has an infectious and a cardiopulmonary component (non-infectious). These components probably interact with each other, and with hypothermia, to induce the fading-puppy/kitten syndrome, as shown in Figure 3. Hypothermic neonates are more susceptible than other neonates to invasion by pathogens.[20] Effects of hypothermia and its management are described on page 3-10.

The neonate receives about 90% of its transferred immunity from colostrum.[20] Therefore, with hypothermia and/or insufficient ingestion of colostrum, infection is more likely. Early ingestion of a sufficient volume of colostrum is also important because initial fluid intake contributes

significantly to the neonate's immediate postnatal circulatory volume. Inadequate intake could result in circulatory insufficiency and cardiopulmonary failure. Concurrent infection could also depress cardiopulmonary response. Every effort should be made to see that neonates nurse from the mother as soon after birth as possible to assure that adequate immunity and circulatory volume are established. Frequently, neonates are denied access to adequate colostrum or milk because of an inability to suckle, especially if they are premature, weak, or hypothermic. Also, agalactia may be present as a result of underdeveloped mammary glands, mammary gland edema, mastitis, metritis, or septicemia. There may simply be too many in the litter or a bitch or queen might die. In cases where the neonates are normal but undernourished, additional food should be given as described for orphans (page 3-18).

During the neonatal period, most illnesses, including the fading-puppy/kitten syndrome, are characterized by dehydration, hypoglycemia, and hypothermia. Regardless of the cause of illness, the management of sick neonatal puppies or kittens should include the correction of these 3 factors.

Keep the neonates warm (as described for raising orphans, page 3-19) to avoid the consequences of hypothermia (page 3-10) Usually, at rectal temperatures below 34.5°C (94°F), neonates will not nurse, and if they do, it is ineffective. Affected neonates cry and may die in a few hours if untreated. Care should be taken to warm them slowly (at 30°C or 85°F). Rapid warming increases oxygen requirements for peripheral tissues while the slow respiratory and cardiac rates preclude adequate tissue oxygenation. If heart rate or respiratory rate are decreased (see page 3-10 for normal rates), give oxygen. If possible, maintain the sick neonate in an environment of 40% oxygen. Warming should be done over 1-3 hours depending on the degree of chilling. Mothers will often reject hypothermic neonates but readily take them back once they are warmed.

Hypoglycemia and dehydration occur quickly when the neonate is not eating. These conditions can be treated, or prevented, by administering subcutaneously 1 ml/30 g body weight of a mixture of equal parts of 5% glucose and Ringer's lactate solutions. Administer orally 1 ml/30 g body weight of a nutrient-electrolyte solution (e.g. Life-Guard, Norden's) every 15-30 minutes until the animal responds. Do not feed a milk formula if their body temperature is below 35°C (95°F).

Neonates are frequently hypoprothrombinemic. This condition should be corrected in the sick neonate by administering 0.01-0.1 mg of vitamin K_1 (Synkavet, Hoffman LaRoche). Specific diseases commonly affecting the neonate and their treatment are described in detail elsewhere.[49,50]

FIGURE 3

CAUSES OF THE FADING PUPPY/KITTEN SYNDROME[20]

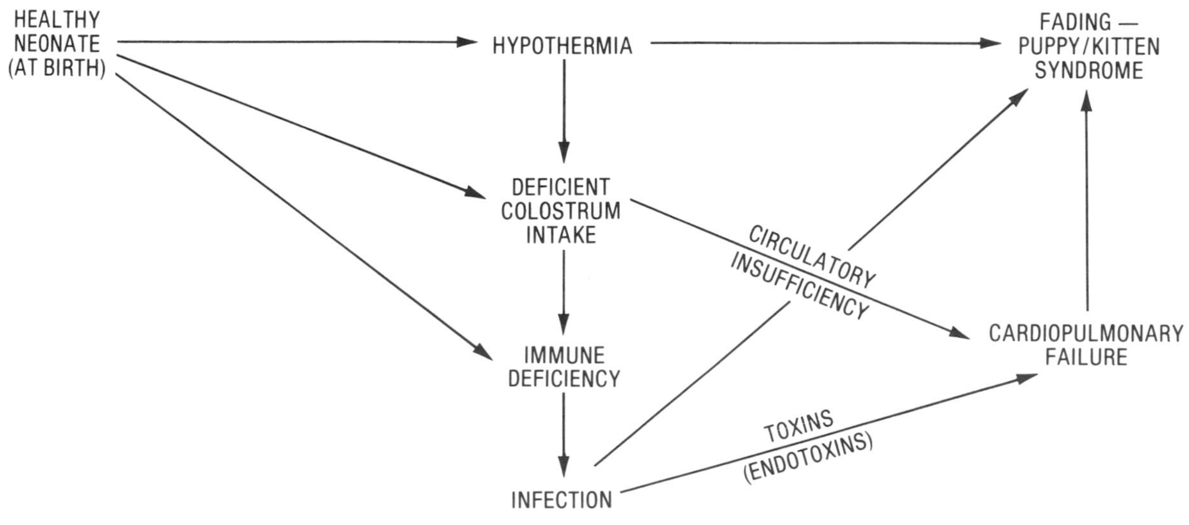

FEEDING
THE AGED DOG OR CAT

The objective in the feeding and care of the older dog or cat is to extend and improve the quality of life. To accomplish this objective:

1. Ameliorate existing problems
2. Eliminate or decrease clinical signs of disease
3. Slow or prevent the development and the progression of disease
4. Maintain optimal body weight

Proper feeding and exercise are important in accomplishing these objectives. Adequate physical activity is important for the older animal to maintain muscle tone and lean body mass, to enhance circulation, and to improve waste elimination.

The average life span is 12 years for dogs and 14 years for cats. Dogs have been reported to live as long as 29 years and cats as long as 36 years. Longevity can be increased with better care throughout life and, particularly, with proper nourishment in the latter years. For example, a properly fed, confined cat at 16 years of age is at the same stage of aging, physiologically, as an 8-year-old, intact, free-roaming cat.

The dog and cat at 1 year of age are at the same physiologic stage of life as a 15-year-old person, at 2 years of age the same as a 24-year-old person, and each successive year for the animal is equivalent to 4 years for people. For example, the dog or cat at 9 years of age is equivalent to a 52-year-old person; i.e. 24 for the first 2 years + [(9 years – 2) × 4] = 24 + 28 = 52. However, large breeds of dogs reach maturity more slowly and their life span is shorter. For giant dog breeds, a better estimate of their equivalent age to people is at 1 year of age they are equivalent to a 12-year-old person, and each successive year is equivalent to 7 years for people. For nutritional purposes most dogs and cats should be considered aged at 7 years, and giant breeds of dogs aged at 5 years.

As shown in Table 7, aged animals experience numerous body changes that result in altered utilization of certain nutrients, as well as decreased tolerance to nutrient excesses or deficiencies and abrupt dietary changes. Because they are less active, older animals require fewer calories. Because of changes in smell, taste, the oral cavity, and digestive system, the food should be highly palatable and digestible. Reduced protein, phosphorus, and sodium intakes are extremely important for older animals because of renal and cardiovascular changes (Table 7). Increased intake of vitamins A, B_1, B_6, B_{12}, and E are indicated because of changes in the digestive system and metabolism with aging, and to counteract some of the aging processes. An increased intake of unsaturated fatty acids and zinc helps to maintain skin and coat of aged dogs and cats. Increasing dietary lysine may help prevent a decrease in tissue lysine that decreases immunocompetence. Administration of vitamin C (50-100 mg/day/dog, orally) may be helpful in the old, arthritic dog.[52] In contrast to aging people, aged dogs have been shown to digest and retain calcium and phosphorus as well as, or better than, young dogs.[7]

Diets designed to meet these altered nutritional needs should be fed to the aged dog. Most commercial dog foods are formulated for the growing puppy and do not contain the nutritional alterations aged dogs need. Be sure that the dog or cat is maintained at its proper weight. Because of the decrease in energy needs that accompanies aging, obesity is often a problem in many older pets. Obesity should be corrected by feeding a high-fiber/low-calorie reducing diet as described in Chapter 6. Obesity should be prevented by feeding a diet moderately high in fiber and moderately restricted in protein, sodium, and phosphorus such as a maintenance diet for the inactive dog (Table 2, page 3-5). In contrast, some older dogs and cats have a decreased appetite and decreased digestive-absorptive ability, resulting in a loss of body weight. These animals should be fed at frequent intervals a palatable high-calorie diet intended for the older animal (Table 2, page 3-5). With aging, the senses of smell and taste are diminished.[63] These conditions reduce food intake so that it may be necessary to feed canned or moistened dry food, warmed, or a food with a strong odor.

Maintaining good oral hygiene is important in ensuring adequate food intake and utilization. Brushing the teeth with a toothbrush and sodium bicarbonate or even wiping the teeth daily with a rag is helpful. If the teeth contain a slimy tartar or extensive plaque, or if gingivitis is present, paint the teeth and gums with 2% tincture of iodine (dogs only—not cats).

Food intake may also be reduced because of decreased salivary secretion. If the older pet's mouth is dry, add 2 drops of ophthalmic 2% pilocarpine solution to the food. This helps prevent choking on the food. If food lodges in the animal's esophagus during eating, relieve the blockage by jerking the front legs up. Decrease the occurrence of esophageal choke by adding methiscol to the food.[52] If this fails to prevent this form of choke, add urecholine to the food.[52]

TABLE 7

CHANGES THAT OCCUR WITH AGING[52]

Metabolism

Decreased sensitivity to thirst————————————Dehydration
Decreased thermoregulation ——————————————Decreased tolerance to cold or heat
Immunologic competence decreased ———————————Increased susceptibility to infectious disease
Decreased rate of drug metabolism ——————————Decreased drug tolerance
Decreased amount or depth of sleep —————————Irritability
Decreased activity and metabolism (~ 20%) ——————Decreased energy need results in obesity

Special Senses

Olfaction decreased

Taste perception decreased

Hearing decreased

Visual acuity decreased

Decreased food intake which may
result in loss of weight and condition

Oral Cavity

Dental calculus, periodontal disease, periodontitis, and loss of teeth. Decreased salivary secretion. Gingival hyperplasia and hypersensitivity. Oral ulcers. These changes may result in inadequate food intake, constipation, vomiting, or decreased appetite.

Digestive

Decreased liver function, intestinal absorption, and colon motility, which may cause constipation. Achlorhydria. Flatulence.

Endocrine

Decreased thyroid function, which may decrease basal metabolic rate. Atrophy, cysts and fibrosis of pituitary gland. Adrenal gland fibrosis. Decreased pancreatic endocrine function, which may result in diabetes mellitus.

Integument

Loss of elasticity, thickened, dry, thin hair coat, hyperplasia of sebaceous glands causing decreased sebum and increased waxy secretions that do not cover the hair, graying of muzzle, brittle nails and hypersensitivity resulting in skin reddening.

Urinary

Decreased total renal function, blood flow and glomerular filtration rate, and number of functional nephrons, which results in an increase in all of these parameters in the remaining functional nephrons, leading to further nephron damage resulting in polyuria, polydypsia, incontinence, pollakiuria, nocturia. Prostatic hypertrophy.

Reproductive

Testicular tumors and atrophy. Mammary gland nodules and neoplasia. Lengthened estrous cycle, loss of libido, and decreased conception rates. Hyperplastic cystic endometritis.

Musculo-Skeletal

Loss of muscle mass and tone. Bone cortex becomes thinner, more dense and brittle, and more subject to fracture. Osteoarthritis. Signs of scurvy. Intervertebral disk lesions. Spondylosis. Posterior ataxia.

Cardio-Vascular

Decreased cardiac output, increased peripheral resistance and hypertension leads to congestive heart disease. Valvular thickening. Coronary arteriosclerosis and myocardial necrosis. Hyaline, calcium, and fibrin increase, and collagen decreases, in blood vessels. Decreased erythrocytes, hemoglobin, and plasma albumin, and increased globulin and fibrinogen, occur.

Respiratory

Obstructive lung disease and chronic bronchitis are common. Lung vital capacity and efficiency decreases, and lung weight, respiratory rate and residual air capacity increases. Fibrosis and emphysema may occur as elastic fibers are replaced by fibrous tissue.

Nervous

Neurotransmitter changes occur. The number of cells in the brain, nerves, plexuses, ganglia and spinal cord decrease. Decreased reactivity to stimuli and partial loss of memory and sensation (vision, hearing, taste and smell) may result. Thickened meninges and ossification of the dura result in irritability and disorientation.

*As in any biologic system there is much individual variation. Any individual animal with aging may show only a few of these changes, and the age at which they occur, and their severity, is quite variable. Some of the changes have opposite effects. For example, obesity as a result of decreased metabolic rate or decreased thyroid function may occur in one animal, whereas in another, loss of weight and condition due to decreased food intake may occur as a result of decresed sense of smell, taste or thirst, salivary secretion, digestive system function, and teeth and oral cavity changes.

If the animal is overly lethargic, a testosterone-estrogen combination has been reported to be helpful and more beneficial than anabolic steroids.[52] If the animal exhibits an increased sensitivity to cold, a thinning of the coat or other indications of reduced thyroid function, studies of thyroid function should be conducted (see page 6-4). If thyroid function is reduced, give thyroid hormone. Older dogs often need a dosage 2-4 times greater than do younger dogs.[52] If the older dog has urinary incontinence, but is not polyuric because of decreased renal function, administering 100 mg/dog 2-3 times daily of a metrazole-estrogen combination (Pentaline Titrozole, Summit Hill) may be helpful.[52]

The major non-accidental causes of death in dogs and cats are cancer, renal failure, and heart failure; therefore, all older animals should be carefully evaluated periodically for the presence of these diseases. Ideally, this should be done in conjunction with an annual physical examination.

Early detection and proper nutritional management will slow or prevent the progression of renal damage. A water-deprivaton test, which is one of the earliest practical tests in detecting decreased renal function, should be conducted in the older dog or cat (see page 8-22). If the test results are not normal, proper nutritional management for renal failure should be instituted. The aspects of nutritional management of renal failure is a diet low in protein, phosphorus, and sodium (see Chapter 8). However, in contrast to these recommendations, it has been suggested that older dogs should be fed a high-protein diet because: 1) a higher protein diet is needed by the older dog than the young mature dog to recover from a protein deficiency in the same amount of time, 2) protein requirements are increased in animals with renal failure, 3) increased protein intake increases renal blood flow and glomerular filtration rate, and these are decreased in the animal with reduced renal function, 4) the amino acid tryptophan is need for cerebral activity and function, and 5) the kidney's production of the amino acid arginine may be reduced in the older animal because of decreased renal function. All five of these statements have been well proved and would seem to provide support for recommending a high-protein diet for older dogs. However, **these statements are taken out of context.** When they are viewed in conjunction with the total body of research evidence on dietary protein and the progression of renal failure, the teliologic conclusion is that a diet that contains restricted, but adequate, amounts of a high biologic-value protein, is indicated for the older dog (and cat) (see Chapter 8).

The fact that the older dog needs a higher protein intake to replace body protein stores in the same amount of time as the younger dog has no relationship to protein needs of the older animal. Instead it demonstrates that the older animal has a decreased ability to tolerate dietary deficiencies or excesses. The dog (and quite likely the cat) with renal failure requires more protein but has less tolerance to protein in excess of the requirement. Feeding diets containing reduced amounts (10-16% in diet dry matter for the dog and 26-28% for the cat) of high-quality, high-digestible protein has been demonstrated in several species, including geriatric dogs, to slow a progressive decrease in renal function.[10,16] Studies have also demonstrated that restricting protein intake increases longevity and the onset of age-associated renal lesions.[34] In addition, increased renal perfusion, known for some time to occur in dogs as a result of increased protein intake,[65] has recently been shown to cause renal damage and the progression of renal failure.[6,30] For a thorough discussion of these topics, see Chapter 8.

The amino acid tryptophan is the precursor for serotonin. Serotonin synthesis depends on the amount of available tryptophan. Serotonin is a neurotransmitter which, if deficient, would be expected to adversely affect cerebral activity and function. This is the basis for speculation that feeding a higher protein, and therefore, a higher tryptophan diet, may improve spontaneous physical activity, alertness, and responsiveness of the older dog or cat. However, in rats with renal disease the plasma tryptophan concentration was 26 μM/L when a 24% protein diet was fed, but was 55 μM/L on a 6% protein diet.[40] In this study, feeding a lower protein diet increased plasma tryptophan concentration. As suggested, an increase in plasma tryptophan may be beneficial; however, this occurred as a result of feeding a low (not a high) protein diet. Increasing protein intake had the opposite effect.

Much of the amino acid arginine needed by the animal is synthesized in the kidney. Thus, it has been speculated that with reduced renal function, as is commonly present in older animals, renal arginine production may be decreased and, therefore, dietary needs increased. However, in immature uremic rats with a 90% decrease in renal function, there was no difference in growth rate, food intake, brain or muscle arginine concentration; in brain, muscle, kidney or liver protein content; or in health when an 18% protein diet with and without arginine was fed.[75] In addition, plasma arginine concentration did not differ between uremic and normal rats fed either the argi-

nine-supplemented or arginine-free diet. Renal arginine concentration was higher in uremic rats than normal rats with or without arginine in the diet. Thus the presence of renal failure does not appear to affect the arginine requirement.

The third most common non-accidental cause of death in dogs and cats is heart failure, which results in decreased exercise tolerance and pulmonary or peripheral edema, and ascites. If these, or any indication of decreased cardiac function are present, a diet restricted in sodium should be fed. As suggested in Chapter 11, initiate dietary sodium restriction with a diet moderately restricted in sodium (Prescription Diets Canine k/d or Feline k/d, Hill's). Prescription Diets Canine h/d or Feline h/d, (Hill's) should be used when severe sodium restriction is desired.

In **summary,** many studies support the concept that reducing the older animal's protein, phosphorus, and sodium intake is beneficial. Reducing the intake of these nutrients before clinical renal failure occurs helps prevent renal function from decreasing to the point that failure does occur. The recommendation to feed older animals diets reduced in these nutrients is a manifestation of the same philosophy that advocates using vaccines to prevent infectious diseases, rather than allowing them to occur and then treating with medications. Prevention is the best treatment. This is particularly true for diseases commonly seen in older animals, such as renal failure, where once the damage occurs it cannot be reversed.

FEEDING FOR PHYSICAL EXERTION, OR ENVIRONMENTAL OR PSYCHOLOGIC STRESS

Working dogs are exposed to a variety of stressful situations including:
1. Ambient temperature extremes
2. Racing
3. Hunting
4. Police and sentry duty
5. Guiding the blind
6. Touring the show circuit

These stresses increase a dog's requirement for energy as well as non-energy nutrients. These different situations result in variable combinations of physical and psychologic stress. However, ideal diets for these assorted forms of stress should have a similar nutrient profile. Psychologically stressed dogs usually require more nutrients. Often

they also have some degree of appetite suppression and, therefore, their food intake is limited. Physically stressed dogs have even greater increases in nutrient requirements, but usually have normal or enhanced appetites. However, the amount of dry matter that can be consumed is limited by gastrointestinal capacity, and the fact that excessive dry matter intake interferes with maximum physical performance.[14,43] Thus, palatable, nutritionally-dense, highly-digestible diets are desirable for both psychologic and physical stress.

STRESS/PERFORMANCE DIETS

Stress/performance diets should contain a minimum of 1900 kcal of metabolizable energy/lb of dry matter (4.2 kcal/g) and the digestibility and nutrient content shown in Table 2 (page 3-5). Some commercial stress/performance diets contain over 2300 kcal/lb of dry matter (5.1 kcal/g).[14] To attain a high energy density these diets are high in fat (over 23% on a dry matter basis) and their dry matter must be greater than 82% digestible. Fat is high in energy density and digestibility, providing about 2.5 times more available calories than any other nutrient. In addition, all of the non-energy nutrients should be balanced to the higher energy density of these diets. Diets which are high in calories result in less food being consumed to meet the animal's energy needs, relative to diets of lower energy density. Therefore, unless the non-energy nutrient content is increased accordingly (Table 2, page 3-5), fewer non-energy nutrients are ingested and a deficiency of one or more non-energy nutrients could occur. The higher the energy density of a diet the less of that diet needed to supply the animal's energy needs and, therefore, the higher the percentage of non-energy nutrients in the diet must be to meet the animal's needs for these nutrients.

An alternative to using a good-quality stress/performance-type diet is to supplement other diets with 1 tablespoonful (15ml) of fat or vegetable oil per cup of dry food. This will increase the caloric density of the diets by about 30%. There are disadvantages to this approach, including: 1) it is less convenient than feeding commercially prepared stress/performance diets, 2) it will decrease diet palatability for some dogs, and 3) the supplementation may be done improperly, including intermittent, insufficient, or excessive supplementation. Intermittent and/or insufficient addition of fat would result in a diet less beneficial for stress or performance. Excessive fat supplementation may result in inadequate intake of non-

energy nutrients, particularly with maintenance-type diets. This would also limit the desired diet response when feeding that diet and could be harmful if done for a prolonged period of time. Also, average-quality commercial maintenance- and growth/lactation-type diets are less digestible than properly formulated commercial stress/performance-type diets. A diet high in digestibility is very important for endurance-type physical performance.[14]

The importance of diet in one form of stress, i.e., exhaustive physical activity, is emphasized by a study in which four diets (three commercial and one experimental) were compared by the endurance performance of Beagle dogs on a treadmill (Table 8).[14] Exhaustion occurred at the equivalent of 15 miles when the dogs were fed a regular commercial dry diet (Purina), and at approximately 20 miles when they were fed highly-digestible/high-energy diets. Digestible fat intake was positively correlated with endurance performance. There was no significant association between digestible protein intake and performance. These results underscore the necessity of feeding an energy-dense (high fat), highly digestible diet for physical stress.

It has been contended that high-protein diets are beneficial for physical performance in the dog,[1,44] even though the results of studies such as those shown in Table 8 do not support this position.[14] The contention is based, in part, on another study that noted a difference in the hematocrit in severely stressed racing sled dogs fed a higher level of protein (Table 9).[1] Both diets fed were energy dense, high fat diets. This study

did not measure performance but monitored a variety of hematologic parameters. The study was hampered by an episode of parvovirus-induced diarrhea. The only variables which showed a difference between diets were erythrocyte indices. A higher hematocrit in the dogs fed the experimental diet may have been due to its higher fat and, therefore, energy density, its lower carbohydrate content, or its higher protein content. If it is due to higher protein, as these investigators contend, it may have been because of increased erythropoiesis, decreased erythrocyte destruction (or loss), or greater dehydration. Increased protein utilization for energy increases urinary and insensible water losses, because of increased urinary urea excretion and increased body heat production.[67] However, the difference in hematocrit between these two groups of dogs may not have been due to any of these differences in the diets. In addition, the higher hematocrit may be detrimental (because of increased blood viscosity) or have no effect on performance. The relationship between hematocrit, or what is referred to as "sports anemia," and performance is uncertain.

Sports anemia has been reported in human and animal athletes.[57,70] There is a question as to whether the anemia is relative or absolute. It is well documented that endurance athletes, both canine and human, manifest a larger total blood volume, and that endurance training is accompanied by an increase in plasma volume.[46,57] Thus, a decrease in hematocrit could result from an elevated plasma volume which is not matched by a proportional elevation of red cell mass. Thus, sports "anemia" could be present with

TABLE 8

DIETARY EFFECTS ON CANINE PERFORMANCE[14]

Diet Dry Matter* (%)	Diets**			
	Purina	Alpo	Science Diet	Exp.
Digestibility	78	85.6	81.5	86.7
Protein	22.9	48.7	30.5	45.4
Fat	12.8	28.3	33.1	41.9
Soluble Carbohydrate	52.7	11.1	26.4	4.4
Performance				
Average Exhaustion Time (minutes)	103.7	136.1	137.6	138.6
Average Exhaustion Distance (miles)	15.5	20.4	20.6	20.8

*Percent digestibility or nutrient in the diet as fed divided by the % dry matter of the diet.

**Diets: Purina Dog Chow (Ralston Purina), Alpo Beef Chunks Dinner (Allen Products), Science Diet Maximum Stress (Hill's), and Experimental Diet Ex-1 (Allen Products).

TABLE 9

HEMATOCRIT IN RACING SLED DOGS[1]

| Diet | % of Available Energy | | | | Hematocrit (%) |
	Protein	Fat	Carbohydrate	Total	
Commercial	23	57	20	100	35*
Experimental	28	69	3	100	40*

*Difference may or may not have been related to diet. If it is due to diet it may be due to a difference in any of these three nutrients or others. The higher hematocrit may have been because of increased erythropoesis, decreased erythrocyte destruction or loss, or greater dehydration. The higher hematocrit may be beneficial, detrimental or have no effect on physical performance.

total erythrocyte numbers being the same or even elevated. Indeed this has been reported to occur in human athletes.[57] As these studies demonstrate, more definitive work is needed before currently recommended dietary protein levels[53] are increased for exercise stress. Currently there are no data, nor logic, to support the use of extra-high protein diets for physical stress.

The study described in Table 8 indicated that carbohydrate intake was negatively correlated with endurance. This correlation depends somewhat on the fact that carbohydrate displaced fat from the poor performing diet, rather than a direct negative effect of dietary carbohydrate. The importance of carbohydrate in a stress-type diet is unclear. In one study, three different diets containing 0, 23 or 38% of energy from carbohydrate (39, 32 and 28% from protein, and 61, 45 and 34% from fat, respectively) were fed to racing sled dogs through a 28-week training period.[23] No difference in performance was noted between diets. However, the dogs fed the diet containing no carbohydrate were prone to diarrhea.[43] These workers have subsequently recommended that the "ideal" racing sled dog diet contain carbohydrate as 17% of the calories.[43] However, the three stress/performance type diets used in the study described in Table 8 provided from 3 to 20% of the energy as carbohydrate but performed identically.[14] A multitude of studies in man indicate that dietary carbohydrate is important for performance.[54,60] However, to be effective, the carbohydrate must be highly digestible and must not limit the energy density or protein content of the diet.

Vitamins are often considered by layman to be the magical dietary ingredient for performance. In fact, the advertising for countless multivitamin products touts their ability to increase resistance to disease, increase performance, promote "high energy-potency," and to treat alleged nutritional deficiencies associated with stress.[35] However, there is no objective scientific evidence to indicate that vitamin supplementation during stress improves performance, if good-quality, balanced diets are being ingested in adequate amounts.[77] For example, large doses of vitamin C have been advocated for relief of various stress conditions; but none of 10 well-designed studies demonstrated any beneficial effects of vitamin C supplementation on aerobic or anerobic capacity, endurance performance, strength, or mechanical efficiency.[77]

Many other studies using good methodology have examined the effects of dietary supplementation with vitamins A, D, E, B$_1$, B$_2$, B$_6$, or B$_{12}$, without finding any improvement in physical performance from their administration.[77] Although there is no known research that has investigated the effect of supplementation with biotin, folic acid, or pantothenic acid on physical stress, there is evidence that niacin supplementation may even be contraindicated for this purpose.[77] Certainly the excessive intake of vitamins A and D may contribute to the development of several health problems (see Table 13, page 1-23). It appears that **vitamin supplementation is unnecessary for a stressed dog consuming adequate amounts of a well-balanced diet.** The necessary vitamins are in the food.

Adequate water intake is the most important dietary consideration. This is particularly true for dogs working in conditions of high ambient temperatures. Loss of water as perspiration is minimal in dogs, even those that are thermoregulating in hot environments. However, significant water is lost by evaporation from the tongue and the upper and lower respiratory surfaces.[18] In addition, respiratory water losses can increase 10- to 20-times during exercise.[21] In compensating for heat, dogs primarily lose water. Even in species that sweat significantly, such as man and ruminants, the most important constituent lost is water, because their sweat is hypotonic to their plasma. In contrast, sweat from horses is hypertonic to plasma; there-

fore, electrolyte considerations are more important in this species.[18]

Even very mild dehydration (hypohydration) has been shown to induce several detrimental effects, including circulatory instability, reduced physical work capacity, decreased strength, possible renal ischemia, and hyperthermia.[21] With increased thermoregulatory strain, the duration over which maximum aerobic work can be maintained is reduced significantly.[21] The generation of excessive body temperature during exercise may even be a limitation to the performance of racing sled dogs in arctic environments.[43] Thermoregulation, as well as cardiovascular response during exercise, may be enhanced by the expansion of the plasma volume (sports anemia) that occurs during training.[21]

Besides obtaining exogenous water, the body has several mechanisms for compensating moderate water loss associated with exercise, thereby avoiding the potentially detrimental affects of hypohydration. Metabolic water is produced during the combustion of energy-providing nutrients, as discussed in Chapter 1 (page 1-2). The metabolism of 100 kcal of energy yields 10-16 ml of water, depending on the percentage utilization of protein, soluble carbohydrate, or fat. A considerable amount of water is also bound to glycogen (3-4 g water/g glycogen). As glycogen is used, this water is released. The total amount of water released can be considerable. The water and glucose obtained from glycogen use emphasizes the importance of assuring adequate glycogen stores prior to endurance exercise.[21]

Drinking water should be made available at frequent intervals, particularly for dogs working in high temperatures. Animals should be encouraged to drink early in the exercise period. If hypohydration is allowed to develop, the sensation of thirst may be reduced and the animal may be reluctant to drink, further aggravating the hypohydration and, as a result, performance.[19,32] Cold water (4-10°C, 40-50°F) is preferred. It is not only more palatable than warm water, it empties from the stomach more rapidly. Cold water helps cool the body.[19]

Diet dry-matter digestibility should be greater than 82%. Besides providing fewer usable nutrients, diets of low digestibility will result in expenditure of additional energy for physical activity because of increased gastrointestinal bulk. In the study described in Table 8 (page 3-26) the extra fecal bulk resulting from the diet with the lowest digestibility amounted to about 150 g/day.[14,43] This is equivalent to about a 7 kg handicap for a race horse.[43] Since the amount of energy needed for physical activity is dependent on the weight times the distance that weight is moved, the longer distance run by the sled dog than the race horse makes it an even greater handicap for the dog (150 g for 100 miles = 15 kg-miles for the dog versus 7 kg for 1 mile = 7 kg-miles for the horse). On a body-weight basis the difference would be magnified about 16 times.

FEEDING DURING WEATHER EXTREMES

Extreme weather conditions impose a number of nutritional considerations. Arctic temperatures may increase caloric requirements above the amount a dog can obtain from conventional foods. Despite rapid heat loss, dogs can maintain normal body temperatures by increasing their metabolic rate and hence their heat production (and energy utilization). In extremely cold environments (subfreezing wind-chill factor), increases of 70-80% in metabolizable energy intake for maintaining body weight are not uncommon.[15] However, subfreezing temperatures are uncommon in the conditions under which most dogs are kept. Even those housed outside usually have some sort of shelter which ensures that the temperature of the dog's immediate environment seldom falls below freezing. Under these circumstances, food intake should be increased approximately 25%. In one study, it was found that lowering ambient temperature from 15°C (59°F) to 8.5°C (47°F) resulted in a 25% (range 12-43% in 5 dogs) increase in metabolizable energy intake while body weight remained unchanged or dropped slightly (4%).[4]

Dietary energy needs also increase with high environmental temperature and humidity. Tropical climates increase the calories expended for cooling and reduce the dog's desire to eat. Thus, more calories are required in fewer grams of diet. In tropical climates, 60-80 lb guard dogs require as high as 140 kcal/kg body weight/day to maintain their body weight, as compared to the average requirement of 55-60 kcal/kg for similar-sized dogs in temperate climates. Glycogen stores have been shown to become depleted much more rapidly in individuals working in hot climates.[9] In order to supply an adequate energy intake for guard dogs in tropical climates, the caloric density of the food must approach 2000 metabolizable kcal/lb of food dry matter. High-fat diets generate less meal-induced heat, which would theoretically be better in tropical climates, particularly as compared to low-fat, high-protein diets.[67] In addition, water requirements must be met continuously, as discussed previously (page 3-27).

FEEDING RACING DOGS

Skeletal muscle fibers are divided into three main types on the basis of physiologic and biochemical characteristics. Physiologically there are fibers that contract relatively slowly (slow-twitch) and those that contract more quickly (fast-twitch). Biochemically, the slow-twitch fibers are oxidative, i.e. energy for contraction is generated by aerobic pathways. These fibers use fatty acids and/or glucose for fuel, and are somewhat diet responsive. Fast-twitch fibers can be subdivided into oxidative or glycolytic. Fast-twitch glycolytic fibers utilize anaerobic pathways to generate energy for contraction, using stored glucose and high-energy phosphate compounds (e.g. adenosine triphosphate [ATP]). The proportions of the various fiber types in any given muscle vary between individuals. There is a relationship between muscle fiber composition and the type of athletic performance for which an individual is best suited. Generally, slow-twitch fibers predominate in endurance athletes and fast-twitch fibers predominate in speed/strength athletes.[22] Awareness of the predominate fiber type present in an individual, and the type of work to be performed, allows for a more logical approach to optimal nutrition.

Racing dogs may be involved in sprinting (Greyhounds) or endurance events (sled dogs). Greyhounds have been genetically selected for sprint performance and, as a result, have a greater percentage of fast-twitch glycolytic muscle fibers than other breeds.[22] These animals engage in brief, intense, anaerobic type work, averaging velocities of 36-38 mph for 30-40 seconds. The sled dog performs at the opposite end of the spectrum and epitomizes endurance activity in the canine athlete. Racing sled dogs average approximately 20 mph for 25-30 **miles** and may repeat this feat on successive days.[43] Human sprinters and short-distance runners place considerably more emphasis on training, than diet. This same emphasis would appear to be appropriate for canine sprinters. However, sprinting dogs should be fed stress/performance-type diets (Table 2, page 3-5 that contain a reasonable amount of highly digestible carbohydrate (25-30% on a dry-matter basis). Diet selection and feeding management appears to be particularly important for endurance performance.[14] Endurance racers should also be fed stress/performance-type diets (Table 2, page 3-5).

Muscle and liver glycogen stores are important determinants of performance in sprinting athletes and of stamina in endurance athletes.[17,32] Because of this relationship, a technique known as glyco-gen loading (glycogen packing or supercompensation) has received much attention.[17] With this technique, glycogen stores are first depleted by exhaustive exercise and restricting dietary carbohydrate, then repleted by rest and high dietary carbohydrate intake. Like most physiologic processes, there is an overshoot so that following this regimen, muscle glycogen is increased above controls.[71,72] However, there is good evidence that the exercise component is the most important factor in inducing the glycogen-loading phenomenon, if the athlete is continuously ingesting adequate dietary carbohydrate.[17] Furthermore, it has been shown that endurance is improved by increasing the availability of free fatty acids and that this effect is mediated by a slowing of glycogen depletion.[17] Glycogen depletion is slowed by long-term adaptation to a low carbohydrate diet. This limits oxidation of glycogen with **no** adverse effect on performance.[17] In contrast, short-term (3-7 days) adaptation to a low-carbohydrate diet can result in reduced glycogen stores, and impaired performance. Thus it appears that avoiding glycogen depletion during physical exertion by slowing glycogen depletion is much more important than glycogen packing. Studies in the horse also support this concept.[71,72] Therefore, the continued use of a commercial stress/performance-type diet, low in carbohydrate and high in fat, energy density, and digestibility. (Table 2, page 3-5) in conjunction with an appropriate exercise schedule, is recommended to assure maintenance of adequate muscle and liver glycogen and, as a result, optimal performance.

Ingesting carbohydrates that elicit a sharp rise in plasma insulin should be avoided before (0.25-4 hours) exercise. Increased insulin levels, coupled with enhanced insulin sensitivity associated with exercise, may result in hypoglycemia. Insulin also interferes with the mobilization of free fatty acids and glycerol from adipose stores, depriving muscle of an important fuel. As a result, a greater reliance on muscle glycogen would occur that would more rapidly deplete glycogen stores and decrease performance. The ingestion of carbohydrates near the start of, and during, endurance exercise does not cause such an insulin response and may prolong endurance exercise.[17] Thus, do not feed from 0.25-4 hours before endurance activity, but (if practical) do feed small amounts just before and frequently during prolonged endurance activity.

Studies have also shown that muscles that were depleted of glycogen during treadmill running showed the greatest rates of glycogen resynthesis for up to the first 4 hours after exercise. The increased synthesis of glycogen coincided with

enhanced glucose transport and insulin sensitivity, which was back to pre-exercise levels, four hours after exercise.[17] The early post-exercise period is also important for protein metabolism. While protein requirements are not greatly altered with exercise, most protein metabolic activity as a result of exercise (increased catabolism and increased synthesis) occurs after, rather than during, exercise.[13] Thus, feeding during the early post-exercise period is beneficial in rapidly repleting diminished glycogen stores, and in replenishment and repair of body proteins.

Many of the aforementioned studies have been conducted in human subjects, some in dogs, and a few in horses. Until more definitive work is done in the dog, these data have to suffice and serve as the basis of recommendations for feeding dogs for physical exertion and stress.

In summary, racing dogs of all types should be fed a stress/performance-type diet (Table 2, page 3-5) continuously throughout the training and racing period. Racing sled dogs may consume 3-4 times maintenance amounts of food, whereas sprinters require considerably less (approximately 1-2 times maintenance).[43] Drastic dietary changes and supplementation should be avoided. To avoid inappropriate hyperinsulinemia, racing dogs should probably not be fed during the last 0.25 to 4 hours before racing and should ideally be re-fed within the first 4 hours after a race to assure glycogen and protein repletion. Frequent water consumption should be encouraged, particularly during hot weather (see page 3-27). Endurance racers could be fed small amounts (less than 10% of their daily requirement) and allowed to drink immediately prior (15 minutes or less) to a race and intermittently during a race, preferably using the same stress/performance diet to which they are accustomed. **However, food intake during exercise appears to be of little value to performance except in events lasting two hours or longer.**[8] Feeding during racing may not be practical in many situations. However, feeding within the first four hours after the race may assure glycogen replenishment and optimum protein response in endurance dogs, and is feasible. The dogs used in the first successful dogsled trip (without resupply) to the North Pole since Peary (1909)[68] were fed this way. They received approximately 2 lb of a mixture of 75% commercial stress/performance-type diet (Maximum Stress Diet, Hill's) and 25% pemmican (dried beef and lard), once daily every evening within 1 hour of cessation of physical activity.[69]

FEEDING HUNTING DOGS

The contemporary hunting dog is commonly asked to indulge in a very stressful form of endurance performance: i.e. a seasonal, intermittent endurance activity for which they are often underconditioned and improperly fed. Many of these animals are pets or are kept in a kennel and hunt only a few weekends each year. Therefore, most of the time they do not require a stress/performance-type diet. However, it is advisable to treat these animals more like the racing sled dog, during the hunting season, switching them from a maintenance diet to a stress/performance-type diet (Table 2, page 3-5), 1-3 weeks prior to hunting. The amount fed should be proportionate to the dog's workload (see Table 1, page 1-6).

The timing and frequency of feeding may be very important for hunting dogs, probably more so than for racing dogs. Hunting dog hypoglycemia (functional hypoglycemia) is seen most commonly in hyperactive dogs, 1-2 hours after beginning a hunt. This form of hypoglycemia has been thought to be a form of glycogen storage disease (Type III or Cori's Disease) due to a deficiency of the glycogen debranching enzyme, amylo-6-phosphatase[5] (see page 7-60 for a discussion of these diseases). While this etiology is possible, hunting dog hypoglycemia is more likely a feeding management problem exacerbated by underconditioning and a nervous temperament (physically and psychologically stressed). The dog may also have a metabolic predisposition to hypoglycemia. High ambient temperatures are probably also a risk factor. The hunting dog should be fed as advised for endurance activity. Feeding the total daily ration from 0.25 to 4 hours prior to hunting can result in increased plasma insulin levels at the time exercise begins. The elevated insulin, coupled with the exercise-induced enhanced insulin sensitivity, can cause a rapid fall in blood glucose. In human subjects, the hypoglycemia persists until the end of the exercise and causes significantly greater rates of glycogen utilization.[17] In addition, high insulin levels inhibit mobilization of free fatty acids and glycerol, which subsequently reduces fat oxidation by working muscles and lowers hepatic precursors available for glucose production. This puts an additional burden on glycogen stores.[28] In one study a subgroup of people was identified who had a tendency to develop hypoglycemia during endurance exercise.[11] Feeding **during** exercise improved their glycemic status and performance.

Training is an important factor in preventing

exercise-induced hypoglycemia. The proportion of fat and carbohydrate used differs markedly between trained and untrained individuals. In trained individuals, fat is the primary fuel, and muscle and hepatic glycogen depletion are slower than in untrained individuals.[28] Glycogen sparing has been reported to occur in all three muscle fiber types (slow-twitch, fast-twitch oxidative, and fast-twitch glycolytic) in trained animals exposed to graded exercise. In trained animals the slower rate of glycogen utilization in either slow-twitch and fast-twitch oxidative fibers is due primarily to an exercise-induced increased ability to oxidize fat. The slower rate of glycogen utilization by fast-twitch glycolytic fibers of trained animals suggests that there is greater recruitment of this fiber type in untrained individuals. Fast-twitch glycolytic fibers are recruited as oxidative fibers become fatigued, or during strenuous exercise when the excitatory input by motor neurons exceeds the capacity of oxidative fibers to respond.[28] As a result of these effects, untrained dogs are more likely, than physically conditioned dogs, to experience hypoglycemia during intense physical activity. Also, glycogen depletion occurs more rapidly in individuals exercising in hot environments.[9]

In summary hard-working hunting dogs should be fed a stress/performance-type diet (Table 2, page 3-5) beginning 1-3 weeks prior to conditioning and conditioned for at least 3 weeks prior to hunting. They should be fed their usual amount of this same diet at least four hours before entering the field. Immediately prior to the beginning of the hunt (within 15 minutes), and at each opportunity (approximately every 2 hours at rest stops, lunch etc.) encourage water consumption and feed small amounts (approximately 10% of the daily requirement) of the same stress/performance diet. Feeding larger amounts during exercise may predispose to bloat (see page 7-23). Feed the remainder of the daily requirement (see Table 1, page 1-6) within 1-4 hours after the hunt.

FEEDING OTHER WORKING DOGS

Police and sentry dogs, guide dogs, dogs for hearing-impaired people, and show dogs may experience prolonged psychologic stress coupled with variable ambient temperature and less exercise stress as compared to racing or hunting dogs. As a result, these dogs may have more appetite suppression than other working dogs. Therefore, they require a very palatable, highly digestible, nutrient-dense stress/performance-type diet (Table 2, page 3-5). These dogs will vary widely as to the amount needed to maintain body weight and should be fed to maintain optimal condition. They may require more than maintenance amounts even if they are not exercising heavily (Table 1, page 1-6). Depending on the situation, criteria discussed for temperature extremes, racing dogs, or hunting dogs, may be applicable. Again, adequate water intake is important because water deprivation negatively influences appetite. A review of the factors affecting palatability (see page 2-2) may be helpful in maintaining food intake in dogs that are psychologically stressed.

REFERENCES

1. Adkins TO, Kronfeld DS: Diet of racing sled dogs affects erythrocyte depression by stress. Can Vet J 23:260-263 (1982).

2. Alexander JW, Stinnett JD: Changes in immunologic function. In Surgical Nutrition Editor JE Fischer, Little, Brown and Co, Boston, Mass pp 535-549 (1983).

3. Baines FM: Milk substitutes and the hand rearing of orphaned puppies and kittens. J Small Anim Practice 22:555-578 (1981).

4. Blaza SE: Energy requirements of dogs in cool conditions. Canine Practice 9:10-15(1982).

5. Bordens JW: Glycogen storage disease in puppies. Vet Med/Small Anim Clin 61:1174-1176 (1976).

6. Brenner BM, Meyer TW, Hostetter TH: Dietary protein intake and the progressive nature of kidney disease: The role of hemodynamically mediated glomerular injury in the pathogenesis of progressive glomerular sclerosis in aging, renal ablation and intrinsic renal disease. New England J Med 307:652-659 (1982)

7. Cornell Daynemouth Lab for Canine Nutrition as reported in Cornell Univ College of Vet Med Annual Health Newsletter I(3):6 (1983)

8. Costill DL: Carbohydrate nutrition before, during, and after exercise. Fed Proc 44:364-368 (1985).

9. Costill DL: Fats and carbohydrates as determinants of athletic performance. In Nutrition and Athletic Performance. Editors W Haskell, T Scala, J Whittam, Proc Conf Nutr Determinants Athlet Perf pp 16-28 (1981).

10. Cowgill LD, Spangler WL: Renal insufficiency in geriatric dogs. Vet Clin of N Amer 11:727-747 (1981)

11. Coyle EF: Effects of glucose polymers feedings on fatigability and the metabolic response to prolonged strnuous exercise. In: Nutrient Utilization During Exercise. Editor EL Fox, Ross Laboratories, Columbus, OH pp 43-44 (1983).

12. Dodge JA: Production of duodenal ulcers and hypertrophic pyloric stenosis by administration of pentagastrin to pregnant and newborn mammals. Nature 255:285 (1970).

13. Dohm GL: Protein metabolism in exercise In: Nutrient Utilization During Exercise. Editor EL Fox, Ross Laboratories, Columbus, Ohio pp 8-13 (1983).

14. Downey RL, Kronfeld DS, Banta CA: Diet of Beagles affects Stamina J Amer Anim Hosp Assoc 16:273-277 (1980).

15. Durrer JL, Hannon JP: Seasonal variations of intake of dogs living in an arctic environment. Amer J Physiol 202:375-378 (1962)

16. Edney ATB: Observations on the effects of feeding a low protein diet to dogs with nephrites. J Small Anim Pract 11:281 (1970)

17. Evans WJ, Hughes VA: Dietary carbohydrates and endurance exercise. Amer J Clin Nutr 41:1146-1154 (1985).

18. Fettman MJ: Fluid and electrolyte Metabolism during heat stress. Comp Cont Ed 8:391-397 (1986).

19. Fink WJ, Greenleaf JE: Fluid intake and athletic performance. W Haskell, J Scala, J Whittam. In Nutrition and Athletic Performance. Proc Conf Nutr Determinants Athletic Perf pp 33-66 (1981).

20. Fisher EW: Neonatal diseases of dogs and cats. Brit Vet J 138:277-284 (1982).

21. Gosolfi CV: Water and electrolyte metabolism in exercise, In Ross Symposium on Nutrient Utilization During Exercise, Editor EL Fox, Ross Laboratories, Columbus, OH pp 21-25 (1983).

22. Guy PS, Snow DH: Skeletal muscle fibre composition in the dog and its relationship to athletic ability. Res Vet Sci 31:244-248 (1981).

23. Hammel EP, Kronfeld DS, Ganjam VK, Dunlap HL: Metabolic responses to exhaustive exercise in racing sled dogs fed diets containing medium, low and zero carbohydrate. Amer J Clin Nutr 30:408-418 (1977)

24. Hartly WJ, et al: Goitre and low copper status in a litter of meat fed pups. New Zealand Vet J 11:5 (1963).

25. Hazewinkel HAW, Goedegebuure SA, Poulos PW, Wolvekamp WthC: Influences of chronic calcium excess on the skeletal development of growing Great Danes. J Amer Anim Hosp Assoc 21:377-391 (1985).

26. Hedhammar A, Wu F, Krook L, et al: Overnutrition and skeletal disease. An experimental study in growing Great Dane dogs. Cornell Vet 64 (Supple 5):1-160 (1974)

27. Hedhammer A: Nutrition as it relates to skeletal disease. Proc 4th Kal Kan Symp pp 41-44 (1980).

28. Hickson RC: Carbohydrate metabolism in exercise, In: Nutrient Utilization During Exercise Editor EL Fox, Ross Laboratories, Columbus, OH pp 1-8 (1983).

29. Holme DW: Practical use of prepared foods for dogs and cats. In Dog & Cat Nutrition. Editor ATB Edney, Pergamon Press, New York, NY pp 47-59 (1982).

30. Hostetter TH, Helmut GR, Brenner BM: Compensatory renal hemodynamic injury: a final common pathway of residual nephron destruction. Amer J of Kidney Dis 1:310-314 (1982).

31. Houpt KA, Wolski TR: In Domestic Animal Behavior, publisher Iowa State Univ Press (1982)

32. Jezyk PF: Metabolic diseases-an emerging area of veterinary pediatrics. Comp Cont Ed 5:1026-1032 (1983).

33. Johnson EA: Pediatrics. Auburn Vet 31, No 3 (1975)

34. Johnson JE, Barrows CH: Effects of age and dietary restriction on the kidney glomeruli of mice: Observations by scanning electron microscopy. Anatomical Rec 196:145-151 (1980).

35. Jukes TH: In Nutrition, Metabolic and Clinical Applications. Editor RE Hodges, Plenum Press, New York, NY (1979).

36. Kallfelz FA: DVM pp 12-13 (May 1979).

37. Kane E, Morris JG, Rogers QR, et al: Zinc deficiency in the cat. J Nutr 111:488-495 (1981)

38. Kasstrom H: Nutrition, weight gain and development of hip dysplasia. An experimental investigation in growing dogs with special reference to effect of feeding intensity. Act Radiol (Suppl 334):135-179 (1975).

39. Kendall PT, Burger IH: The effect of controlled and appetite feeding on growth and development in dogs. Proc 3rd Kal Kan Symp pp 60-63 (1979).

40. Kihlberg R, Sterner G, Wennberg A, Denneberg T: Plasma free amino acid levels in uremic rats given high and low protein diets or intravenous infusion of amino acid solutions. J Nutr 112:2058-2070 (1982).

41. Konrad, Bagshaw: J Comp Physical Psychol 70:157-164 (1970) as reported by Hart BL: Feline behavior. Feline Pract 2(6):6-8 (1972)

42. Kronfeld DS: Nature and use of commercial dog foods. J Amer Vet Med Assoc 166:487-493 (1975).

43. Kronfeld DS: Feeding dogs for hard work and stress. In Dog and Cat Nutrition. Editor ATB Edney, Pergamon Press, New York, NY pp 61-73 (1982).

44. Kronfeld DS, Hammel EP, Ramberg CF, Dunlap HL: Hematological and metabolic response to training in racing sled dogs fed diets containing medium, low or zero carbohydrates. Amer J Clin Nutr 30:419-430 (1977).

45. Leare AA, et al: Proc Int Symp Nutrition of Dog and Cat. Hanover, Germnay (1978).

46. Mackintosh IC, Dormehl IC, van Gelder AL, du Plessis M: Blood volume, heart rate, and left ventricular ejection fraction changes in dogs before and after exercise during endurance training. Amer J Vet Res 44:1960-1962 (1983).

47. Meyer H, Hommerich G, Schoon M: Experimenteller zinkmangel bei ausgeevachsenen hunden. Kleintierpraxis 31:21-28, 1986.

48. Mohrman RK: Supplementation . . . why/why not. Chapt F-10, In Nutrition and Management of Dogs and Cats. Vet Services, Ralston Purina Co, St Louis MO (1979)

49. Mosier JE (Editor): Canine Pediatrics—Vet Clinics of N Amer WB Saunders Co, Philadelphia, PA Vol 8 no. 1 (1978).

50. Mosier JE: Causes and treatment of neonatal deaths. In Current Vet Therapy VI. Editor RW Kirk, WB Saunders Co, Philadelphia, PA pp 44-49 (1977).

51. Mosier JE: Nutritional recommendations for gestation and lactation in the dog. Vet Clinics of N Amer 7:683-692 (1977)

52. Mosier JE: Canine and feline geriatrics. Proc Amer Anim Hosp Assoc pp 153-160 (1978).

53. Nutrient Requirements of Dogs. National Research Council, National Academy of Sciences, Washington, DC (1974).

54. Nutrition and Athletic Performance. Editors W Haskell, J Scala, J Whittam, Proc Conf on Nutr Determinants in Athletic Perf, San Francisco, CA (1981).

55. Oftedal OT: Lactation in the Dog: Milk composition and intake by puppies. J Nutr 114:803-812 (1984).

56. Olsson SE: Osteochondrosis—A growing problem to dog breeders. Gaines Progress pp 1-11 (Summer 1976).

57. Pate RP: Sports anemia and its impact on athletic performance. In Nutrition and Athletic Performance. Editors W Haskell, J Scala, J Whittam, Proc Conf Nutr Determinants in Athletic Perf pp 202-216 (1981).

58. Resnick S: Effect of an all-meat diet on hip formation in dogs. Vet Med/Sm Anim Clin 69:739-743 (1974).

59. Romsos DR, Belo PS, Bennink MR, et al: Effects of dietary carbohydrate, fat and protein on growth, body composition and blood metabolite level in the dog. J Nutr 106:1452-1464 (1976).

60. Ross Laboratories: Nutrient Utilization During Exercise Editor FL Fox, Columbus, OH (1983).

61. Ross MH: Length of life and caloric intake. Amer J Clin Nutr 25:834-838 (1972).

62. Ross MH, Bras G: Food preference and length of life. Science 190:165-167 (1975).

63. Schiffman SS: Taste and smell in disease. New Engl J Med 308(21):1275-1279 (1983).

64. Schulta R: Ambient temperature affects canine immune response. Norden News p 36 (Spring 1984).

65. Shannon JA, Jollife N, Smith HW: The excretion of urine in the dog. IV. The effect of maintenance diet, feeding, etc., upon the quantity of glomerular filtrate. Amer J Physiol 101:625-628 (1932).

66. Sheffy BE: Nutrition and the immune response. J Amer Vet Assoc 180:1073-1076 (1982).

67. Smith RR, Rumsey GL, Scott ML: Heat increment associated with dietary protein, fat carbohydrate and complete diets in salmonids: comparative energetic efficiency. J Nutr 108:1025-1032 (1978).

68. Steger W: North to the Pole. Nat Geographic 170:288-317 (1986).

69. Steger W: Personal communication. Steger International Polar Expedition, 1708 Savoy Ave, Ely, MN 55731, August, 1986.

70. Tobin T, Kamerling SG: Iron: its functions and metabolism in the horse. Eq Sports Med 4(2):1-3 (1985).

71. Topliff DR, Potter GD, Dutson TR, et al: Diet manipulation and muscle glycogen in the equine. Proc Eighth Equine Nutr and Phys Symp pp 119-124 (1983).

72. Topliff DR, Potter GD, Kreider JL, et al: Diet manipulation, muscle glycogen metabolism and anaerobic work performance in the equine. Proc Ninth Equine Nutr and Phys Symp pp 224-229 (1985).

73. Tvedten HW, Carrig CB, Flo GL, Romsos DR: Incidence of hip dysplasia in Beagle dogs fed different amounts of protein and carbohydrate. J Amer Anim Hosp Assoc 13:595-598 (1977).

74. Walsh JH, Grossman MI: Gastrin, New Engl J Med 292:1324-1384 (1975).

75. Wang M, Kopple JD, Swendseid ME: Effects of arginine-devoid diets in chronically uremic rats. J Nutr 107:495-501 (1977).

76. Waterhouse HN, Fritsch CW: Dog food palatability tests and sources of potential bias. Lab Anim Care 17:93-102 (1967).

77. Williams MH: Vitamin supplementation and physical performance. In Nutrient Utilization During Exercise. Editor EL Fox, Ross Laboratories, Columbus, OH pp 26-30 (1983).

78. Wingfield WE: Proceedings Colorado State University Annual Conference for Veterinarians pp 85-88 (1978).

CHAPTER 4

Cats—Feeding and Care

CONTENTS

INTRODUCTION

For maximum health, longevity and quality of life, cats must be properly fed and cared for throughout life. To feed cats properly or to advise others on proper feeding requires: 1) a basic understanding of nutrients and the cat's nutritional needs as discussed in Chapter 1; 2) knowledge of the foods available to provide the nutrients needed, including the advantages, disadvantages, quality, and nutrient content of various foods (both commercial and homemade) as discussed in Chapter 2; and 3) knowledge of how to feed and care for cats during each stage of the life cycle as well as common

errors made in feeding cats, which are described in this chapter.

DIET RELATED ANOMALIES OF CATS

A review of the behavioral, anatomic, physiologic, and metabolic "peculiarities" of cats provides a basis for understanding their special nutritional requirements as compared to dogs.

Cats are not small dogs. Even though both cats and dogs are taxonomically classed as belonging to the order Carnivora, cats naturally exhibit carnivorous feeding behavior whereas dogs are naturally omnivorous (some members of the order Carnivora

are even herbivorous, e.g. Pandas).[11] The omnivorous nature of the canine is further supported by the fact that coyotes in Wyoming prey on sheep flocks; whereas in southern California coyotes are responsible for depredation of melons, peaches, apricots, grapes, plums, and cherries.[21]

The fact that cats are carnivorous in their natural feeding behavior, relative to dogs, is not readily apparent. Cats are primarily solitary hunters (except the African lion) whereas wild dogs hunt in groups. An individual large cat does not have to consume an entire carcass, including entrails, to be satiated. This is in contrast to packs of wild dogs or wolves eating similar game. In fact, the viscera of prey are often one of the first parts consumed by wolves.[10] Since herbivores are common prey, gastrointestinal contents of prey are generally of plant origin. Hence, a certain amount of plant material is included in the diet of animals ingesting entrails. Also, coyotes have been reported to comsume droppings of herbivorous prey[13] and domestic dogs will readily consume herbivore feces. In contrast, lions do not generally eat entrails. However, when forced to do so, lions have been seen to first empty the ingesta from the entrails by expressing the contents with their tongue.[8] Both wild and domestic cats usually consume the head of their prey first and leave the entrails. There may be more than wry humor in Kliban's "Momcat" poem:

> "Love to eat them mousies,
> mousies what I love to eat.
> Bite they little heads off . . .
> nibble on they tiny feet."[7]

The fact that the cat is indeed a strict carnivore is supported by several unique anatomic features including:

1. **Teeth and jaws**—Cats have fewer premolars and molars than dogs and their carnassial teeth are more specialized for cutting. The jaw of the cat is restricted in latero-medial and craniocaudal mobility. Thus, cats have little provision for grinding food, only cutting and shearing. They are designed to eat animal tissue. The dentition and greater jaw mobility of dogs indicates use of a more varied diet, including plant tissue.[16]

2. **Facial structures**—Cat's eyes are particularly adapted for hunting. They are positioned in the front of the face and are very sensitive to movement. Their ears are upright and face forward as well.[16] Cats have prominent specialized facial tactile hair. These adaptations evidently aid in nocturnal pursuit of prey and function to protect the eyes.[17]

3. **Limbs**—Cats (excluding cheetahs) have retractable claws designed to secure animal prey.[16] The claws of dogs play only a secondary role in capturing prey.

Cats also have several physiologic and metabolic characteristics that are common to true carnivores and are distinct from dogs:

1. **Energy metabolism**—Interestingly, the energy metabolism of cats is somewhat comparable to that of ruminants. For instance:

   a. The livers of most animals have two active enzyme systems, hexokinase and glucokinase, for converting glucose to glucose-6-phosphate (this conversion is necessary before glucose can be used by the liver). The glucokinase system operates only when the liver receives a large load of glucose from the protal vein. The **natural** diets of both cats and ruminants contain only small amounts of soluble carbohydrate. Therefore, when consuming their natural diets, the portal system of cats or ruminants delivers very little absorbed glucose to the liver. Both felines and ruminants have very low activity of liver glucokinase. Omnivores such as people, dogs, and rats have high hepatic glucokinase activity.[9,11]

   b. Both cats and ruminants naturally ingest soluble carbohydrates (lactose or milk sugar) prior to weaning but as adults are designed to rely primarily on gluconeogenesis from glucogenic amino acids, propionic acid (a volatile fatty acid), lactic acid, and glycerol for maintenance of blood glucose. In omnivorous animals, maximal gluconeogenesis occurs in the post-absorptive state. In cats and ruminants, gluconeogenesis occurs in the absorptive phase immediately following a meal. In ruminants gluconeogenesis is primarily from propionic acid, whereas in cats glucose is produced from glucogenic amino acids.[9]

2. **Protein metabolism** is unique in the cat and is manifested by the unusually high maintenance requirement for protein as compared to the dog (see Table 9, page 1-16). The cat's protein requirement for growth is only 50% higher than the dog's, whereas it is twice that of the dog's for adult maintenance. The higher protein requirement of cats is not due to an exceptionally high requirement for any specific amino acid (see Table 6, page 1-13); instead it is caused by a high activity of enzymes in the liver (transaminases and deaminases) that remove the amino groups from the amino acids so the resulting keto acids

can be used for energy or glucose production. Unlike omnivores (e.g. dogs) and herbivores, the cat cannot decrease the activity of these enzymes when it is fed a low-protein diet. It seems that the cat's strict adherence to a diet of animal tissue resulted in a lack of evolutionary pressure to accommodate lower protein diets. As a result, these enzyme systems are constantly active so that a fixed amount of dietary protein is always catabolized for energy.[9,11] The gluconeogenic enzymes in the liver of the cat appear to be permanently turned on as well, unlike most other species, including the dog.[11] In addition, an alternative gluconeogenic pathway common in the liver of flesh-eating animals is active in the cat. This pathway uses **serine** as a glucose precursor. Serine is a non-essential amino acid found in large amounts in muscle, milk, and egg.[5] Cats also have a special need for two amino acids:

a. **Arginine**—As discussed on page 1-13, arginine deficiency in the cat causes one of the most dramatic responses of any nutrient deficiency. Feeding a diet devoid of arginine may result in hyperammonemia in less than one hour. Within 2-5 hours affected cats exhibit severe signs of ammonia toxicity and may die.[9] The reason for the cat's high sensitivity to arginine deficiency is that the cat cannot synthesize sufficient ornithine or citrulline for conversion to arginine, which is needed for the urea cycle. Thus, after the cat eats an arginine deficient diet, the highly active protein catabolic enzymes in its liver produce ammonia, but without arginine the urea cycle cannot convert the ammonia to urea and ammonia toxicity occurs.[9] Because the cat's natural diet consists of animal tissue high in protein (including arginine), the flexibility required in the protein metabolism of species (e.g. dog) eating diets more variable in protein content has not evolved. However, an arginine deficiency will not occur unless the cat is fed an experimental diet specially formulated to be deficient in arginine.

b. **Taurine**—Taurine is a β-amino sulfonic acid (see page 1-13) required dietarily by cats because they cannot synthesize sufficient amounts from cystine as can other animals (including dogs). A chronic taurine deficiency can cause central retinal degeneration and blindness in cats. Plant products are poor sources of taurine (see soybean meal, Table 7, page 1-13).

3. **Fat metabolism**—Cats have the ability to digest and utilize high levels of dietary fat (as is present in animal tissue). They have a special need for **arachidonic acid** since they cannot make it from linoleic acid as can the dog.[9] Animal source fats are high in arachidonic acid (see Table 10, page 1-18). The domestic cat is not the only carnivore that lacks the ability to convert linoleic to arachidonic acid. The lion, the turbot (a carnivorous fish), and even the mosquito have similar inabilities to synthesize arachidonic acid. This metabolic peculiarity appears to be correlated with species that are strict carnivores, regardless of their position on the phylogenetic tree.[9]

4. **Vitamin metabolism** in cats differs from that of dogs in the following ways:

a. Cats do not convert **tryptophan** to **niacin**.[9] As a result, the niacin requirement of cats is four times higher than that of dogs.[14,15] Animal tissue is high in niacin.

b. The prosthetic group of all transaminases is **pyridoxine** (vitamin B_6).[19] As has been discussed, flesh-eaters, such as cats, derive considerable energy from dietary protein. Because these animals have high transaminase activity, it is logical to expect that their pyridoxine turnover, and therefore requirement, would be higher than that of omnivores. The pyridoxine requirement of the cat is about 4-times higher than that of the dog.[14,15]

c. **Vitamin A** occurs naturally only in animal tissue. Vitamin A precursors (e.g. β-carotene) are synthesized by plants. Omnivorous and herbivorous animals can convert β-carotene to vitamin A; cats lack this ability.

Much can be learned about an animal's nutritional requirements simply by analyzing its **natural** diet. None of the so-called metabolic "peculiarities" of the cat are really peculiar. They are what one would expect in a true carnivore.

Cats' water needs also differ from those of dogs, not because of their feeding behavior (carnivorous vs omnivorous); but instead because of their ancestors' adaptation to environmental extremes. The modern domestic cat (*Felis domesticus*) is thought to have been derived from the African wild cat (*F. lybica*), a small desert cat native to north Africa.[20] Being descendants of desert animals, domestic cats can form a more concentrated urine than dogs, and as a result survive with less water intake. However, this adaptation to water conservation may also contribute to the cat's susceptibility to the feline urologic syndrome[9] (described in Chapter 9). The weaker thirst drive of the cat results in a water intake that is often too low to prevent crystal-

lization of struvite (ammonium-magnesium-phosphate) crystals in the urine.[9] If fed a typical commercial dry cat food, cats will drink about 1.5 to 2 ml of water per gram of dry food eaten. This proportion (2:1) is near the proportion of water (67%) in the animals that are prey for carnivores. Thus, cats need or drink very little water if they are fed only canned food.[9] Canned foods have a 3:1 water/dry matter ratio (75% water). Cats do, however, drink during both the day and night whereas dogs normally drink only during the day.[9]

Regardless of what or how the cat is fed, all cats should have water easily available at all times. The **only** exceptions to this rule are: 1) when diagnostic tests, such as a water-deprivation test, are being conducted, 2) in the management of some diseases, and 3) before certain surgical procedures. Some cats like fresh water every day; others prefer water that has been left in the bowl several days. The procedure that results in the greatest water consumption should be used. Increased intake of drinking water results in an increase in urinary water excretion and thus a decreased risk of FUS.

METHODS OF FEEDING

There are three commonly used methods of feeding: 1) free-choice feeding, 2) time-restricted meal feeding, and 3) food-restricted meal feeding. In the free-choice method, more food is always available than the cat will consume; thus, the cat can eat as much as it wants, whenever it chooses. With time-restricted meal feeding, the cat is given more food than it will consume within a specified period of time, generally 5-30 minutes; whereas with food-restricted meal feeding, the cat is given a lesser amount of food than it would eat if the amount fed were not restricted. Both types of meal feeding are repeated at a specific frequency, such as once or twice a day. Some people use only one method, but others use a combination of all three feeding methods, such as free-choice feeding a dry or soft-moist food and meal-feeding a canned food or specific food(s) (meat, table scraps, etc.).

Each feeding method has advantages and disadvantages. The main advantage of free-choice feeding is that it takes the least amount of work, thought, and knowledge on the part of the owner and ensures that the cat receives an adequate amount of food. Unless obesity becomes a problem, or only canned foods are fed, free-choice feeding is usually the easiest and best method.

Since dogs naturally hunt in packs, they generally eat voraciously and their feeding behavior can be affected by the presence of other dogs or people (inhibited-type eaters). Cats are solitary hunters and generally eat alone. As a result, most cats are non-voracious, non-inhibited eaters, and when food is always available, they nibble at it frequently. Most cats fed free-choice, regardless of the form of food (dry, soft moist or canned), will eat every few hours—24 hours a day.[12] In a study in which 20 cats were fed either a dry or canned cat food free choice, the amount consumed each 5-8 hour period throughout the day and night was the same, except in the afternoon during the summer when it was decreased by about 50% compared to the other periods. This fairly constant frequency of intake occurred with each of the 20 cats studied and with each of several different dry and canned cat foods fed. Results of other studies have shown that cats fed free-choice will eat 10-20 times during a 24 hour period.[9] This appears to mimic natural feeding patterns. Mice, being the domestic cat's most common prey,[2,3] provide about 30 kcal each.[17] If an active 3.5-kg cat expends approximately 300 kcal of metabolizable energy per day (3.5 x 85 kcal/kg, see Table 1, page 1-6), it would require at least 10 mice and, therefore, 10 meals per day. However, when a cat is meal-fed, food is available and, therefore, consumed only during that period.

If more than one cat is being fed, they should have separate bowls (as well as litter pans), and their bowls should be placed apart. If dogs are present, the cat's bowl should be placed where it can be reached by the cat, but not the dog. Many cats, particularly females (intact or neutered), are erratic eaters, consuming little food for one or several days and then consuming a large amount the next day. If the diet is changed during the time when little food is being consumed, one may mistakenly assume that the decrease in food consumption occurred because the cat did not find the previous food palatable. This belief is strengthened if food consumption increases when the diet is changed. However, these fluctuations in food consumption may have nothing to do with the palatability of the diets, but instead may simply be due to the normal erratic eating behavior of the cat or the novelty of a new diet.

Most healthy, mature, non-lactating house cats can consume enough of a good-quality cat food to meet their needs when meal-fed once daily. However, unless obesity is a problem, free-choice feeding is recommended. Free-choice feeding or feeding at least 3 times a day is preferred during periods of increased caloric need such as growth, reproduction, and lactation. Because of the limited capacity of its gastrointestinal tract, the cat may be unable to consume enough food to meet its needs during these periods when it is meal-fed once a day or fed a low-energy food. Excessive caloric intake during lactation or growth is not a problem in cats.

TABLE 1

APPROXIMATE FOOD REQUIREMENT* AND GROWTH RATE OF THE CAT

Life Cycle Stage	Body Weight (lbs)	(kg)	Dry (cups)**	Soft-Moist (cups)**	(1.5 oz pkgs)	Canned (oz)	(g)
Mature non-lactating:	6	2.7	0.7	0.8	1.9	8	227
	8	3.6	0.8	1.0	2.3	9	255
	10	4.5	1.0	1.1	2.6	10	284
	12	5.5	1.1	1.3	3.0	12	338
	14	6.4	1.2	1.5	3.3	13	377

Gestation (last 3 weeks): 1.25 times above amount.

Peak lactation: 2-3 times above amount.

Nursing kittens: Should weigh 90–110 g at birth and gain 50–100 g weekly from birth to 5–6 months of age. Encourage solid food consumption beginning at 3–4 weeks of age.

Weaned kittens:

Age (months)+ Female	Male	(lbs)	(kg)	Dry (cups)**	Soft-Moist (cups)**	(1.5 oz pkgs)	Canned (oz)	(g)
1	1	1	0.5	0.4	0.5	1.0	4.2	117
2	2	2	0.9	0.6	0.7	1.6	6.6	186
3	3	3	1.4	0.8	1.0	2.3	9	259
4.5	4	4	1.8	0.9	1.1	2.5	9.9	281
6	5	5	2.3	1.0	1.2	2.7	10.6	301
8	6.5	6	2.7	1.1	1.3	3.0	12	340
10	8	7	3.2	1.2	1.4	3.1	12.5	354
	10	10	4.5	1.2	1.5	3.3	13.2	374

*The amount needed by any individual cat may vary as much as 50% above or below the amounts given (see Figure 4, page 1–10). Thus, unless obesity is a problem do not restrict the cat to these amounts; feed all they will eat. Amounts given are based on the energy content of average quality cat foods as shown in Table 9, page 2–22.

**An 8 oz (volume) measuring cup holding 3–3.5 oz (weight) of dry cat food or 3.5–5 oz of soft-moist cat food.

+The age at which these weights are reached varies. Usually the larger the parents and the more calories consumed (from a nutritionally well-balanced diet), the larger the kittens' size. The amount of food needed/unit body wt decreases with increasing age. For example, the 3 lb kitten that is 2 months old needs more, and the 3 lb kitten that is 4 months old needs less, than the amounts given for the 3 lb kitten that is 3 months old.

Frequent consumption of a highly digestible food, high in caloric density, is also beneficial for cats with small intestinal or hepatic dysfunctions, pancreatic exocrine insufficiency, and any cause of debilitation, suboptimal body weight, anorexia, or increased dietary needs.

Regardless of the method of feeding used, it is best to feed on a regular schedule, and to avoid table scraps and feed a ration-type cat food (any form; canned, soft moist or dry). Table scraps, like other supplements, may unbalance a balanced diet (see page 2-11). A ration-type cat food is one that contains several energy- and protein-supplying food ingredients rather than just one or two.

Any single food item, such as tuna fish or cat food consisting of primarily or exclusively a single food item (as do some of the canned gourmet cat foods), should not constitute more that 25% of the cat's diet. Many cats fed a diet consisting primarily of a single food item will develop a fixed food preference and may refuse to eat anything else. Even if the food is nutritionally complete and adequate, a fixed food preference is undesirable. It causes difficulty in changing a cat's diet as may be required in different situations, including the management of many diseases. A fixed food preference is prevented by feeding a ration-type cat food containing varied sources of protein and calories. If a ration-type cat food is fed, a variety of foods need not be fed since each product already contains a variety of food items. The cat by nature is a good eater. **Finicky cats are made, not born.**

AMOUNT TO FEED

The amount of food required by the average cat can be determined from the cat's caloric needs and the caloric density of the diet, as shown in Tables 1-5, Chapter 1. The approximate amount of the three forms of average-quality cat food needed is given in Table 1. These values are helpful only in determining the starting amount to feed an individual cat, or the approximate amount of food needed by a group of cats. These amounts, or those given by the manufacturer of a particular cat food, should not be used for other than these purposes. There is much variation between individual cats in the amount of food needed to maintain optimal body weight (see Figure 4, page 1-10).

The proper amount to feed a cat is whatever amount is needed to maintain optimal body weight and condition. Weight and condition are optimal when the ribs cannot be seen but there is no excess of subcutaneous fat. In most cats, excessive subcutaneous fat is most noticeable as an "apron" along the ventral abdomen. A mature cat should be weighed weekly during the time when the quantity to feed is being established. After the appropriate quantity is established, the cat's body weight should be monitored monthly. Changes of more than 5-10% from the ideal should be accompanied by a change in the amount fed. Most cats voluntarily control their energy intake quite well[9] and will eat the proper amount, if a sufficient quantity of a good quality cat food is available and it is not too palatable. Thus, unless obesity is a problem, do not restrict the amount of food offered to cats.

MAINTENANCE

FEEDING

The mature non-reproducing cat in which obesity is not a problem may be fed a good-quality maintenance-type dry, soft-moist or canned food (Table 2), either free choice or meal-fed.

If only meal-feeding is used, a minimum of twice-daily feeding is recommended unless the duration of the meal is more than 2 hours. Factors useful in determining the quality of a commercial cat food are described beginning on page 2-16.

If obesity is a problem, a properly balanced high-fiber/low caloric dense food should be fed. The food should contain less than 10% fat and more than 15% fiber in its dry matter* (Prescription Diet Feline r/d, Hill's, or Recipe 10, Appendix Table 3). For a complete discussion of obesity, see Chapter 6.

Development of dental tartar is highly variable between individual cats. If dental tartar is a problem, clean the teeth and feed a dry food. The abrasive effect of the dry food decreases tartar accumulation, as has been observed over many years with hundreds of cats in our cattery.

If urolithiasis, cystitis, or the feline urologic syndrome (FUS) is a problem or concern, a diet, providing no more than 20 mg of magnesium/100

---

*The amount of a nutrient in the food dry matter equals the amount of that nutrient in the food as fed, divided by the food dry-matter content. For example, a canned food containing 2.5% fat, 5% fiber and 75% moisture as fed would contain 2.5% ÷ (1–0.75) or 10% fat, and 5% ÷ (1–0.75) or 20% fiber in its dry matter.

TABLE 2

DIET CHARACTERISTICS RECOMMENDED FOR CAT FOODS

| Situation | Energy (metabolizable kcal/g dry matter) | Digestibility[b] | Nutrients in Diet Dry Matter[a] (%) | | | | | | |
			Protein	Fat	Fiber	Calcium[c]	Phosphorus[c]	Sodium	Magnesium[d]
Maintenance	≥ 3.75[e]	>75[e]	> 25	> 10[e]	< 5[e]	0.5–0.9	0.4–0.8	0.2–0.5	< 0.10
Growth Gestation Lactation	≥ 4.5	> 80	> 35	≥ 17	< 5	1.0–1.8	0.8–1.6	0.3–0.7	< 0.12
Old Age	≥ 3.75[e]	> 80[e]	25–35	> 15[e]	< 5[e]	0.5–0.8	0.4–0.7	0.2–0.4	< 0.10

[a]To determine the amount of nutrient in the dry matter, divide the values preferably obtained by laboratory analysis or if unavailable the values given in the guaranteed analysis by the dry matter content of the food which is 1 − (% moisture in the food ÷ 100). The nutrient percentages given apply to a diet with the specific dry matter energy density listed. For diets of greater energy density, adjust the nutrient percentages accordingly (see Table 9, page 1–16).

[b]% digestibility = [(food dry weight necessary for maintaining body weight − stool dry weight) ÷ (food dry weight necessary for maintaining body weight)] × 100.

[c]The amount of calcium should be greater than the amount of phosphorus.

[d]Or not over 5% ash in a dry or soft-moist food if the magnesium content is not known (see page 9–11).

[e]≥ equal to or greater than, > greater than and < less than. If excess body weight is a problem, not more than 3.5 kcal ME/g, 10% or less fat and 15% or more fiber in the diet dry matter, and a lower digestibility are recommended.

kcal of metabolizable energy, and that maintains the urine pH below 6.4, should be fed exclusively (see Table 13, page 9-27). A diet of this type prevents this disease in most cats. For a complete discussion of this common disease, see Chapter 9.

Feeding aged cats is discussed in Chapter 3, page 3-22.

NON-FEEDING CARE

In addition to proper feeding, other factors are important in maintaining the health and well-being of cats. Frequent grooming is recommended, particularly for long-haired cats. It helps keep loose hair off of furniture and decreases the development of hairballs in the cat's gastrointestinal tract, which may cause vomiting and/or obstruction (see Chapter 7 for a complete discussion of this problem). A comb works best for long-haired cats. If the fur is tangled, use scissors and cut parallel with, not perpendicular to, the hair.

Most cats do not require baths. Baths wash away protective natural oils. If a cat needs to be cleaned, sprinkling cornstarch onto the coat and brushing it out is usually adequate. If a bath is necessary, use warm water in a warm room and use a very mild shampoo intended for cats. If the cat is afraid of water, allowing it to cling to a window screen placed in the tub may be helpful.

Cats should have access to a scratching post. They use it as much for exercise as for sharpening their claws. Provide a soft piece of wood. It is better not to cover the post with carpet. Many cats will not differentiate between the carpet on a scratching post and the carpet in the house.

Cats should be given a physical examination annually. Booster vaccinations, teeth cleaning, and treatment for both external and internal parasites should be done as needed.

REPRODUCTION AND GROWTH

FEEDING AND CARE BEFORE BREEDING AND DURING PREGNANCY

Before breeding, the procedures described in the previous paragraph should be conducted. It is important that the queen be given booster vaccinations at this time so that she has good immunity. This greatly assists in preventing infectious diseases in her kittens. In addition, it is important that the queen be free of internal and external parasites and be in good health before she is bred. She should be at optimal body weight and

FIGURE 1

BODY WEIGHT AND FOOD INTAKE DURING GESTATION AND LACTATION IN THE QUEEN

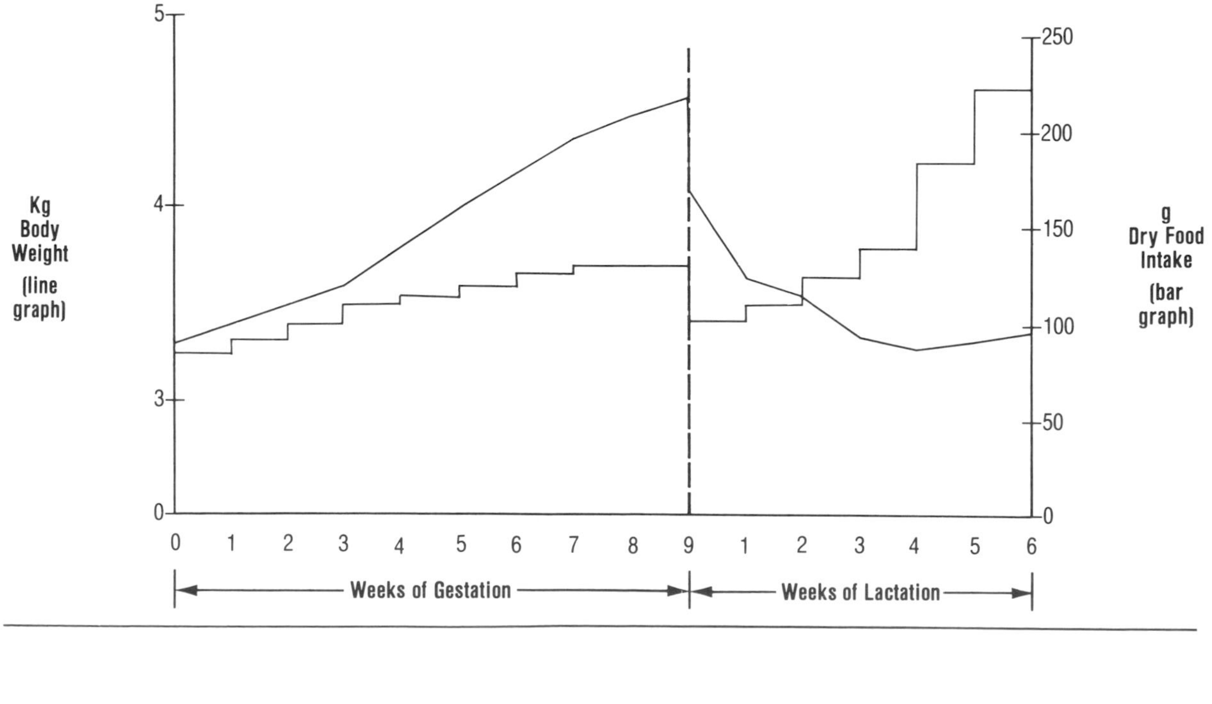

fully mature, which for most cats is 10-12 months of age. Generally, it is better to wait until at least the second estrus before breeding the cat. Pregnancy before maturity may decrease her mature size. Prior to breeding she should be fed a good-quality maintenance-type cat food (Table 2, page 4-6).

Gestation lasts for 63-65 days (9 weeks), although it may be as variable as 58-70 days. Larger breeds often have a gestation period closer to 70 days.[1] The kittens can usually be palpated by the 3rd to 4th week of pregnancy. A diet intended for reproduction (growth/lactation-type diet, Table 2, page 4-6) may be fed throughout gestation but is particularly important during the last 3-4 weeks of gestation. The amount of food needed increases gradually during gestation (Figure 1) so that at parturition the queen needs about 25% more food to prevent utilization of her own body tissues. Unlike bitches (Figure 1, page 3-8), the queens gain weight linearly during gestation (Figure 1). The earlier weight increase in the queen is apparently due to an increase in body fat, because postgestational body weight does not immediately return to pregestational weight (Figure 1) as it does in bitches (Figure 1, page 3-8). This additional body fat is helpful and, for large litters, probably necessary in providing the energy needed for milk production. Without this extra fat, as well as a good diet, the queen may be unable to produce sufficient milk to support her young.

During the last week of gestation, most cats will appear restless. At this time, if the queen is not being kept in a cattery, she should be introduced daily to the maternity box until she becomes familiar with it. This box will be used for queening and nursing.

A maternity box can be made from a cardboard carton. The box (with a top) should be large enough for the queen to stretch out and stand up, with plenty of room to spare. An entrance cut 3-5 inches up from the bottom allows her to get in and out, but keeps the kittens inside. The top on the box should be left attached on one side so that it can be opened for easy access but otherwise is dark inside. The bottom should be covered with a rug, blanket or clean rags. The box should be placed in a quiet, warm, draft-free location away from usual family activity.

CARE DURING QUEENING

The queen should be left alone during labor. Between labor contractions she may walk around and drink some water. Veterinary attention is needed if she has strong contractions for more than 2 hours and no kittens appear. Normal birth of 4 kittens takes 2-3 hours. The placenta is attached to the umbilical cord and should be passed after each kitten. The queen normally tears the sac from around the kitten, nips the umbilical cord with her teeth, and eats the afterbirth. She will usually clean the kittens' nostrils of mucus and lick the kittens dry. It is rare for a queen not to perform these procedures perfectly. However, she may stop if there is interference. Some queens may even cannibalize their kittens if there is too much human involvement at this stage, particularly if the kittens are handled and acquire a human odor.

Anyone who might have been present during the entire delivery should keep track of the number of afterbirths to make certain that all have been passed. A retained afterbirth usually results in uterine infection and systemic toxicity which, if not properly treated, may be fatal. A dark red or reddish-brown discharge after queening usually means all afterbirths have been expelled. A bright red discharge may indicate hemorrhage. Discharge of any other color, particularly brown or greenish, which generally appears 48-72 hours after queening, indicates a retained afterbirth or kitten, or a uterine infection. In these cases, the queen often eats less and is lethargic.

NEONATAL KITTEN CARE

Like all newborn animals, kittens should receive adequate amounts of colostrum shortly after birth to enhance immunity and resistance to infectious diseases. Early ingestion of adequate amounts of colostrum also appears to be important because initial fluid intake contributes significantly to immediate postnatal circulatory volume. Lack of intake could cause circulatory failure. The fading-kitten complex (see page 3-20) is sometimes considered to have two separate causes: infectious and non-infectious (which includes cardiopulmonary failure). Thus, early ingestion of adequate colostrum would help prevent both major causes of the fading-kitten complex.[4] Holding the kitten up to a nipple soon after queening is completed helps assure colostrum intake. The greater the infectious challenge the more important it is that adequate amounts of colostrum be ingested soon after birth. Thus, in addition to adequate intake of colostrum, the kittens' environment should be kept scrupulously clean. Cattery-raised kittens should be isolated from other cats until 1 week after they have been given their first vaccinations. These procedures greatly assist in reducing parasite infestations and the chance of bacterial or viral diseases.

After the first few days of life, the kittens should be handled daily, but only for a few minutes. This has been shown to be beneficial both physiologi-

cally and psychologically.[6,12] Except for this minimal amount of daily handling, they should be left alone to eat and sleep. Their eyes will open between 10-16 days, and their ears will begin to function between 15-17 days of age. Normal body temperature is about 35°C (95°F) for the first 2 weeks of life. Kittens have no shivering reflex for the first 6 days and, therefore, must depend on an external heat source, such as the queen, to sustain normal body temperature. The body temperature of the kitten drops rapidly in an environmental temperature of less than about 30°C (86°F). Unless kept warm, a kitten quickly becomes hypothermic, metabolism is reduced, and death ensues (see Figure 3, page 3-21).

At 6 days of age, kittens can shiver and begin to be self-sustaining. Between the second and fourth weeks of life, their body temperature rises to 36-37°C (97-99°F). After the fourth week, it is near adult body temperature. By 2-3 weeks of age, kittens begin to walk, which helps to stimulate and maintain a higher body temperature. The environmental temperature should be at least 21°C (70°F) for a queen and her kittens for the first few weeks of life. If a kitten is separated from the queen and littermates, the environmental temperature should be maintained as described for orphans (page 3-19).

Neonatal kittens have little subcutaneous fat. Their energy source is almost entirely glycogen, which is rapidly depleted after birth and not restored until after several days of nursing. If the kitten does not receive adequate nourishment, it soon becomes dehydrated, cold, weak, and debilitated and its survival is threatened. To prevent death of newborn kittens, keep them in a sufficiently warm environment, weigh them daily, and initiate supplemental feeding if they do not gain weight (see page 3-18 for these procedures). Weighing the kittens at birth, and then daily for the first 2 weeks of life, followed by every 3 days until they are a month old, is a good management practice. Periodic weight checks should be made thereafter. A gram scale should be used (it is one of the best investments a breeder can make). A steady weight gain and normal stools are the best indications of the adequacy of the diet and maintenance of good health.

Kittens at birth should weigh 90-110 g and should gain approximately this amount weekly (50-100 g) from birth to 5-6 months of age. Growth rate will slow as they approach maturity, which is usually attained at 10-14 months. The growth rate, however, varies between individuals. The bigger the kitten's parents and the more calories consumed, the faster the growth rate. Males tend to grow faster and become larger than females (Table 1, page 4-5).

FEEDING LACTATING QUEENS AND NURSING KITTENS

During lactation it is very important that both the queen and nursing kittens be encouraged to eat as much as possible of an excellent-quality growth/lactation-type cat food (Table 2, page 4-6). This will ensure adequate milk production by the queen and optimal growth of the kittens. The ability of a diet to support adequate lactation, while allowing the queen to maintain optimal body weight, is the ultimate test for a cat food's quality and adequacy for growth and reproduction.

In one study a dry cat food containing 21% fat was compared to a leading-selling kitten diet containing 12% fat. Relative to the 12% fat diet, the 21% fat diet resulted in:

1. 10% higher birth weights
2. 40% greater kitten survival rate
3. Higher weight gain of kittens
   a) 30% greater from birth to weaning
   b) 17% greater from 6-22 weeks of age, even though one-third less of the high-fat diet was consumed by the kittens.

In addition, five qualified individuals who did not know the kittens were being fed different diets evaluated the kittens eating the high-fat diet as being in better physical condition, including skin and coat appearance, attitude, and bone and muscle development. These results demonstrate the dramatic nutritional differences between reproduction and maintenance in cats. Cat foods adequate for adult maintenance are frequently inadequate for optimal reproductive performance.

Nutritional deprivation during pregnancy can compromise immunologic competence of the offspring. There is even evidence that severe malnutrition during pregnancy can adversely affect immunocompetence not only in the offspring from that pregnancy, but also in those offspring's subsequent young, even though they are fed adequately. Evidently the reticuloendothelial system is highly vulnerable to nutritional and metabolic derangement during its period of formation and development.[18]

The lactating queen needs 2-3 times more dietary energy than she did for maintenance (Table 1, page 1-6), and thus more food (Figure 1, page 4-7). Without adequate nutrients, her milk production will be decreased. Inadequate milk is the most common cause of death of kittens. Kittens not receiving adequate milk cry and become restless, their abdomens contract, and they fail to gain the normal

10-15 g/day. Excessive crying of kittens probably indicates hunger, cold, or both. Gently squeeze the mother's teats to determine if she is producing milk. If the kittens are not getting enough milk from their mother, supplement their diet by feeding a kitten milk replacer as described in the feeding and care of orphan kittens and puppies (page 3-18).

The kittens should be encouraged to begin eating solid food at 3 weeks of age. This can be accomplished by mixing enough milk with the solid food to make a gruel. Add just enough milk to make the food mushy, not sloppy. Smear some of the gruel on the kittens' lips, being careful not to get it in their nostrils. In licking the gruel off their lips, the kittens usually find they like the taste. Once they are eating the gruel, gradually decrease the amount of milk mixed with the food until the kittens are eating only the solid food. Throughout lactation and growth, feed free-choice or at least 3 times daily so both the queen and kittens can eat as much as they desire.

FEEDING AND CARE
DURING WEANING

The queen will usually begin weaning the kittens when they are 6-10 weeks old. Unless necessary, it is best not to wean the kittens until they are at least 6 weeks old and preferably 8-10 weeks old. Cats that were weaned at 2 weeks of age are slower to learn and are more suspicious, cautious, and aggressive.[6,12] There is little behavorial difference between those weaned at 6 and 12 weeks of age.[6,12]

By 8-10 weeks of lactation, milk production of most queens has decreased so they have little discomfort at weaning time as a result of excess milk production. However, if the queen has been uncomfortable during previous lactations due to excessive distention of the mammary glands, this can be reduced by restricting the queen's food intake before and during weaning. This is accomplished by separating the queen from the litter the day before weaning and withholding all food from the queen that day. Reunite the queen and kittens during the night and remove the food from both. Completely wean all kittens the next day, and then gradually increase the amount fed the queen so that by several days after weaning she is receiving the amount of food needed for **maintenance.**

FEEDING WEANED KITTENS

Following weaning, the kittens should continue to be fed all they will consume of a good-quality growth/lactation-type diet (Table 2, page 4-6). If poor-quality foods with low digestibility are fed, the resulting high intake will further reduce the digestibility of the food. Thus, the kittens do not receive sufficient digestible nutrients to meet their needs. The kittens will have a "pot-bellied" appearance, slow growth, poor muscle and skeletal development, decreased resistance to infectious diseases, and frequently diarrhea. Feeding a good-quality food will eliminate these problems.

A good-quality growth/lactation-type diet should have the nutrient levels listed in Table 2 (page 4-6). However, simply meeting these requirements does not assure that the food will support optimal growth because the amount of nutrients in the diet tells nothing about the diet's palatability, nutrient availability, or protein quality. Thus, in addition to these nutrient levels, ensure that feeding tests of the food have shown it to be nutritionally adequate for growth (see Table 7, page 2-17 for indications of pet food quality).

The average amount of food needed during growth and the cat's growth rate are shown in Table 1 (page 4-5). However, do not restrict kittens to these amounts. Feed them all the food they will consume. Excessive caloric intake and excessive growth rate or obesity are not problems in growing kittens. Selection of a ration-type diet is best, as discussed on page 4-5.

Once the diet has been selected, feed only that diet. Supplementation with meat, table scraps, or other items can create dietary imbalances and finicky eaters.

Supplementation with protein, minerals, or vitamins is not necessary and, in fact, is contraindicated. High-quality growth/lactation-type cat foods are nutritionally balanced. They have adequate levels of all nutrients cats need for growth. Extra protein or vitamin/mineral supplements only upset the balance of nutrients in the food.

If the owner or veterinarian previously has seen clinical signs of nutritional imbalance in cats consuming a particular brand of food, the proper action is to change to a better-quality nutritionally-adequate diet rather than attempt to supplement a diet that has proved to be imbalanced (see supplement discussion page 2-11). The prophylactic use of vitamin/mineral supplements in conjunction with a good-quality balanced cat food is unnecessary and can be harmful.

COMMON FEEDING ERRORS

Supplements that provide specific nutrients such as calcium, phosphorus, vitamin A, and vitamin D are sometimes given to cats, particularly during growth or reproduction. Unfortunately, these are usually given by well-meaning, but misinformed, cat owners. If a poor-quality or nutritionally deficient cat food is being fed, it is highly unlikely that supplementation will correct the food's deficien-

cies. Low digestibility or specific nutrient excesses (which can be harmful) are common problems with poor-quality diets. Thus, rather than attempt to supplement a questionable food, switch to a good one. Then do not alter it with unnecessary, and occasionally harmful, supplementation.

Vitamin A and D toxicities are much more common than deficiencies because of unnecessary supplementation with these vitamins and high-potency fish oils. Excessive amounts of most minerals decrease the absorption of other minerals and may result in mineral imbalances in the diet. A number of supplements, such as B-complex vitamins and vitamins C and E, are not known to be harmful to the cat. However, there are no data based on controlled studies to suggest that additional quantities of these vitamins above the normal cat's requirements are beneficial.

Another common error made in feeding cats is feeding primarily or exclusively a single food item. Frequently the food fed is meat, fish, or a glandular organ such as liver or kidney. The cat becomes addicted to the food and refuses to eat anything else. Although many of these foods are excellent sources of protein in a balanced diet, they are very unbalanced nutritionally when fed as the greater part of the diet (see page 2-3) and will cause a number of nutritional diseases. Therefore, they should not make up more than 25% of the cat's total diet and preferably not more than 10%. Meat, liver, and kidney are all very low in calcium and will cause extensive skeletal malformation as a result of nutritional secondary hyperparathyroidism if fed in excess (see page 12-7 for a complete discussion of this problem). The viscera of some fish contain thiaminase, which is an enzyme that destroys thiamin (vitamin B_1). This loss of vitamin B_1 causes cerebral cortical necrosis resulting in convulsions and brain damage and a condition called Chastek Paralysis (see page 12-13). Cooking destroys this enzyme. Some fish oils contain excess quantities of unsaturated fatty acids and are low in antioxidants such as vitamin E. This imbalance causes pansteatitis (see pages 1-19 and 12-13).

Milk is occasionally fed to cats and is an excellent food, provided it does not cause diarrhea. If diarrhea occurs, reduce the amount of milk fed. Some cats past weaning do not have an adequate amount of the intestinal enzyme lactase to digest the milk sugar lactose. If more lactose is consumed than the cat is able to digest, diarrhea results (see page 7-42).

Unless they are finely ground, bones should not be fed to cats. Poultry and fish bones can splinter and damage the throat or gastrointestinal tract. Chewing large bones can cause broken teeth.

Feeding dog foods to cats is one of the most common feeding errors. Perhaps dog foods are fed to cats because they are less expensive than cat foods, but this problem arises most often when dogs and cats are fed together. Most cat foods are higher in fat and protein than dog foods and are more palatable for dogs than are dog foods. Thus, if dogs have access to both dog and cat foods, they will eat the cat food, which forces the cat to eat the dog food. The owner may even quit offering cat food. Although some dog foods meet nutrient requirements for cats, most do not and, as a result, will cause nutritional problems in cats. As discussed (page 4-1), cats have several important metabolic differences from dogs. Problems in the cat that result from these differences can all be prevented or corrected by feeding diets containing more animal-source foods and less plant-source foods. This does not mean that cats cannot utilize plant-source foods or that these foods should not be in the diet. What it does mean is that the diet must contain adequate amounts of animal-source foods. The practical reasons why dog foods cause nutritional problems in the cat are:

1. The cat has a much higher protein requirement than the dog (Table 9, page 1-16). The effects of inadequate protein intake are described on page 1-17.

2. Cats require taurine in the diet, whereas dogs do not. Inadequate taurine results in central retinal degeneration and blindness (see page 1-14 for a further explanation of this effect).

3. Cats cannot convert the fatty acid linoleic acid to arachidonic acid as can the dog and other animals, and therefore, cats must consume preformed arachidonic acid, which is present only in animal tissues (see page 1-18). If cats do not have an adequate intake of this nutrient, they develop a dry, lusterless coat or, if the cat is severely deprived, emaciation and spots of moist dermatitis develop (see page 1-18 for a more complete discussion of fatty acid deficiency).

4. Cats cannot convert β-carotene, present in plants, to vitamin A as can dogs, and therefore they must consume preformed vitamin A, which is present only in animal tissues (see Table 13, page 1-23 for the effects of vitamin A deficiency).

5. Cats cannot convert the amino acid tryptophan to the B vitamin, niacin, as can dogs; thus cats require more niacin in the diet (see Table 13, page 1-23 for effects of niacin deficiency).

6. Cats require higher levels of pyridoxine (vitamin B_6) (see Table 13, page 1-23 for effects of pyridoxine deficiency).

SUMMARY

In summary, to ensure the best possible nutrition for cats and to alleviate all of the problems caused by the most common feeding errors:

1. Feed a good-quality cat food that has been proven by feeding trials to be nutritionally adequate (see page 2-20) and that contains a number of different food items.

2. Select the food designed for the purpose for which it is being fed (Table 2, page 4-6).

3. Do not supplement the diet.

4. Do not feed dog food to cats.

5. Do not feed as more than 10-25% of the cat's total food intake (preferably do not feed them at all), any single food item or cat food consisting of a single food item (as do some gourmet cat foods).

6. Do not restrict the cat's food intake unless obesity is a problem.

REFERENCES

1. Colby ED, Stein BS: The reproductive system. In Feline Medicine. Editor PW Pratt. American Veterinary Publications, Inc. Santa Barbara, CA pp 511-554 (1983).

2. Coman BJ, Brunner H: Food habits of the feral house cat in Victoria. J Wildlife Mgmt 36:848-842 (1972).

3. Everhard T: Food habits of Pennsylvania house cats. J Wildlife Mgmt 18:284-286 (1954).

4. Fisher EW: Neonatal diseases of dogs and cats. Brit Vet J 138:277-284 (1982).

5. Fruton JS, Simmonds S: Amino acids as structural units of proteins. In General Biochemistry. John Wiley & Sons, Inc. New York, NY pp 45-84 (1958).

6. Hart BL: Feline behavior. Feline Pract 2 (6):6-8 (1972).

7. Kliban W: Cat. Workman Publishing Co, New York, NY (1975).

8. Leyhausen P: Cat behavior: The Predatory and Social Behavior of Domestic and Wild Cats. Garland Press, New York, NY pp 6-53 (1979).

9. MacDonald ML, Rogers QR, Morris JG: Nutrition of the domestic cat, a mammalian carnivore. Ann Rev Nutr 4:521-562 (1984).

10. Mech DL: The Wolf: The Ecology and Behavior of an Endangered Species. Natural History Press, Garden City, NY pp 181-192 (1970).

11. Morris JG, Rogers QR: Nutritional implications of some metabolic anomalies of the cat. Amer Anim Hosp Assoc Proc, pp 325-331 (1983).

12. Mugford RA: External influences on the feeding of carnivores. In the Chemical Senses and Nutrition. Editor MR Kare, O Maller. Academic Press, New York, NY pp 25-50 (1977).

13. Munro JA: Observations of birds and mammals in central British Columbia. Occasional Papers, British Columbia Provincial Museum, Victoria BC 6:120-123 (1947).

14. Nutrient Requirements of Cats. National Academy of Sciences, Washington DC, pp 1-49 (1978).

15. Nutrient Requirements of Dogs. National Academy of Sciences, Washington DC, pp 1-71 (1974).

16. Prescott CW: Feeding the cat. Proceedings No 53, The University of Sydney, Post Graduate Committee in Veterinary Science, Refresher Course for Veterinarians. Sydney NSW, Australia, pp 604-638 (1980).

17. Reinke SI, Ihrke PJ: The skin. In Feline Medicine. Editor PW Pratt. American Veterinary Publications Inc. Santa Barbara, CA pp 555-604 (1983).

18. Sheffy BE: Nutrition and the immune response. J Amer Vet Med Assoc 180:1073-1076 (1982).

19. Stryer L: Amino acid degradation and the urea cycle. In Biochemistry. WH Freeman and Co, San Francisco, CA pp 407-429 (1975).

20. The Book of the Cat. Summit Books, New York, NY (1980).

21. Young SP, Jackson HT: Economic status: food habits. In The Clever Coyote. Wildlife Management Institute Publication. University of Nebraska Press, Lincoln NE pp 124-162 (1978).

CHAPTER 5

Anorexia, Inanition, and Critical Care Nutrition

CONTENTS

SUMMARY OF MANAGEMENT RECOMMENDATIONS

1. Evaluate the patient to determine if undernutrition is a problem associated with the disease process and, therefore, nutritional support is indicated (Table 4, page 5-15). In general, recent weight loss of more than 10% (or body weight below optimal) that is not caused by dehydration, or a history of anorexia for more than 3-5 days, is sufficient evidence that nutritional support is needed. The earlier nutritional support is instituted, the better the response.

2. Correct fluid, acid-base, and electrolyte status (as described beginning on page 5-16) before nutritional support is started.

3. Choose the most appropriate type of nutritional support (Figure 7, page 5-19).
   a. **"If the gut works, use it!"** First, try to stimulate the animal's appetite by feeding a very palatable food. A high protein, high fat canned cat food (e.g. Prescription Diet Feline p/d or Feline c/d, Hill's or the 3-6.5 oz can gourmet foods) is palatable for most dogs and cats. Warming the food to, but not above, body temperature volatilizes odors and encourages voluntary consumption (Figure 1, page 2-3). Cleaning the nose, if plugged, and petting and coaxing may help. If unsuccessful, try placing food in the mouth (Figure 8, page 5-21). If still unsuccessful, tube-feed. Figures 9-15 (pages 5-22 to 5-29) and Tables 8-15 (pages 5-26 to 5-34) describe methods of tube placement and feeding protocols.
   b. If the gut does not work, that is, if giving food via the gastrointestinal tract is contraindicated (for reasons described on page 5-35), feed intravenously (as described beginning on page 5-35).

4. For feeding via the gastrointestinal tract, a blenderized diet (Tables 10 and 13, pages 5-29 and 5-33) or commercially prepared liquid diets for people (Tables 11, 12 or 13), page 5-30, 5-31, and 5-33) is adequate for nearly all patients.

5. If intravenous feeding is necessary, mix 1 part of 8.5% amino acids plus electrolytes with 1 part of 25% glucose the first day; thereafter, replace the 25% glucose with 1 part of 50% glucose. A B-vitamin supplement should be included in the mixture. This mixture should suffice for 1-2 weeks of feeding in the absence of severe metabolic abnormalities.

6. Determine energy needs as shown in Figure 6 (page 5-13) or Table 3 (page 5-12). Divide the energy requirement by the energy density of the diet to determine daily food dosage. Feed enterally according to recommended protocol (Table 14, page 5-34). Feed intravenously according to protocol on page 5-37. Regardless of the method of feeding, begin by providing 1/3 to 1/2 the animal's energy needs. Increase this gradually to the total amount needed by the third day.

7. If the patient is being fed intravenously, urine or blood glucose concentration should be monitored because hyperglycemia is a common complication. If urine glucose is 3+ or greater, administer insulin or decrease the rate of administration. Any discontinuance of intravenous feeding must be done gradually over 2-3 hours to prevent rebound hypoglycemia. Once the patient is stable, body weight should be determined daily. Significant day-to-day changes are usually caused by alterations in fluid content rather than lean body mass. Urine glucose, body temperature, heart and respiratory rates, and clinical status should be recorded daily and should direct further laboratory evaluation to explain any abnormalities observed (Table 18, page 5-38).

8. Regardless of the method of feeding used, unless specific contraindications exist, voluntary food consumption should be encouraged. Intensive intervention is often necessary for only 2-4 days to stimulate an anabolic response sufficient for the animal to begin eating voluntarily. If a method of tube feeding is used where the animal can eat with the feeding tube in place, the animal can be "weaned" from nutritional support as voluntary intake increases.

9. Avoid undesirable practices that may adversely affect the nutritional status of hospitalized patients (Table 5, page 5-16).

INTRODUCTION

For centuries historians have recorded that famine often precedes disease. Hippocrates recognized the importance of proper nutrition for sick patients in the 5th century B.C.[68] However, only within the last two decades has the medical community come to appreciate the relationship of undernutrition to problems such as ineffective wound healing (soft tissue and orthopedic), decubitus ulcers, inadequate immune and nonimmune defense mechanisms, decreased tolerance to cancer therapy, muscle weakness, and multiple organ system dysfunctions. As a result of this recent awareness, exciting advances have been made in diets, delivery systems, and patient monitoring. This "new" branch of clinical nutrition is referred to as "critical care nutrition," and is generally associated with the nutritional support of patients that are postsurgical, traumatized, septic, burned, or that have cancer. The principles and techniques described in this chapter are also applicable to other diseases (e.g. renal or hepatic failure) affecting patients that have some degree of appetite suppression and require nutritional support.

ANOREXIA, INANITION, INJURY, AND DISEASE

A review of the regulation of food intake and the normal adaptive responses to food deprivation provides a basis for: 1) understanding what happens when even short-term food deprivation is complicated by injury or disease, and 2) for determining when, and how, to provide nutritonal support.

REGULATION OF FOOD INTAKE

Appetite is the desire for food and is often used synonomously with hunger. Satiety is the opposite of hunger. It means that hunger has been satisfied. The body is normally in a state of hunger, which is intermittantly relieved by eating.

There are appetite and satiety centers in the brain. The lateral hypothalamus is the hunger center. Stimulation of this area causes an animal to eat voraciously. The ventromedial hypothalamus is the satiety center. Stimulation of this area causes complete satiety. Many neuroendocrine and metabolic factors affect these centers and therefore control appetite (Figure 1). Several of these factors are discussed on page 6-12. In addition, the special senses of taste and smell are involved in the regulation of food intake.

Taste is mediated through taste buds and free nerve endings. The cells that comprise the taste buds are constantly being renewed from dividing epithelial cells surrounding the taste buds. Buds are located on the tongue, soft palate, pharynx, larynx, epiglottis, cranial esophagus, and even on the lips and cheeks of some species. Gustatory information received from the buds is projected by cranial nerves to several areas of the brain including the lateral hypothalamus.[116]

Olfaction occurs via axons of bipolar neurons that course through the small holes of the cribriform plate of the ethmoid bone and form connections in the olfactory bulb. As with taste, there are olfactory projections to the hypothalamus.[116]

The flavor of food results from chemical stimulation of the taste buds, free nerve endings in the nose, mouth and throat area, and olfactory neurons. "Taste" disorders are often the result of deficiencies in olfaction. Disorders of taste or smell can impair appetite and occur due to:

1. Age, which decreases the senses of taste and smell. The number of taste buds declines with age and olfaction is usually the first sensory system to show an age effect.

2. Damage to neural connections due to surgery or traumatic head injury. Accidental blows to the head can shear the fine olfactory nerves that pass through the cribriform plate and are a common cause of anosmia (inability to smell) in people.

3. Impaired renewal of taste buds and olfactory epithelium. Decreased chemosensory cell turnover is consistent with the decreased cell renewal that has been reported to occur in small intestinal epitheluim as a result of food deprivation, radiation therapy, uremia, vitamin B_{12} deficiency, and therapy with methotrexate. Many endocrine factors also lead to depressed cell proliferation in small-bowel epithelium. These factors and many of the conditions and drugs listed in Tables 1 and 2 probably impair regeneration and functioning of taste buds and olfactory cells in the same manner that they

FIGURE 1

FACTORS INVOLVED IN APPETITE CONTROL*

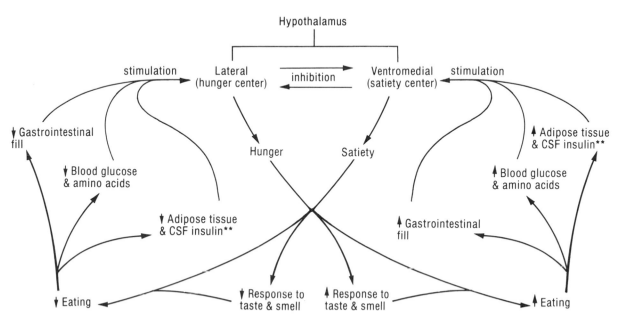

*Lateral and ventromedial parts of the hypothalamus inhibit each other, and together form a central control for appetite regulation. Active neurons in the lateral hypothalamus initiate hunger and increased responsiveness to taste and olfaction, which increase eating. Increased eating increases blood glucose, etc. (as shown on right side of the diagram), which activates the ventromedial neurons that inhibit the lateral neurons. Opposing regulatory activity is shown on the left, where active ventromedial hypothalamic neurons depress hunger, taste and olfactory responsiveness. This decreases eating, etc., which promotes activity in lateral neurons to increase appetite.[75]

**CSF insulin = cerebrospinal fluid insulin, which appears to regulate the amount of stored body fat; whereas, plasma insulin primarily regulates plasma glucose concentration (see page 6–12).

impair the regeneration of intestinal epithelium. Since the turnover time of taste bud and olfactory cells is approximately 10 days, a return to normal taste functioning after the interruption of mitosis requires a minimum of 10 days and usually much longer.[116]

4. Modification of receptor cells as a result of a chronic change in local environment, such as an alteration in saliva or the fluids bathing the olfactory mucosa which can be caused by drugs or metabolic agents such as urea.[116]

Normally satiety occurs after an animal's caloric needs have been met. Loss of the desire for food before caloric needs have been satisfied is called anorexia. Besides alterations in taste or smell, anorexia can be caused by numerous medical problems including organic disease, inflammation, trauma, and neoplasia. Pain, fear, and other components of emotional stress also inhibit the desire for food.[116,117] If anorexia persists, nutritional depletion occurs. Nutritional depletion may also

occur as a result of facial or oral injuries, or obstruction or dysfunctions of the gastrointestinal tract, liver, or pancreas so that the animal is incapable of ingesting, chewing, swallowing, digesting, or absorbing food.

EFFECTS OF FOOD DEPRIVATION

Starvation is the long-continued deprival of food. Inanition is the condition which results from complete lack of food, no matter what the duration. Several important adaptive responses to food deprivation occur before an animal would be considered to be "starving."

Food deprivation in normal animals causes a lowering of blood glucose values and a resultant decrease in insulin secretion. An insulin-responsive thyroxine-deiodinase system converts thyroxine (T_4) to triiodothyronine (T_3), the more active of the two thyroid hormones.[54,55] As blood insulin values decline in response to the relative hypoglycemia induced by food deprivation, the conver-

TABLE 1

DISORDERS AFFECTING* SENSES OF TASTE AND SMELL IN PEOPLE[116]

Disorder	Taste	Smell
Head trauma	A/D	A/D
Burn	A/D/D	
Cancer	A/D	
Radiation therapy	A/D/D	
Chronic renal failure	A/D/D	A/D
Hepatic cirrhosis	A/D	A/D
Viral hepatitis (acute)		A/D/D
Diabetes mellitus	A/D	A/D
Adrenal cortical insufficiency	IDDR	ID
Cushing's syndrome	A/D	A/D
Hypothyroidism	A/D/D	A/D/D
Hypertension	A/D	
Allergic rhinitis		A/D
Nasal polyposis		A/D
Sinusitis		A/D
Bronchial asthma		A/D
Influenza-like infections	A/D/D	A/D/D
Zinc deficiency	A/D	
Niacin deficiency	A/D/D	
Cobalamin deficiency		A/D

*A/D denotes absent or diminished; A/D/D absent, diminished or distorted; and IDDR, increased detection but decreased recognition.

TABLE 2

DRUGS AFFECTING SENSES OF TASTE AND SMELL IN PEOPLE[116,117]

Classification	Drug
Amebicides	Metronidazole
Antiepileptic drugs	Phenytoin
Anesthetics (local)	Benzocaine, procaine hydrochloride, tetracaine hydrochloride
Antihistamines	Chlorpheniramine maleate
Antimicrobial agents	Amphotericin B, ampicillin, cephalosporins, chloramphenicol, gentamicin, griseofulvin, kanamycin, lincomycin, neomycin, nitrofurantoin, sulfonamides, streptomycin, tetracyclines
Antineoplastic agents	Doxorubicin, methotrexate, azathioprine, vincristine sulfate
Antirheumatic, analgesic-antipyretic, antiinflammatory agents	Allopurinol, colchicine, levamisole, D-penicillamine, phenylbutazone
Antithyroid agents	Propylthiouracil, thiouracil
Diuretics and anti-hypertensive agents	Captopril, furosemide, thiazides
Opiates	Codeine, morphine
Sympathomimetic drugs	Amphetamines, ephedrine
Others	Digitalis glycosides, estrogens, iron sorbitex, oral antidiabetic agents, vitamin D

sion of T_4 to T_3 is diminished. The reduction in T_3 levels lowers the basal metabolic rate (BER, see page 1-5). This system attempts to balance the animal's energy expenditure with energy intake.

Most tissues can use energy-providing nutrients other than glucose. However, blood cells, renal medullary cells, and nervous tissue have an obligatory glucose requirement. Besides decreasing insulin secretion, inanition-induced hypoglycemia stimulates glucagon secretion. Glucagon stimulates hepatic glycogenolysis and glucose release. Glucagon also stimulates hepatic gluconeogenesis from glucogenic amino acids, lactic acid, glycerol, etc. Glycerol and fatty acids are released from fat stores due to the lipolytic effects of glucagon and the relative inactivity of insulin.[108] The liver uses the fatty acids for the energy needed for gluconeogenesis and releases ketone bodies as a partial end-product of fatty-acid metabolism. As a result, blood levels of fatty acids, ketone bodies, and glucose rise. Thus, the tissues that specifically require glucose are satisfied and continue to function. However, the glucose is derived primarily

from amino acids (body protein), and results in an initial rapid decline in body protein, as shown in Figure 2. During the first few days of food deprivation the rising blood levels of ketones cause enzymatic changes in peripheral tissues, including brain and heart, that increases their use of ketone bodies for energy and decreases their use of glucose.[83] This transition decreases the use of amino acids for glucose production, thereby preserving body proteins. As shown in Figure 2, the transition phase occurs during the first week of food deprivation and is associated with a reduction in body protein utilization and an increase in the use of body fat. Following the transition phase, stored fat becomes the main body fuel (until it nears depletion). This fact has important implications regarding selecting the diet to feed for inanition, starvation, injury, or disease (see page 5-29).

Because the principal functions of adipose tissue are energy storage, insulation, and protection of internal organs, the progressive loss of body fat during starvation does not result in loss of critical

FIGURE 2

DISAPPEARANCE OF ENERGY NUTRIENT STORES DURING FOOD DEPRIVATION[60]

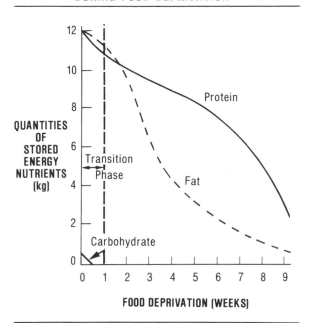

QUANTITIES OF STORED ENERGY NUTRIENTS (kg)

Transition Phase

Protein

Fat

Carbohydrate

FOOD DEPRIVATION (WEEKS)

body functions. For this reason, loss of body fat does not seriously threaten survivability until the fat stores are almost completely depleted. However, even after the transition phase, when the body is using fat as its main fuel, moderate protein losses continue (Figure 2), primarily to produce glucose. Body protein use is not random. Various proteins are more labile than others. Approximately one-half of the body proteins are relatively inactive, metabolically (stable). They provide structural support in the form of bones, ligaments, tendons, and cartilage. The other half are more labile and are present primarily in plasma, viscera, and muscle.[83] These proteins are more labile because they are metabolically active and are in a dynamic state of synthesis, breakdown, and resynthesis. Since the constituent amino acids of the labile proteins are in more constant flux, they are easier to siphon off into other metabolic pathways such as for new glucose production. As a result, during a period of food deprivation, a loss of function occurs earlier in tissues and systems that contain more labile proteins. Early tissue and organ changes as a result of inanition-induced protein depletion include (in the general order of occurrence):

1. **Liver and plasma proteins**—During the first 2-3 days of food deprivation there is a rapid loss of liver protein and liver protein synthesis

falls dramatically.[83] Essentially all of the albumin and fibrinogen and 80% of the globulins (except gamma globulins) are formed by the liver.[60] Plasma albumin and transferrin (a beta globulin) usually decrease during food deprivation,[18,83] and are used as indicators of nutritional status (see page 5-15).

2. **Gastrointestinal tract**—The small intestine is very active metabolically and its mass decreases substantially during prolonged deprivation of food. Gastric emptying and intestinal transit times are prolonged. Eventually there is flattening of the intestinal villi, a reduction of absorptive surface area, and a lowered disaccharidase (especially lactase) activity. Carbohydrate and fat digestion are impaired sooner than is protein digestion.[83]

3. **Kidney**—The kidney loses little mass during starvation but other important changes occur rather early. The kidney becomes an important gluconeogenic organ during the first few days of food deprivation. Urinary calcium and phosphorus excretion are high and there is a decreased ability to excrete acid.[83] As a result, the body has less ability to respond to acid-base abnormalities.

4. **Host defenses**—With inanition, the ability to mount adequate responses to challenges by various infectious agents via immune and non-immune defense mechanisms is altered including:

   a. Variable depression of humoral immunity. The ability to synthesize antibodies (usually IgA) and interferon is impaired.[1,83,121]

   b. Depression of cell-mediated immune response with low total lymphocyte counts due to reduction of T-lymphocytes[1,83,121]

   c. Decreased barrier function of skin and mucosal surfaces[1,83]

   d. Decreased inflammatory response[1,83]

   e. Depression of the levels of most complement proteins (except C_4) resulting in decreased chemotactic response and abnormal opsonization[1,83,121]

   f. Decreased leukocyte motility and bactericidal activity.[83]

   As a result of these changes, it becomes apparent that the physiologic state of an individual can be more important than the pathogenicity of, and/or the intensity of exposure to, an infectious agent, in determining whether an infection fails to occur, occurs but runs an abortive course, or evolves into overt disease.[42]

5. **Pulmonary system**—Partial food deprivation for only 10 days has been shown to lead to a significant diminution of the hypoxic ventilatory response (42% of control) in people.[83] Thus another component of acid-base control is compromised. Short-term food deprivation has also been shown to reduce lung elasticity.[83]

6. **Cardiac function**—The heart, like the kidneys and lungs, influences acid-base metabolism both metabolically and physically: metabolically by using lactic acid as a fuel; physically by perfusing tissues, maintaining oxygen delivery and removing acidic end products of metabolism. However, adaptation to food deprivation results in a decreased ability of the heart to use lactic acid as an energy source.[83] Also cardiac function is impaired and cardiac failure is common.[83] People deprived of food for 10 days and then subjected to submaximal treadmill work promptly exhibited abnormal electrocardiograms.[29]

7. **Skeletal muscle**—Food deprivation depresses synthesis and increases degradation of muscle protein. This may be due to decreased insulin levels associated with inanition (see page 5-4). Insulin normally stimulates amino acid transport into muscle and regulates muscle protein synthesis. In people, hand-grip strength is one of the most sensitive parameters of nutritional status and reflects loss of muscle function due to muscle protein degradation.[69] However, muscle protein loss occurs more slowly than other changes,[83] therefore, **by the time muscle atrophy or weakness is clinically obvious, food deprivation-induced alterations of other tissues may be well underway.**

As the period of food deprivation is extended, use of the labile proteins continues and finally accelerates as the body's fat stores are depleted and protein is forced to resume the role of primary energy source (Figure 2). As a result, critical body functions are rapidly lost. Terminally there is diarrhea; the wall of the small intestine is so thin that it is almost transparent. With a loss of 40-45% of lean body mass, intercostal muscle and diaphragm failure often occur. Pneumonia is common at this stage.[82] In human beings dying of starvation, the heart is atrophied to one-half its normal size. The tissue showing the least starvation-induced change is bone.[83]

Rather than simply extending the period that an animal can live without food, the adaptations that occur during food deprivation preserve reversibility and protect reproductive capacity for as long as possible. These adaptations have to some degree been dictated by evolution, through which the successful continuation of a species is due in part to its ability to reproduce.[83]

The metabolic and physiologic effects of food deprivation are primarily due to decreased intake of energy and protein. Thus, starvation, or prolonged food deprivation, is often referred to as protein-calorie malnutrition (PCM). However, most PCM victims also suffer from varied and multiple deficiencies of minerals and vitamins because there is inadequate intake of food that includes these nutrients as well.

RESPONSE TO INJURY AND DISEASE

Responses to food deprivation differ in many ways from the endocrine, metabolic, and physiologic responses to injury, infection, and disease. With inanition, body tissues and systems assume the posture of energy economy. However, cancer as well as injuries due to trauma, infection, or burn, induce changes that are in direct contradiction to energy-economy.

With **trauma,** metabolic and physiologic alterations are mediated by a general neuroendocrine stress response that is common to stressful stimuli, such as surgery, burn injury, cold, or emotional stress.[107] There is an acute phase and an adaptive phase of this stress response. The acute phase varies in duration and intensity, depending on the severity of the stress. The adaptive phase follows the acute phase and lasts for several days (see Figure 5, page 5-11). During the acute phase, simultaneous sympathetic nervous stimulation and release of catecholamines, adrenocorticoids, glucagon, growth hormone, and antidiuretic hormone induce a number of metabolic and physiologic responses, including:

1. Suppression of insulin secretion, resulting in hypoinsulinemia

2. Hyperglycemia through inhibition of insulin secretion and stimulation of glycogen breakdown and new glucose production. The glucose provides a readily available fuel for muscles for the generalized "fight or flight" response.[107] Also, fibroblasts in wounds use considerable glucose and metabolize much of it anaerobically to lactic acid in early phases of repair. Oftentimes injured animals are glucose-intolerant and insulin-resistant, which has important implications with regards to diet constituents (page 5-29).

3. Increased proteolysis to supply amino acids for glucose production and wound healing. A number of studies suggest increased break-

down of serum albumin and muscle protein after severe injury.[26,84]

4. Increased protein synthesis for tissue repair
5. Increased lipolysis to provide fatty acids for use by muscle and liver and glycerol for glucose production
6. Increased rate and depth of respiration[107]
7. Increased heart rate and shunting of blood from storage areas (e.g. spleen and splanchnic bed) to brain and muscles. Cardiac output may be increased 2-3 times normal.[107] As new vascular beds develop in wounds, cardiac demands are further increased.
8. Hypertension
9. Piloerection and hyperhydrosis (sweating)

Infection often accompanies trauma (i.e. wounds, surgery, burns) but may occur separately. A toxic response ensues as a result of an invasive infection and resorption of necrotic tissue. Lysosomal enzymes are released, as well as specific chemical mediators including histamine, kinins, prostaglandins, and serotonin. These substances amplify the previously mentioned responses to trauma. In addition fever, induced by interleukin-1 (endogenous pyrogen) released from phagocytic cells, causes an increase in energy expenditure estimated at 13% per degree celcius rise in body temperature.[107] This polypeptide also stimulates the increased degradation of muscle protein (proteolysis) that occurs during fever.[9] Another phagocytic cell product, leukocyte endogenous mediator (LEM) is released and causes the liver to produce acute-phase globulin proteins. Thus, energy-expensive protein synthesis is further stimulated. Endotoxins released from dead gram-negative bacteria trigger coagulation cascades[98] and induce profound effects on carbohydrate metabolism ranging from hyperglycemia to hypoglycemia and lactic acidosis.[47,64]

Cancer induces altered host metabolism. Neoplastic tissue is very competitive with the host for energy and nitrogen supplying nutrients. Also, many tumors use glucose anaerobically and therefore are metabolically inefficient, placing a disproportionate energy burden on the host,[30] and in the process generate increased amounts of lactic acid.

THE NEED TO FEED

As a result of the metabolic and physiologic changes induced by injury, infection, or cancer, the affected animal that appears on the outside to be resting quietly actually has the internal milieu of a dynamo. Unlike the starving animal, which has down-regulated its

metabolic rate to conserve energy, the injured/ diseased animal must recover from trauma, repair wounds, mount an immune response, or compete with cancer in order to survive. These processes require much cellular work and energy. Thus, **when injury, infection, or cancer are combined with food deprivation, they result in an accelerated form of starvation.** The adverse effects of food deprivation (page 5-6) occur much more rapidly; therefore, the ability to respond to in insult (e.g. maintenance of fluid, electrolyte, and acid-base status, defense mechanisms, and wound healing) is quickly and profoundly compromised. The importance of proper nutritional support for recovery from trauma, sepsis, and burn is well documented. [2,6,34,48,84,112,113] With proper feeding, the acute phase of the stress response is shortened, the adaptive phase occurs sooner (Figure 5, page 5-11), and body protein function is preserved. Feeding early has been shown to prevent 40% of the increased metabolic rate that occurs in traumatized animals.[10]

Aggressive nutritional support of cancer patients may not prolong life, but does improve the quality of life, the response to therapy, the recovery from therapy, and the patient's immunocompetence.[30,92] Besides anorexia and the metabolic burden that neoplasias impose, cancer therapies result in tissue injury and subsequent need for their repair. In addition, surgery, chemotherapy, and radiotherapy may result in decreased food intake for prolonged periods.[30] Appropriate nutritional support is an essential component of proper cancer therapy. The effects of both inanition and nutritional support on the response to injury and/or disease is summarized in Figure 3.

NUTRIENT PRECENDENCE AND REQUIREMENTS

During a period of inadequate food intake the body gives priority to certain functions as well as the nutrients required to perform them. The nutrient with the highest priority is water. The body goes to great extremes to conserve water. During a shortage of water, animals will decrease their water requirement by reducing food intake and decreasing physical activity,[110] and will decrease water losses by reducing urine volume. Reduction in urine quantity also may minimize other nutrient losses by this route.[99,100] During periods of inadequate food and water intake, signs and effects of water deficiency appear first.

The energy-supplying nutrients (carbohydrates, fats and proteins) have the second highest priority. Energy-supplying nutrients must be provided in

FIGURE 3

EFFECT OF FOOD DEPRIVATION AND NUTRITIONAL SUPPORT ON RESPONSES TO INJURY OR DISEASE

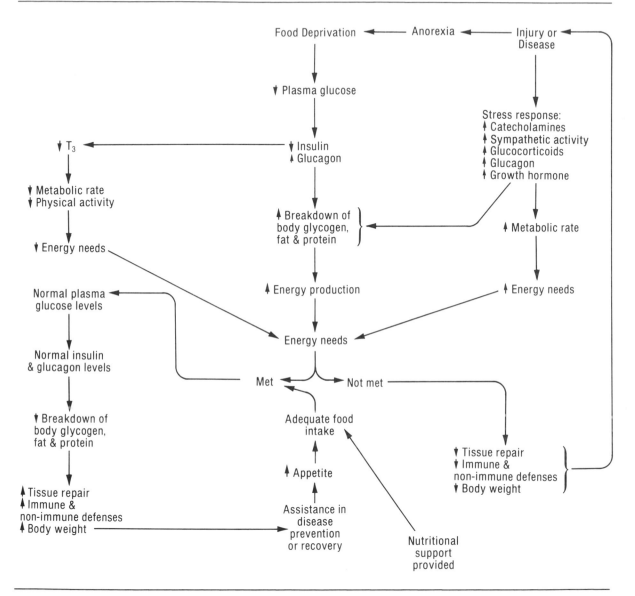

sufficient amounts or body tissues are used for energy with a resultant loss of function. Besides providing energy, protein is involved in a myriad of other functions. These functions, and therefore protein, have the third highest priority. Even if energy intake is adequate, protein deficiency suppresses growth, alters a variety of tissue functions, and retards wound healing.[84,132] During periods of food deprivation, signs and effects of energy deficiency occur prior to, and are more severe than, signs of protein deficiency.

Unless there is a disease-related increase in the loss of minerals and vitamins, clinical signs and effects of deficiencies of these nutrients, during periods of inadequate food and water intake, occur later than do signs of water, energy or protein deficiency.[59] Therefore, these nutrients, which are often given early in the course of many clinical conditions due to their ease of administration, are usually the **least** important ones to give therapeutically.

WATER REQUIREMENTS

For sick as well as healthy animals, water should always be available unless it is contraindicated, as in initial management of vomiting (see page 7-21). If water consumption is insufficient to prevent dehydration, water should be supplemented as described for fluid and electrolyte therapy (page 5-16).

Water is the nutrient animals require in the largest amount. An animal can survive loss of all of its glycogen, almost all of its storage fat, and nearly one-half of its protein; yet the acute loss of 10-15% of its water may result in death.

The animal's water needs are supplied by drinking water, water in the food consumed, and water resulting from energy metabolism called "metabolic water." Metabolic water normally provides about 10% of the total daily water requirement.[5] An average of 13 ml of water is produced per 100 kcal of energy metabolized.[5] The amount of water consumed as drinking water increases as the amount of water consumed in the food decreases.

Food deprivation eliminates the water obtained from food, changes the amount an animal drinks, and greatly decreases total water intake.[99,100] Figure 4 shows the effect of fasting on the amount of water consumed as drinking water and the total water intake for dogs previously fed a canned or a dry food. Total water intake decreases dramatically in both groups, but the change in the amount drunk is quite different. The response of dogs previously fed a canned diet is shown in panel A (Figure 4). Because the previous water intake by most of these dogs was obtained primarily from the food, only a small amount was drunk. During fasting, water in the food is no longer available, so the amount consumed as drinking water **increases.**

The response of dogs previously eating a dry food is shown in panel B (Figure 4). These dogs obtained little water from the food, so a large amount was drunk. During fasting, less water is needed, and the amount of water drunk **decreases.** Thus, when the previous food consumed was dry, the amount of water drunk during fasting is **less** than it was before fasting; whereas, when the previous food consumed was canned, the amount of water drunk during fasting is **more** than it was before fasting. This is true even though the total amount of water drunk during fasting is the same, regardless of the animal's previous diet.

The influence of previous diet on the amount of water consumed as drinking water can be important diagnostically. The owner reporting that a dog is not eating but is drinking twice as much

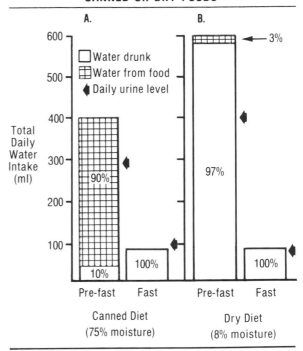

FIGURE 4

EFFECT OF FASTING ON THE AMOUNT OF WATER CONSUMED IN THE FOOD AND DRUNK BY BEAGLE DOGS PREVIOUSLY CONSUMING CANNED OR DRY FOODS

water, may be describing the normal response of a dog that has stopped eating a canned food. However, the dog that had been eating dry food may appear almost to stop drinking during periods of anorexia. These effects emphasize the importance of including a complete diet history as part of the anamnesis.

Water loss follows three different routes: 1) urinary, 2) fecal, and 3) "insensible losses" by evaporation from the respiratory tract, mucous membranes, and skin. In addition to the normal routes, water loss can occur because of vomiting, excessive salivation, and hemorrhage. In normal animals, water intake and excretion are closely balanced.[24] Approximately 7% of total water intake is excreted in the feces,[5] 70% in the urine, and the remainder as insensible losses.

Many diseases can alter the amount of water lost from any of the normal routes. With anorexia, in the absence of diarrhea, fecal water loss becomes minimal because stool output is greatly reduced. Decreased water intake is compensated for by increased renal reabsorption of water and production of a concentrated urine.[104] When water intake exceeds requirements, excesses are eliminated via the urine. In sick animals with normal kidneys,

these mechanisms greatly assist in compensating for inaccuracies in estimating fluid replacement needs.

Water requirements for dogs average 65-110 ml/kg/day, being larger the smaller the dog. Cats require 65-80 ml of water/kg/day. **The water requirement in milliliters for healthy animals approximately equals their energy requirement in kcal** (see Table 1, page 1-6, and page 1-2). This relationship is reflected in the energy density of milk (Table 4, page 3-18) and is convenient to remember when dosages for liquid diets (either enteral or parenteral) are being determined.

ENERGY REQUIREMENTS

Energy requirements are divided into basal (BER), resting (RER), and maintenance requirements (MER).

They are discussed in detail beginning on page 1-5. Basal energy requirements are those of an animal lying quietly in the post-absorptive state in a thermoneutral environment. Resting energy requirements include BER plus energy expended for recovery from physical activity. Resting energy requirements may vary from the same as BER to as much as 25% greater. Maintenance energy requirements are those needed for nutrient digestion and absorption, and normal physical activity. The MER is approximately twice BER for the dog and 1.4 times BER for the cat.

As discussed earlier (page 5-8), many factors affect the injured or diseased animal's caloric need. Most sick animals are inactive and anorectic and therefore do not have the normal maintenance needs for physical activity. These decreases in

FIGURE 5

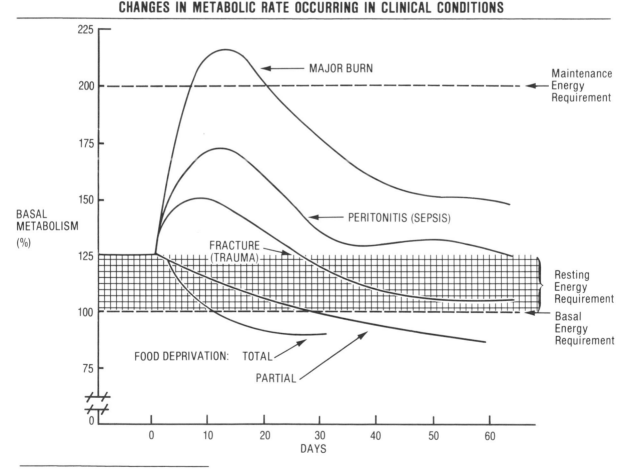

CHANGES IN METABOLIC RATE OCCURRING IN CLINICAL CONDITIONS

For example, the peak calories needed by the patient with peritonitis is about 75% more than is needed for the basal energy requirement, but is still 25% below that needed for maintenance activity.

Peaks indicate the acute phase of the generalized stress response. The adaptive phase follows (see page 5-11). Although this information is from people, it is probably applicable to animals.

caloric needs are partially offset by additional caloric needs related to the various injury or disease processes. As shown in Figure 5, injuries, infections, and burns all increase caloric needs in proportion to their severity.[63,83]

To determine the caloric needs of an ill patient, an estimate of the effect of the disease process on energy expenditure must be made. **It is important to note that BER rather than MER is the basis for calculating the energy needs of the injured or diseased patient** (see page 1-6). Use of MER results in a 1.4- to 2-fold food "overdose" and can cause metabolic (page 5-40) and gastrointestinal problems (page 5-34). The BER for dogs or cats weighing over 2 kg can be calculated:

$$BER \ (kcal/day) =$$
$$30 Wt_{kg} + 70 \quad (\text{see page 1-6}).$$

Calculation of the BER of all dogs or cats, regardless of body weight is calculated:
$$BER \ (kcal/day) =$$
$$70(Wt_{kg}^{0.75}) \quad (\text{see page 1-5}).$$

As indicated in Table 3 and Figure 6, a patient resting in a hospital cage expends about 25% more calories than needed for its BER, post-surgical needs are from 25-35% greater than BER,[63,107] trauma or cancer increase needs by about 35-50%,[63,92,96,107] infection from 50-70%,[63,107,119] and burn from 70-100% greater than BER.[63,96,107] The percent increase in energy needs listed for post-surgery, trauma, cancer, infection, and burn include the 25% allocated for cage rest. Using these values the sick animal's approximate water, caloric and protein needs can be estimated (Table 3 or Figure 6). These amounts establish minimal nutritional goals. Nutritional support should attempt to reach the goal for the animal's water needs within the first day, whereas goals for energy and protein should be reached within 48 hours after therapy begins (see page 5-8). These amounts of energy and protein may be well below those needed to restore body mass lost during the course of the disease. However, the immediate aim of nutritional support is to meet the animal's energy requirement and thereby attempt to halt disease-induced catabolism. Repletion of body substance may in most instances be deferred until the disease process is under control.

PROTEIN REQUIREMENTS

Protein makes up 15-20% of body weight and is second only to water in abundance in the body.[105] In the normal animal, protein synthesis, breakdown and resynthesis occur constantly. As discussed (page 5-6), the rate at which a protein turns over varies according to its metabolic activi-

TABLE 3

ENERGY REQUIREMENT OF INJURED OR DISEASED DOGS OR CATS*

Status**		Mathematical Factor**
Dogs and cats over 2 kg***		
BER (metabolizable kcal/day)	=	$(30 \ Wt_{kg} + 70)$
All dogs and cats***		
BER (metabolizable kcal/day)	=	$70 \ (Wt_{kg}^{0.75})$
Cage rest	=	$1.25 \times BER$
Post surgery	=	$1.25{-}1.35 \times BER$
Trauma	=	$1.35{-}1.5 \times BER$
Cancer	=	$1.35{-}1.5 \times BER$
Sepsis	=	$1.5{-}1.7 \times BER$
Major burn	=	$1.7{-}2.0 \times BER$

*For examples see pages 5-32 and 5-38.

**For discussion on derivation of these factors see page 5-12.

***For discussion of origin of these formulas see page 1-5.

ty. In the process, many constituent amino acids are reused. Because the reutilization of amino acids is not completely efficient, some nitrogen is constantly lost from the body.[127] The more rapid the protein's turnover rate, the more rapidly the amino acids must be replaced.[133] Dietary proteins normally provide amino acids and nitrogen to replace these daily losses. In the anorectic animal not receiving nutritional support, these losses are not replaced. Nitrogen is being excreted while none is taken in; thus, the animal is in negative nitrogen balance. Normal dogs, when adapted to inanition, lose nitrogen equivalent to 1.2-1.6 g protein/kg body weight/day.[38,105] However, losses are greater at the onset of anorexia (see Figure 2, page 5-6). With injury or disease, this initial increased rate of loss may continue, that is adaptation does not occur, which may lead to large nitrogen losses.

As previously discussed (page 5-5), during early stages of food deprivation, plasma glucose levels are maintained at the expense of readily mobilizable or labile proteins in plasma, liver, and the intestinal tract.[50] After the first few days of food deprivation, muscle proteins begin to be catabolized as well. Severely stressed patients, such as those with trauma, major burns, or sepsis, may be unable to provide sufficient amino acids for wound healing and immune function.[127] In addition, when presented, animals with chronic disease (e.g. cancer) may be protein-depleted because of inappetence and decreased food intake in the face of ongoing or increased nitrogen losses caused by the disease process.

FIGURE 6

MINIMAL WATER, ENERGY, AND PROTEIN NEEDS OF INJURED OR DISEASED DOGS AND CATS*

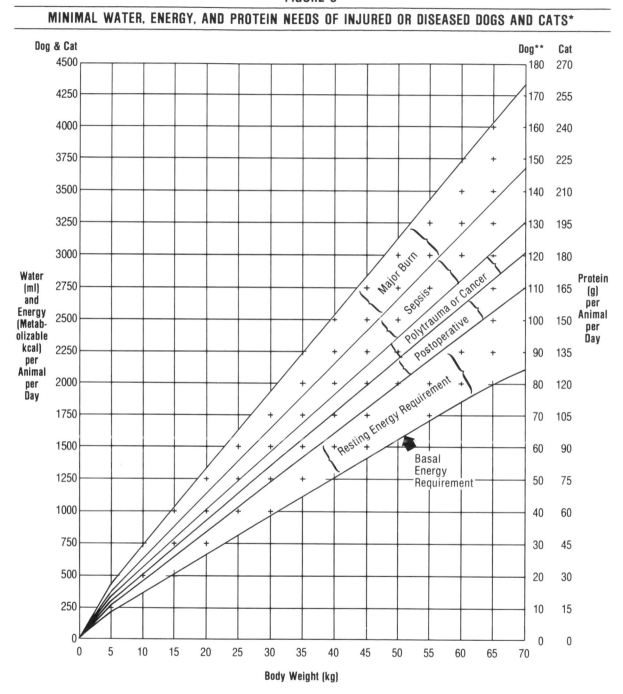

*These amounts, as determined for people, are the minimum needed for the patient resting in the hospital and are below that necessary to restore body mass. In most cases, nutritional support is necessary for only a few days and repletion of body mass may be deferred until anorexia terminates. For long-term nutritional support, these amounts should be increased sufficiently to maintain optimal body weight.

See pages 5-32 and 5-38 for examples.

**These amounts (4 g protein/100 kcal) are for moderate protein loss. For extensive protein loss in the dog use amounts listed for cats (6 g protein/100 kcal).

Also direct protein losses may occur with:
1. Hemorrhage
2. Protein-losing enteropathy, which may occur with or without diarrhea
3. Protein loosing nephropathy, which may occur with or without azotemia
4. Persistent vomiting
5. Draining wounds
6. Severe burns

Calculation of precise protein needs in disease is difficult. This is because of uncertainties concerning the patient's previous nutritional status and the effect of the disease on protein metabolism and severity of the insult. In a number of conditions such as surgical trauma, soft-tissue wounds, fractures, infections, or burn, protein is lost extensively during the acute phase of the injury or disease, while losses decrease during convalescence (adaptive phase, see Figure 5, page 5-11). In addition, during the acute phase, there is preferential use of branched-chain amino acids (leucine, isoleucine, and valine) as an energy source.[94,123,136,139]

Basal protein requirements may increase 2-3.5 times, depending on the severity of the disease.[12,85] Decreased efficiency of utilization results in protein needs for the dog of at least 4 g protein/100 kcal (calorie/nitrogen ratio of approximately 150:1) or about 16% of dietary energy as protein with the quality of egg. For the cat, or for managing extensive protein loss in the dog, this ratio should be increased to at least 6 g/100 kcal (calorie/nitrogen ratio of approximately 100:1, or about 24% of dietary energy as protein). If proteins of lower quality or digestibility are fed, amounts must be increased proportionally. Kidney diseases and some liver diseases are special cases which require careful use of limited amounts of high quality dietary protein (Table 13, page 5-33). The protein needs of the sick animal can be estimated from Figure 6 (page 5-13). However, the most practical approach to meeting the protein needs of the injured or diseased patient is the same as that recommended for physiologic states (page 1-16). Select a high-quality commercially-prepared diet containing the appropriate amount of protein balanced to the energy density of the diet. Then feed the selected diet to meet the patient's estimated energy requirement. Adherence to this approach simplifies and optimizes dietary management.

MINERAL AND VITAMIN REQUIREMENTS

The minerals and vitamins needed by injured or diseased animals are provided in the foods that supply dietary energy and protein. Additional mineral and vitamin needs depend on the type, duration, and severity of the disease process as well as the method of feeding and the diet being fed. Supplementation with several minerals and vitamins should be considered during extended periods of exclusive intravenous feeding. Zinc supplementation should be considered in anorectic patients, especially those with gastrointestinal disease where losses may be increased.[137] Zinc is important because of its role in protein synthesis, immune function, phagocytic activity, taste, and smell.[109] Zinc deficiency delays wound healing. However, zinc supplementation does not enhance wound healing if no deficiency exists.[74] Urinary excretion of zinc rises sharply after trauma.[74] Supplementation with 1 mg of elemental zinc/kg /day should be adequate until voluntary intake resumes (zinc sulfate, $ZnSO_4 \cdot 7H_2O$ contains 23% elemental zinc). Selenium supplementation should be given to patients receiving long-term intravenous feeding (see Table 11, page 1-20).[91] Patients being fed adequate amounts of high-quality blenderized enteral diets designed for the dog or cat (Tables 10 and 13, pages 5-29 and 5-33) should not need zinc supplementation.

Vitamin B complex supplementation may also be beneficial in the anorectic animal. Little research, however, has been conducted on the effect of various diseases on vitamin requirements. The work that has been done indicates that at least a few of the water-soluble vitamin (ascorbic acid, riboflavin, pyridoxine, and folic acid) requirements are increased with injury or disease associated stress.[72,84] Vitamin K supplementation should be considered for cases where intensive antibiotic therapy is being employed, because antibiotics may decrease intestinal bacterial synthesis.[72,84] All vitamins should be supplemented to animals on prolonged, exclusive intravenous feeding.[72,91] It is recommended that mineral and vitamin intake during disease be at least as much as that needed for maintenance (Tables 11 and 13), pages 1-20 and 1-33). Feeding good-quality enteral diets designed for managing injury/disease-induced stress should provide adequate minerals and vitamins in most situations. Thus, administration of additional vitamin/mineral supplements usually is not required.

PATIENT SELECTION FOR NUTRITIONAL SUPPORT

Nutritional assessment is an important part of the evaluation of all patients. **Certainly not all patients require nutritional support.** Such support is not necessary for well-nourished animals undergoing elective surgical procedures that do

not result in extensive trauma, i.e. where hypermetabolism and inappetance are not anticipated. Identification of patients needing nutritional support is based on history, physical examination, laboratory evaluation, and common sense. Important historical information includes: 1) types and amounts of all foods eaten, 2) appetite and frequency of feeding, 3) recent weight changes, 4) presence of gastrointestinal dysfunctions including any difficulty in chewing or swallowing food, and 5) type and dosage of any medication being given should also be considered. "Medications" could range from nutritional supplements to drugs that alter protein metabolism such as corticosteroids, immunosuppressants, certain antibiotics, and antitumor agents. Also, many drugs alter sensations of taste and smell or directly affect appetite (Table 2, page 5-5).[7,63,116,117] Factors which generally indicate a need for nutritional support are listed in Table 4.

The extent to which the animal is under- or overweight is evaluated during the physical examination. Lack of subcutaneous fat, or presence of muscle wasting or edema are indications of chronic

TABLE 4

INDICATIONS FOR NUTRITIONAL SUPPORT[17]

From History:

1. Recent loss of greater than 10% of usual body weight or below optimal body weight
2. Recent surgery or trauma
3. Restricted food intake or infusion of simple intravenous solutions for more than 3–5 days
4. Increased losses caused by:
   a. Nausea, vomiting, diarrhea, or malabsorption from any cause
   b. Surgical absence of portions of the gastrointestinal tract
   c. Draining abscesses, wounds or burn
5. Increased nutrient needs caused by:
   a. Extensive burns, infection, trauma, or recent surgery
   b. Fever
6. Use of antinutrient or catabolic drugs, such as:
   a. Corticosteroids, immunosuppressants, anticancer agents, and antibiotics
7. Cancer or other chronic disease or organ dysfunction

From Physical Examination:

1. General appearance—cachexia, edema
2. Skin—thin, dry, scaly, easily pluckable hair, decubital ulcers, non-healing wounds
3. Musculoskeletal—muscle weakness and atrophy, growth retardation, bone or joint pain, metaphyseal swelling
4. Organ systems—hepatomegaly, splenomegaly, ascites, small bowel distention, lymphadenopathy, tumors, pregnancy

malnutrition. Obese anorectic patients should be carefully examined as obesity can mask lean-tissue depletion. All normal body processes depend on adequate nutrition for normal function. For this reason, clinical signs specific for malnutrition do not occur.

Many laboratory parameters are affected by food deprivation, but few are specific indicators of malnutrition.[81] A decrease in plasma albumin concentration[18,97,103] or albumin/globulin ratio, transferrin concentration,[18,97] and total lymphocyte count may indicate poor nutritional status. Prealbumin and retinol-binding protein have shorter half-lives and are also used in human medicine as an indication of nutritional status.[57] Fibronectin (a plasma opsonic protein) also appears to be a sensitive index of nutritional status in human patients. However, except for plasma albumin, globulin, and total lymphocyte counts, all of these tests are expensive and difficult to perform and are not used clinically in dogs or cats.[34] It has been reported that animals found to have a preoperative albumin concentration below 2.0 g/dl have a higher rate of wound dehiscence, seroma formation, and infection as compared to animals with a normal plasma albumin concentration. Providing preoperative nutritional therapy for 2-3 days decreased the incidence of these postoperative problems.[34] Plasma albumin concentrations of less than 20%, between 20-40%, and greater than 40% below normal are used in human medicine to indicate mild, moderate, and severe protein depletions, respectively.[59]

The plasma half-life of albumin in dogs is 8.2 days,[41] which is a short enough time for decreases to occur before nutritional depletion is severe. Plasma albumin concentration may also be decreased as a result of decreased production caused by liver disease, or as a result of increased loss such as occurs with protein-losing enteropathy or nephropathy.

A decrease in the plasma albumin, like all plasma concentrations, is lessened or masked by dehydration. In addition, the plasma albumin concentration (like the blood urea nitrogen concentration [BUN]) decreases with decreasing dietary protein. This will occur even though dietary protein and calorie intake are adequate. For example, a diet containing 8-10% of a high-quality/highly-digestible protein in its dry matter will meet the normal dog's protein requirement but will result in a plasma albumin concentration of 2 to 2.5% and a BUN of 1-6 mg/dl (as compared to 3-3.5 and 10-25 mg/dl when a 25-40% protein diet is being consumed). Thus, the protein content of the diet, as well as the state of hydration, must be con-

sidered in evaluating the plasma albumin concentration.

Total lymphocyte count may be depressed by protein depletion. Even if the total number of lymphocytes is in the normal range, functional abnormalities may be present—a condition which adversely affects immune function.[23] Stress and immunosuppressive drugs can also decrease lymphocyte numbers. **Although laboratory parameters are sometimes helpful, changes indicative of nutritional status occur after other changes detectable from the anamnesis and physical examination.**

Undernutrition may not be a factor when the patient is admitted but may become apparent during hospitalization. Undesirable hospital practices that may cause undernutrition are listed in Table 5. These should be avoided, and the patient managed as shown in Figure 7 (page 5-19).[86] However, **regardless of the animal's previous nutritional status or its laboratory values, an animal that is sick and not eating should be fed as soon as possible, unless a specific contraindication exists.**[101,103] Studies indicate that early feeding significantly improves response.

Guinea pigs with thermal injuries fed within 2 hours after receiving the injury had statistically lower metabolic rates, greater small intestine weight and mucosa thickness, and lower plasma cortisol levels compared to guinea pigs not fed until 72 hours post-injury.[95] Thus, early feeding resulted in a diminished stress response and sparing of visceral protein breakdown. In human trauma patients significant improvement in nitrogen balance was demonstrated in patients given nutritional support within 18 hours postoperatively as compared to patients that experienced less trauma but were not given nutritional support for 5 days.[97] In addition, septic complications occurred in 29% of the late-fed group compared to none in the early-fed group. Many studies have demonstrated reduced postoperative weight loss, improved nitrogen balance, increased protein synthesis, accelerated wound repair, and improved immunocompetence in patients given early postoperative nutritional support.[103] In addition, providing nutritional support early allows installation of feeding tubes or catheters at a time when the patient may already be undergoing surgery and anesthesia, obviating the need for additional stressful procedures. Therefore, rather than waiting until obvious laboratory or clinical signs of undernutrition have been manifested (Table 4, page 5-15), scientific evidence and common sense dictate that for optimal response, nutritional support should be provided as early as possible, preferably as soon as the patient's fluid, electrolyte, and acid-base status have been stabilized.

FLUID AND ELECTROLYTE THERAPY

Because of the primary importance of proper fluid balance, this equilibrium must be reestablished as the first step of nutritional support. There are three primary goals of fluid therapy:[93]

1. Rehydration or treatment of shock
2. Electrolyte replacement
3. Normalization of acid-base status

Feeding should begin only after these three goals are accomplished.

The oral route is preferred for fluid and electrolyte administration. Contraindications for this route include vomiting or conditions so acute or severe that mesenteric blood flow is inadequate for fluid absorption to occur (8% or greater dehydration—Table 6). For best results, fluids used for oral administration should be formulated to take advantage of the synergistic effect that sodium, glucose, bicarbonate, and certain amino acids have on the absorption of each other and, therefore, water. When properly formulated, these fluids result in the maximum rate of absorption (e.g. Life-Guard, Norden).

TABLE 5

UNDESIRABLE PRACTICES AFFECTING THE NUTRITIONAL STATUS OF HOSPITAL PATIENTS

1. Failure to record weight daily or more frequently in acute cases.
2. Rotation of staff at frequent intervals and diffusion of responsibility for patient care.
3. Prolonged administration of glucose and electrolyte solutions without added nutritional support.
4. Failure to observe, measure, and record the amount of food consumed.
5. Withholding food because of multiple diagnostic tests.
6. Failure to recognize and treat increased nutritional needs brought about by injury or illness.
7. Performance of surgical procedures without first making certain that the patient is optimally nourished, and failure to give nutritional support after surgery.
8. Failure to appreciate the role of nutrition in the prevention of and recovery from infection; unwarranted reliance on drugs.
9. Delay of nutritional support until the patient is in an advanced state of depletion which is sometimes irreversible.
10. Limited availability of laboratory tests to assess nutritional status and a failure to use those that are available.

TABLE 6

ESTIMATING DEGREE OF DEHYDRATION[a]

Percentage of Dehydration	Physical Findings
< 5	No abnormalities present.
6	Slightly doughy inelasticity of skin so that it remains in a pinched position longer than normal.[b]
8	Definite inelasticity of skin; capillary refilling time 2-3 sec.[c], slight enopthalmos, mouth and mucous membranes dry.
10-12	Severe skin inelasticity; capillary refilling time greater than 3 sec.; marked enopthalmos; cold extremities; shock in debilitated animals; involuntary muscle twitching; tachycardia generally present.
12-15	Marked shock; imminent death.

[a]Liters of fluid needed to correct the dehydration equals the percent dehydration times kilograms of body weight.

[b]Best evaluated over the dorsal midline of the lumbar region and not loose skin, such as on the neck. A cachectic animal's skin, even without dehydration present, loses elasticity; whereas an obese animal tends to retain its skin elasticity even when dehydration is severe. In cats, dry oral mucous membranes may be the only noticeable sign of dehydration until it is severe enough to cause sufficient peripheral vasoconstriction to result in a clinically detectable decrease in the temperature of the extremities. However, open-mouthed breathing, such as occurs with nasal congestion or discharge, quickly results in dry membranes even though body hydration may be normal.

[c]Normal capillary refilling time is 1½ to 2 seconds.

If fluids cannot be given orally, they may be administered either subcutaneously or intravenously. In any case, it is important that fluids be warmed to body temperature before they are administered (for reasons described on page 9-21). Subcutaneous administration of fluids may be used alone or in conjunction with oral or intravenous fluid therapy. However, if the animal is more than 6% dehydrated (Table 6), at least one-half of the existing deficit must be given intravenously to increase blood volume and circulation to, and therefore absorption from, the subcutaneous tissues. In addition, fluids should not be given subcutaneously if subcutaneous edema is present.

Fluids given subcutaneously should be sterile, contain nearly isotonic concentrations of electrolytes, and contain not more than 2.5% glucose (glucose is not an electrolyte). It is best not to give more than 20-30 ml/kg at one time, and to administer it in several sites. The rate at which fluid is administered subcutaneously is dictated only by the patient's comfort. Fluids administered subcutaneously are absorbed over 6-8 hours unless peripheral vasoconstriction is present.

Fluids must be given intravenously if:

1. Dehydration is 8% or more
2. Fluid losses are occurring faster than they can be absorbed from the intestinal tract or subcutaneous tissues
3. Shock or symptoms of altered plasma electrolyte concentrations are present or of concern
4. The gastrointestinal tract cannot be used or subcutaneous edema is present
5. A hypertonic solution is needed to induce diuresis or treat for edema

The rate of intravenous fluid administration must be adjusted for each situation. In the majority of the cases, one-half of the fluid deficit may be given during the first 1-3 hours, and the remainder over the next 8-24 hours.

An estimate of the fluid deficit may be made from the presence of the signs given in Table 6. The percent dehydration multiplied by the body weight, in kilograms, yields the liters of fluid deficit present. The first concern in fluid therapy is to replace this deficit. Once this is accomplished, if continued fluid administration is needed, the amount given should be sufficient to replace continuing losses and thus maintain body weight. The fluids most commonly used and indications for their use are given in Table 7.

For patients that are dehydrated because of anorexia, an extracellular replacement fluid (ECRF) such as Ringer's lactate with O-5% glucose added is generally best for correcting the initial deficit. An ECRF contains electrolytes at the same concentration as is normally present in the extracellular fluid (ECF). Thus, administration of an ECRF will alter neither normal ECF electrolyte concentrations nor acid-base status. The animal's acid-base status may be determined and corrected as described on page 9-21.

If acidosis is present, it may be corrected by adding sodium bicarbonate to the fluid being administered. If the fluid contains calcium, adding bicarbonate will result in the formation of calcium carbonate, which makes the fluid cloudy. The calcium carbonate that forms will settle out as a white precipitate. Several hours are required for this reaction to become visible. No problems are created if the fluid is administered before this occurs.

If alkalosis is present, Ringer's solution or isotonic saline solution should be administered. These solutions do not contain bicarbonate or bicarbonate precursors (such as lactate, acetate, or citrate) and have a higher chloride content than

TABLE 7

SOLUTIONS AND ADDITIVES FOR FLUID AND ELECTROLYTE THERAPY

Solutions	Content	Metab kcal/L	Route of Administration and Usual Uses
Ringer's Lactate, Acetate or Bicarbonate	Same as ECF or plasma	9	Parenteral ECF (extracellular fluid) replacement
Ringer's	ECF without a bicarbonate producer	0	Parenteral ECF replacement and acidification
Isotonic Saline	0.9% NaCl	0	Parenteral ECF replacement and acidification with hyperkalemia present
Isotonic Dextrose	5% glucose	170	IV for hypertonic dehydration
Hypertonic Dextrose	20% glucose	680	IV for osmotic diuresis, hypoglycemia and to provide energy
Maintenance Fluid	5% glucose, 20–40 Na,K,Cl & HCO_3 and 0–5 Ca,P & Mg mEq/L	170	Parenteral replacement of non-pathologic losses in anorexia
Protein Hydrolysate, 10%	Hypertonic	400	IV feeding, usually given mixed with equal parts of 50–70% glucose solution
Total Parenteral Feeding Fluid	10–25% glucose, 5% amino acids, maintenance level of electrolytes, B vitamins	600–1200	IV feeding
Oral Nutrient-Electrolyte Fluid	1–6% glucose, 0–3% amino acids and maintenance to plasma concentrations of electrolytes	600–2000	Oral fluid therapy
Additives			**Added to solutions as needed for**
Dextrose	50% glucose	1700	Osmotic diuresis, hypoglycemia and energy
Jam and Jelly Pectin	4 g glucose/tsp	4/g	Oral source of energy, particularly beneficial for animals with enteritis
Sodium Bicarbonate (7.5%)	1 mEq $NaHCO_3$/ml	0	Parenteral alkalinizer
Baking Soda	4 g $NaHCO_3$/tsp	0	Oral alkalinizer
Potassium Chloride	1 or 2 mEq/ml	0	Parenteral correction of potassium deficiency
Potassium Gluconate	0.75 mEq K^+/ml	0	Oral correction of potassium deficiency
Salt Substitute	4 g KCl/tsp	0	Oral correction of potassium deficiency
Lite Salt	2 g NaCl & 2 g KCl/tsp	0	Oral correction of potassium, sodium and chloride deficiency
Calcium Gluconate 10%	466 mEq Ca^{++}/L (9.3 mg/ml)	0	IV correction of hypocalcemia
Calcium Gluconate 23%	1070 mEq Ca^+/L (21.4 mg/ml)	0	IV correction of hypocalcemia

the ECF. Thus, their administration lowers the ECF bicarbonate concentration and, therefore, will tend to correct metabolic alkalosis. Rarely is it necessary, or of benefit, to give solutions more acidifying than Ringer's solution or isotonic saline solution, such as those containing ammonium chloride. However, frequently 10-20 mEq/L of potassium chloride must be added to the fluid administered to the alkalotic animal. This is done to correct a total body potassium deficit, with or without hypokalemia. As hydrogen ions are conserved by the alkalotic animal, potassium and sodium are excreted in the urine. In addition, much potassium, sodium and chloride are lost in vomitus—vomition being the main cause of meta-

bolic alkalosis (see page 7-15 for a discussion of the acid-base status of the vomiting animal).

If additional non-feeding fluids are needed after the animal's initial fluid and electrolyte deficits and acid-base alterations are corrected, an oral nutrient electrolyte fluid is best (Life-Guard, Norden); or if the fluids are to be given intravenously, a maintenance fluid (Table 7) should be used. Normal sodium, potassium, and chloride requirements are 19-25 mEq of each per 1000 kcal or per liter of fluid.[65] These amounts, as well as 5% glucose (which provides enough calories to prevent fasting-induced ketosis but less than 20% of caloric needs) are provided by a maintenance fluid. Additional electrolytes, as indicated by plasma concen-

trations or signs, should be added to the fluid as needed.

ENTERAL FEEDING

Feeding should begin after fluid volume, electrolyte, and acid-base abnormalities have been corrected. Animals may be fed via the gastrointestinal tract (enteral nutrition) or intravenously (total parenteral nutrition). Factors suggesting which method of feeding to use are given in Figure 7.

The basic rule of critical-care nutrition is **"if the gut works, use it!"**, and the gut works a large percentage of the time.[67] Feeding via the gastrointestinal tract is the simplest, fastest, easiest, safest, least expensive, most physiologic, and best method of feeding; it should be used whenever possible. When compared to parenteral feeding, enteral feeding is less likely to induce hepatic lipidosis,[89] results in increased secretory IgA production,[4] and improved resistance to infectious challenge.[77] When the gut does work, the animal may be induced to eat (appetite stimulation), force fed, or tube fed (via an orogastric, nasogastric, pharyngostomy, gastrostomy, or enterostomy tube).

The simplest method, for which there are no contraindications, should be tried first. If it is not completely effective, continue using it in conjunction with other feeding methods. Frequently, a number of feeding methods used together are effective in providing sufficient nutrients to meet the animal's needs; whereas, any single procedure alone may not be totally effective. For example, first try to stimulate the anorectic animal to eat voluntarily. If this is not completely successful force feed, tube feed, or both, while continuing attempts to stimulate voluntary food intake. If these procedures are not adequate, administer at least some of the needed nutrients intravenously while continuing to feed orally. Regardless of which feeding method or combination of feeding methods is used, caloric intake should be sufficient to maintain body weight.

If the animal is undernourished, a diet adequate (particularly in protein) for growth should be fed, unless a diet of this type in contraindicated by the presence of other conditions such as uremia. Lean body mass can be restored more rapidly with less food and fewer calories by using a higher-protein growth/lactation-type diet rather than a maintenance-type diet (Table 2, page 3-5 or Table 2, page 4-6).[3,50]

When the animal is fed via the gastrointestinal tract, giving small amounts at frequent intervals is best. The animal should be fed at least 2-3 times daily and in some cases 4-6 times daily. Small

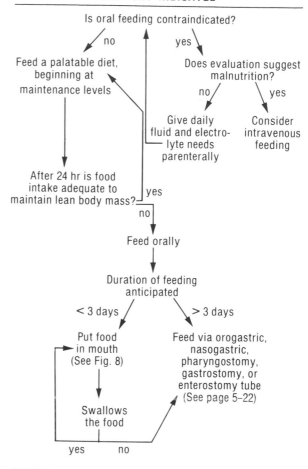

FIGURE 7

DETERMINING THE TYPE OF NUTRITIONAL SUPPORT INDICATED

amounts fed at frequent intervals result in increased utilization of nutrients and often enhance the animal's appetite sufficiently to initiate voluntary eating.

APPETITE STIMULATION

A number of techniques may be used to induce animals to eat. Some animals may not eat when hospitalized. At home, in a familiar surrounding with lots of tender loving care provided by family members, these pets may eat more readily. Thus, do not hospitalize undernourished or anorectic animals unless it is necessary. Many animal owners are willing and able to perform feeding and treatment procedures if properly instructed. Animals should be hospitalized if their owners cannot give them proper care at home, if diagnostic procedures are to be conducted, or veterinary supervision is necessary.

Staying with an animal when food is offered may encourage it to eat. Because hospitalized animals are in unfamiliar surroundings, among strangers, and often being subjected to unpleasant diagnostic procedures and treatments, fear-induced inhibition of food intake is a frequent problem. Petting, in conjunction with vocal reassurance, may be all that is necessary to induce eating. Mixing a highly palatable canned food (e.g. Science Diet Mixit, Hill's) with the usual food will often increase palatability enough to induce the dog or cat to eat. Warming the food to body temperature (but not more) will enhance its aroma and also directly improves palatability (see Figure 1, page 2-3). If necessary, cleaning the animal's nose to improve its ability to smell the food may be helpful, particularly for cats. Intranasal instillation of 5% saline drops can be used for this purpose.

If the foregoing procedures fail, try a different food. Some cats prefer a dry food or a canned gourmet food (see page 2-2). Most dogs greatly prefer a good-quality cat food. Prescription Diets Feline p/d and Feline c/d (Hill's) have been used successfully to induce anorectic dogs to eat. If this is not successful, try a canned nutritionally complete gourmet-type cat food or meat-type dog food such as Alpo Beef Chunks Dinner (Alpo Pet Foods) or Mighty Dog (Carnation). An animal that will not eat from a bowl, may take food if hand-fed. If these methods are unsuccessful and hospitalization is necessary, the owner can be asked to come in to feed the animal. One or two days are usually sufficient.

Once the animal begins eating, it usually continues voluntarily. Additional factors affecting food acceptability and palatability that might be helpful are described on page 2-2.

Animals that are sick or anorectic for more than a few days may have potassium, zinc, or B-vitamin deficiencies. A potassium deficit causes lethargy and anorexia. A zinc deficiency decreases the sense of taste and smell and may cause anorexia. If the animal is anorectic, fully hydrated, and not anuric, and if the plasma potassium concentration is less than 4 mEq/L, add 1-2 mEq of potassium chloride/kg of body weight to the food or a nutrient-electrolyte fluid given orally. This may be done by giving 1/4 teaspoon (1 g)/5-10 kg body weight of salt substitute (KCl) which is available in most grocery stores. Giving vitamin B-complex and 1 mg of elemental zinc/kg body weight/day may also be helpful in stimulating voluntary food consumption (see page 5-14 for zinc source and percentages). Giving potassium, zinc and B-vitamins may be helpful in some cases and, when they

are given as described, are not harmful (for vitamin dosages, see Table 13, page 1-23).

Drugs may also be used to stimulate the appetite. Benzodiazepines have been used for this purpose in a variety of species.[7] Diazepam (Valium, Roche) stimulated food intake in experiments with cats and puppies given oral doses of 2 and 14 mg/kg of body weight, respectively.[40] Diazepam is commonly used clinically for this purpose in both dogs and cats. Almost all cats that are physically able will eat immediately after intravenous administration of 0.1-0.5 mg/cat of diazepam.[63] Food must be available when the drug is given. Oral administration of 1-2 mg/cat will maintain appetite stimulation in most cats.[126] Oxazepam (Serax, Wyeth) also has transiently stimulated appetite in cats, but to a greater degree than diazepam. The recommended oral dose is approximately 2 mg/cat (1/8 of a 15-mg tablet). An appetite response is apparent within 30 minutes. Appetite stimulation with diazepam or oxazepam should be used on a temporary basis only (approximately 2 days or less). Corticosteroids and anabolic steroids are also occasionally administered to stimulate food intake. Although they may improve appetite in some cases, because of their other effects, they are not recommended.

FORCE FEEDING

If all attempts fail to induce the animal to eat voluntarily, it may be force-fed. A convenient method of force-feeding is shown in Figure 8. Placing food into the pharyngeal area stimulates the swallowing reflex, which causes the food to be swallowed. This method usually meets with little resistance from ill or debilitated animals. However, when the animal has reasonable control of its activity, the method often meets with less than full cooperation. But, some animals that refuse to eat voluntarily swallow food placed in their mouth, particularly when this is done in small quantities gently and with petting and vocal reassurance. A highly digestible, palatable and caloric-dense diet should be used. A good high-fat (20% or greater in the food dry matter) cat diet such as Prescription Diets Feline p/d or Feline c/d (Hill's) works well for both dogs and cats.

Semisolid oral calorie supplements such as Nutrical (Evsco) are available in tubes. These products, used by some veterinarians to supply supplemental nourishment, have several shortcomings: 1) the labels warn they should not be given for long periods because they are not complete and balanced, 2) the labels may not indicate the energy density of the product or how much to give, 3) because of their toothpaste-like consistency, it is

FIGURE 8
A METHOD OF FORCE FEEDING

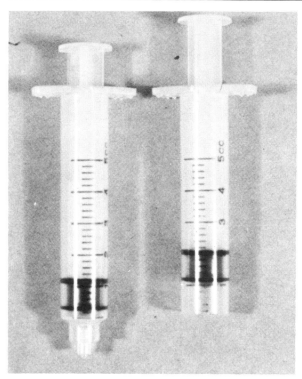

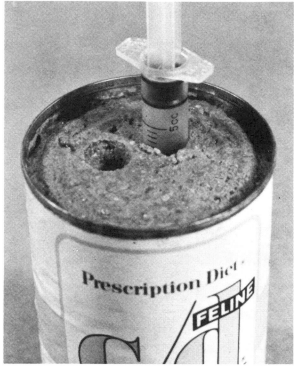

STEP 1
Cut off the end of a syringe and smooth the edges so they will not cut the animal's mouth. A 5-ml syringe works well for cats, and a 10-ml syringe for dogs.

STEP 3
Place the filled syringe into the animal's mouth and eject the core of food.

STEP 2
Push the open end of the syringe into the food, allowing the plunger to rise as the food fills the barrel. Remove the syringe with a gentle twist, retrieving a core of food. Use a high-fat, caloric-dense food such as Prescription Diets Feline p/d or Feline c/d (Hill's) for either dogs or cats. One 10-ml core of this food provides 25 kcal or the approximate daily requirement for 1 lb. body weight.

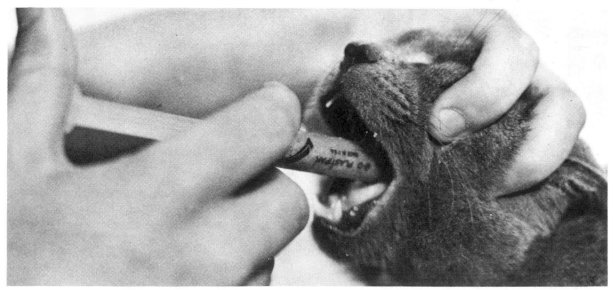

difficult and time consuming to administer adequate quantities, and 4) they provide little water.

Human baby food meats can be used as nutrient supplements for anorectic animals. These products are palatable for many sick pets but may produce diarrhea in some. Administration of baby food meats or egg yolks may be helpful in restoring voluntary food consumption, but these products are not nutritionally balanced and should not be given as a sole diet for more than 2-3 days. They are also considerably more costly than the nutritionally balanced pet foods recommended.

If force-feeding is successful, it may be used for as long as necessary. However, force-feeding can be a slow, tedious process. If feeding is necessary for more than a few days, tube-feeding should be considered.

TUBE FEEDING*

In many instances, tube feeding is much faster, easier, less stressful to the patient, and more successful than force feeding. Animals that resist force-feeding, or that are too depressed to be successfully force fed, may be tube fed.

The dog and cat may be tube fed via orogastric, nasogastric, pharyngostomy, gastrostomy, or enterostomy routes. The least invasive methods are orogastric and nasogastric. Diets for tube feeding, diet dosages, and recommendations for feeding frequency are described on pages 5-29, 5-32 and 5-32, respectively.

Feeding Tube Placement

Orgastric Intubation—Orogastric tube feeding is generally used for 2-3 days duration in an animal whose disposition is such that intubation can be accomplished with minimal restraint and stress. Use a soft-rubber urinary catheter (8-12 French for cats and small dogs, 12-24 French for larger dogs). Mark the tube for depth of placement as shown in Figure 9. Lubricate the tube with water or a tasteless lubricant. Open the animal's mouth just far enough to introduce the tube (Figure 10) and pass it over the tongue, keeping the head in a normal position (Figure 11). Limited restraint and opening the mouth just far enough to introduce the tube will minimize the animal's objections. When the animal swallows, advance the tube down the esophagus to the premeasured mark. Instill 5-10 ml sterile

*Appreciation is expressed to Charles A. Buffington DVM, MS, Department of Physiological Sciences, School of Veterinary Medicine, University of California, Davis, CA 95016 for his assistance on this chapter, particularly this section.

FIGURE 9

INTUBATION PROCEDURES

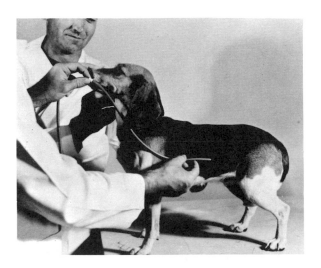

Premark tubes with a marker or piece of tape, prior to insertion as follows: For accurate gastric placement, insert to the level of the 9th intercostal space. Deeper insertion may result in a doubling over of the tube which could induce esophageal trauma when removed. For indwelling nasal or pharyngeal tubes, caudal-esophageal rather than gastric placement is preferable for minimizing gastric reflux and esophagitis. For accurate caudal-esophageal placement, insert the tube no deeper than the 7th intercostal space. When rib location cannot readily be determined (e.g. obesity), use 90% (gastric) or 75% (caudal esophagus) of the distance from the tip of the nose to the last rib.

water to assure that the trachea has not been intubated.[63]

Nasogastric Intubation—A nasogastric tube may be left in place for extended periods of time (several weeks or longer) and is usually well-tolerated if properly inserted.[25,36,51] The animal can eat or drink with the tube in place. A number of different types of tubes, as given in Table 8 may be used for nasogastric indubation. Polyvinyl tubes are the least expensive and work quite well; however, they will harden if left in the stomach for longer than two weeks. For this reason it is important that polyvinyl tubes not be inserted too deeply. If they are too long, they may double back, harden, and be difficult to remove without traumatizing the stomach or esophagus. If a polyvinyl tube is to be used for longer periods, it should be changed weekly, or it can be positioned in the caudal esophagus (see Figure 9). Alternatively, polyurethane or silicone tubes, which are

FIGURE 10

OROGASTRIC INTUBATION PROCEDURES

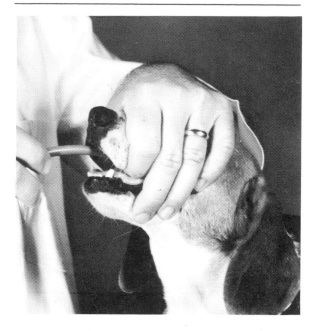

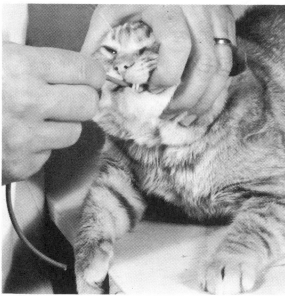

Restrain the animal's head by grasping it with the free hand and inserting the index finger into the mouth. At the same time fold the lip inward over the premolars. The index finger acts as a spacer to establish the proper gap between the incisors. The three other fingers should be used to prevent the mandible from opening too wide and prevent chewing on the index finger or catheter. An alternative procedure to prevent the animal from chewing or biting the tube is to insert into the animal's mouth a disposable syringe case with the closed end cut off and smoothed, or a roll of tape, through which the tube may be passed. If necessary the mouth, with these in place, may be tied shut.

FIGURE 11

OROGASTRIC INTUBATION PROCEDURES

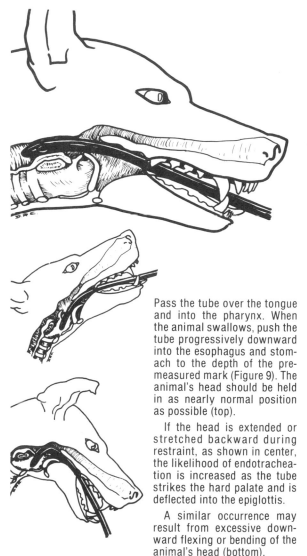

Pass the tube over the tongue and into the pharynx. When the animal swallows, push the tube progressively downward into the esophagus and stomach to the depth of the pre-measured mark (Figure 9). The animal's head should be held in as nearly normal position as possible (top).

If the head is extended or stretched backward during restraint, as shown in center, the likelihood of endotracheation is increased as the tube strikes the hard palate and is deflected into the epiglottis.

A similar occurrence may result from excessive downward flexing or bending of the animal's head (bottom).

resistant to gastric acid, can be used. The size of tube to use is given in Table 9 (page 5-26).

The use of a stylet, either wire or nylon, may add rigidity to tubes that are too flexible. A 15° angle 2 cm from the tip of the stylet makes the tube easier to pass. If stylets are used they should be lubricated for easier withdrawal. They should not extent beyond the tip of the nasogastric tube or they could traumatize the mucosa. Inadvertant endotracheal intubation with a nasogastric tube guided by a wire-stylet has resulted in pulmonary damage, including pneumothorax and pneumonia, in people [130]

For nasogastric intubation, the appropriate tube is selected (Tables 8 and 9, page 5-26), premeasured, and marked (Figure 9, page 5-22). The nasal cavity should be desensitized and the tube inserted as shown and described in Figure 12, and illustrated in Figure 13. As the tube is passed under the maxilloturbinate bone (Figure 13) some resistance may be encountered. As the ventral meatus narrows because of ventral expansion of the maxilloturbinate (Figure 13). If the tube does not pass ventrally, it will continue caudally through the dorsal or middle meatus and lodge against the ethmoidal turbinates at a level between the middle and caudal thirds of the nasal cavity. If this occurs, withdraw the tube and readvance it ventromedially. Once the tube successfully passes under the maxilloturbinate it can be readily advanced through the nasopharynx into the pharynx. At this point, proper positioning of the animal's head is essential (Figure 11) to prevent endotracheal intubation, which can easily occur. Many dogs show absolutely no distress or discomfort with the tube in the trachea. The tube is advanced to the premeasured mark (Figure 9, page 5-22). If a stylet has been used, it should now be removed. Prior lubrication of the lumen of the tube allows for easy removal of the stylet after insertion of the tube has been completed. Occasionally dogs or cats may shake their head and sneeze while the tube is being inserted.

Esophageal, rather than tracheal, tube location should be assured by oral examination (visual and/or digital, dog), injecting air through the tube while ascultating for gurgling sounds over the desired location (caudal portion of the thorax for caudal esophageal placement and cranial left paralumbar region for stomach placement). If the tube appears to be in the esophagus, inject 5-10 ml of sterile water or saline solution through the tube while ascultating for gurgling sounds from the tracheobronchial tree and observing for coughing. If uncertainty remains, obtain a lateral thoracic radiograph. Radiography can also assure desired depth of tube in the gastrointestinal tract.

After confirming proper tube placement, the tube should be attached to the skin of the muzzle and face using 3-0 or 4-0 nonabsorbable suture swaged on a cutting needle. The first suture should be placed as close as possible to the external nares. Tape "butterflies" can be used (Figure 14). In the cat, the tube must not touch the whiskers. Surprisingly, if the suture is passed quickly through the skin, no local anesthesia is necessary and the procedure meets with little or no resistance from the patient. It is preferable to attach the catheter to the animal's facial skin at 4-8 cm intervals and to direct the tube caudally over the forehead and the dorsum of the neck. An Elizabethan collar is essential to prevent the animal from removing the tube. Be sure the cone of the collar extends far enough cranially. When the tubes are not in use, keep them capped to prevent gastric accumulation of air.

FIGURE 12
NASOGASTRIC INTUBATION PROCEDURES

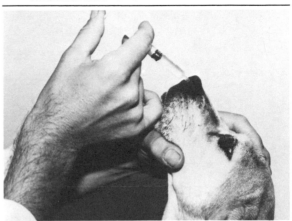

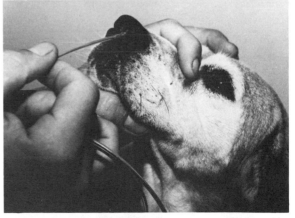

Instill into a nostril a topical anesthetic, such as 4 or 5 drops of 0.5% proparacaine HCl (Ophthetic, Allergan Pharmaceuticals, or Opthaine, Squibb) for the cat, and 0.5-1 ml of 2% lidocaine HCl for the dog. Elevate the animal's head so that the anesthetic runs into the nostril. Maintain this position for 2-3 minutes before attempting intubation.

Lubricate the tip of the tube with 2% lidocaine jelly (Xylocaine Jelly 2%, Astra). In **dogs**, direct the lubricated tube dorsomedial to the alar fold. After the tip is inserted 1-2 cm into the nostril, direct the tube ventro-medially. If turbinates are encountered, withdraw all but the last 1-2 cm and re-insert until the tube passes without resistance. In **cats**, there is no ventrolateral protruberance at the base of the nasal vestibule so the tube is inserted initially in a ventromedial direction and advanced through the ventral meatus, nasopharynx, pharynx, and esophagus. Tracheal intubation is unlikely as long as the head is maintained at the normal angle, as shown in Figure 10 (page 5-23).

FIGURE 13

PARASAGITTAL SECTION OF CANINE SKULL SHOWING PROPER ROUTING OF NASOGASTRIC TUBE

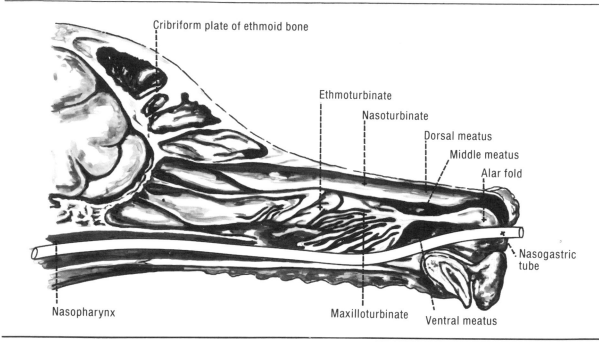

FIGURE 14

NASOGASTRIC TUBE FIXATION AND PROTECTION

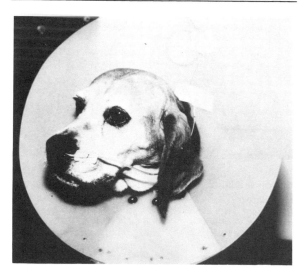

Secure the tube to the external nares by a cruciate suture placed through a tape butterfly. The tube should be placed as close as practical to the nasal planum. The tube should be secured to the skin with sutures every 4–8 cm and the end taped to an Elizabethan collar. An Elizabethan collar is necessary to prevent the dog from removing the tube. Routing the tube over the forehead and dorsum of the neck, rather than along the side of the face as shown, also helps prevent the animal from removing it.

To avoid plugging, be sure to thoroughly flush the tube after each feeding. When the nasogastric tube is no longer required, remove the fixation sutures and withdraw the capped tube using gentle traction.[36,51,63] Complications with nasogastric feeding include tube removal by the patient, airway aspiration of food, or gastric reflux. Occasionally a dog or cat cannot be successfully intubated nasogastrically.[36]

Pharyngostomy Tube Placement—Tube placement via a pharyngostomy can be used for patients with disease,[115] trauma, or surgery of the maxillary, mandibular, or facial region, or with impaired swallowing secondary to neuromuscular disorders.

Pharyngostomy tube placement is adequately described elsewhere.[32,78,115] Care must be taken when using pharyngostomy tubes as the technique is not without problems. Potential complications include infection, hemorrhage, and airway aspiration.[32,79]

Gastrostomy Tube Placement—Tube gastrostomies have previously been limited to situations where the mouth, pharynx, or esophagus had to be bypassed. There were two approaches available: percutaneous and surgical. These procedures have been well described elsewhere.[31,63]

Recently another percutaneous approach has been developed and used successfully in people,[52,53] dogs,[13] and cats. The technique is more rapid,

TABLE 8

TUBES FOR NASOGASTRIC FEEDING

Composition	Sizes (French x cm length)	Tip Weight	Name	Manufacturer
Polyvinylchloride*	5x16	no	Infant	
	5x42	no	feeding	National Catheter Co.
	8x42	no	tube	
	3½x12	no		
	5x16, 5x36	no		Argyle, division of Sherwood
	8x16, 8x42	no		Medical
	10x42	no		
Polyurethane	5x20, 5x36	no	Indwell	
	8x42			
	6x31	no	Entron	Biosearch Medical Products
	8x36, 8x43	yes	Entriflex	
Silicone	5x15, 8x15	no	Nutrifeed	American Pharmaseal
	6x42, 8x42	yes		
	6x36	yes	Keofeed	Ivac Corporation
	7.3x36, 7.3x42			

*Will harden if left in stomach for more than 2 weeks.

TABLE 9

SIZE OF NASOGASTRIC TUBES TO USE

Animal Wt (kg)	Tube Size (French)
< 5	3.5-5*
5-15	5-8
> 15	8-10

*A 19-21 gauge butterfly catheter (Abbott Labs) also may be used.

safer, and simpler than the gastrostomy procedures mentioned above. These advantages have broadened the application of this technique to include patients that would have been managed with pharyngostomy or even nasogastric tubes. The procedure does require the use of an endoscope. The tubes used are large enough to allow feeding of blenderized diets, even in small dogs and cats (Tables 10 and 13, pages 5-29 and 5-33).

Insertion of the tube in dogs can usually be done under neuroleptanalgesia (Innovar-Vet, Pitman-Moore). Ketamine induced anesthesia (Vetalar, Parke-Davis) is adequate for tube placement in cats. Place the animal in right lateral recumbency and clip and prepare a small area (10 cm × 10 cm) behind the last rib on the left side for aseptic surgery. Make a small (4 mm) stab incision through the skin. Pass a fiberoptic endoscope orally into the stomach and inflate the stomach with air until it presses against the abdominal wall. Position the illuminated tip of the endo-

scope, which can be seen from the exterior, under the skin incision. Push an 18 gauge Medicut intravenous cannula (Sherwood Medical Industries) through the stab incision into the stomach (Figure 15A) next to the tip of the endoscope which is used to support the stomach wall from the inside. Confirm the presence of the cannula and the needle stylet within the stomach lumen with the endoscope, and remove the stylet. Pass heavy suture (#1 or #2) into the stomach via the cannula. Grasp the end of the suture with a snare on the endoscope (Figure 15B). Withdraw the endoscope (and attached suture) from the stomach through the mouth. Remove and save the cannula. The suture now extends through the abdominal wall, into the stomach, cranially through the esophagus and exits the oral cavity. Pass the end of the suture protruding from the mouth retrograde through the cannula previously removed from the abdomen (Figure 15C).

A French Pezzar mushroom-tip catheter (Bardex, Bard Urological Division, C.R. Bard Inc., Murray Hill NJ), from 16-24 French in size, is used for the tube gastrostomy (Figure 15C). Cut off a 2 cm piece of the flared end of this catheter, opposite the mushroom tip. Make a stab incision through the center of the 2 cm piece of tubing and fit it over the cut end of the mushroom catheter and push it down to the mushroom (Figure 15C). This serves as a flange to keep the catheter from pulling out when insertion is complete. Further modify the cut end of the mushroom catheter by removing two "v" shaped pieces, which allows the cut end

FIGURE 15

PERCUTANEOUS GASTROSTOMY TUBE PLACEMENT USING AN ENDOSCOPE[13]

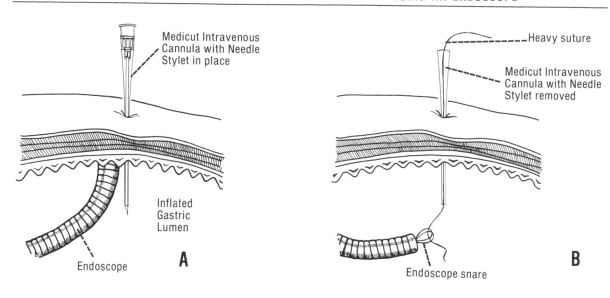

Medicut Intravenous Cannula with Needle Stylet in place

Inflated Gastric Lumen

Endoscope

A

Heavy suture

Medicut Intravenous Cannula with Needle Stylet removed

Endoscope snare

B

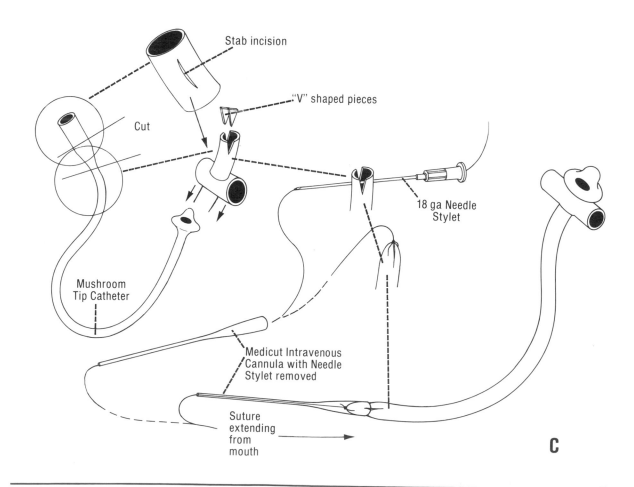

Stab incision

"V" shaped pieces

Cut

18 ga Needle Stylet

Mushroom Tip Catheter

Medicut Intravenous Cannula with Needle Stylet removed

Suture extending from mouth

C

FIGURE 15—Continued

GASTROSTOMY TUBE PLACEMENT[13]

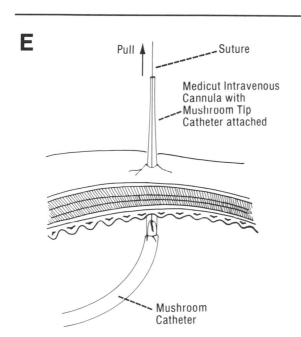

D

Medicut Intravenous
Cannula with Mushroom
Tip Catheter attached

Pull
Suture

E

Pull ↑ — Suture

Medicut Intravenous
Cannula with
Mushroom Tip
Catheter attached

Mushroom
Catheter

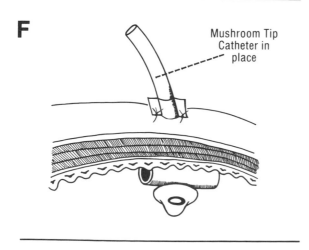

F

Mushroom Tip
Catheter in
place

to be tapered (Figure 15C). Pass the 18-gauge needle stylet (saved from the medicut intravenous cannula) through the modified end of the mushroom catheter, just back from the "v's" (Figure 15C).

Pass the tip of the suture, extending from the mouth and through the cannula retrograde through this needle and remove the needle from the mushroom catheter, leaving the suture passing through the mushroom catheter. Then tie the suture across the cut end of the mushroom catheter with a square knot and stretch the tied end of the mushroom catheter by pulling on the suture. Pass the cannula down the suture over the stretched end of the mushroom catheter (Figure 15C). The tapered cannula acts as a dilator for the mushroom catheter. Liberally lubricate the cannula and the attached mushroom catheter. Apply traction to the end of the suture protruding from the abdominal wall and pull the cannula/mushroom tube caudally through the esophagus (Figure 15D), into the stomach and out through the abdominal wall stab incision (Figure 15E). Remove the cannula from the mushroom catheter. Pull the tube through the abdominal wall until the inner flange rests against the gastric mucosa (Figure 15F). Use the endoscope to confirm the position of the mushroom tip. Suture the exteriorized portion of the mushroom catheter to the skin. Cap the catheter and cover with a bandage. An Elizabethan collar is advised. Clients can usually manage the feeding of these patients at home.

When the patient is ready for oral alimentation the tube can be removed (although oral feeding can be done with the tube in place). For removal of the tube from dogs, apply traction to the tube and cut it off at skin level. Push the remaining mushroom tip into the stomach. It will pass in the feces within 48-72 hours.[13] Alternatively, in either dogs or cats, the mushroom tube can be pulled through the inner flange and out through the abdominal wall. The inner flange can be retrieved with endoscopy or will pass in the feces. Most cats will not pass the mushroom tip. Therefore, it must be removed from cats with endoscopy. With experience, this percutaneous gastrostomy method requires 5-10 minutes to complete. The gastrocutaneous fistula will close spontaneously in 1-2 weeks.[63]

Enterostomy Catheter Placement—Catheter enterostomy (duodenostomy or jejunostomy) feeding is indicated to maintain nutritional support when any portion of the gastrointestinal tract cranial to the duodenum cannot or should not be used for alimentation.[33,39,88,103,118] Ideally these

catheters are placed at the time of abdominal surgery. The technique for enterostomy tube placement has been adequately described elsewhere.[63,103]

Diets for Tube Feeding

Liquid diets for tube feeding should supply all necessary nutrients while inducing a minimum of digestive and metabolic disturbances. The nutrients should be in forms that are easily digested, readily assimilated, and efficiently utilized. Ideally the food should be of a quality sufficient to allow its administration to animals with gastritis, enteritis, or colitis without additionally irritating the gastrointestinal tract. However, most liquid diets for tube feeding produce soft stools. Because these diets bypass the oral cavity, they need not be highly palatable. **The diets should be balanced so that they simultaneously supply the correct amounts of all nutrients (including water) when they are fed to meet the patient's caloric requirement.** If excessive fluid losses or dehydration are present, additional water should be given along with any liquid diet. Methods for estimating the degree of dehydration and the amount of fluid needed to correct it are given in Table 6 (page 5-17). The amount of water needed to compensate for losses can be calculated from changes in body weight.

Two basic types of liquid diets are used for tube feeding: 1) blenderized diets and 2) commercially prepared human diets. Both have specific advantages and disadvantages.

An excellent blenderized liquid diet for orogastric-, nasogastric-, pharyngostomy-, or gastrostomy-tube feeding for either dogs or cats can be prepared as described in Table 10. This diet contains all nutrients required by recuperating dogs or cats and has many advantages over human liquid diets. These include:

1. This blenderized diet is higher in protein and fat and lower in carbohydrate than commercially prepared human liquid diets. This may be an advantage in animals that are injured or septic or that have cancer.[19] Protein requirements are increased in patients in these situations (page 5-12). They use increased amounts of fat for fuel (page 5-5), and sometimes are carbohydrate-intolerant (page 5-8). High-fat diets are also more desirable for patients with respiratory disease. Fat metabolism results in a lower respiratory quotient (amount of carbon dioxide produced per unit oxygen used) than does metabolism of glucose.

2. The protein in the diet contains approximately 20% branched-chain amino acids. Branched-chain amino acids are desirable in recouperative diets.[35] Preferential use of these amino acids occurs during sepsis and following trauma (see page 5-14).

3. Many of the human liquid diets contain medium-chain triglycerides. These may induce hepatic lipidosis if given long term to cats (page 1-17).

4. There is less diarrhea and fewer loose stools associated with the use of the blenderized diet than with human liquid diets.

5. The blenderized diet may be administered in fewer feedings per day than the human liquid diets (Table 14, page 5-34)

6. The blenderized diet is approximately 50% less expensive than either the human liquid diets or blenderized human baby foods.

TABLE 10

BLENDERIZED TUBE FEEDING DIET FOR DOGS AND CATS*

½ can (224 g) Prescription Diet Feline p/d**
¾ cup (170 ml) water

Blend for 60 seconds at high speed. Strain twice through a kitchen strainer (approximately 1 mm mesh). Yields 390 ml. Administer an amount sufficient to meet the animal's energy needs, as given in Figure 6 (page 5-13) or Table 3 (page 5-12). Divide the amount into 2 or 3 feedings/day. See Table 15, page 5-34, for the maximum amount that can be given at each feeding.

ANALYSIS

	As Fed	Dry Matter
Moisture %	83	0
Protein %	7.4	44.2 or 33% of calories
Fat %	5.0	29.6 or 55% of calories
Carbohydrate %	2.8	17.0 or 12% of calories
Calcium %	0.19	1.1
Phosphorus %	0.13	0.8
Sodium %	0.10	0.6
Metabolizable energy	0.8 kcal/ml	4.76 kcal/g

*Recommended for orogastric, nasogastric, pharyngostomy, or gastrostomy feeding (but not enterostomy). Administer through tubes size 8 French or larger that have an opening at the tip (end port). Additional ports on the sides are optional. Tubes with only side ports will plug with this diet. Failure to follow all instructions may result in plugging of the feeding tube. Straining removes particulates but has no effect on nutrient content. See page 5-32 for example problem using this diet.

Use Feline, **not Canine, Prescription Diet p/d. Use of the canine diet results in a liquid which is too viscous for tube feeding.

TABLE 11

HUMAN LIQUID DIETS

PRODUCT (Company)	Caloric Density (Kcal/ml)	Osmolality (mOsm/L)	Nutrients (% of total kcal)			Electrolytes (mEq/L)		
			Protein	Fat	Carbohydrate	Sodium	Potassium	Chloride
Meal Replacement Diets:								
Osmolite HN (Ross)	1.06	310	Casein (16.7)	Corn Oil & MCT (30)	Hydrolysed Cornstarch (53.3)	39.5	38.6	40.1
Isocal HCN (Mead-Johnson)	2.0	690	Casein (15)	Soy Oil & MCT (40)	Corn Syrup (45)	35	36	34
Ensure Plus HN (Ross)	1.5	650	Casein (16.7)	Corn Oil (30)	Hydrolysed Cornstarch & Sucrose (53.3)	50.2	45	44.8
Elemental Diets:								
Vital HN (Ross)	1.0	460	Hydrolysate of Whey, Meat, and Soy, and Essential Amino Acids (16.7)	Safflower and MCT Oil (9.3)	Hydrolysed Cornstarch & Sucrose (74)	16.7	29.9	18.8
Criticare HN (Mead-Johnson)	1.54	650	Hydrolysed Casein (30%) & Amino Acids (70%) (14)	Safflower Oil (3)	Malto-dextrins & Modified Cornstarch (83)	27.5	33.8	29.6
Vivonex HN (Norwich-Eaton)	1.0	810	Crystalline Amino Acids (17)	Safflower Oil (0.8)	Glucose & Oligosacch-arides (82.2)	33.5	17.9	52.3

7. Once the patient's appetite is regained, the patient can be hand fed the same food used in the blenderized diet, directly from the can, obviating the need for a diet change.

A variety of high-quality commercially prepared human liquid enteral diets are available and their number is increasing. Two decades ago similar commercial veterinary products were marketed. They were later withdrawn because veterinarians lacked interest in them.[99,100] These products were ahead of their time. Several human liquid diets that can be used for injured or diseased dogs or cats are listed in Tables 11, 12, and 13. Most of the products fall into one of three groups: 1) meal-replacement diets, 2) peptide or elemental diets, and 3) nutrient additives, sometimes referred to as "feeding modules." Most are available at pharmacies or human hospitals.

Meal-replacement diets (also called "polymeric diets") are for use in patients with almost normal gastrointestinal function. These products are mixtures containing protein (usually casein, soy, or egg albumin), fats (about 30% of calories), and carbohydrates in high molecular-weight forms to reduce osmolality to approximately 350 mOsm/L. These are low-lactose and low-residue products that are adequate for most clinical situations.[76] They are similar in application to the blenderized diet (Table 10) because they can be fed via orogastric, nasogastric, pharyngostomy, and gastrostomy routes. Although they are not designed for enterostomy feeding, they have been used successfully via this route in dogs and cats.[103] Meal-replacement type human liquid diets can be fed through smaller tubes than the blenderized diet (smaller than 8 French) and are less likely to plug tubes. However, they must be fed more frequently (Table 14, page 5-34). Diarrhea is common in dogs and cats given these diets. The diets cost from 2 to 2.5 times more to feed than does the blenderized diet. Even so, they are a relatively inexpensive form of therapy.

In peptide and elemental diets, proteins are present in the form of peptides or amino acids. Carbohydrates are in the form of smaller oligo-saccharides or monosaccharides. These diets are

usually low in fat and may contain part of the fat as medium-chain triglyceride oil (MCT) (see page 1-17 for a discussion of MCT). Because small molecular weight nutrients are included, the osmolality of these solutions is 450-850 mOsm/L. Elemental diets are designed to be fed via an enterostomy catheter. They require minimal digestion. When fed by this route they cannot be bolus-fed but must be fed by continuous infusion, i.e. pump or gravity flow (see Table 14, page 5-34). These diets are recommended for human patients with abnormal gastrointestinal function, e.g. inflammatory bowel disease and pancreatic insufficiency.[45] In this regard they may also be useful for animals. Feeding elemental diets to dogs prior to radiation therapy has afforded protection to the intestine from the acute phase of radiation injury; therefore, these diets may also have specific prophylactic value during cancer treatment.[90]

Nutrient additives or feeding modules are con-centrated sources of one nutrient; i.e. protein, fat, or carbohydrate (Table 12). These modules may be added to diets to increase specific component concentrations or to reduce the required volume of diet needed.[124] These products may also increase the osmolality of the formulation. However, if the solutes are readily absorbable, a hypertonic fluid is absorbed more rapidly than an isotonic fluid.[21,22]

Appropriate dietary management of gastrointestinal, hepatic or renal failure patients is an essential part of therapy for these diseases as described in Chapters 7 and 8. In situations where these patients are anorectic they may require tube feeding. Table 13 lists blenderized diet formulas and human liquid diets (meal-replacement type) for managing anorectic dogs or cats with these diseases.

Procedures for Tube Feeding

The tube feeding protocol recommended is summarized in Table 14 (page 5-34). The first step

TABLE 12

NUTRIENT ADDITIVES FOR LIQUID DIETS*

Product (Company)	Kcal	Osmolality (mOsm/L)	Nutrient Source			Electrolytes (mEq/L)	
			Protein	Fat	Carbohydrate	Sodium	Potassium
Protein:							
Pro-mix (Navaco)	4/g	—	Whey			7	410
Casec (Mead-Johnson)	4/g	—	Casein			7	30
Propac (Organon)	4/g	—	Whey			10	13
Fat:							
Microlipid (Organon)	4.5/g	80		Safflower Oil			
MCT Oil (Mead-Johnson)	7.7/g	—		Fractionated Coconut			
Vegetable Oil	9.4/g	—		Corn, Safflower, Soy, etc.			
Carbohydrate:							
Polycose (Ross)	4/g 2/ml	850			Hydrolysed Cornstarch	25	5
Moducal (Mead-Johnson)	4/g 2/ml	725			Maltodextrin	15	6
Sumacal (Organon)	4/g	—			Maltodextrin	4	< 1
Corn Syrup	2.9/ml	—			Primarily Maltose	30	1
50% Glucose	2/ml	2800			Glucose	0	0
Jam and Jelly Pectin	4/g	—			Glucose	0	0

*Also see additives, Table 7, page 5–18.

in any method of feeding is to select the proper diet. Selection criteria for tube feeding diets should include:

1. Energy density (usually about 1 kcal/metabolizable energy/ml—range 0.6 to 2.0 kcal/ml)

2. Desired percentage of calories from carbohydrate, fat, and protein (see page 5-29 for considerations).

3. The diet should be complete and balanced. All non-energy nutrients (water, protein for non-energy purposes, minerals, and vitamins) balanced to the energy density of the diet. This greatly simplifies feeding. When this type of diet is fed, all that is needed is to feed the proper amount to meet the patient's energy requirement and the requirements for all nutrients will automatically be met.

4. Animals requiring tubes smaller than size 8 French cannot be fed a blenderized diet because the tubes may plug.

5. Osmolality—Isoosmotic diets (approximately 350 mOsm/L) are best suited for orogastric, nasogastric, pharyngostomy or gastrostomy bolus feeding. However, hyperosmotic diets, if readily absorbable, can be given via these routes.[21,22] Hyperosmotic diets (450-850 mOsm/L) are usually fed via continuous infusion through an enterostomy tube (page 5-31).

The second step is to determine the daily food dose. If a properly balanced diet has been selected, this step is simple:

1. Estimate the animal's daily energy requirement in kcal, either by calculation (Table 3, page 5-12) or from a nomogram (Figure 6, page 5-13).

2. Divide the energy requirement by the energy density of the diet. The answer is the total daily amount to be fed.

For diets that have an energy density of 1 kcal/ml—the volume to feed in ml is numerically the same as the animal's energy requirement in kcal (see example problem).

The third step is to initiate feeding. The goal is to have the patient on the total food dosage as soon as possible with minimal metabolic and gastrointestinal complications. To accomplish this gradually increase the amount of liquid diet given as described in Table 14. This protocol allows for a rapid but careful transition and continues to meet the animal's water requirement.

The final step is to determine feeding frequency (number of feedings per day). Frequency recommendations depend on:

1. Type of diet—blenderized diets usually can be fed fewer times per day (2-3 times/day) than the human liquid diets (3-5 times/day).

2. Route of feeding—with orogastric-, nasogastric-, pharyngostomy-, or gastrostomy-tubes, animals can be fed multiple boluses per day (e.g. 1-5 times/day). Bolus feeding is easily done with a 60 ml plastic "dose syringe" (60 ml Catheter Tip Syringe, Monoject). With indwelling tubes (i.e. nasogastric, pharyngostomy, gastrostomy, or enterostomy) a constant infusion (maximum 15 ml/kg/hr) over several hours per day is ideal but is necessary only with enterostomy feeding (page 5-31). Interrupted or cyclic feeding is more physiologic and results in increased visceral protein production.[106] Enterostomy patients should not be bolus fed. When the constant feeding is used, start the infusion slowly (5 ml/kg/hr for the first hour) and gradually increase the infusion rate (10 ml/kg/hr for the second hour, and 15 ml/kg/hr thereafter).

3. Gastric and digestive/absorptive capacity— The amount of fluid given orally that the normal dog and cat can tolerate at one time without obvious discomfort or regurgitation is given in Table 15 (page 5-34).[44,128]

Tube Feeding Example

A 10-kg dog with a severe infectious disease has not eaten for 4 days. There are no contraindications to enteral feeding so a nasogastric tube is inserted.

1. Because the dog weighs 10 kg, an 8 French or larger tube can be used (Table 9, page 5-26) and the blenderized diet (Table 10, page 5-29) is selected. The energy density of this diet is 0.8 kcal/ml.

2. The daily food dose is determined by estimating the dog's daily energy requirement and dividing it by the energy density of the balanced diet:

   a. The dog's energy requirement is estimated, using BER and injury/disease factors (Table 3, page 5-12). It could be also obtained from the nomograph (Figure 6, page 5-13).

$$\text{BER (metabolizable kcal/day)} = 30 \text{ Wt}_{kg} + 70$$
$$\text{BER} = (30)10 + 70 = 370 \text{ kcal/day}$$
$$\text{Severe sepsis} = 1.7 \times \text{BER} = 1.7 \times 370 = 629 \text{ kcal/day}$$

   b. The daily energy requirement is divided by the energy density of the diet (0.8 kcal/ml) to obtain the daily food dose.

TABLE 13

TUBE FEEDING DIETS FOR DOGS AND CATS WITH RENAL, HEPATIC, OR GASTROINTESTINAL DISEASE

Clinical Condition	Liquid Diet	Metabolizable Energy Density[a] (kcal/ml)	Protein (g/500 ml)
	BLENDERIZED DIETS[b]		
Canine:			
Renal failure	Canine k/d + water	0.62	9.5
Advanced renal failure	Canine u/d + water	0.66	6.4
Hepatic failure	Canine k/d + water	0.62	9.5
Gastrointestinal disease	Canine i/d + water	0.57	16.7
Feline:			
Renal failure	Feline k/d + water	0.90	19.6
Hepatic failure	Feline k/d + water	0.90	19.6
Gastrointestinal disease	Feline c/d + water	0.62	27.5
	HUMAN LIQUID DIETS		
Canine:			
Renal failure	Travasorb Renal (Travenol)	1.35	11.5
Hepatic failure	Travasorb Hepatic (Travenol)	1.10	14.5
Gastrointestinal disease	Feed elemental diets (Table 11, page 5-30)		

[a]Administer an amount sufficient to meet the animal's energy needs as given in Figure 6 (page 5-13) or Table 3 (page 5-12). Divide this amount by the number of daily feedings recommended in Table 14 (page 5-34). See Table 15 (page 5-34) for the maximum amount that can be given at each feeding.

[b]For each diet, blend at high speed for 60 seconds, ½ can (224 g) of Prescription Diet (Hill's) indicated plus 10 oz (284 ml) of water. Then strain the blended mixture twice through a 1 mm mesh strainer. The resulting liquid diet will pass through a size 8 French tube or larger. The tube must have an opening at the tip (end port). Additional side ports are optional.

629 kcal/day ÷ 0.8 kcal/ml = 787 ml/day

3. Blenderized diets can be fed 2-3 times per day (Table 14, page 5-34). However, this dog has not eaten for 4 days and some degree of gastric contraction and diminished digestive function is anticipated. Thus, multiple small feedings are desired. A feeding frequency of 3 times per day is chosen.

787 ml/day ÷ 3 feedings/day = 262 ml/feeding
262 ml ÷ 10 kg = 26 ml/kg which is approximately 25% of normal gastric capacity (Table 15, page 5-34) and therefore should be well tolerated.

4. The initial feeding regimen (Table 14, page 5-34 calls for dilution of the diet for the first two days.

   a. Day 1—1/3 the amount of blenderized diet needed plus 2/3 water:
   1/3 (787 ml) of blenderized diet + 2/3 (787 ml) of water =
   262 ml diet + 525 ml water =
   787 ml of diluted diet/day
   787 ml diluted diet ÷ 3 feedings/day =
   262 ml/feeding

   b. Day 2—2/3 the amount of diet needed plus 1/3 water:
   2/3 (787 ml) of blenderized diet + 1/3 (787 ml) of water =

525 ml diet + 262 ml water =
787 ml diluted diet/day
787 ml diluted diet ÷ 3 feedings/day =
262 ml/feeding

   c. Day 3—787 ml undiluted diet ÷ 3 feedings/day

   d. After adapting to the blenderized diet, feeding frequency can often be reduced to 2 feedings/day.

5. The dog should be offered unblended diet frequently to determine when voluntary eating starts and the nasogastric tube can be removed. At that time the dog should be fed the amount of food needed for maintenance (Table 1, page 1-6).

Problems and Complications with Tube Feeding

Three types of problems may occur when tube feeding is being used: mechanical, gastrointestinal, and metabolic. Mechanical problems are those related to placement and maintenance of the feeding tube. When a tube is placed in the caudal esophagus, stomach, or duodenum, its proper placement may be assured by radiography. Tube placement should be checked before feeding. Regurgitation and aspiration may ensue from improper tube placement or too rapid administra-

TABLE 14

TUBE FEEDING PROTOCOL FOR DOGS AND CATS

Initial Feeding Regimen:

Day	Diet
1	1/3 amount needed* + 2/3 water
2	2/3 amount needed* + 1/3 water
3 on	Full amount needed* (no additional water)

Feeding Frequency: (times/day)**

Route	Blenderized Diets (Tables 10 and 13)	Human Liquid Diets (Table 11)
Orogastric	2-3	3-5
Nasogastric	2-3	3-5 or continuous
Pharyngostomy	2-3	3-5 or continuous
Gastrostomy	2-3	3-5 or continuous
Enterostomy	Not Recommended	continuous

*Amount needed to provide the animals' energy requirement as calculated from Table 3 (page 5-12) or determined from Figure 6 (page 5-13). Thus, the first day the animal would receive one-third of the amount of the undiluted liquid diet needed to meet its energy needs plus twice that volume of water. More water should be given if the patient is dehydrated or has greater than normal water losses. See example page 5-32.

**The total daily amount to be fed is divided by the number of feedings per day to determine amount to feed per feeding. Bolus feeding is easily done with a 60 ml plastic "dose syringe" (60 ml Catheter Tip Syringe, Monoject). Continuous feeding is by infusion pump or gravity flow (page 5-31). Do not exceed volumes listed in Table 15 at any one feeding. See example page 5-32.

tion of food. Tubes may become occluded if coarse food materials are infused or if the tube is not flushed adequately after use.

Esophagitis may occur from nasogastric or pharyngostomy tubes, usually from the use of a tube having too large a diameter.[78] Smaller tubes have the further advantage of allowing the animal to begin to eat voluntarily with the tube in place. However, too small a tube prevents the use of blenderized diets.

Other problems associated with pharyngostomy tubes include regurgitation of the tube and infection at the pharyngostomy site. Good nursing care should make infection unlikely at the site of tube entry. No food material should be allowed to collect at the pharyngostomy site, and the tube should be kept tightly capped when not in use.

Most of the gastrointestinal problems caused by tube feeding are caused by too rapid administration of the solution, or administration of poorly absorbed solutes or solutions of too high osmo-

lality. When nutrient solutions enter the duodenum too rapidly, they can cause vomiting, cramps, and diarrhea by overwhelming the normal neural and endocrine gastrointestinal mechanisms. Solutions too hypertonic, particularly those containing poorly or slowly absorbed constituents, cause rapid fluid and electrolyte movement into the intestinal lumen, which leads to intestinal distention and cramping. These problems are prevented by using a more conservative feeding protocol that includes initial reduction of the concentration of the liquid diet (Table 14).[32]

Metabolic problems include rapid absorption of glucose which results in hyperglycemia and osmotic diuresis at blood glucose concentrations above 180 mg/dl. At blood glucose concentrations above 900 mg/dl, a non-ketotic hyperosmolar coma may occur in the dehydrated dog (although this is rare). The most common metabolic complications reported in a human survey of tube fed patients were hyperglycemia (29%), hyponatremia (31%), hyperkalemia (40%), and hypophosphatemia (30%). Only hyperglycemia was thought to result from the therapy as opposed to the disease process.[131] Hyperglycemia can be detected by monitoring urine glucose concentrations at regular intervals. It can be managed by reducing feeding rate or giving insulin (0.5-1 IU/kg of NPH insulin subcutaneously in the dog, 0.25 IU/kg in the cat).[46]

TABLE 15

MAXIMUM STOMACH CAPACITY OF DOGS AND CATS*

	Body Weight (kg)	Stomach Volume** (ml/kg body wt)
Dogs[32,44,128]	All	90
Cats[27]	0.5-1	100
	1-1.5	70
	1.5-4	60
	4-6	45

*These amounts are maximum amounts for **normal** animals. Many animals tolerate less. Animals anorectic for more than 2 days have decreased stomach capacity and small intestinal digestive and absorptive capacity (page 5-6).[135] These animals should initially be given one-half or less of these amounts at any one time. The amount given should be gradually increased over several feedings. Adherence to recommendations in Table 14 will accomplish this. In all cases, fluids given orally should be given over a several minute period to allow gastric dilation to occur.

**Amount of water that will produce vomiting or distress.

INTRAVENOUS FEEDING*

When animals cannot be supported by nutrient intake via the gastrointestinal tract, intravenous feeding (total parenteral nutrition [TPN]) should be used. Otherwise, intravenous feeding has the same indications as enteral feeding (page 5-19). Intravenous feeding should be considered in lieu of enteral feeding if one or more of the following conditions is present:

1. Inadequate digestive or absorptive capacity
2. Intestinal obstruction or ileus
3. Uncontrollable vomiting
4. High risk of aspiration because of unconsciousness or neurologic deficit
5. Inability to tolerate food orally for any reason
6. Need for complete bowel rest to minimize the effects of digestive disease and allow healing of gastrointestinal tract lesions, acute pancreatitis or hepatitis

All of the dog's and cat's nutritional requirements can be met with intravenous feeding, and it is a valuable medical/surgical adjunct.[62] However, it requires extensive staff time and care and is expensive. The cost of the intravenous feeding fluid alone approaches $30/1000 kcal (enough for a 20-kg septic dog for 1 day). In addition, if the animal is malnourished, treatment must be initiated carefully. Transition from a compensated, often balanced hypometabolic state to a normometabolic or anabolic state, if made too rapidly, can cause death. Therefore, the refeeding of a severely malnourished patient must be progressive and initiated only after all fluid, electrolyte, and acid-base alterations have been corrected with the administration of fluid, electrolytes, and 5% glucose (page 5-16).

EQUIPMENT NEEDED AND CATHETERIZATION FOR INTRAVENOUS FEEDING

Because of the high osmolality of intravenous feeding solutions, they should be administered via a central venous catheter. The administration of high osmolality fluids into a peripheral vein will result in phlebitis, formation of thrombi and emboli, and eventual occlusion of the vein. Thus, the first step needed for feeding the animal intravenously is the insertion of a central venous

*Appreciation is expressed to Aunna C. Lippert, DVM, Veterinary Clinical Center, Michigan State University, East Lansing, MI 48824, for her assistance with this section.

TABLE 16

CATHETERS FOR INTRAVENOUS FEEDING

Application	Size		Brand* Name
	Gauge	Length	
Cats/Small Dogs	19	8 inches	Intracath
	20	8 cm	L-Cath
Medium Dogs	19	8 inches	Intracath
	18	12 cm	L-Cath
Large Dogs	19	12 inches	Intracath
	18	25 cm	L-Cath

*Other catheters may be equally well suited. These are recommended: Intracath (Vialon), Deseret Medical Inc., Division of Parke-Davis and Co., Sandy, UT 84070 and L-Cath (polyurethane), Luther Medical Products, Inc., Santa Ana, CA 92705)

catheter. Ready-made commercial catheter sets for this purpose are listed in Table 16.

Prior to inserting the catheter into the external jugular vein, the area is prepared as it would be for any aseptic surgical procedure. Inadequate skin preparation significantly increases catheter-related infection.[15,134] Catheter-related infection may be reduced by tunneling the end of the catheter subcutaneously prior to entry into the jugular vein.[2] This procedure supposedly eliminates the direct entry of bacteria into the vein from the skin surface.[8] Because feeding solutions are an excellent medium for microbial growth, exacting aseptic techniques should be used in the insertion, maintenance, and use of the intravenous catheter.[134]

For ambulatory patients, tightly coiled latex tubing (Extendex tubing, W. A. Baum Co., Copiaque, NY or Medical Supply, Boulder, CO) coupled with a swivel adapter (Becton-Dickinson) allows reliable fluid flow without restricting the patient's freedom of movement. They are incorporated into the system with Luer-Lok adapters (Becton-Dickinson). However, changes in the diameter of the tubing as it is extended and retracted make the use of screw clamps over the tube unreliable for regulating fluid flow. A 2-way or 3-way stopcock (Becton-Dickinson) may be used for reliable control of flow rate. For inactive patients standard intravenous infusion sets can be used with a buret interposed to control flow. The addition of a 0.22 micron filter (Millipore Co) in the line assists in preventing bacterial contamination, but cannot be used with intravenous lipids. Some institutions are no longer using in-line filters.[66]

Purchase of an intravenous infusion pump should

be considered if intravenous feeding is to be done regularly. It greatly simplifies fluid delivery. The cost of the pump is further justified by the saving in time and labor that it provides.

SOLUTIONS FOR INTRAVENOUS FEEDING

The major components of intravenous feeding solutions are amino acids and glucose. Lipids may also be included. Amino acid solutions with added electrolytes are most convenient for general use. They minimize many of the "hypo-electrolyte" problems that may occur as a consequence of the normal anabolic response to feeding (see Table 19, page 5-40). The number of required solution additions is reduced, lessening the chance of bacterial contamination. Two such products currently available are 8.5% Aminosyn (Abbot) and 8.5% Travesol with electrolytes (Travenol).

In one study of human subjects, a premixed amino acid-electrolyte solution was satisfactory in 83% of all cases, and only additional potassium was needed in 16%.[120] In addition to standard amino acid concentrations of 4.5-10%, special formulations for use in liver disease (Hepatamine, McGraw), and kidney disease (Nephramine, McGraw and Aminosyn-RF, Abbott) are available. Even if the amount of amino acids in some feeding solutions is less than that required in normal dogs and cats, and these solutions contain no taurine which is needed by cats, problems from these deficiencies bear little practical significance in most clinical cases because of the length of time intravenous feeding is used.

Glucose is the most readily available and widely used source of calories included in intravenous feeding solutions. It is inexpensive, compatible with almost all solutions, and is a primary biochemical energy substrate. Glucose is commercially available in concentrations ranging from 5-70%. The 50% and 70% solutions are most commonly used in preparing intravenous feeding solutions. The osmolality and energy density of various glucose solutions and fat emulsions are listed in Table 17. Other carbohydrates such as fructose or xylitol are not recommended. Fructose is expensive and may cause lactic acidosis in severely ill patients.[138] Xylitol may cause liver and kidney damage.[49,122] Ethanol is a more concentrated energy source (7 kcal/g as compared to 3.4 for glucose), but only small amounts (generally less than 3%) may be used without causing depression. In addition, ethanol causes lactic acidosis and inhibition of gluconeogenesis in people[73] and interferes with the response to trauma.[11,14,87]

TABLE 17

SOLUTIONS FOR INTRAVENOUS FEEDING

Solution	Osmolality (mOsm/kg)	Calories (kcal/ml)
5% dextrose	278	0.17
10% dextrose	556	0.34
50% dextrose	2780	1.7
10% lipid emulsion*	280	1.1
20% lipid emulsion	330	2.0

*Lipid emulsions include Intralipid (Cutter), Travamulsion (Travenol), Liposyn (Abbott), Soyacal (Lyphomed).

Lipid emulsions may also be used to provide calories (Table 17). Fat emulsions have been extensively tested in dogs[61,70] and have been used clinically.[111] Generally the recommendation is that they be used to provide not more than 40-60% of the patient's caloric needs. These products are expensive ($25-40/1000 kcal). The rationale for use of fat as a source of calories includes:

1. Easier management of patients being fed intravenously.[111] The use of fat as a major calorie source greatly reduces the amount of glucose needed. This decreases the insulin response to feeding which reduces hyperglycemic-hypoglycemic episodes.

2. Lipids may be better utilized than glucose in severely ill patients and patients with respiratory complications (page 5-29), although this has been difficult to demonstrate.[102]

3. Lipids provide essential fatty acids. However, dogs have been shown to grow normally when fed intravenously without the use of lipids. Growth is a time when essential fatty acid requirements would presumably be relatively great.[43]

4. Lipids provide a concentrated source of calories in an isotonic fluid (Table 17). This is helpful for patients requiring fluid restriction (such as in congestive heart failure or oliguric renal failure). The lower osmolality of the lipid emulsion solutions also permits their infusion into peripheral veins without inducing phelebitis.[111]

Contraindications to the use of lipid emulsions include pathologic hyperlipemic conditions, severe liver disease, and bleeding diathesis.[80] After the infusion of a fat emulsion, transient hyperlipidemia invariably occurs. Some patients may have difficulty clearing lipids from the blood. When lipid emulsions are given daily, ideally serum triglyceride concentration should be determined on

the third day of therapy before giving lipids that day, and preferably at least 4 hours after the previous day's administration of lipids was stopped. If plasma triglyceride concentration exceeds 300 mg/dl, consider decreasing the amount of lipid being given. Febrile responses may be observed following intravenous infusion of fat emulsions. Chills, vomiting, obscure pain, sleepiness, dyspnea, cyanosis, and allergic reactions reportedly occur sometimes in people given fat emulsions.[66]

Trace minerals currently recommended for intravenous feeding of people include zinc, copper, chromium, manganese. and selenium.[58,91,122] With the possible exception of zinc losses from bowel secretions, trace mineral deficiencies during short periods of intravenous feeding are unlikely unless the animal was seriously depleted before treatment. Trace mineral additives for intravenous feeding are available (M.T.E.-4,Travenol and Multiple Trace Metal Additive, Abbott).

The amino acid solutions with electrolytes do not contain calcium. For long-term feeding, 5 ml of 23% (or 11 ml of 10%) calcium gluconate/L can be added. However, one must ensure solution compatibility. Calcium and phosphorus may precipitate if their sum exceeds 45 mEq/L (90 mg/dl); sodium bicarbonate and magnesium can also precipitate calcium.[58] To avoid adverse interactions, blood products and drugs (excepting insulin and glucocorticoids) should not be administered in the intravenous feeding solution.

Vitamin requirements for sick animals are not well established, but in most cases an adequate regimen would include daily administration of a vitamin B-complex preparation in the intravenous feeding solution, and weekly oral or intramuscular administration of folate, vitamin B_{12}, and the fat-soluble vitamins A,D,E,and K.[72]

The least possible number of additions to the intravenous feeding solution and rigid adherence to aseptic technique during solution preparation are essential to avoid problems of contamination.[134] Solutions should be prepared in a clean, low traffic-flow area (such as a surgery room). The area and all apparatus used for transfers should be thoroughly disinfected and rinsed with 70% isopropanol before solutions are mixed.[56] Both glucose and amino acids containing electrolytes are available in 500-ml volumes in 1-liter bottles so that only one transfer is necessary. They may also be mixed in a buret. Delivery from a buret has the additional advantage of safety. Inadvertent administration of excessive amounts of TPN solution is precluded. Ideally, fat emulsions are given through a separate peripheral vein catheter. However, they can be "piggybacked" to a central venous system.

ADMINISTRATION OF INTRAVENOUS FEEDING SOLUTIONS

Dogs can be maintained on a mixture of equal volumes of 8.5% amino acids containing electrolytes and 50% glucose solutions. The resulting solution contains approximately 0.85 kcal/ml. The amount needed to meet the animal's energy needs can be calculated as shown on Table 3 (page 5-12) or obtained from the nomogram (Figure 6, page 5-13). This mixture contains approximately 1800 mOsm/L and must be infused slowly via a central vein. Feeding should be initiated with more dilute solutions, which may be prepared by mixing amino-acid and glucose solutions in a burette. For the first day's feeding, mix equal parts of an 8.5% amino acid solution with a 25% glucose solution. If there are no complications the second day, mix equal parts of the same amino-acid solution with a 50% glucose solution. Urinary glucose should be carefully monitored as the glucose concentration in the feeding solution is increased to avoid hyperglycemia in excess of 200 mg/dl.

Once the solution is mixed, it should be administered immediately. Delayed administration after additions have been made to the solution allows time for bacterial growth. Feeding solutions are excellent media for microbial growth; therefore, exacting aseptic techniques are necessary to prevent sepsis.[134] The catheter site should be cleaned, an antimicrobial ointment applied, sterile gauze placed over the skin opening, and the site wrapped daily. The intravenous feeding apparatus, from the tip of the catheter to the solution bottle, must be considered a closed system and should not be used for monitoring central venous pressure or for administering blood or medications.[37,134] All junctions should be cleaned with povidone-iodine or 70% isopropanol before they are connected and at any time they are disconnected. Administration sets should be changed every 48-72 hours or whenever they become contaminated.

The catheter should not be used for taking blood samples. Fibrin tags, which frequently form on the end of the catheter, may be aspirated into the catheter, occluding the catheter if blood is drawn into it. When not in use, the catheter should always be filled with a heparinized saline solution.

Because of the high levels of nutrients in the intravenous feeding solutions, their rate of administration must be changed slowly. Providing one-half of the of the intravenous feeding solution needed the first day and increasing to the full amount needed the second day (if no complications occur) is advocated. The flow should deliver the desired daily amount over a 24 hour period. If the rate of administration falls behind do not give a bolus to catch up. Increase the rate gradually. With animals that have difficulty regulating blood glucose, care should be taken to ensure constant flow. The reason for this precaution is the possibility that rebound hypoglycemia could occur if the infusion is abruptly interrupted. The high glucose concentration in the intravenous feeding solution causes hyperglycemia while it is being administered. Hyperglycemia stimulates insulin secretion which results in hyperinsulinemia. If administration of the intravenous feeding solution is stopped abruptly, because of the hyperinsulinemia, the blood glucose concentration will fall rapidly. Therefore, when intravenous feeding is discontinued, it should be done gradually over a period of 3-4 hours. This is recommended for either termination or interruption of intravenous feeding.

Growing dogs being fed intravenously have been disconnected (via gradual reduction) for 1.5 hours daily with no reported problems.[42] Similar periodic interruption of infusion in adult dogs was without observable adverse effect.[20] In some cases, it may be possible to give the desired daily amount of feeding solution over 8-12 hours. This would be achieved by progressively increasing and then decreasing the rate of administration over 2-3 hours. This type of cyclic feeding has been shown to have advantages if done correctly.[106] However, administration over 8-12 hours requires high delivery rates which may not be compatible in a glucose-intolerant injured, septic, or burned canine or feline patient and is not currently recommended.

Animals fed intravenously should be closely monitored as described in Table 18. Trends are more important than individual values. Most important is careful attention to clinical signs. The cause for any deterioration of the animal's condition must be rapidly diagnosed if intravenous feeding is to be an asset, rather than a liability, to therapy. The more sick the animal, the more thorough and frequent the monitoring must be.

EXAMPLE OF INTRAVENOUS FEEDING

A 10-kg dog with a severe infectious disease is unable to tolerate food orally; intravenous feeding using a glucose-amino acid solution is desired.

1. As determined from Table 3 (page 5-12) (see example problem page 5-32):

   a) The BER for a 10 kg dog is 370 kcal/day.

   b) However, as shown in Table 3, an infectious

TABLE 18

GUIDELINES FOR MONITORING THE ANIMAL BEING FED INTRAVENOUSLY

Parameter Monitored	Monitoring Frequency	Rationale for Monitoring
Body weight	Daily	Large fluctuations indicate fluid imbalance
Temperature, pulse and respiration	Daily	Identification of inflammation or infection
WBC count and differential	Twice weekly	Identification of infection or inflammation
Plasma glucose concentration	Daily until stable, then twice weekly	Control of blood glucose levels
Urine glucose presence	Every 6 hours until stable, then daily	Identification of hyperglycemia
Plasma concentrations of Na, K, Cl, bicarbonate, Ca and P	Daily until stable, then twice weekly	Alterations may occur (See Table 19, page 5–40)
Plasma protein and albumin concentrations	Weekly	Indication of response to therapy
ALT (SGPT), SAP, BUN	Weekly	Liver function may be affected (See Table 19, page 5–40)
Blood ammonia concentration	As needed if signs of elevation occur	Large increases suggest too rapid administration of a protein hydrolysate solution containing free ammonia

disease increases these needs by 50-70%, depending upon the severity. In this case 70% is arbitrarily chosen because the dog is seriously ill. Therefore, this dog needs 629 kcal (1.7 × 370 kcal).

c) As described on page 5-14, approximately 4 g of protein/100 kcal are needed, and therefore 25 g of protein are needed daily (629 kcal/day × 4 g protein/100 kcal).

d) Alternatively energy and protein needs can both be obtained from Figure 6 (page 5-13). This nomogram indicates that the 10-kg dog with sepsis needs approximately 630 kcal and 25 g of protein/day.

2. Glucose provides 3.4 metabolizable kcal/g. Therefore, a 50% glucose solution provides 1.7 kcal/ml.

$$\frac{3.4 \text{ kcal}}{\text{g glucose}} \times \frac{50 \text{ g glucose}}{100 \text{ ml}} = 1.7 \text{ kcal/ml}$$

3. This dog needs 370 ml of a 50% glucose solution daily to meet its caloric requirement.

$$\frac{(629 \text{ kcal/day needed}) \times 1 \text{ ml of } 50\% \text{ glucose solution}}{1.7 \text{ kcal}} = 370 \text{ ml/day}$$

4. This dog needs 294 ml of an 8.5% amino acid (protein) solution (AA sol) daily to meet its protein needs.

$$\frac{(25 \text{ g protein/day needed}) \times 100 \text{ ml AA sol}}{8.5 \text{ g protein}} = 294 \text{ ml/day}$$

5. Thus, the dog's nutritional needs could be met by giving 370 ml of a 50% glucose solution and 294 ml of an 8.5% amino acid solution.

6. A simpler method is to calculate the amount of 50% glucose solution required to satisfy energy needs and give an equal volume of 8.5% amino acid solution. This would provide 370 ml times 8.5% or 31 g of protein daily; slightly more than the estimated requirement.

7. The amount of electrolytes needed for maintenance is included in the amino acid solution. Plasma electrolyte concentrations, particularly potassium and phosphorus, should be monitored; if they fall below normal, additional electrolytes should be added to the fluid.

8. Vitamin B complex should be given daily in at least the amount needed for maintenance (Table 13, page 1-23).

9. If feeding is to be continuous, a rate of about 30 ml/hr is required (740 ml ÷ 24 hr). Ten milliliters should be given the first hour, 20 the second and then 30 ml/hr until feeding is to be stopped; at which time the feeding rate should be tapered off in the same manner. In addition, during the first 24 hours, equal parts of 25% (rather than 50%) glucose solution and 8.5% amino acid solution should be used. This would allow the patient to gradually adapt metabolically.

COMPLICATIONS OF INTRAVENOUS FEEDING

Many complications can occur with intravenous feeding. These include: 1) catheter-related problems, 2) mechanical difficulties, 3) sepsis, and 4) metabolic abnormalities.

The most common catheter-related problems are occlusions and thrombophlebitis. Thrombus formation may be caused by the type of catheter material, vascular damage during catheter insertion, and local infection.[16,20,125] Blood hemoglobin may be a predictor of thrombosis related to the central venous catheter. A study in people showed that if a patient's initial blood hemoglobin concentration was greater than 12.7 g/dl before catheterization, there was increased risk of catheter related thrombosis during intravenous feeding for one week or more.[71] Technique, attention to catheter care, and **using the catheter only for infusion of the feeding solution** will minimize catheter-related problems. The catheter should not be used to obtain blood samples, except those taken to check for catheter sepsis. Occlusion of the catheter can be cleared by irrigating the catheter with heparinized saline solution. Interruption of flow can also result from mechanical problems related to kinked lines and clogged filters. If filters are used, they should be changed daily.

The following procedure should be followed for evaluating all patients showing signs of sepsis during intravenous feeding:[28,114]

1. Identify all potential causes for sepsis and manage them appropriately.

2. Draw blood from a peripheral vein for culture.

3. If sepsis secondary to a contaminated intravenous solution is suspected, replace the administration apparatus and solution bottle.

4. If no source for persistent fever is found after 24 hours, blood for cultures may be drawn both via the feeding catheter and a peripheral vein. Technique must be meticulous because taking a sample via the feeding catheter could result

in contamination and subsequent development of catheter-related sepsis, if it is not already present.

5. If peripheral blood cultures are positive but blood taken via the feeding catheter is negative, the catheter is probably not the cause of sepsis.

6. If fever persists and cultures are negative, cli-

nical concern regarding potential intravenous feeding-line induced sepsis may be further evaluated by changing the catheter.

7. If the blood cultures are positive for *Staphylococcus* spp., if only the blood taken via the feeding tubing is positive, or if other clinical evidence implicates the feeding tubing as the site of entrance for sepsis, a new catheter should

TABLE 19

METABOLIC COMPLICATIONS OF INTRAVENOUS FEEDING AND THEIR MANAGEMENT[129]

Complication	Characterized by	Usual Cause	Treatment
Ammonia Toxicity	Elevated blood ammonia. Lethargy. Seizures. Coma.	Hepatic dysfunction.	Slow or discontinue infusion.
Hypochloremic Metabolic Acidosis	Acidosis with increased serum chloride and often sodium.	Excessive renal or gastrointestinal losses of base. Infusion of hydrogen ions. Cationic greater than anionic amino acid concentration in feeding solution. Excessive chloride in feeding solution.	Decrease chloride and increase bicarbonate, acetate or lactate content of feeding solution
Hyperglycemia	Elevated blood glucose. Glycosuria (3 to 4+). Polyuria.	Glucose intolerance. Too rapid initiation of feeding. Infection, or diabetes mellitus.	Decrease rate of infusion. Search for infection. Consider insulin administration.
Hyperosmolar Nonketotic Dehydration	Hyperglycemia. Dehydration. Increases in serum osmolality and serum sodium. Seizures or Coma.	Failure to recognize initial hyperglycemia.	Give insulin and a mixture of equal volumes of isotonic saline rather than the feeding solution. Closely monitor plasma glucose, osmolality, sodium, and potassium, and urine glucose.
Hypoglycemia	Hypothermia. Lethargy. Peripheral vasoconstriction.	Too rapidly stopping intravenous feeding.	Immediately begin dextrose infusion. Monitor plasma glucose and potassium
Hypokalemia	Muscular weakness. Cardiac arrhythmias. Increased digitalis sensitivity.	Excessive gastrointestinal or urinary potassium losses, or inadequate potassium in feeding solution.	Increase potassium concentration in feeding solution and monitor plasma potassium.
Hypomagnesemia	Weakness. Convulsive seizures with or without tetany.	Insufficient magnesium in feeding solution, or excessive gastrointestinal or renal losses.	Increase magnesium in feeding solution. In an emergency, give magnesium sulfate solution intramuscularly.
Hyponatremia	Lethargy. Confusion.	Excessive gastrointestinal or urinary sodium losses, or inadequate sodium in feeding solution.	Increase sodium concentration in feeding solution and monitor plasma sodium.
Hypophosphatemia	Paresthesia. Hyperventilation. Lethargy.	Usually caused by inadequate inorganic phosphate in feeding solution. Concentrated glucose infusion may precipitate syndrome.	Add phosphate to feeding solution. In an emergency give potassium phosphate slowly, mixed well with 5% dextrose solutions. (Note: rapid correction of hypophosphatemia may cause hypocalcemic tetany.)
Pre-renal azotemia	Depression. Increased BUN.	Dehydration or calorie:nitrogen imbalance	Correct dehydration. Give insulin if patient is hyperglycemic. Increase nonprotein calories.

be inserted at a new site. Generally 24 or more hours of specific antibiotic therapy is indicated before intravenous feeding is reinstituted.

8. Confirmation of the catheter as the septic focus is made by obtaining a positive culture from the catheter tip.

Many metabolic problems can be caused by intravenous feeding; the most common, along with their management, are given in Table 19. A decrease in plasma electrolyte concentrations, particularly of phosphorus and potassium, is not usually related to disease, but instead is caused by the cellular uptake of these ions as anabolism begins to normalize body homeostasis. Deficiencies should be corrected by adding additional quantities of these electrolytes to the feeding solution (see Table 7, page 5-18 for sources of additives).

CONCLUSIONS

Anorexia is common and occurs with many diseases. It is important to recognize, however, that anorexia is much more than a non-specific sign of disease. Absence of food intake, even for a few days, in conjunction with disease or trauma adversely affects all body systems, making it more difficult for the animal to resist the effects of the disease, to recover, and to respond to therapy.

Few contraindications exist to feeding patients, and a broad range of procedures to ensure adequate nutrient intake are available. Products for feeding anorectic dogs and cats are available in forms ranging from standard commercial diets to the most elemental forms of the nutrients, e.g. amino acids, glucose and lipids. The variety of products and the many methods available for delivering them provide sufficient combinations to ensure that nutrient deprivation need not add insult to the injury of the disease.

Finally, it is emphasized that supplemental nutrition is adjunctive therapy. For example, without antibiotics, all the food in the world will not cure a septic animal. Neither will all the antibiotics in the world save the starving animal. Both forms of therapy are necessary. Nutritional intervention has been shown to reduce the number of disease-related complications and shorten the acute phase of injury and healing time. When the limitations are understood and the advantages weighed against the potential complications, nutritional support can make an important contribution to what is the goal of therapy: rapid and complete recovery of the patient.

REFERENCES

1. Alexander JW, Stinnett JD: Changes in immunologic function. In Surgical Nutrition. Editor JE Fischer, Publisher Little, Brown and Co, Boston, MA pp 535-549 (1983).

2. Allen TA: Specialized nutrition. Proceedings Amer Acad Vet Int Med pp 2-55 to 2-64 (1986).

3. Ilison JB: Calorie and protein nutrition. Ann NY Acad Sci 69:1009-24 (1958).

4. Alverdy J, Chi HS, Sheldon GF: The effect of parenteral nutrition on gastrointestinal immunity: The importance of enteral stimulation. Ann Surg 202:681-684 (1985).

5. Anderson RS: Water balance in the dog and cat. J Sm Anim Pract 23:588-598 (1982).

6. Archibald J, Holt JC, Sokolovsky V: The body's response to trauma. In Management of Trauma in Dogs and Cats. American Veterinary Publications, Santa Barbara,CA pp 21-33 (1981).

7. Baile CA, McLaughlin CL: A review of the behavioral and physiological responses to elfazepam, a chemical feed intake stimulant. J Anim Sci 49:1371-1395 (1979).

8. Baker JC, Lippert AC: Total parenteral nutritional therapy in the calf. Comp Cont Ed (in press, 1986).

9. Baracos V, Rodemann HP, Dinarello CA, Goldberg AL: Stimulation of muscle protein degradation and prostaglandin E^2 release by leukocytic pyrogen (interleukin-1). New Engl J Med 308:553-558 (1983).

10. Basu TK, Dickerson JWT, Parke DV: The effect of diet on rat plasma corticosteroids and liver aromatic hydroxylase activity. Biochem J 125:16-23 (1971).

11. Bengmark S, Goransson G, Idvall J, Zoucas E: Increased bleeding during liver resection in ethanol-intoxicated rats. Thrombos Haemostas 43:185-232 (1980).

12. Blackburn GL, Baltej SM, Pierce EC: Nutrition in the critically ill patient. Anesthesiology 47: 181-194 (1977)

13. Bright RM: Percutaneous tube gastrostomy with and without endoscopy. Proceedings, Amer Acad Vet Int Med pp 2-65 to 2-69 (1986).

14. Brodner RA, Van Gilder JC, Collins WF Jr: Experimental spinal cord trauma: potentiation by alcohol. J Trauma 21:124-129 (1981).

15. Burrows CF: Inadequate skin preparation as a cause of intravenous catheter-related infection in the dog. J Amer Vet Med Assoc 180:747-749 (1982).

16. Burrows DF: Inadequate skin preparation as a cause of intravenous catheter-related infection in the dog. J Amer Vet Med Assoc 180:747-749 (1982).

17. Butterworth CE Jr: Some clinical manifestations of nutritional deficiency in hospitalized patients. In Nutritional Assessment—Present Status, Future Directions and Prospects. Editor SM Levenson, Report of the Second Ross Conference on Medical Research, Columbus, OH Ross. Laboratories, pp 2-3 (1981).

18. Buzby GP, Mullen JL, Matthews DC, et al: Prognostic nutritional index in gastrointestinal surgery. Amer J Surg 139:160-167 (1980).

19. Buzby GP, Mullen JL, Stein TP, et al: Host-tumor interaction and nutrient supply. Cancer 45:2940-2948 (1980).

20. Carter JM, Freedman AB: Total intravenous feeding in the dog. J Amer Vet Med Assoc 171:71-76 (1977).

21. Case GL, Lewis LD, Phillips RW, Click JL: Effects of osmolality of liquid nutrient diets on meal passage and nutrient absorption in Yucatan miniature swine. Amer J Clin Nutr 1868-1878 (1981).

22. Case GL, Phillips RW, Lewis LD, Connolly B: Effects of osmolality of liquid nutrient diets on plasma equilibration of water and carbohydrate in Yucatan miniature swine. Amer J of Clin Nutr 34:1861-1867 (1981).

23. Chandra RK, Scrimshaw NS: Immunocompetence in nutritional assessment. Amer J Clin Nutr 33:2694-2697 (1980).

24. Cizek LJ: Long term observations on the relationship between food and water ingestion in the dog. Amer J Physiol 197:342-346 (1959).

25. Clark CH: Fluid therapy. In Feline Medicine and Surgery. Editor EJ Catcott, 2nd ed, Publisher Amer Vet Publ, Santa Barbara, CA pp 601-619 (1975).

26. Clowes GHA Jr, George BC, Villee CA Jr, Saravis CA: Muscle proteolysis induced by a circulating peptide in patients with sepsis to trauma. New Engl J Med 308:545-552 (1983).

27. Collette WL, Merriwether WF: Oral Alimentation of cats. Vet Med Sm Anim Clin 59:839-845 (1964).

28. Colley R. Wilson J, Kapusta E, et al: Does fever mean infection in central total parenteral nutrition? J Parent Ent Nutr 3:32 (1979).

29. Consolazio CF, Nelson RA, Johnson HL, et al: Metabolic aspects of acute starvation in normal humans: Performance and cardiovascular. Amer J Clin Nutr 20:684-695 (1967).

30. Copeland EM III, Dudrick SJ, Daly JM, Ota DM: Nutritional changes in neoplasia. In Surgical Nutrition. Editor JE Fischer, Publisher Little, Brown and Co, Boston, MA pp 515-534 (1983).

31. Crane SW: Placement and maintenance of a temporary feeding tube gastrostomy in the dog and cat. Comp Cont Ed for Pract Vet 2:770-776 (1980).

32. Crowe DT, Downs MD: Pharyngostomy complications in dogs and cats and recommended technical modifications: experimental and clinical investigations. J Amer An Hosp Assoc 22:493-503 (1986).

33. Crowe DT Jr: Enteral nutrition for the critically ill or injured patient, Part 1. Paper presented at Vet Crit Care meetings, Las Vegas, NV (1982).

34. Crowe DT Jr: Nutritional support for the seriously ill or injured patient: an overview. J Vet Emerg Crit Care 1:1-7 (1985).

35. Crowe DT Jr: Tube feeding diets for nutritional support of the critically ill or injured patients. J Vet Emerg Crit Care 1:8-18 (1985).

36. Crowe DT Jr: Use of a nasogastric tube for gastric and esophageal decompression in the dog and cat. J Amer Vet Med Assoc 188:1178-1182 (1986).

37. Daly JM, Long JM: Intravenous hyperalimentation techniques and potential complications. Surg Clin of NA 61:583-592 (1981).

38. deBruijne JJ: Biochemical observations during total starvation in dogs. Int J Obesity 3:239-247 (1979).

39. Delany HM, Carnevale NJ, Gauvey JW: Jejunostomy by a needle catheter technique. Surgery 73:786-790 (1973).

40. Della-Fera MA, Baile CA, McLaughlin CL: Feeding elicited by benzodiazepine-like chemicals in puppies and cats: structure-activity relationships. Pharm, Biochem and Beh 12:195-200 (1980).

41. Dixon FJ, Mairer PH, Deichmiller MP: Half-lives of homologous serum albumins in several species. Proc Soc Exp Biol Med 83:287-288 (1953).

42. Dubos RJ: The micro-environment of inflammation or Metchnikoff revisited. Lancet 2:1-5 (1955A).

43. Dudrick SJ, Wilmore DW, Vars HM, Rhoads JE: Long-term total parenteral nutrition with growth, development, and positive nitrogen balance. Surgery 64:143-142 (1968).

44. Evans HE, Christensen GC (eds): The digestive system. In Anatomy of the Dog, Publisher WB Saunders Co, Philadelphia, PA, pp 476.

45. Fairfull-Smith R, Abunassar R, Freeman JB, Maroun MD: Rational use of elemental and nonelemental diets in hospitalized patients. Ann Surg 192:600-603 (1980).

46. Feldman EC: Diseases of the endocrine pancreas. In Textbook of Veterinary Internal Medicine. Editor SJ Ettinger, Publisher WB Saunders Co, Philadelphia, PA, 1615-1649 (1983).

47. Filkins JP: Insulin like activity (ILA) of a macrophage mediator on adipose tissue glucose oxidation. J Reticuloendothel Soc 25:591-595 (1979).

48. Fischer JE (ed): Surgical Nutrition. Little, Brown and Co, Boston, MA (1983).

49. Fischer JE, Freund HR: Central Hyperalimentation. In Surgical Nutrition. Editor JE Fischer, Publisher Little, Brown & Co, Boston, MA, 663-702 (1983).

50. Fisher H: Nutritional aspects of protein reserves. In Newer Methods in Nutritional Biochemistry. Editor AA Albanese, Publisher Academic Press, New York, NY, 101-124 (1967).

51. Ford, RB: Nasogastric intubation in the cat. Comp Cont Ed for the Anim Hlth Tech I:29-33 (1980).

52. Gauderer MWL, Ponsky JL: A simplified technique for constructing a tube feeding gastrostomy. Surg Gyn Obstet 152:83-85 (1981).

53. Gauderer MWL, Ponsky JL, Izant RJ: Gastrostomy without laparotomy: a percutaneous endoscopic technique. J Pediatr Surg 15:872-875 (1980).

54. Gavin LA, McMahon FA, Moeller M: Carbohydrate in contrast to protein feeding increases the hepatic content of active thyroxine-f'-deiodinase in the rat. Endocrinol 109:530-536 (1981).

55. Gavin LA, Moeller M: The mechanism of recovery of hepatic T₄-5'-deiodinase during glucose refeeding: role of glucagon and insulin. Metabol 32:543-551 (1983).

56. Giovanoii R: The manufacturing pharmacy; solutions and incompatibilities. In Total Parenteral Nutrition. Editor JE Fisher, Publisher Little, Brown & Co, Boston Ma, 27-53 (1976).

57. Goode AW: The Scientific basis of nutritional assessment. Brit J Anesth 53:161-182 (1981).

58. Grant JD: Handbook of total parenteral nutrition. Publisher WB Saunders Co. Philadelphia, PA (1980).

59. Grant JP, Custer PB, Thurlow J: Current techniques of nutritional assessment. Surg Clin of N Amer 61(3):437-463 (1981).

60. Guyton AC: Dietary balances, regulation of feeding; obesity and starvation. In Textbook of Medical Physiology. Publisher WB Saunders Co, Philadelphia, PA pp 899-906 (1981).

61. Hakansson I: Experience in long term studies of nine intravenous fat emulsions in dogs. Nutr 10:54-76 (1968).

62. Hakansson I, Holm I, Wretlind A: Studies of complete intravenous alimentation in dogs. Nutr 8:1-24 (1966).

63. Hand MS, Crane SW, Buffington CA: Surgical nutrition. In Manual of Small Animal Surgical Therapeutics. Editors CW Betts, SW Crane, Publisher Churchill Livingstone. New York,NY pp 91-115 (1986).

64. Hand MS, Fettman MJ, Chandrasena LG, Phillips RW: The effects of various endotoxin doses on Yucatan miniature swine. Part I. Hemodynamic, metabolic, and lethal consequences. Am J Phys 244: E385-E398 (1983).

65. Harrison JB, Sussman HH, Pickering DE: Fluid and electrolyte therapy in small animals. J Amer Vet Med Assoc 137:637-645 (1960).

66. Heizer W and Nutrition Support Service Staff: Intravenous Feeding. Physicians Handbook for Adult Patients. N Carolina Memorial Hosp, Univ N Ca, Chapel Hill NC pp1-41 (1984).

67. Heymsfield SB, Bethel RA, Ansley JD, et al: Enteral hyperalimentation: an alternative to central venous hyperalimentation. Ann Int Med 90:63-71 (1979).

68. Hippocrates. Aphorisms. Hippocrates with an English Translation. Editor WHS Jones, Publisher Heineman, London (1931).

69. Hunt DR, Rowlands BJ, Johnston D: Hand grip strength—a simple prognostic indicator in surgical patients. J Parent Ent Nutr 9:701-704 (1985).

70. Izzo RS, Leissing N, Woods E, et al: The effects of intravenous administration of 10% travamulsion fat emulsion to Beagle dogs for 91 consecutive days. J Parent Ent Nutr 7(3):257-265 (1983).

71. Jacobson S, Brismar B: Blood hemoglobin: a possible predictor of central venous catheter-related thrombosis in parenteral nutrition 9:471-473 (1985).

72. Jeppsson B. Gimmon Z: Vitamins. In Surgical Nutrition. Editor JE Fischer. Little Brown and Co. Boston, MA pp 241-281 (1983).

73. Karran SJ, Alberti KGMM: Carbohydrates in parenteral nutrition. In Practical Nutritional Support. Editors SJ Karran, KGMM Alberti, Publisher John Wiley & Sons, New York, NY, pp 94-105 (1980).

74. Kay RG, Knight GS: Trace metals. In Surgical Nutrition. Editor JE Fischer. Little, Brown and Co, Boston, MA pp 283-329 (1983).

75. Klemm R: Behavioral physiology. In Dukes Physiology of Domestic Animals. Editor MJ Swenson, Cornell University Press, Ithaca NY pp 687-706 (1984).

76. Koretz RL, Meyer JH: Elemental diets - facts and fantasies. Gastroenterology 78:393-410 (1980).

77. Kudsk KA, Carpenter G, Petersen S, Sheldon GF: Effect of enteral and parenteral feeding in malnourished rats with E coli-hemoglobin adjuvant peritonitis. J Surg Res 31:105-110 (1981).

78. Lant: GC Pharyngostomy tube installation for the administration of nutritional and fluid requirements. Comp Cont Ed for Pract Vet 3:135-142 (1981).

79. Lant GC, Cantwell HD, Van Vleet JF, et al: Pharyngostomy tube induced esophagitis in the dog: an experimental study. J Amer Anin Hosp Assoc 19:207-212 (1983).

80. Law DH;: Current concepts in nutrition: total parenteral nutrition. New Engl J Med 297:1104-1107 (1977).

81. Levenson SM (ed): Nutritional Assessment - present status, future directions, and prospects Report of the Second Ross Conference on Medical Research, Columbus, OH, Ross Laboratories (1981).

82. Levenson SM, Crowley LV, Seifter E: Starvation. In American College of Surgeons, Manual of Surgical Nutrition. WB Saunders Co, Philadelphia, PA pp 236-266 (1975).

83. Levenson SM, Seifter E: Starvation: metabolic and physiologic responses, In Surgical Nutrition. Editor JE Fisher, Publisher Little Brown and Co, Boston, MA pp 423-478 (1983).

84. Levenson S, Seifter E, Van Winkle W Jr: Nutrition. In Fundamentals of Wound Management. Editors TK Hunt and JE Dunphy. Appleton-Century-Corfts, New York, NY pp 286-363 (1979).

85. Long CL, Schaffel N, Geiger JW, et al: Metabolic response to injury and illness: estimation of energy and protein needs from indirect calorimetry and nitrogen balance. J Parent Ent Nutr 3:452-456 (1979).

86. MacBurney M, Wilmore DW: Rational decision-making in nutrition care. Surg Clin of N Amer, pp 571-582 (1981).

87. Malt SH, Baue AE: The effects of ethanol as related to trauma in the awake dog. J Trauma 11:76-86 (1971).

88. Markowitz J, Archibald J, Downie HG (eds): Jejunostomy. In Experimental Surgery Including Surgical Physiology. Publisher Williams and Wilkins, Baltimore, MD, pp 241-243 (1954).

89. McArdle AH, Palmason C, Morency I, Brown RA: A rationale for enteral feeding as the preferable route for hyperalimentation. Surgery 90:616-623 (1981).

90. McArdle AH, Wittnick C, Freeman CR, Duguid WP: Elemental diet as prophylaxis against radiation injury. Arch Surg 120:1026-1032 (1985).

91. McGee CD, Ostro MJ, Kurian R, Jeejeebhoy KN: Vitamin E and selenium status of patients receiving short-term total parenteral nutrition. Amer J Clin Nutr 42:432-438 (1985).

92. Meguid MM, Gray GE, Debouis D: The use of enteral nutrition in the patient with cancer. In Enteral and Tube Feeding. Editors JL Rombeau, MD Caldwell, Publisher WB Saunders, Philadelphia, PA pp 303-337 (1984).

93. Michell AR: The pathophysiological basis of fluid therapy in small animals. Vet Rec 104:542-548 (1979).

94. Mizock B: Septic shock. A metabolic perspective. Arch Intern Med 144:579-585 (1984).

95. Mochizuki H, Trocki O, Dominioni L, et al: Mechanism of prevention of postburn hypermetabolism and catabolism by early enteral feeding. Ann Surg 200:297-310 (1984).

96. Molnar JA, Bell SJ, Goodenough RD, Burke JF: Enteral nutrition in patients with burns or trauma. In Enteral and Tube Feeding. Editors JL Rombeau, MD Caldwell. WB Saunders Co, Philadelphia, PA pp 412-433 (1984).

97. Moore EE, Jones TN: Nutritional assessment and preliminary report on early support of the trauma patient. J Amer College Nutr 2:45-54 (1983).

98. Moore JN: Endotoxemia: part II. Biological reactions to endotoxin. Comp Cont Ed 3:S392-S400 (1981).

99. Morris ML, Collins DR: The problem of anorexia. Vet Med/Small Anim Clin 62:1075-1080 (1967).

100. Morris ML, Collins DR: Anorexia in the dog. Vet Med/Small Anim Clin 62:753-759 (1967).

101. Mullen JL, Crosby LO, Rombeau JL (eds): Symposium on surgical nutrition. Surg Clin of N Amer 61(3) (1981).

102. Nordenstrom J: Utilization of exogenous and endogenous lipids for energy production during parenteral nutrition. Acta Chir Scand Suppl 510 (1982).

103. Orton EC: Enteral hyperalimentation administered via needle catheter-jejunostoma as an adjunct to cranial abdominal surgery in dogs and cats. J Amer Vet Med Assoc 188:1406-1411 (1986).

104. Osborne CA, Finco DR, Low DG: Pathophysiology of renal disease, renal failure and uremia. In Textbook of Veterinary Internal Medicine. 2nd ed. Editor SJ Ettinger, Publisher WB Saunders Co, Philadelphia, PA 1733-1792 (1983).

105. Payne PR: Assessment of the protein values of diets in relation to the requirements of the growing dog. In Canine and Feline Nutritional Requirements. Editor D Graham-Hones, Publisher Pergamon Press, London, 19-31 (1965).

106. Pinchcofsky-Devin RD, Kaminski MV: Visceral protein increase associated with interrupt versus continuous enteral hyperalimentation. J Parent Ent Nutr 9:474-476 (1985).

107. Popp MB, Brennan MF: Metabolic response to trauma and infection. In Surgical Nutrition. Editor JE Fisher, Publisher Little, Brown and Co, Boston, MA pp 479-513 (1983).

108. Porte D Jr, Halter JB: The endocrine pancreas and diabetes mellitus. In Textbook of Endocrinology. Editor RH Williams, Publisher WB Saunders Co, Philadelphia, PA pp 716-843 (1981).

109. Prasad A: Zinc in human nutrition. Publisher CRC Press, Boca Raton, FL (1979).

110. Prentiss PG, Wolf AV, Eddy HE: Hydropenia in cat and dog: ability of the cat to meet its water requirements solely from a diet of meat or fish. Amer J Physiol 196:625-632 (1959).

111. Renegar WR, Stall SG, Bojrab MJ, Simpson ST: Parenteral hyperalimentation—the use of lipid as the prime calorie source. J Amer Anim Hosp Assoc 15:411-415 (1979).

112. Rombeau JL, Caldwell MD (eds): Enteral and Tube Feeding. WB Saunders Co, Philadelphia, PA (1984).

113. Rombeau JL, Caldwell MD (eds): Parenteral Nutrition. WB Saunders Co, Philadelphia, PA (1984).

114. Ryan JA, Abel RM, Abbott WM, et al: Complications of catheters in total parenteral nutrition. New Engl J Med 290:757-761 (1974).

115. Sanford TD, Colby ED, Kealy R: Tube pharyngo-esophagostomy and liquified diet in the treatment of feline upper respiratory disease. Feline Pract 15:35-38 (1985).

116. Schiffman SS: Taste and smell in disease. New Eng J Med 308(21):1275-1279 (1983).

117. Schiffman SS: Taste and smell in disease. New Eng J Med 308(22):1337-1343 (1983).

118. Scott, HG, Ivy AC: Jejunal alimentation: an experimental study in dogs. Amer J Surg 93:1197-1201 (1931).

119. Selivanov V, Sheldon GF: Enteral nutrition and sepsis. In Enteral and Tube Feeding. Editors JL Rombeau, MD Caldwell. WB Saunders Co, Philadelphia, PA pp 403-411 (1984).

120. Seltzer MH, Asaadi M, Coco A, et al: The use of a simplified standardized hyperalimentation formula. J Parent Ent Nutr 2:28-30 (1978).

121. Sheffy FE, Williams AJ: Nutrition and the immune response. J Amer Vet Med Assoc 180:1073-1076 (1982).

122. Shils ME: Parenteral nutrition. In Modern Nutrition in Health and Disease. Editors RD Goodhart, ME Shils, Publisher Lea and Febiger, Philadelphia, PA, pp 1125-1152 (1980).

123. Siegel JH, Cerra FB, Coleman B, et al: Physiological and metabolic correlations in human sepsis. Surgery 86:163-193 (1979).

124. Smith JL, Heymsfield SB: Enteral nutrition support: formula preparation from modular ingredients. J Parent Ent Nutr 7:280-288 (1983).

125. Spencer KR: Intravenous catheters. Vet Clin of N Amer 12:533-543 (1982).

126. Stein B: The cat versus its gastrointestinal tract. Ohio Vet Med Assoc, Annual Meeting, Feb (1984).

127. Stein TP, Buzby GP: Protein metabolism in surgical patients. Surg Clin of N Amer 6:519-527 (1981).

128. Teeter SM, Collins DR: Intragastric intubation of small animals. Vet Med Sm Anim Clin 61:1067-1076 (1966).

129. Travenol Laboratories, Fundamentals of nutritional support. Deerfield, IL (1981).

130. Valentine RJ, Turner WW: Pleural complications of nasoenteric feeding tubes. J Parent Ent Nutr 9:605-607 (1985).

131. Vanlandingham S, Simpson S, Daniel P, Newmark SR: Metabolic abnormalities in patients supported with enteral tube feeding. J Parent Ent Nutr 5:322-324 (1981).

132. Viteri FE, Torun B: Protein-calorie malnutrition. In Modern Nutrition in Health and Disease. Editors RD Goodhart, ME Shils, Publisher Lea and Febiger, Philadelphia, PA, pp 697-720 (1980).

133. Wedge JH, DeCampos R, Kerr A, et al: Branched chain amino acids, nitrogen excretion and injury in man. Clin Sci Mol Med 50:393-399 (1976).

134. Williams WW: Infection control during parenteral nutrition therapy. J Parent Ent Nutr 9:735-746 (1985).

135. Williamson RC: Intestinal adaptation: structural, functional and cytokinetic changes. New Engl J Med 291:1393 & 1444 (1978).

136. Wolfe RR, Shaw JHF: Alanine-urea-glucose interrelationships in normal and septic man. Circ Shock 13:64 (1984).

137. Wolman SL, Anderson GH, Marless EB, Jeejeebhoy KN: Zinc in total parenteral nutrition requirements and metabolic effects (Alimentary tract) Gastroenterology 76:458 (1979).

138. Woods HF, Alberti KGMM: Dangers of intravenous fructose. Lancet 2:1354-1357 (1972).

139. Woolf LI, Groves AC, Duff JH: Amino acid metabolism in dogs with E. Coli bacteremic shock. Surgery 85:212-218 (1979).

CHAPTER 6

Obesity

CONTENTS

SUMMARY OF MANAGEMENT RECOMMENDATIONS

1. Emphasize to the client who owns puppies the importance of preventing excess fat deposition in the puppies during growth in order to prevent obesity throughout their life (see page 6-31).

2. Follow all recommendations given. Chances of success are reduced with each procedure omitted.

3. Have prepared materials available for the client to take home describing the effects of obesity, the steps required for successful weight reduction, and a graph for recording the animal's weight versus time (may copy pages 6-34 and 6-35).

4. At each visit compare the animal's weight to its previous weights.

5. If the animal is more than 15% above optimum body weight (determined as described on page 6-5):

   a) Inform the client of the degree of obesity present.

   b) Review with the client the prepared materials describing the effects of obesity (Tables 7 and 8, and Figure 1, pages 6-7, 8 and 9), and the resulting increase in mortality (Table 1, page 6-3).

   c) Emphasize that weight reduction will lessen the chances of these detrimental effects, improve their pet's appearance and health, decrease future health-care costs, and prolong their pet's life.

   d) Suggest that a weight-reduction program be started immediately.

6. Evaluate the patient thoroughly to determine the presence of conditions other than obesity that require therapy (See page 6-4).

7. Estimate optimum body weight, set it as the goal for weight reduction, and estimate the time required to reach this goal (Tables 11 and 12, pages 6-22 and 23).

8. Instruct the client to:

   a) Feed a nutritionally balanced, high-fiber (more than 15% in dry matter), low-fat (less than 10% in dry matter) diet that is 35-45% for dogs and 20-30% for cats lower in caloric density than the animal's previous diet (Table 15, page 6-26). Some cats and dogs reduce to, and then maintain, optimum weight even when a diet of this type is always available (Table 14, page 6-25). Although weight loss will be slower than when a restricted amount is fed, this approach may be tried first. If the resulting weight loss is not satisfactory, the amount fed should be restricted to provide 60-65% of caloric requirements for maintenance at optimum (not obese) weight (Table 13, page 6-23).

   b) Feed at least three times daily.

   c) Keep the animal out of the room when food for the family is being prepared or eaten.

   d) Feed absolutely nothing other than the specified amount of the proper dietary food. If clients insist on giving their pets snacks, have them give a nugget or cube of the dry form of the reducing diet and record the exact amount of everything fed.

   e) Take the animal for two 10- to 15-minute walks daily unless a specific medical reason exists for not doing so. Gradually increase the distance covered in the same length of time but ensure that the animal never becomes unduly stressed or dyspneic.

   f) Weekly, weigh the animal and record its weight on a graph versus time (see example, page 6-35).

   g) Return the animal and the graph every 2-3 weeks. If necessary, adjust the amount being fed to produce a 2-4% weekly weight loss.

   h) Insure that the cat eats. Both obesity and fasting, particularly by obese cats, may result in hepatic lipidosis and death.

9. If weight loss at the desired rate does not occur, hospitalize the animal and adjust the amount fed to produce weight loss, thus showing the client that the goal can be reached.

10. When optimum weight is reached, give the client the choice of feeding more reducing diet or changing to a low-calorie maintenance diet (such as Prescription Diet w/d, Hill's) fed in a restricted amount. Frequently the weight-reducing diet can be fed free-choice, whereas the amount of other diets must be restricted to prevent recurrence of obesity.

11. To prevent recurrence, instruct the client to:

    a) Continue weighing the animal at least once a week, mark the weight on the graph and, if necessary, adjust the amount fed to maintain optimum weight.

    b) Bring the animal and the graph back in one month and again three to four months later.

    c) Continue ensuring that the animal is exercised daily and fed a restricted calorie diet.

INCIDENCE

Obesity is the most common nutritional disease of dogs, cats, and people in a prosperous society (Tables 1 and 2), exceeding by far all deficiency diseases combines.[54] Obesity is considered present when body weight is 15% more than optimum; health problems begin increasing at this weight (Table 1).[46,88,139] In affluent societies 25% of adult people and 24-44% of dogs are obese, whereas only 2-3% of dogs are thin.[14,53,54a,117,128] In a recent study 24.3% of dogs seen at veterinary practices were above and 15.4% were below optimum body weight.[54a] In cats the incidence of obesity in 1972 was reported to be 6 to 12%,[53] but the current incidence is probably much greater, due largely to the increased palatability and popularity of dry cat foods and the more common practice of feeding free-choice.

The incidence of obesity increases with age (Table 2).[27,128] This increase occurs up to age 45 in men, but throughout life in women.[27] In people, body fat increases throughout life—from 15% at puberty to about 30% in men and 40% in women. However, lean body mass decreases; thus, on the average, body weight increases only 10-15%.[27] This same trend also occurs in dogs and cats. Both the decrease in lean body mass and physical activity that occur with increasing age reduce expenditure of energy. As a result, an aged animal's caloric need at rest is about 20% less than that needed by a young, active adult. However, the increase in body fat and decrease in lean body mass that occur with aging can be lessened by physical activity.[27]

Obesity in dogs is more common in females than males up to 12 years of age (Table 2) and is about twice as high in neutered as non-neutered dogs of either sex (Table 3).[4,54a,128] Conversely, only about one-half as many neutered as non-neutered dogs of both sexes are underweight (Table 3). In order of incidence Labradors, Cairn Terriers, Cocker Spaniels, Dachshunds, Shetland Sheepdogs, Basset Hounds and Beagles had the greatest tendency to obesity.[54a] German Shepherds, Greyhounds, Yorkshire Terriers, Dobermans, Staffordshire Bull Terriers, Lurchers, Whippets, Boxers and Sealyhams were the breeds least likely to become obese.[54a,117,139]

Obesity is more prevalent in dogs belonging to owners who are overweight (44% vs 25%) and middle-aged or older (36% vs 20%).[117] This is most

TABLE 1

INCREASED MORTALITY AND INCIDENCE OF DISEASE IN OBESE PEOPLE[27,178]

	% Above Desirable Body Weight*				
	10–19	20–29	30–45	50–60	100
Men—% of All	18	14	5	----	----
Women—% of All	13	24	----	7	----
	% Higher at That Body Wt.				
Mortality**	9	25	65	230	1200
Heart Disease	----	25	75	----	----
Stroke	----	15	90	----	----
Diabetes	----	110	200	----	----
Digestive Diseases	----	60	275	----	----

*Desirable body weight is the weight for a specific age and sex associated with the lowest mortality among persons covered by life insurance.

**Increased incidence of mortality and disease as compared to people of the same sex and age who are at desirable body weight. This increase is higher in younger than in older adults.

TABLE 2

INCIDENCE OF OBESITY IN DOGS[117]

Sex (Not Neutered)	n	% Obese at the Years of Age Shown				
		All Ages	1–4	5–7	8–11	Over 12
Male	537	23	12	30	34	41
Female	463	32	21	37	41	40

TABLE 3

EFFECT OF NEUTERING ON THE DOG'S BODY WEIGHT*

| Sexual Status | Percent of Dogs of Each Sexual Status that are | | | % of Population** |
	Under Wt.	Optimum Wt.	Over Wt.	
Male				
Intact	18.3	65.1	16.6	45.8
Neutered	11.5	51.0	37.5	3.9
Female				
Intact	15.7	62.4	21.9	29.3
Neutered	8.1	46.5	45.4	17.0
All Dogs	15.4	60.3	24.3	

*Adapted from reference 54a by dividing the percent of dogs of each sexual status at that weight by the percent of the total population which are of that sexual status.

**All dogs seen at 11 veterinary practices in England and Scotland from June 1 to Nov. 30. 1983; a total of 8268 dogs.

likely due to inadequate exercise. Increased food intake may also be a factor. Older overweight persons are more likely to exercise less and, as a result, to exercise their pets less. These people may also have a greater tendency to feed home-cooked meals, table scraps, treats or snacks. Dogs fed these items are more likely to be overweight than those fed only prepared pet foods (30% vs 20%).[117]

DIAGNOSIS

DIFFERENTIAL DIAGNOSIS

Obesity is obvious and easily diagnosed. However, before a diagnosis is made, a complete physical examination should be performed to determine the possible presence of edema or ascites, which may be mistaken for obesity. Also, these or other conditions associated with obesity (hyperadrenocorticism, hypothyroidism, congestive heart failure, and diabetes mellitus) may be present and require treatment. Diagnosis and management of heart failure are discussed in Chapter 11. As shown in Table 4, either or both fasting hyperglycemia and sustained hyperglycemia following the administration of glucose is diagnostic for diabetes.[118]

The major clinical signs useful in differentiating hyperadrenocorticism and hypothyroidism from simple obesity are given in Table 5. If there is any question as to their presence, adrenocortical function tests and thyroid stimulating hormone (TSH) stimulation tests should be conducted.

Commercial kits for accurately measuring serum thyroxine (T4) and triiodothyronine (T3) concen-

TABLE 4

TYPES OF DIABETES MELLITUS IN DOGS[118]

| Type | Insulin | Plasma Glucose (mg/dl) | | Plasma Insulin Concentration | | | |
| | | | | Fasting | | Challenge+ | |
		Fasting	Challenge+	Non-Obese	Obese	Non-Obese	Obese
I*	Dependent	>150	>150	0	0	0	0
II	Non-Dependent	>150**	>150	Normal	Increased	No Increase	
III	Decreased Postprandial Secretion	<150	>150	Near Normal		Subnormal Increase	

+45–60 min. after intravenous administration of 500 mg glucose/kg body wt.

*Characterized by sudden onset of clinical signs and, in contrast to human beings, most commonly manifests in mature or aged dogs.

**In contrast, in people it is generally normal and this form manifests in adults. > indicates greater than and < less than.

TABLE 5

CLINICAL SIGNS IN SIMPLE OBESITY, HYPERADRENOCORTICISM AND HYPOTHYROIDISM[46,132,141,150]

Symptoms	Simple Obesity	Hyperadrenocorticism	Hypothyroidism
Polydipsia-Polyuria	no	usually	no
Polyphagia	no	usually	no
Absence of Estrus	no	generally	occasionally
Alopecia, dry, dull hair and "dandruff"	no	generally diffuse & bilateral	generally
Hyperpigmentation	no	occasionally	occasionally
Increased sensitivity to cold	no	no	occasionally
Increased fasting plasma cholesterol concentration	no	occasionally	usually
Major fat deposits	trunk	abdomen	trunk
Abdominal enlargement	no	usually	no
Lethargy	occasionally	usually	usually

trations by radioimmunoassay are available.* Resting plasma T4 and T3 concentrations are below normal in most dogs and cats (60-80%) with hypothyroidism (below 1.0 μg T4/dl in both species, or 40 or 10 mg T3/dl in dogs or cats, respectively). However, many non-thyroidal disorders, including uremia, hepatic disease, hyperadrenocorticism and diabetes mellitus can also reduce either or both T4 and T3 concentrations. In addition, both are commonly less than normal in animals treated with Dilantin, phenobarbital, glucocorticoids, phenylbutazone and lithium. The most reliable means for distinguishing primary hypothyroidism from other causes of low thyroid hormone concentrations is the TSH stimulation test.**

Single plasma cortisol concentration values are of little use in diagnosing hyperadrenocorticism. Many factors alter these values, and values in both normal and affected animals overlap. Both ACTH-stimulation and dexamethasone-suppression tests are necessary to confirm the diagnosis of hyperadrenocorticism.†

---

*Micromedic T3 and T4 Radioimmunoassay Kit, Micromedic Systems, Horshaw PA; and T3 and T4 Diagnostic Kit, Nuclear Medical Labs, Irving, TX.

**An increase of less than 0.2 μg T4/dl and 10 mg T3/dl eight hours after intravenous administration of 0.25 U/kg to dogs and 1 U/kg to cats of TSH (Dermathycin, Coopers Animal Health Inc.) is diagnostic of hypothyroidism.

†A plasma cortisol concentration of 1.4 μg/dl or greater eight hours after intramuscular administration of 0.01 mg of dexamethasone/kg, or greater than a three-fold increase in plasma cortisol concentration two hours after intramuscular or intravenous administration of 20 units/dog or 10/cat of ACTH gel (Acthar, Armour Pharmaceutical Co) or 0.25 mg/dog of synthetic ACTH (Cortrosyn, Organon Inc). The dexamethasone suppression test should be done before the ACTH stimulation test. If results of either test are abnormal, hyperadrenocorticism is present.

ASSESSING DEGREE OF OBESITY

Degree of obesity can be accurately determined by comparing the animal's present weight to its non-obese weight such as that generally associated with the first year or so of maturity. The animal's non-obese weight may be found in veterinary or family records. With few exceptions, a healthy non-obese domestic cat weighs 3.5-4.5 kg (8-10 lb). Some domestic shorthair cats with large frames may be slightly heavier. However, cats of common domestic breed weighing more than 5.5 kg (12 lb) are likely to be overweight. For dogs, as shown in Table 6, comparison to a standard weight is not generally helpful because body builds vary widely, even among dogs of the same breed and sex.

If the animal's optimum weight is not known, the most practical means of assessing the degree of obesity is the amount of adipose tissue overlying the ribs and the amount of fat along the ventral abdomen. Although this assessment is subjective and will undoubtedly vary among individuals making this judgment, it is adequate for most clinical situations. The animal is too thin if its ribs are easily seen, normal if they are readily felt without any appreciable layer of subcutaneous fat, and obese if they cannot be easily palpated. To assess the fat overlying the ribs, stand behind the dog. Place both thumbs on the dorsal midline with fingers spread over the ribs. With thumbs pressing on the dorsal vertebral processes and fingers on the ribs, slide the hands gently backwards and forwards. Ideally, a moderately thin layer of fat should be felt. Visibly protruding bones usually suggest that the animal is too thin. A cushion of fat that cloaks the edges of the ribs and allows only a smooth wavy feel to the chest indicates that the dog is obese. Generally most

TABLE 6

OPTIMUM BODY WEIGHT OF MATURE DOGS — Kg (lb)* [6.139]

Giant Breeds—Ht	66-79 cm	(26-31 in)
Bloodhound	36-50	(80-110)
Borzoi	34-48	(75-105)
Bull Mastiff	45-59	(100-130)
Great Dane	52-66	(115-145)
Great Pyrenees	41-57	(90-125)
Irish Wolfhound	48-61	(105-135)
Komodor	34-48	(75-105)
Kuvaszok	34-55	(75-120)
Mastiff	77-89	(170-195)
Newfoundland	50-68	(110-150)
Rottweiler	32-45	(70-100)
Saint Bernard	68-82	(150-180)
Scot Deerhound	34-50	(75-110)

Large Breeds—Ht	58-64 cm	(23-25 in)
Afghan Hound	23-27	(50-60)
Alaskan Malamute	34-39	(75-85)
Amer Foxhound	27	(60)
Belgian Sheepdog	27	(60)
Bernese Mtn Dog	30	(66)
B&T Coon Hound	27	(60)
Bluetick Hound	27-32	(60-70)
Bouvier des Flandres	32	(70)
Boxer	32	(70)
Briard	32	(70)
Ches Bay Retriever	25-34	(55-75)
Collie	23-34	(50-75)
Curly Coat Retrv	32	(70)
Doberman Pinscher	32	(70)
English Foxhound	32	(70)
English Setter	30	(66)
Eskimo	34	(75)
Flat-Coat Retrv	27-32	(60-70)
German Shepherd	27-39	(60-85)
German Short-Haired Pointer	21-32	(45-70)
Golden Retriever	27-34	(60-75)
Gordon Setter	21-36	(45-80)
Greyhound	27-32	(60-70)
Irish Setter	27-32	(60-70)
Irish Water Spaniel	21-29	(45-65)
Kuvasz	32	(70)
Labrador Retriever	25-34	(55-75)
Old Engl Sheepdog	30	(66)
Otterhound	27-32	(60-70)
Pointer	27	(60)
Redbone Hound	30-32	(65-70)
Rhodes Ridgeback	18-27	(40-60)
Saluki	27	(60)
Schnauzer—Giant	34	(75)
Standard Poodle	25	(55)
Vizsla	21-30	(45-65)
Weimaraner	25-38	(55-85)

Medium Breeds—Ht	43-56 cm	(17-22 in)
Airedale Terrier	23	(50)
Amer Water Spaniel	11-20	(25-45)
Border Collie	18-23	(40-50)
Brittany Spaniel	14-18	(30-40)
Bulldog	18-23	(40-50)
Bull Terrier	23	(50)
Chow Chow	27	(60)
Clumber Spaniel	16-29	(35-65)
Dalmatian	21	(45)
Engl Spring Span	20-25	(45-55)
Field Spaniel	16-23	(35-50)
Harrier	21	(45)
Keeshond	18	(40)
Kerry Blue Terrier	15-18	(33-40)
Norweg Elkhound	23	(50)
Puli	16	(35)
Samoyed	25	(55)
Schnauzer—Std	16	(35)
Siberian Husky	16-27	(35-60)
Staffordshire Terrier	21	(45)
Sussex Spaniel	16-21	(35-45)
Welsh Spring Span	17	(37)
Wire-Haired Pointing Griffon	25	(55)
Whippet	5-12	(10-28)

Toy Breeds—Ht	13-28 cm	(5-11 in)
Affenpinscher	3.6	(8)
Australian Terrier	5.5-6.5	(12-14)
Brussels Griffon	3.5-5.5	(8-12)
Chihuahua	1-3	(2-6)
Dachshund—Mini	3.6	(8)
Engl Toy Spaniel	4-5.5	(9-12)
Fox Terrier—Toy	1.8-3.4	(4-7)
Italian Greyhound	4.1	(9)
Japanese Spaniel	3.6	(8)
Maltese	2-3	(4-6)
Manchester Terrier	2.5-5.5	(5-12)
Mexican Hairless	5.5	(12)
Miniature Pinscher	3.6	(8)
Norwich Terrier	5-5.5	(11-12)
Papillon	5	(11)
Pekingese	4.1	(9)
Pomeranian	2-3	(4-6)
Poodle—Toy	3.2	(7)
Silky Terrier	3.5-4.5	(8-10)
Yorkshire Terrier	3.2	(7)

Small Breeds—Ht	30-41 cm	(12-16 in)
Basenji	10-11	(22-24)
Basset Hound	11-25	(25-55)
Beagle	8-14	(18-30)
Bedlington Terrier	10-11	(22-24)
Border Terrier	5.5-7	(12-15)
Boston Terrier	6-11	(13-25)
Cairn Terrier	6-6.5	(13-14)
Cocker Spaniel	11.5	(25)
Dachshund	9	(20)
Dandie Dinmont	8-11	(18-24)
Engl Cocker Span	12-15	(26-34)
French Bulldog	8-13	(18-28)
Fox Terrier	7-8	(16-18)
Irish Terrier	11-12	(25-27)
Lakeland Terrier	7.7	(17)
Lhasa Apso	6.8	(15)
Manchester Terrier	5.5-10	(12-22)
Poodle—Miniature	7.3	(16)
Pug	6-8	(14-18)
Schipperke	6.8	(15)
Schnauzer—Mini	6.8	(15)
Scottish Terrier	8-10	(18-22)
Sealyham	9-10	(20-22)
Shetland Sheepdog	7.3	(16)
Shih Tzu	5.5-7	(12-15)
Skye Terrier	11.4	(25)
Smooth Fox Terrier	7.7	(17)
Spitz	7.3	(16)
Welsh Corgi	8-11	(18-24)
Welsh Terrier	8-10	(18-22)
West Highland White Terrier	7.3	(16)
Whippet	9.1	(20)
Wire-Haired Fox Terrier	7.7	(17)

*Amount varies depending on body size and build. Males are larger than females. For dogs of mixed or unknown breed, use weight of dog of similar height at shoulder and of a breed similar in appearance.

breeds should have an hourglass shape when viewed from above; this means there should be some indentation behind the rib cage. Light fleshiness over the hips, and a trim firm abdomen also indicate good body condition.

Additional physical characteristics that may be present in obese dogs or cats include:

1. The abdomen is pendulous or protrudes on the sides when the animal is viewed from above.
2. Enlarged fatty areas on either side of the tail-head and over the hips
3. A waddling walk instead of a normal gait
4. Sluggishness

A healthy pet of normal weight and body condition is alert and interested in its surroundings. Weight/height, weight/height squared, weight/height cubed, height/weight to the $\frac{1}{3}$ power, relative weight (weight of a subject compared to the average weight of a subject of the same height and sex), and skin-fold thickness have been shown to correlate highly to the degree of obesity in human subjects,[34] but these correlations have not been demonstrated in either dogs or cats. Skin-fold thickness does not correlate to the degree of obesity in dogs or cats as it does in people. This is because the skin of dogs and cats can be readily lifted from the subcutaneous tissue. Some additional criteria may be used for research purposes but are rarely used clinically to determine the degree of obesity in dogs, cats or other animals. These include:

1. Body density[27]
2. Total body potassium content[27]
3. Total body water content[27]
4. Uptake of fat-soluble inert gases[34,61]
5. 24 h urinary creatinine or 3-methylhistidine excretion[125]

6. Near-infrared interactance[36]
7. Tomography[78]
8. Ultrasound[78]
9. Total body electrical conductivity or impedance[112,145]

Total body electrical conductivity or impedance, ultrasound, and near-infrared interactance appear to be the only methods practical for use in most clinical situations.[78,111,112] However, none of these procedures is currently used clinically in veterinary medicine and their accuracy in dogs or cats is not established.

EFFECTS

Many people consider the overweight pet less pleasing and less healthy in appearance. The obese pet's general response and physical activity are often diminished. Obesity can shorten the pet's life and predispose to or cause medical problems. As shown in Table 7, circulatory, locomotion, skin, reproductive and neoplastic diseases are 40-74% greater in overweight dogs than those at optimum body weight. Mortality in human beings at any age is 9, 25, 65, 230 and 1200% higher in individuals that are 15, 25, 40, 55, or 100% overweight, respectively (Table 1, page 6-3).[27,178]

Increased mortality in obese people results primarily from increased heart disease, stroke, diabetes, and diseases affecting the digestive system. In contrast, mortality from lung cancer is least among people that are overweight and greatest in lean or underweight individuals.[67] As a result of these diseases, mortality is higher in both underweight and overweight people than in those of optimum body weight.[67] Thus, both inadequate and excess body weight are harmful.

TABLE 7

EFFECT OF BODY WEIGHT ON DISEASE INCIDENCE IN DOGS

Disease	Percent of Population* Affected	% Above (+) or Below (−) That Occurring at Optimum Body Wt**	
		Under Wt	Over Wt
Circulatory	3.1	+104	+74
Locomotion	9.0	+ 42	+57
Skin	18.6	− 20	+40
Reproductive	3.9	+ 12	+64
Neoplasia	1.8	+ 6	+50

*All dogs seen at 11 veterinary practices in England and Scotland from June 1 to Nov. 3, 1983; a total of 8268 dogs.[54a]

**Equals (% at that wt with that disease − % at optimum wt with that disease) ÷ (% at optimum wt with that disease). % at that wt with that disease = (% of population at that wt with that disease, as given in [54a] × 8268) ÷ % of total population at that wt as given in [54a] × 8268).

TABLE 8

HEALTH CONCERNS AND EFFECTS OF OBESITY

Above Ideal Wt (%)	Health Concerns	Effects	
10	Not critical if it doesn't worsen.	Diabetes mellitus	↑ renal & heart disease
20–30	Predisposes to numerous problems.	Hypertension ──────────▶	
40–50	Problems imminent or present.	Decreased immunocompetence	
60–70	Serious problems usually present.	Increased dermatosis	
80–100	Death not far off without weight loss.	Impaired GI function ─────▶	↑ constipation, flatulence, & ulcers
		Decreased reproductive efficiency	
		Increased dystocia	
		Increased surgical risk & difficulty	
		Increased neoplasia	
		Locomotion problems	
		Interference with diagnostic procedures	
		Less pleasing appearance	

The degrees of increased mortality and incidence of most diseases that occur with increasing obesity in dogs and cats are not known. However, one would expect, except for atherosclerotic diseases, the same trends as in people. The health problems that may occur and their severity, based on degree of obesity, are given in Table 8. A number of problems caused by or predisposed to by obesity in turn cause or predispose to obesity. The result is the vicious cycle shown in Figure 1.

Obesity occurs with or predisposes to any one or combination of the following factors:

1. **Joint or locomotion problems.** More than 24% of overtly obese dogs have serious locomotion problems.[54] Causes include arthritis, herniated intervertebral disks, and ruptured anterior cruciate ligaments caused by carrying excessive weight. As shown in Table 7, the incidence of locomotion problems is 57% higher in overweight dogs and 42% higher in those that are underweight than in those at optimum body weight. The greater the deviation from optimum body weight the greater the incidence of locomotion problems. In one study the incidence of locomotion problems was 160% greater in grossly obese dogs than those at optimum body weight, but it was only 27% greater in moderately overweight dogs.[54a] The incidence was 63% greater in very thin dogs than in those at optimum body weight, whereas it was 39% greater in dogs moderately underweight.[54a] The higher incidence of locomotion problems with increasing deviation below optimum body weight may be due to decreased muscle mass.

2. **Respiratory difficulties,** particularly with exercise. These problems are caused by the increased oxygenation required for the excessive tissue and additional mass against the chest wall, which increases respiratory effort, reduces respiratory efficiency and may lead to alveolar hypoventilation.[178] As a result, dyspnea, impaired endurance, and fatigue occur. These effects are reversed after weight loss. In one study of obese children, only a small weight loss (approximately 5%) increased lung capacity 300 ml and increased aerobic capacity 34.5%.[155]

3. **Hypertension** is exacerbated by obesity[178] and is reduced with weight loss.[148,155,175] Over feeding causes sympathetic stimulation.[199] This in turn contributes to the increased incidence of hypertension and cardiovascular disease in obese individuals.[199] Hypertension increases the risk of development and progression of renal, heart and peripheral vascular diseases.[43]

4. **Congestive heart disease.** Hypertension and the greater cardiac workload required to perfuse the increased tissue present with obesity are imposed on a heart that may already be weakened by fatty infiltration. Thus, obesity can be involved in the development and progression of congestive heart disease. As shown in Table 7 the incidence of circulatory diseases is almost twice as high in dogs that are either overweight or underweight as it is in dogs at optimum body weight. The greater the deviation from optimum body weight, the greater the incidence of circulatory diseases. In one study the incidence of circulatory diseases was

348% greater in grossly obese dogs than in those at optimum body weight; it was only 35% greater in moderately overweight dogs.[54a] The incidence was 243% greater in very thin dogs than in those at optimum body weight, whereas it was 87% greater in moderately underweight dogs.[54a] With obesity, cardiomegaly, cor pulmonale, circulatory congestion, edema, ascites, and hypervolemia may occur.[178] All of these factors are reversed with weight loss.[181] Weight reduction has been shown to reduce left ventricular mass in overweight hypertensive people. It is also important in treating for hypertension and preventing left ventricular hypertrophy.[114] The most important measure for controlling cardiovascular disease in the obese patient is correction of obesity.[178]

5. **Decreased hepatic** function due to hepatic lipidosis, and in people, increased gallbladder disease.[178]

6. **Impaired reproduction efficiency** in both obese males and females is common in many species. With obesity, plasma testosterone concentration lessens[27] and the viability of sperm is impaired. This impairment is due to inability to maintain proper testicular temperature because the testes are insulated by excessive scrotal fat. As shown in Table 7 the incidence of reproductive problems was 64% higher in dogs that were overweight, and 12% higher in those that were underweight, than in those at optimum body weight.

7. **Increased dystocia**

8. **Decreased heat tolerance** due to the insulating properties of excessive subcutaneous fat, which contributes to increased irritability.

9. **Increased dermatosis.** As shown in Table 7 the incidence of skin problems was 40% higher in overweight dogs than in dogs at optimum body weight. The incidence of skin problems was lowest in dogs below optimum body weight.

10. **Increased neoplasia.** Incidence of neoplasia was 50% higher in overweight dogs than in those at optimum body weight (Table 7).

11. **Increased surgical risk and difficulty**[54,109,178] because of:[158]
    a) Uptake of anesthetic agents by adipose tissue, thus necessitating a higher dose of the anesthetic
    b) Decreased hepatic or renal metabolism or excretion of anesthetic agents
    c) Compromised pulmonary function
    d) Increased risk of wound infection and dehiscence

FIGURE 1

CAUSES AND THE VICIOUS CYCLE OF OBESITY

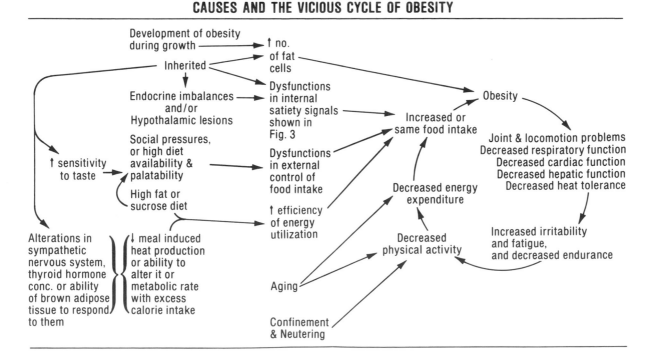

e) Increased thrombophlebitis and pulmonary embolism

12. **Interference with diagnostic procedures** such as auscultation and palpation.

13. **Increased constipation, flatulence, and ulcers** due to impaired gastrointestinal function.

14. **Lowered resistance to infectious diseases.** Altered cell-mediated immunity has been demonstrated in genetically obese mice.[31] Mortality from canine distemper occurred 20% sooner and was 17.5% higher in dogs 20% overweight than in those at optimum body weight.[133] Anorexia, bacteremia, icterus, and weight loss from bacterial infections are also more severe in obese dogs than those of normal weight.[186]

15. **Impaired release of growth hormone** from the pituitary which returns to normal with weight loss.[27,187]

16. **Increased adrenocortical secretion** with no change in plasma cortisol concentration.[25]

17. **Increased risk of metabolic bone disease** and vitamin D deficiency, probably because of reduced exposure to ultraviolet radiation, has

been demonstrated in grossly obese human subjects.[35]

18. **Less pleasing appearance** to most people.

19. **Increased risk and severity of diabetes mellitus.** About 80% of the 8 to 10 million diabetic people in the United States are diabetic because they are overweight.[66] Although similar statistics are not available for dogs or cats, similar trends occur and control of diabetes is improved by weight loss.[119] Even though hyperglycemia may not exist, either glucose intolerance or hyperinsulinemia, or both, is present in 61% of obese dogs.[119] The greater the degree of obesity and the longer its duration, the more severe the glucose intolerance and hyperinsulinemia.[119] Basal insulin concentration and the total amount of insulin secreted are correlated with adiposity; the fatter the individual the greater the amount of insulin secreted and the higher the basal insulin concentration.[13,191] Both decrease if the individual loses weight.

These effects occur because of the increased adipose tissue mass accompanying obesity. Insulin regulates the release of free fatty acids from adipose

FIGURE 2

DIABETES—OBESITY INTERACTIONS

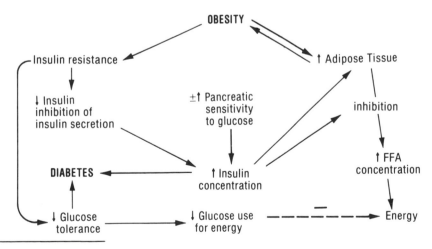

Insulin inhibits the release of free fatty acids (FFA). The increased adipose tissue associated with obesity offsets this inhibition and FFA levels increase. These greater FFA levels increase the use of FFA for energy, which reduces the use of glucose for energy. A resistance to insulin in obese individuals reduces glucose tolerance. This further impairs the use of glucose for energy and lessens insulin's inhibition of insulin secretion, both of which increase the secretion and levels of insulin. Increased pancreatic sensitivity to glucose may also be present in some obese-prone individuals. This further increases insulin secretion and levels. Increased insulin enhances lipogenesis, worsening obesity; i.e. it increases fat deposition which, as described, intensifies hyperinsulinemia. These factors result in diabetes mellitus; i.e. hyperinsulinemia and decreased glucose tolerance, which if sufficiently severe, causes hyperglycemia.

TABLE 9

PROGRESSION OF CANINE DIABETES[119]

| Stage of Diabetes | Plasma Concentration | | | |
| | Glucose | | Insulin | |
	Fasting	Challenge*	Fasting	Challenge*
1st	Normal	Normal	Normal	Normal
2nd	Normal	Normal	Increased	Increased
3rd	Normal	Increased	Increased	Increased
4th	Increased	Increased	Increased	Increased

*Change after glucose administration.

tissue. Thus, if normal and obese individuals had the same insulin levels, free fatty acid levels would be higher in obese individuals because of their greater adipose tissue mass.[14] Free fatty acids displace glucose for production of energy. This results in increased glucose levels that stimulate greater insulin secretion. Increased insulin slows lipolysis, thereby decreasing release of free fatty acids from adipose tissue. This creates the paradox of obese individuals having higher free fatty acid values and higher insulin concentration than considered normal, even though insulin decreases lipid utilization.[62] As illustrated in Figure 2, the resultant hyperinsulinemia enhances lipogenesis, increasing obesity. Obesity further aggravates the hyperinsulinemia.

Increased plasma insulin concentration inhibits insulin secretion both in obese and non-obese subjects.[55] However, with obesity there occurs a resistance to insulin's effect on peripheral tissues, the liver, and the pancreas.[21,55,98,127] As a result, there is less suppression of insulin secretion by insulin feedback. In response to similar blood glucose concentrations, rats genetically predisposed to obesity have been shown to secrete three to four times more insulin than normal, both before and during the obese state.[103] Therefore, a genetic predisposition for insulin hypersecretion is an additional factor that may be responsible for the prevailing hyperinsulinemia that occurs with obesity (Figure 2).[55] These factors lead to diabetes which, as shown in Table 9, appears to develop in stages and is reversed with weight loss.[13,39,119] Increased pancreatic sensitivity to glucose may cause obesity. Hyperinsulinism would result, and insulin not only enhances fat deposition but may also cause hyperphagia as a means of maintaining euglycemia in the presence of chronic hyperinsulinemia.[103]

Obesity is the most important factor accounting for the variations in insulin responses among all types of diabetes in dogs, as well as within each type.[118] Substantial evidence supports the importance of weight control and avoidance of obesity in the healthy dog, and in the management of all types of diabetes.[118] Dogs and people with non-insulin-dependent diabetes can often dispense with insulin therapy and always decrease insulin dosage after return to optimal body weight.[15,118] The different types of diabetes are described in Table 4 (page 6-4).

CAUSES

The cause of obesity is simple: Intake of dietary energy exceeds expenditure of energy. Body weight in the mature animal increases 1 g for each 7-9 kcal ingested in excess of that expended.[64] Therefore, if the dog or cat consumes only 1% more calories than needed, it will be almost 25% overweight by middle age. The factors responsible for causing a positive energy balance and, as a result, obesity are not simple. Some dogs and cats are "easy keepers." They become overweight while consuming amounts of food just adequate to maintain optimum weight in their kennel mates. A number of both physiologic and environmental factors affect energy intake, energy expenditure and body weight. Appropriate alterations in these factors, as shown in Figure 1 (page 6-9), cause obesity. The primary concept to derive from the following discussion of the causes, stages and types of obesity is that obesity is not due simply to a gluttonous appetite or, lack of willpower by a pet or its owner. Instead, it is a disease which, like other diseases, results from alterations in normal physiologic functions. To achieve a high degree of success in treating obesity, it must be treated as a disease, not simply as a problem induced by an overindulgent animal or owner which can be corrected with an admonition to reduce the amount fed.

FACTORS AFFECTING FOOD INTAKE

Food intake is regulated by peripheral and central internal controls as well as external factors. Internal controls include: 1) mechanical stimulation of the gastrointestinal tract, 2) hormonal responses to sight, smell and ingestion of food, and changes in the concentrations of various metabolic substrates in body fluids, 3) body stores of glycogen and fat, and 4) possibly ovarian and testicular hormones. These signals, as well as those from external factors, are integrated by the brain; food intake is modified accordingly.

Satiety Signals

The internal controls of food intake ensure that adequate energy is always available for cellular functions. Accomplishing this objective requires that enough food be ingested periodically to meet current energy needs and to maintain an energy reserve for times when food is unavailable. Food intake is adjusted through negative feedback on the body's normal state of hunger and the corresponding drive to seek food.[179] This perpetual drive to eat is intermittently held in check by inhibitory impulses generated by the presence of food in the gastrointestinal tract, and by the flow of the products of digestion into the liver and systemic circulation.[179] After these impulses, called satiety signals, have become sufficiently attenuated, the desire to eat returns.[2] The amount of food eaten is further controlled by the amount of energy supplying nutrients, fat and glycogen, stored in the body.

Because the body's basic condition is hunger, there is a resistance to a lower set point of body weight, body fat content, or fat-cell size. There is much less resistance to elevation of these set points. Any dysfunction or diminution in any one of the body's many satiety signals, either internal or external, allows the body's basic condition of hunger and perpetual drive to eat to go unchecked. The result is positive energy balance and, eventually, obesity.

No single satiety signal can induce satiety. Every link in the chain depends on the link immediately distal to it. Thus, the mouth will not signal satiety if ingested food is being drawn from the stomach via a gastric fistula. The stomach does not signal satiety if there is a duodenal fistula, and the small intestine does not signal satiety if the liver is depleted of glycogen and, therefore, has a reduced capacity to maintain blood glucose concentration.[179]

In addition to these peripherally stimulated satiety signals, there are satiety signals from the central nervous system (CNS). They are stimulated by meal-induced changes in hormones, peptides, or nutrient concentrations in body fluids and energy stored in the body. These are illustrated in Figure 3.

The stomach generates two kinds of satiety signals: distention and nutrient content.[49] Degree of gastric distention is relayed to the brain via the vagus. A number of peptides released from cells in either or both the gastrointestinal tract or the brain in response to food ingestion also regulate food intake.[107,123,164,195] These peptides, which stimulate satiety, include cholecystokinin, bombesin, pancreatic glucagon, and somatostatin. Peptides that inhibit satiety are the endogenous opioids, dynorphin, enkephalins, and beta endorphin. Appropriately altered sensitivity to or secretion of these substances would contribute to excessive food intake and result in obesity. Genetically obese rats and mice have been shown to have a decreased sensitivity to cholecystokinin, which is evident at three to five weeks of age, and to have three times more beta endorphin in their pituitaries.[123] Excess secretion of, or response to, the appetite-stimulating effects of endogenous opioids appear to be responsible for the overconsumption of palatable foods by genetically obese and stressed subjects.[195] In addition, pituitary dynorphin concentration in obese mice has been shown to be twice that of lean littermates.[195] Whether dysfunctions of these types occur in dogs and cats is not known. In addition, the control of food intake may differ among species. For example, in the wolf, in contrast to other species studied, high doses of cholecystokinin do not affect food intake.[129]

Meal-induced increases in the insulin concentration or the insulin/glucagon ratio also stimulate CNS satiety signals that inhibit food intake, thus playing a role in controlling body weight and fat content.[107] The size of the fat depot appears to be regulated by the concentration of insulin in the cerebral spinal fluid (CSF).[179] The CSF insulin concentration is an integral over time of the concentration of insulin in plasma without its daily fluctuations.[191] Both basal- and glucose-stimulated insulin secretion increase as fat cells get larger and decrease as fat cells get smaller.[179] As a result, CSF insulin concentration rises with the degree of obesity and becomes less with weight loss.[191] Insulin in the CSF appears to have access to brain receptors not directly accessible to plasma insulin. Insulin receptors directly accessible to the plasma would be involved with regulating plasma glucose concentration and fuel needs of the body, the insulin receptors accessible to the CSF would be involved with regulating body adiposity.[191] This control has been

FIGURE 3

SATIETY SIGNALS

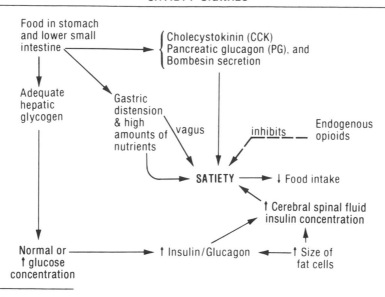

A number of signals, rather than a single one, are needed to induce satiety. Thus, obesity induced by excess food intake may occur as a result of any one of the following: 1) reduced amounts of satiety-inducing substances (CCK, bombesin or PG) or response to them; 2) increased amounts of, or sensitivity to, satiety-inhibiting substances, e.g. endogenous opioids; 3) dysfunction in the satiety center (ventral medial hypothalamus); 4) decreased insulin/glucagon response to fat-cell size; or 5) decreased awareness of, or response to, satiation.

confirmed by infusing insulin into the CSF over a period of several weeks. When this was done, food intake and body weight decreased in a dose-dependent manner.[191] Conversely, when antibodies to insulin were infused, food intake and body weight increased. These effects occurred without changes in the concentration of insulin in the plasma.

Thus, the CSF insulin concentration appears to modulate the response of the brain's satiety system to gut-generated satiety signals, adjusting food intake upward when fat cells get smaller and downward when they get larger. As a result, when fat stores are reduced to less than the usual amount by a decrease in the size of the body's fat cells, the animal increases its food intake and may reduce its expenditure of energy in order to restore the preexisting quantity of fat. Conversely, when fat in excess of normal results from an increase in the size of the body's fat cells, the animal reduces its food intake and may expend more energy by producing more body heat. The level of fat storage an animal maintains may relate to such factors as the survival value built in by past evolutionary experience and the number of fat cells, which in turn may be influenced by both genetics and previous body fat

content. However, failure to transport sufficient insulin to critical brain sites or a deficient brain insulin receptor response, would result in excess fat deposition, as has been shown in a strain of obese rats.[191]

Additional dysfunctions in internal satiety signals known to predispose to or cause obesity include:[121]

1. Emotional trauma

2. Hypopituitarism

3. Lesions involving the satiety center which appears to be the ventral medial hypothalamus. Its bilateral destruction results in hyperphagia and obesity. In contrast, the destruction of the lateral hypothalamus decreases food intake and may cause total aphagia; whereas its stimulation increases food intake.[25]

4. Failure of the satiety center to develop (Prader-Willi syndrome)

5. Endocrine imbalances. These include:
   a) Insulinoma
   b) Diffuse hyperplasia of the pancreatic islets associated with type II diabetes (see Table 4, page 6-4)
   c) Chromophobe adenoma of the pituitary

d) Hyperadrenocorticism

e) Hypothyroidism

The increase in body fat content that occurs with endocrine imbalances is usually limited.[27] All of these factors combined are responsible for less than 5% of obesity in people.[23] A higher prevalence in either dogs or cats is doubtful.[46]

The major causes of obesity in dogs and cats are generally believed to be factors affecting either or both external satiety signals or energy expenditure. However, little investigating has been done on the role and prevalence of alterations in internal satiety signals as a cause. External factors that affect food intake include social pressure, availability and palatability of food.

Social Pressures

Social pressures that affect food intake include competition between animals and a desire to please. Frequently, feeding two animals together results in more food intake by both than would occur if they were fed separately. This may occur because the animal's natural instinct is to consume as much food as quickly as possible before other animals get it. In some instances the dog, and less frequently the cat, may eat because it is rewarded for doing so. A treat is offered, the animal eats it and is rewarded by being petted, noticed or spoken to. In turn, the animal is fed because the owner thinks feeding pleases the animal and shows it how much it is loved. This love and care could be demonstrated without the feeding. For the sake of the animal true caring and concern is demonstrated by not overfeeding. **The obese dog or cat is often a helpless victim of its owner's compulsions.**

People overfeed pets for many reasons, including:

1. Treating pets like people

2. Cultivating and then indulging an animal's taste for highly palatable foods

3. Force of habit such as feeding several times daily or feeding the same quantity regardless of the animal's need

4. Interpreting hunger and eating as a sign of health

5. Guilt feelings, perhaps because the animal has been left alone

6. Ignoring calories from treats and other food consumed outside of meal time

These factors do not generally exist in a kennel environment. As a result many dogs kept in kennels can be allowed free access to dry food without becoming obese.[88]

Dietary Factors

The more palatable the diet, the more efficiently it is utilized and the higher its caloric density, the more likely obesity is to occur. The primary emphasis by most pet food manufacturers is on increasing the palatability of their products. This occurs because, provided the diet does not make the animal obviously sick or cause loose stools, palatability is the main criterion pet owners use in selecting a pet food sold in the grocery store. Optimal nutrient content for maintaining animals in excellent health and extending their life is, unfortunately, not considered by most consumers. Because of this emphasis by both consumer and manufacturer, palatability of pet food continues to increase and so does obesity. Factors affecting palatability are discussed in Chapter 2.

Obese or obese-prone individuals have been shown to be highly responsive to food palatability but abnormally unresponsive to the awareness of satiety.[134] This results in overconsumption of a particularly good-tasting food beyond physiologic requirements, and underconsumption of a bland or tasteless food by the obese animal. Therefore, fluctuations in the amount of food consumed as a result of changes in food palatability is much greater for the obese-prone individual than for those not prone to obesity.[134]

One factor that increases palatability of diet for most dogs and cats is fat.[88,92] Fat also increases the caloric density of the diet. Fat is higher in caloric density, more digestible, and is used and stored as fat by the body more efficiently than either protein or carbohydrate. Only 4-15% of the caloric content of either dietary fat or carbohydrate is lost as heat in their utilization, as compared to 30% when dietary protein is used for energy.[165] Less energy is lost as heat after a meal high in fat content than after an equal calorie-high carbohydrate meal.[71] These differences arise from the effect of these nutrients on the heat-producing brown adipose tissue.[71] Obese human subjects have been shown to produce less heat in response to ingested fat, but not carbohydrate or protein.[171] In addition to lower heat production from ingested fat, only 3% of the energy content of ingested fat is lost when it is stored as body fat; whereas 23% of the energy content of dietary carbohydrate and protein are lost when they are stored as body fat.[45,86] Thus, high-fat diets can induce obesity even without increased caloric intake.[7,126] However, increasing dietary fat usually raises caloric intake because diet palatability and caloric density are increased. Thus, when consumed in excess, fat is more likely to result in obesity than are carbohydrate or protein, even when the diets are

isocaloric. Studies have shown that fat stored in the body comes mainly from dietary fat and that the energy expended in response to food intake is determined primarily by dietary carbohydrate.[45]

Obesity is also more likely to occur when the diet is high in sugar. Sugar or sucrose is a disaccharide consisting of glucose and fructose. Glucose is utilized less efficiently than fructose, i.e. heat production after consumption of glucose is higher.[70] In one study the increase in oxygen utilization after a glucose meal was 57% higher than after a fructose meal.[70] Thus, because of the fructose content of sugar, sugar is utilized more efficiently than starch, which is a polysaccharide consisting of only glucose. Therefore, even when consumed in isocaloric amounts, the animal is more likely to become obese when eating a high-sugar diet than when eating a high-starch diet. Increased dietary sugar, like fat, also increases diet palatability for most dogs,[74,87,88] further enhancing the likelihood that obesity will occur when a high-sugar diet is fed. The effect of sugar on the palatability of diets for cats varies considerably.[10,11,88]

EFFECTS OF NEUTERING

Neutering approximately doubles the incidence of obesity in dogs and cats of each sex (Table 3, page 6-4).[4,54a] This may be because neutering increases caloric intake, decreases energy expenditure, or both. It is frequently attributed to a decrease in energy expenditure without a compensatory decrease in food intake.[110] Neutering has been shown to reduce roaming and therefore physical activity in both sexes of dogs and cats.[77,85] Regardless of the animal's age when neutered, roaming and other objectionable behavior are curtailed, although inactivity and lethargy do not occur.[76,85] Less roaming decreases energy expenditure. However, as a creature of habit, the animal will often continue to eat the same amount as before neutering. The owner, also a creature of habit, continues to feed the same amount. As a result, energy intake exceeds energy expenditure and body weight increases. As in the aged animal, the positive energy balance is not due to increased energy intake, but is due instead to an uncompensated reduction in energy expended. Neutering before puberty has been shown to decrease the incidence of obesity in the bitch.[4]

A decrease in physical activity unmatched by a decrease in caloric intake undoubtedly contributes to an incidence of obesity greater in neutered dogs and cats than in non-neutered animals. However, both an increase in food intake and an increase in the efficiency of energy utilization may also be responsible. Ovariohysterectomized dogs have been shown to eat more and, as a result, to gain more weight than sham-operated controls.[87] This most likely results from an absence of estrogen. Estrogen has been shown to depress food intake in several species of animals.[40,172] In another study, 16 of 32 intact male cats were randomly selected and castrated. All 32 were fed the same diet ad libitum and were housed together in separate cages. During the period from 1 to 17 months after castration, the castrated cats ate slightly less (0.3 g/kg body wt/day) yet gained more weight (145 vs 18 g/cat).[51] This increased efficiency of energy utilization by the castrated cats may be due to the absence of testicular testosterone.

BODY ENERGY USE

Body weight and fat content are determined by the balance between intake and expenditure of energy. With average physical activity the body's energy expenditure is:[50,86,147]

1. 60-75% for the resting energy requirement (RER), which is the energy expended to maintain normal body functions and homeostasis.

2. 10% for meal-induced heat (MIH), which is the heat produced by the initial energy expended for food utilization (formerly referred to as heat increment or specific dynamic action) and a more sustained diet-induced thermogenesis that occurs for several hours after a meal

3. 30% for physical activity

A sufficient increase in physical activity results in increased caloric intake. However, mild-to-moderate increases in physical activity from sedentary activity have no effect[7,192] or decrease food intake.[23,122] Conversely, there is a zone of physical activity in which caloric intake does not decrease in response to reduced activity; as a result, a decrease in activity to below this level results in obesity.[120,192] For example, severely restricted physical activity produced gross obesity in previously lean rats.[27]

The efficiency of energy utilization for muscular activity is fixed; therefore, the energy utilized for physical activity is affected only by the amount of work performed.[86,147] The greater the body weight, the more work required to move that mass; therefore the more energy needed for physical activity. This is the only difference between obese and lean subjects in the amount of energy needed for physical activity.[86,147] In contrast, both RER and meal-induced heat production may vary with nutritional state and environmental factors.

The RER depends on lean (non-obese) body mass, but most animals can change it by 10-15% in response to the environment. Hibernating animals

may change it even more. The change is called adaptive thermogenesis. During prolonged food deprivation, lean body mass in both obese and lean individuals decreases. As a result there is a progressive decrease in RER and, therefore, the amount of food needed.[86] This decrease in RER benefits survival but progressively slows weight loss in response to caloric restriction. In contrast, during periods of excess caloric consumption both lean body mass and body fat content increase. The increase in lean body mass increases RER.[44,147] The higher the plane of nutrition, the higher the RER for both obese and lean animals.[99] This helps blunt the effect of excess energy intake on fat deposition. Thus, altering RER is one means that assists in maintaining body weight within a certain range; altering meal-induced heat production is another.

Meal-induced heat production can be markedly increased when energy intake exceeds need. In one study a 60% increase in caloric intake increased meal-induced heat production by 270%.[44] As a result, 50% of the excess energy intake was given off as heat. The remaining 50%, however, was stored as body fat. As a result of this effect, the caloric deficit for weight loss is less than the caloric excess necessary for a similar increase in body weight.[136]

Changes in the RER in response to changes in the environment, caloric intake and body fat content, or nutritional state are due primarily to changes in thyroid hormone levels, whereas changes in meal-induced heat production in response to changes in these factors is due to changes in sympathetic nervous activity and its effect on the brown adipose tissue.[44,86] There are two major types of adipose tissue: white and brown. Most adipose tissue in the body is white. Brown adipose tissue constitutes only 1-3% of body weight in rats.[79] White adipose tissue is the body's major means of storing excess energy. Greater than 90% of the body's available energy supply is stored as white adipose tissue.[27] In contrast, the main function of brown adipose tissue is heat production and control of body weight.

Brown adipose tissue lies primarily in the interscapular region and chest, and is named for the color produced by the cytochrome pigments and the high density of mitochondria it contains. It has a rich sympathetic innervation and an extensive network of vascular capillaries. Its metabolic activity is regulated primarily by norepinephrine secreted by its nerve supply. The metabolism of energy-supplying nutrients by brown adipose tissue does not result in the synthesis of body constituents or regeneration of high-energy phosphate compounds (e.g. ATP) which provide the energy necessary for body function; it results instead in the utilization of energy-supplying nutrients for heat production by mitochondrial uncoupling. Brown adipose tissue is the primary site of heat production following food intake, for the maintenance of body temperature in the newborn animal and for adaptation to cold. As a result, increased amounts are found in neonates, cold-adapted and hyperphagic animals.[79] Food ingestion and cold, the two external stimuli that trigger thermogenesis of brown adipose tissue, do so by increasing sympathetic nervous activity to this tissue.[198] Brown adipose tissue adapts to excessive caloric intake by varying the amount of heat produced in response to a meal.

Both white and brown adipose tissue increase in size with increased caloric intake and decrease in size when caloric intake is less than needed. For white adipose tissue this occurs because excess energy is stored as fat or used to provide additional energy. For brown adipose tissue this occurs as an adaptive mechanism. An increase in total amount of brown adipose tissue increases both RER and meal-induced heat, which lessens deposition of excess white adipose tissue and gain in body weight due to excess caloric intake.[176] Conversely, a reduction in total amount of brown adipose tissue results in decreased loss of energy as heat. This increases the efficiency of dietary energy utilization, thus slowing the loss of body weight with restricted caloric intake. Thus, an impairment of function or stimulation of brown adipose tissue would impair the ability to increase RER and meal-induced heat production when excess calories are consumed and, as a result, would predispose to obesity.

Meal-induced heat production is as much as 40-50% less in obese subjects than those of normal body weight in response to a mixed meal.[13,89,160] In obese human subjects, meal-induced heat production has been shown to be absent in response to ingestion of fat, but not to carbohydrate or protein.[171] The impairment of meal-induced heat production is not corrected or normalized but instead is worsened by weight loss.[13,89] In one study in young women who were obese from childhood, meal-induced heat production was 20% below normal before weight loss and 35% below normal after weight loss.[13] Thus, this impairment in meal-induced heat production appears to be a cause, not a consequence, of obesity. Conversely, meal-induced heat production has been shown to be abnormally elevated in a strain of mice that have a lower body fat content, gain less weight, and have a lower feed efficiency than other non-obese strains of mice.[84]

Heat production by brown adipose tissue is stimulated by the release of norepinephrine from its sympathetic neurons. The lower meal-induced

heat production in obese or obese-prone people and animals is due to an impairment of norepinephrine metabolism in brain and brown adipose tissue[91,100,137] and a decrease in epinephrine secretion.[13] A decrease in brown adipose tissue response to norepinephrine (i.e. a norepinephrine resistance similar to the insulin resistance that occurs in obese subjects) has been attributed as the cause of reduced heat production in response to cold exposure and in response to a meal in genetically obese rodents.[116,174] Whereas in obese women, a decrease in norepinephrine secretion has been demonstrated.[13,160] Hypothalamic lesions may induce obesity as a result of a decrease in food ingestion induced hypothalamic stimulation of brown adipose tissue, which occurs via its sympathetic innervation.[79] In one case it was shown that this occurred as a result of a viral infection.[113] The decrease in meal-induced heat production by brown adipose tissue is present prior to the occurrence of obesity; indicating it is a cause, not an effect of obesity.[95]

Alterations in thyroid hormone concentrations or effects also may cause or predispose to obesity. However, brown adipose tissue is considered to play only a small role in the increased RER produced by thyroid hormones.[79] Instead it has been suggested that this increased RER occurs because of increased sodium-potassium-ATPase activity.

Changes in the size of brown adipose tissue and its rate of energy utilization for heat production are stimulated by norepinephrine and, to a lesser extent, thyroid hormones, with norepinephrine producing a rapid response and thyroid hormones a slow adaptive response.[44] These changes in turn alter both RER and meal-induced heat production to help the animal adapt to changes in caloric intake and maintain body weight. Triiodothyronine (T3) is a potent thermogenic hormone. Most of the T3 produced in the body is from conversion of thyroxine (T4) to T3 by non-thyroid gland tissue. In the liver this conversion is stimulated by insulin. Overfeeding increases insulin secretion and, therefore, this conversion; underfeeding decreases it. As a result free T3 levels are directly related to caloric intake.[44] The change in the amount of free T3 helps the animal adapt to changes in caloric intake by altering the RER, thus helping maintain body weight.

Obese, reduced-obese and normal weight subjects appear to have similar total and free T4 plasma concentrations during normal food intake and overeating. Some obese individuals have been shown to produce less free T3 and have lower plasma concentrations.[44,196] In addition, there may be alterations in tissue-binding sites for free T3 that alter its utilization and therefore its inducement of thermogenesis. Overeating normally increases free T3 tissue-binding affinity; thus it induces thermogenesis.[44] The reverse occurs with undereating. A decrease in either free T3 or its tissue-binding affinity lowers both the RER and meal-induced heat production, in this way predisposing to the development or initial stage of obesity. If obesity occurs, lean body mass and body fat content increase. The increase in the lean body mass increases RER.[44,147] This offsets the reduction in RER induced by a decrease in free T3 or its tissue-binding affinity; the static phase of obesity results. These effects lead to the two stages of obesity: an initial phase and a static phase.

STAGES OF OBESITY

During the initial phase of obesity there is a positive energy balance and obesity occurs, resulting in an increase in both lean body mass and body fat. The increase in RER that accompanies the increase in lean body mass speeds the rate at which energy is expended.[39,40] Once this increase offsets the intake of excess energy or the decrease in energy expenditure responsible for initiating obesity, there is a zero energy balance. Body weight is now maintained in the obese state; i.e. the static phase of obesity occurs.

In one study during the static phase of obesity, RER was 35% greater in obese women than lean women.[69] This was offset, however, by a 41% lower meal-induced heat production. Weight loss resulted in normalization of the RER but had no effect on meal-induced heat production. Thus, if the previously obese women ate the same amount of food as those who were never obese, the previously obese women would regain weight until their RER increased enough to offset again their lower meal-induced heat production. Since heat production is reduced and, therefore, efficiency of energy utilization is increased in these individuals, energy balance is reached at a greater body weight than in individuals with normal heat production. A similar situation occurs with hyperphagic obese individuals in whom an increased energy intake causes obesity. Body weight stabilizes at a higher level which allows dissipation of the excess energy as heat due to the elevated RER and the increased energy needed for moving the greater body mass. The body weight at which stabilization, or the static phase of obesity (referred to as the set point) occurs, varies among individuals depending on the cause of obesity.

It is generally believed that during the static phase of obesity the greater the body fat content is, the

lower are caloric requirements, and therefore less food is consumed.[9] On the basis of lean body mass, but not body weight, food intake is less for both obese men and women than it is for lean individuals of the same sex.[9] Even after weight loss previously obese individuals have been shown to require 27% fewer calories to maintain optimal body weight than those that have never been obese.[44] This has been attributed to the reduced production of meal-induced heat in obese or obese-prone individuals[13,89] and decreased physical exertion once obesity occurs. However, no difference has been found in the amount of physical activity between obese and non-obese women,[147] and physical activity of young men and women has been shown to be unrelated to the amount of body fat.[9] In addition, the greater the body weight, the greater the amount of energy needed to move that weight; i.e. the more energy needed to perform the same amount of physical exertion. There are also studies that refute the concept of lower energy needs in obese individuals and instead appear to indicate that the static phase of obesity is characterized by both high energy intake and high energy utilization.[13,89]

TYPES OF OBESITY

Obesity can be classified based on: 1) causes or predisposing factors and 2) the number and size of fat cells. Causes or predisposing factors include anything that increases caloric intake or decreases energy expenditure. Factors that increase caloric intake include any dysfunction in: 1) the body's internal control of food intake or satiety signals including endocrine imbalances, emotional trauma, and lesions involving the satiety center; and 2) dysfunctions in external control of food intake including diet palatability and availability, and social pressures. Factors that decrease energy expenditure and thereby cause or predispose to obesity include: 1) old age; 2) decreased physical activity such as occurs due to confinement, neutering, or locomotion, respiratory or cardiovascular problems; and 3) those that increase the efficiency of energy utilization. The efficiency of energy utilization is increased by a high-fat or sucrose diet, or a decrease in meal-induced heat production or ability to alter it or metabolic rate during periods of excess caloric intake. This may occur as a result of alterations in the sympathetic nervous system, free triiodothyronine concentration or the ability of the brown adipose tissue to respond to them.

These factors as well as an increase in fat cell numbers, all of which cause or predispose to obesity, may be inherited or environmentally in-

duced. They are summarized in Figure 1 (page 6-9). Obesity or a susceptibility to the development of obesity can be genetically transmitted.[91] This transmission may manifest itself in either of two ways:

1. In rare diseases in which there is an inherited defect in the regulation of food intake or energy expenditure that results in obesity independent of any environmental factors. Several that occur in people are the Laurence-Moon-Bardet-Biedl, Alstrom, Morgagni-Morel and the Prader-Willi Syndromes.[25] No similar diseases have been reported to occur in dogs or cats.

2. The inheritance of factors with which the environment interacts to result in the development of obesity.[28] In people inherited factors can account for as much as 65-75% and environmental factors only 25-35% of the differences in body weight between individuals.[26] Although both the inherited and the environmental factors must be present in order for obesity to occur, this indicates that inherited factors may be twice as important.

One mechanism that plays an important role in obesity and is affected by both genetics and environmental factors is the number of fat cells in the body.

In general, all obesity is associated with an increase in the size of fat cells (referred to as hypertrophic obesity), but an increase in numbers of fat cells (referred to as hyperplastic obesity) occurs only in certain types[27] or degrees of obesity.[58] The prognosis for obesity associated with increased fat cell numbers is much poorer than that associated with only increased fat cell size. Hyperplastic obesity carries a poorer prognosis because changes in body fat content in the adult, due either to the development of obesity or to weight loss, are due primarily to changes in fat cell size with little effect on fat cell numbers.[27,80] Fat cells appear to have a minimum size at, or above, which they are maintained. Weight loss due to a decrease in body fat content stops when fat cells reach this size.[16,17] Further weight loss, therefore, requires a decrease in lean body mass. Thus, in order for animals with a different number of fat cells to weigh the same, the one with the greater number of fat cells must have less lean body mass.[182] The lower lean body mass decreases RER and therefore caloric needs. Thus, in order to maintain a similar body weight, the animal with the greater number of fat cells requires less calories.[182] The greater the number of fat cells in the body, the more difficult it is to lose weight and to maintain a lower body weight.[16] The ability to maintain a lower body weight is inversely proportional to the number of fat cells in the body.[16,102]

After the individual matures, the number of fat cells remains relatively constant. In contrast, during growth, changes in body fat content are due to changes in both fat cell numbers and size.[12,58] Although this general concept appears to be valid, there are deviations from it. Fat cell numbers may increase in the adult with aging[32] and with sufficient dietary inducement.[58] In addition, fat cell numbers do not increase during all stages of growth but only during certain stages. The time when this occurs may differ for different fat depots.[12] **To assist in preventing obesity, it is important to prevent an increase in fat cell numbers by not overfeeding during the time when fat cell numbers are increasing.** However, the ages during which the numbers of these cells increase in the dog and cat are not known. Lacking this knowledge, it seems appropriate to assume that increases in fat cell numbers occur at the same relative stages of growth and maturity as it does for other animal species.

Fat cell numbers increase in rats and mice from birth to weaning. In cattle, swine, baboons, and human beings it occurs during childhood and adolescence (11 to 19 months of age in cattle[33]) but not during infancy (birth to 3-8 years of age in children).[56,58,97,109,156] Fat cell numbers in the child are also known to change during the last trimester of pregnancy. Fat cell numbers in newborn infants are reduced by undernutrition, and are increased by diabetes-induced hyperglycemia in the mother during the last trimester of pregnancy.[142] Overfeeding during the time of fat cell hyperplasia increases the number of fat cells present at maturity. Underfeeding at the time of fat cell hyperplasia reduces the number of fat cells present at maturity. Thus, to assist **in preventing obesity in the adult, obesity should be prevented during growth.** If obesity occurs at any age, it should be treated to prevent its many detrimental effects.

MANAGEMENT

In order to be most beneficial to the animal and client, **the veterinarian's emphasis should be on disease prevention—not treatment.** To accomplish this it is important that the animal be maintained at its optimum body weight. For many dogs and cats this means a weight reduction program. Such a program should be recommended for all dogs or cats that are more than 15% over their optimum weight, as health problems begin above this degree of obesity (Table 7 and 8, pages 6-7 & 8).[139]

There are five possible approaches to a weight-reduction program: psychological, exercise, dietary, pharmacological, and surgical. The International Congress on Obesity recommends that for the average human patient psychological support, exercise and diet, should all be used in conjunction since they are closely interrelated and mutually supportive.[184] Neither drugs nor surgery are recommended. Application of these same recommendations to overweight dogs and cats is strongly encouraged. The chances of successful weight reduction and maintenance of near optimum body weight are diminished in proportion to the lack of emphasis given any one of the three components of therapy: psychological encouragement, exercise and diet.

PSYCHOLOGICAL ENCOURAGEMENT FOR WEIGHT REDUCTION

By far the most important requirement necessary for institution and successful completion of a weight-reduction program is to convince all persons associated with the animal that the program is a necessity. Some people do not recognize that their pet is overweight (31% in one study)[117] and will therefore do little to solve the problem unless they are convinced that a problem exists. A permanent record of the animal's weight recorded during previous office visits, allows comparison to the animal's present weight and is quite effective in calling attention to developing obesity. Focusing on the individual pet by name rather than discussing obesity in general may help convince the client that it is his or her pet that is overweight and that the pet will suffer as a result of obesity.[183] Once owners are convinced that their animals are indeed overweight, they must be convinced of the detrimental effects of obesity and the beneficial effects of weight reduction and maintenance. Some owners of overweight pets may not accept the potential for a variety of ailments as sufficient reason to institute a weight-reduction program but will be persuaded by a discussion of the beneficial effects of weight loss for their particular pet.[183] Regardless of the procedure used, complete client cooperation must be obtained. Anything less results in wasted time and effort.

Some veterinarians find it useful to charge one fee, payable in advance, for the entire weight-reduction program. This practice serves two purposes; first, the veterinarian is assured of payment; second, if the owner has just paid to see that his or her pet loses weight, the probability of the client's compliance with instructions, and the ultimate success of the program, is enhanced.

In some cases modification of the client's behavior toward a pet is important in achieving and maintaining this weight loss in the pet. The factors

important for the encouragement and support necessary for reducing overweight pets are discussed in the sections on exercise and dietary management.

EXERCISE FOR WEIGHT REDUCTION

Treatment of obesity requires that caloric intake be less than expenditure. The loss of one pound of adipose tissue requires an energy deficit of approximately 3500 kcal.* This deficit may be produced by decreasing caloric intake or increasing energy expenditure. The only means of significantly increasing energy expenditure is exercise.

Sufficient physical activity increases food intake. However, mild-to-moderate increases in exercise from sedentary activity has no effect on food intake[7,192] or actually decreases it.[23,122] In a six-month study of obese women, exercise 25% above sedentary activity had no effect on ad libitum food intake. It did, however, increase energy expenditure, causing a change in energy balance from a gain of 11 to a loss of 979 kcal/day.[192] This resulted in a weight loss of 0.26 lb/day. This loss is almost exactly the amount that would be anticipated from this caloric deficit (979 kcal/day deficit divided by 3500 kcal/lb of adipose tissue equals 0.28 lb/day). Exercised rats that had free access to a highly palatable diet consumed 15% less food and gained 43% less weight than those not exercised.[39] In another study moderate exercise during growth decreased body fat content to one-half that in sedentary rats.[7] The exercise prevented an increase in body fat content and fat cell numbers induced by feeding a high-fat diet, but not that caused by genetic predisposition.[7]

Exercise not only increases energy expenditure directly, it also increases resting metabolic rate (RMR), which further increases energy expenditure.[106] In contrast, without exercise RMR decreases when caloric intake is restricted.[86] In one study in human subjects who were 15 to 35% overweight, moderate exercise increased RMR 10% and maximum work capacity 12%; there was little change in either of these parameters after weight loss without exercise.[106] These studies emphasize the importance of regular exercise both for weight reduction and prevention of obesity. In contrast to what is occasionally stated,[27] studies demonstrate that postprandial exercise offers no greater benefit than preprandial exercise in increasing energy expenditure.[138,185]

In summary, exercise as part of the weight-control program increases the chances of success[173] and is beneficial for many reasons including:

1. Increased energy expenditure-although the loss of body fat consequent to exercise alone is small.[188]
2. Prevention of a decrease in resting-energy expenditure that would otherwise occur when caloric intake is reduced.[106,173]
3. Reduction in appetite, thus assisting in decreasing caloric intake,[23,39,122] although some other investigators refute this.[144]
4. Prevention of losses in lean body mass and bone minerals that occur when caloric intake is reduced without increased physical activity.[96,194]
5. Decreased insulin need as well as glucose intolerance and hyperinsulinemia that are often present in obese animals.[149]
6. Improvement in cardiovascular function.
7. With increased food intake after weight reduction, continued exercise reduces body fat deposition without compromising the restoration of lean body mass.[146]

As shown in Table 10, expenditure of energy is doubled by a slow walk and tripled by a brisk walk. Two brisk 15-minute walks daily use one-sixth of a 30-lb dog's energy required for maintenance, provide the other benefits described above, and often do wonders for the animal's mental attitude. The animal should be exercised for at least 30 minutes three to five days weekly. However, daily exercise may be more beneficial in instilling exercise as a habit and, thus, ensuring that the animal is exercised. The benefit derived by the person exercising the animal may also be worth mentioning. The exercise should not result in a heart rate that exceeds 85% of maximum.[184] Thus, exercise of minimal intensity may be needed if gross obesity, heart, or pulmonary disease is present.

As weight loss occurs, less energy is expended for the same amount of exercise.[192] Thus, in order to

---

*Adipose tissue is 10-15% water and 85-90% fat. Body fat provides approximately 9 metabolizable kcal/g. Therefore (454 g/lb) x (85% fat x (9 kcal/g of fat) 3473 kcal/lb.

TABLE 10

ENERGY EXPENDITURE WITH EXERCISE[27]

Activity	kcal/min*
Sleep	approx. 1
Resting	1.2–2.5
Walking slowly on level	2.6–4.9
Walking briskly	5–7
Jogging	7–12

*For human subjects.

sustain the same rate of weight loss, exercise must increase progressively. Exercise should continue even after optimum body weight is reached. This reduces deposition of body fat that otherwise occurs when caloric intake is no longer severely restricted.[146] However, if exercise is discontinued it should be terminated gradually. Sudden termination of routine physical exercise by previously obese, obese, or never-obese individuals is associated with rapid weight gain and fat accumulation.[7,140] This phenomenon is evident in many inactive former athletes.

DIETARY MANAGEMENT FOR WEIGHT REDUCTION

Weight reduction can be accomplished successfully in the majority of cases if a systematic program for caloric restriction is implemented. Chances of success are greatest if every step is followed.

1. **Obtain complete client cooperation.** It is important that a complete weight-reduction program be recommended. Compare the probability of success using the following two approaches.

   a) "Mrs. Smith, Fido is overweight. **You** should reduce her."

   b) "Mrs. Smith, Fido weighs 30% more than she should. This will predispose her to cancer, joint, locomotion, respiratory, heart, liver, skin, intestinal and adrenal gland problems. It decreases her resistance to infectious diseases and may precipitate diabetes. To prevent these problems, increase her life-span and her enjoyment of life, as well as reduce your future health-care costs, it is important that **we** institute a weight-reduction program. Let's go through a weight-reduction program and see what **we** need to do to solve this problem and prevent its recurrence."

Use a prepared form containing blank spaces for entry of specific details for the individual animal. The form should describe the detrimental effects of obesity and all procedures and instructions for the weight-reduction program. An example is given on page 6-34. Begin by reviewing with the client the detrimental effects of obesity, emphasizing any that may already be evident. Emphasize that these effects will quite likely increase future health-care costs and inconvenience in caring for the pet. Most people who undertake weight reduction for themselves do so for improved appearance rather than the ultimate health benefits.[24,25,115] Thus, emphasizing improved

appearance as well as health benefits and future reduced health-care costs may be helpful.

Next, using the prepared form, describe to the owner the weight-reduction program step-by-step, filling in the specific details for the particular pet. Be positive! Do not suggest possible problems; doing so greatly increases the likelihood that these problems will be encountered. Provide the client with all information and instructions in writing so that other family members can be informed. Remember, it is not just the client that brought the pet to you that must be informed and convinced of the need for weight reduction; it is everyone involved with the pet.

If the client is not receptive, do not show resentment, frustration, anger or hostility, or you will seriously damage your relationship with the client and lose any chance of helping the animal. Remember, it is the client's animal to do with as he or she chooses. You have done the best you can by suggesting weight reduction. Give clients the prepared form to read. Ask them to consider the weight-reduction program for the health and well-being of their pets and reduction in their pet's future health-care costs. Assure them that if they should later decide to treat the obesity, you will be happy to assist them in doing so. Whether clients choose to take your recommendations or not, they will be impressed with your concern for their pet, as well as future health-care costs. If the client agrees that the animal's weight should be reduced, the following procedures are recommended.

2. **Evaluate the patient thoroughly** to determine the presence of any factors besides obesity for which therapy should be instituted (see page 6-4).

3. **Weigh the animal and set a goal for weight reduction** (see page 6-5). This should be the animal's optimum body weight as you can best determine it. Optimum body weight is often difficult to establish for an obese animal, but your estimate of it can be adjusted later.

4. **Estimate the time required** to reach this goal. People accept many things if they are convinced there is a valid reason for doing them and a chance of achieving success within a reasonable period of time. Chances of success are greatly reduced if there is no fixed goal or any idea regarding the length of time needed to reach that goal. Table 11 shows the time required to reduce weight in a dog not exercised and fed the amount of a low-calorie reducing diet that provides 60% of caloric requirement for maintaining **optimum** body weight. At this degree of caloric restriction body weight lessens at a

steady rate of 3% per week for the first six weeks, then slows to 2% per week after eight weeks. A similar degree of weight loss has been reported when caloric intake was reduced to 50% of that needed to maintain **obese** weight.[128] An estimate of the time required for weight loss can also be calculated as shown in Table 12. The rate of weight loss can be increased by exercise, which is recommended unless severe obesity, cardiac or pulmonary disease, or locomotion problems are present. There is a misconception that initially when a restricted calorie diet is fed, water replaces fat and masks the loss of adipose tissue, and therefore the administration of diuretics aids initial weight loss. Exactly the opposite occurs. With severe caloric restriction there is an accelerated (not a slower) weight loss during the first one to three weeks because of excessive loss of water caused by natruresis and reduction in renal concentrating ability that characteristically accompany early starvation or semi-starvation.[5,27,177] Administration of diuretics increases this loss. These fluid losses are regained later.[5] Therefore, a diuretic is of no benefit to an obese patient. Its only benefit is that results seem to be occurring more rapidly. However, this could be counterproductive because it may lead to discouragement when diuretic-induced fluid losses are regained and, therefore, the rate of weight loss is slowed or body weight may actually increase.

5. **Decrease caloric intake** to 60-70% of that required for maintaining optimum (not obese) body weight (Table 13). For a more complete description of methods for calculating the amount of food needed see page 1-9). Although any degree of caloric restriction may be used, these amounts work well.[27] More stringent caloric restriction results in little increase in the rate of weight loss but increases risk of detrimental effects and begging by the pet.[59] Less stringent restriction causes such a slow rate of weight loss that many pet owners become discouraged with the lack of progress.

6. **Feed three or four times daily** or as often as practical. Feeding increases loss of energy as heat. As a result, small multiple meals result in greater weight loss and reduction of lipogenesis compared to fewer but larger meals containing the same total number of calories.[57] Total oxygen consumption for energy expenditure has been shown to increase 30% when dogs are fed four times per day; it increases only 15% when dogs are fed the same amount of the same diet in one meal per day.[104]

7. **Instruct the client to keep the pet out of the room when food is being prepared or eaten.** Begging and the associated feeding of snacks is thus minimized.

8. **Change the animal's diet to a weight-reduction diet.** Chances for success are greatly diminished and nutritional deficiencies may ensue if the regular diet is fed in reduced amounts.

    Weight-reducing diets are classified as:[27]

    a. Starvation or fasting, which provide less than 10% of caloric needs for maintenance.

    b. Severely calorie-restricted, which provide 10 to 50% of caloric needs for maintenance.

TABLE 11

RATE AND TIME REQUIRED FOR REDUCING WEIGHT OF OBESE DOGS*

Weeks of Caloric Restriction	%/Wk. Decrease in Body Weight	End of Week	mean	range	n	% Over Optimum Body Weight	Weeks to Reach Optimum Weight
		1	2.7	0.4–4.3	6		
		2	5.5	3.2–8	6		
1–6	3	3	9.5	7.4–12	6	15–20	5–7
		4	11.9	10–13	6		
6–8	2.3	5	14.5	12–20	6	20–30	7–9
		6	17	14–22	6		
8–10	2	7	21	18–25	4	30–50	11–13

*Fed a high-fiber low-fat diet (Prescription Diet r/d, Hill's) at 60% of caloric requirements for maintenance at optimum body weight and not exercised.

**Initial body weights were 16–43%, with an average of 28% above optimum.

c. Calorie-restricted, which provide 50 to 75% of caloric needs for maintenance. These may be nutritionally balanced or unbalanced.

1) Balanced weight-reduction diets assure that non-energy nutrient requirements are met, even when energy intake is restricted. These include prepared diets (Prescription Diets r/d, Hill's) and home-made diets (Recipes 4 and 10, Appendix Table 3).

2) Unbalanced weight-reduction diets include very low carbohydrate diets that contain high levels of either protein or fat, and fad or novelty diets that emphasize single food items.

Many fad or novelty weight-reducing diets for human beings have at times enjoyed varying degrees of popularity. Many are nutritionally unbalanced. Among them are grapefruit or Mayo, Beverly Hills, Banting, Dolly Parton, rice, K-28 and macrobiotic diets. These diets rely on the theory that certain foods, nutrients or other substances have unique, previously undiscovered or magical properties to enhance weight loss. Weight loss is achieved by reduction of energy intake, primarily by limiting food choices. Many purport a scientific rationale which is unfounded, and documentation of effectiveness and safety is generally unavailable.[184]

Examples of very low carbohydrate diets for people include the Air Force, Dr. Taller's Calories Don't Count, the drinking man's, Dr. Stillman's and Dr. Atkin's diets. Examples of severely calorie restricted diets include the Last Chance, liquid protein and the Cambridge diets. Claims associated with advocacy of very low carbohydrate diets include those that protein or fat calories will not prevent weight loss, and that the ketonemia that occurs with these diets lessens appetite and allows weight loss to occur even if caloric intake is not reduced.[184]

TABLE 12

CALCULATION OF TIME REQUIRED FOR WEIGHT LOSS

(Obese wt. in lbs.) − (Optimum wt. in lbs.) = Lbs. wt. loss desired

(Lbs. wt. loss desired) × (3500 kcal/lb)* = Kcal of total deficit needed

$$\left[\begin{array}{c} \text{Kcal/lb/day needed for} \\ \text{maintenance (Table 13)} \\ \times \text{ lbs. optimum body wt.} \end{array} \right] - (\text{Kcal/day ingested})** = \text{Kcal/day deficit occurring}$$

$$\left(\begin{array}{c} \text{Kcal of total} \\ \text{deficit needed} \end{array} \right) \div \left(\begin{array}{c} \text{Kcal/day deficit} \\ \text{occurring} \end{array} \right) = \left(\begin{array}{c} \text{Days necessary to} \\ \text{reach optimum wt.} \end{array} \right)$$

*Caloric deficit necessary for the loss of 1 lb of adipose tissue (see page 6-20).

**Amount recommended is the kcal/lb/day for weight reduction given in Table 13 times the animal's optimum body weight.

TABLE 13

CALORIC REQUIREMENTS FOR MAINTENANCE AND WEIGHT REDUCTION

Optimum Body Weight (Kg)	kcal/kg body wt/day needed for*		Optimum Body Weight (Lb)	kcal/lb body wt/day needed for*	
	Maintenance	Wt Reduction		Maintenance	Wt Reduction
Dog:			Dog:		
3	110	70	6	50	30
6	85	55	12	40	25
10	75	50	20	35	22
20+	70	45	50+	30	20
Cat:			Cat:		
2.5–5.5	65	40	6–12	30	20

*Interpolation between these values will give the approximate amount needed for a dog of any size. This will vary between individuals.

Many health-related benefits have also been claimed for all of these diets as well as the novelty diets.[29,135,154,157,197] However, studies of all of these novelty, very low carbohydrate and severely caloric-restricted diets fail to support these claims.[63,94,132,135,143,154,193] In contrast, these diets may be quite harmful and have induced numerous problems including: diminished exercise capacity, fatigue, irritability, depression, vomiting, diarrhea, constipation, electrolyte imbalances, vitamin and mineral deficiencies, dehydration, postural hypotension, hyperuricemia, gout, renal calculi, alopecia, stroke, thrombophlebitis, pulmonary embolism and sudden death from ventricular arrhythmias.[42,59,63,133,135,166,180,184]

Nutritionally unbalanced diets, severely caloric-restricted diets and fasting, even during hospitalization, are rarely prescribed by physicians knowledgeable in managing obesity.[27] All are inherently dangerous.[59] Regardless of caloric intake, nutritionally unbalanced diets may be unhealthy if continued for long periods, and therefore are not recommended.[27,59] Calorie-restricted, nutritionally balanced diets are considered the safest and produce an acceptable rate of weight loss.[27]

In contrast to novelty, nutritionally unbalanced, high-protein low-carbohydrate, or low-protein high-carbohydrate diets, a high-fiber (above 15% in dry matter) low-fat diet (below 10% in dry matter) that satisfies all nutrient needs except energy is quite advantageous for weight reduction. A high-fiber low-fat diet is low in caloric density, prolongs eating time and induces satiety because of gastric distention at a low caloric intake.[42]

Besides their bulk effect, various fractions of dietary fiber alter assimilation and metabolism of energy providing nutrients. Insoluble fiber shortens transit time in the small intestine for nutrient digestion and absorption and, as a result, reduces the efficiency of nutrient assimilation.[3] Wheat bran and other foods rich in insoluble fiber delay glucose absorption and slow starch hydrolysis by insulating it from digestive enzymes.[3] High-fiber diets also decrease availability of dietary fats and proteins.[3]

Because of these effects a high-fiber low-calorie-dense diet is significantly more effective in reducing energy intake as well as the feeling of hunger; therefore, diet compliance and weight loss are increased as compared to low-fiber diets.[42] In one study both obese and non-obese persons had a daily eating time one-third longer but consumed one-half as many calories when fed a high-fiber low-calorie-dense diet.[52] This occurred even though the people were urged to eat all they wanted and both diets were equally palatable and acceptable. Despite the lower energy intake when the low-calorie-dense diet was fed, there was no increase in food intake with days on the diet and, similarly, there was no decrease in food intake with days on the high-calorie-dense diet. The individuals indicated that their hunger was satisfied just as well by the low-calorie-dense diet as the high-calorie-dense diet even though caloric intake was one-half as much. Even when caloric intake is equal, satiety is greater and return of appetite delayed when a high-fiber diet is consumed.[19] As shown in Table 14, these same beneficial effects have also been observed in the cat.

When a high-fiber low-calorie-dense diet (Feline r/d, Hill's) was fed ad libitum, caloric intake was reduced by 45%, even though the cat consumed 10% more of this diet than a low-fiber high-calorie-dense diet (Feline c/d, Hill's). As a result of the lower caloric intake, the cat's body weight decreased by 7.2% during the five weeks the high fiber-low calorie dense diet was fed. Weight loss occurred even though the low calorie diet was always available for the cat to eat as much as it wanted and for this cat was more palatable than the high calorie diet (as determined by the two-pan palatability test described on page 2-4). This study demonstrated that in some animals, even when intake of a palatable diet is not restricted, body weight will return to near optimum within a reasonable period of time if the diet is sufficiently low in caloric density. A high-fiber low-calorie-dense diet is also beneficial because it decreases plasma triglyceride concentration, and rebound hypoglycemia and insulin secretion after a meal.[19] These effects are more pronounced in obese animals.[13,21,98,118]

High cellulose fiber diets (10 and 20%) have been shown to decrease magnesium and zinc absorption in rats.[73] However, the diets caused no negative balance of these minerals and had no effect on phosphorus, calcium, copper or iron absorption. Although iron absorption by the dog is decreased by a high wheat bran diet, this decrease was shown to be due to components of wheat bran other than cellulose (fiber).[60] Adding as much as 9% solka-floc (90% cellulose, 5% hemicellulose, and 5% lignin) to canine diets had no effect on ash, protein, fat or soluble carbohydrate digestibility.[30] Other studies in dogs, however, suggest that high-fiber diets may decrease fat digestibility[168] as has been demonstrated in other animal species.[38,167] Doubling the fiber content of dogs' diets decreased pancreatic lipase secretion 60% from basal levels and 6-to 10-fold after stimulation of secretin.[168] Adding 20% cellulose,[158] 5% pectin,[65] or guar[159] to rat diets has been shown to reduce digestive enzyme activity in intestinal chyme. Fiber not only decreases lipase

TABLE 14

AMOUNT CONSUMED AND BODY WEIGHT OF THE CAT
FED A HIGH- THEN A LOW-CALORIE-DENSE DIET[108]

Diet			Amount Eaten (diets always available)		Body Weight (lb)	
Name	kcal/g	Fiber % in Dry Matter	g/day	kcal/day	Start	End
Feline c/d	1.6	2.7	156	250	----	12.7*
Feline r/d	0.8	21.7	172	138	12.7	11.8**
Change on r/d	50% lower	685% higher	10% more	45% less	----	7.2% loss

*Dry Feline c/d had been fed *ad libitum* for the previous 19 months.

**After feeding canned Prescription Diet Feline r/d (Hill's) *ad libitum* for 5 weeks. Optimum body weight 11–11.5 lb.

secretion, it absorbs digestive enzymes, decreasing their availability for food digestion.[168] Thus, a high-fiber diet is beneficial for weight reduction because fiber decreases both diet caloric density and fat digestibility. In addition, no long-term negative effects associated with eating a high-fiber diet have been demonstrated.[38,73,128] Dietary cellulose is relatively innocuous, causing no deleterious effects unless it is combined with a deficient or poorly balanced diet.[48]

In addition to a high-fiber content, a weight-reducing diet should be low in fat. Reducing dietary fat is beneficial not only because it reduces caloric density of the diet, but also because heat production induced by fat (but not carbohydrate or protein) ingestion may be impaired in obese animals, as has been shown in obese people.[171] If this impairment exists, fat would provide more usable calories than an otherwise isocaloric amount of carbohydrate or protein.

Thus, **the best diet for reducing weight is a nutritionally complete and balanced high-fiber low-fat low-calorie-dense diet.** The diet dry matter should contain more than 15% fiber, less than 10% fat and have a caloric density 35-45% less for dogs and 20-30% less for cats than the diet previously fed the animal. With a diet of this type, the animal can continue eating the same amount of food to which it is accustomed, but in doing so ingest 20-45% fewer calories. As discussed previously (page 6-22) this degree of caloric restriction is recommended for reducing the weight of obese dogs or cats. Diets that meet these criteria are shown in Table 15. Although vitamin supplementation is unnecessary when properly formulated prepared foods are fed, a reluctant client may be convinced to adhere to the weight reduction program if a daily vitamin supple-

ment is prescribed.[183] The weight-reduction diet should be fed in the amount necessary to provide the caloric intake given in Table 13 (page 6-23).

Feeding less of a diet not specifically formulated for weight reduction to decrease caloric intake is not recommended. Success is rare if the animal is kept on its present diet.[110] The reduced food intake does not satisfy hunger as well as the consumption of an equal number of calories in a high-fiber diet.[19,42] As a result, begging and scavenging for food increase. In addition, reducing some diets by the amount needed for achieving sufficient caloric restriction and a reasonable rate of weight loss may cause vitamin, mineral, or protein deficiencies.[4,130]

Regardless of the diet used, **the client must follow instructions explicitly and feed only the specific amount of the food prescribed.** If table scraps, treats, or other foods are included in the animal's diet, reduction of caloric intake sufficient to obtain weight loss is virtually impossible. Remind the owner that giving treats demonstrates a lack of concern for the pet's health and well-being. If the clients feel they cannot resist giving treats, have them give a cube or nugget of the high-fiber low-calorie-dense weight-reduction diet. Other snacks that may be fed if the client cannot resist include air-popper popcorn without oil, butter or salt (25 kcal/cup); and green beans cooked without butter (30 kcal/cup).

Request that the exact amount of everything the animal eats be recorded. This discourages feeding snacks, makes the client aware of the amount of food provided in this manner, and allows you to determine the number of calories consumed. The number of calories in treats can be surprising. They are often overlooked in determining the animal's total caloric intake, or as a reason that weight is

TABLE 15

PET FOODS INTENDED FOR MANAGEMENT OR PREVENTION OF OBESITY

Diet	Form	Company	In Diet Dry Matter			Kcal ME, % Below Avg Comm
			Fat %	Crude Fiber %	Kcal ME/lb	
For Dogs:						
Canine r/d	Can	Hill's	7.0	25	1089	45.5
Canine r/d	Dry	Hill's	7.0	22	1135	36.9
Canine w/d	Can	Hill's	12.1	13.2	1634	18.3
Canine w/d	Dry	Hill's	7.4	16.4	1407	21.8
Science Diet	Can	Hill's	10	8	1540	23
Maint. Light	Dry	Hill's	7	14	1407	21.8
Recipe 4	Homemade	pg. A3-2	12.5	5.1	1614	19.3
Fit-N-Trim	Dry	Purina	8.7	10.6	1405	21.9
Cycle 3	Can	Gaines	14	8	1647	17.6
Cycle 3	Dry	Gaines	10	7	1622	9.9
Alpo Lite	Can	Alpo	18	5	1770	11.5
Less Active	Dry	Iams	14	3	1860	3 above
Avg. Comm.	Can	Many	10–25	2.2	2000	0
Avg. Comm.	Dry	Many	12	3.8	1800	0
For Cats:						
Feline r/d	Can	Hill's	8.4	28.3	1320	32–44
Feline r/d	Dry	Hill's	8.2	18.5	1450	17
Feline w/d	Can	Hill's	16.7	12.4	1680	13-29
Feline w/d	Dry	Hill's	9.4	10.1	1544	11
Science Diet	Can	Hill's	18	7	1770	8-25
Maint. Light	Dry	Hill's	9	7	1590	9
Less Active	Dry	Iams	17	2	1770	2 above
Recipe 10	Homemade	pg. A3-3	11.3	0.1	1950	0–18
Avg. Comm.	Can–ration	Many	14	2.7	1933	0
Avg. Comm.	Can–gourmet	Many	27	1.1	2350	0
Avg. Comm.	Dry	Many	12	2.0	1740	0

being lost slowly or not at all. If treats are fed, the client may believe that the weight-reduction program isn't effective. If an animal is being given only the proper amount of the recommended low-calorie diet and is not losing weight, the cause can be only another source of calories.

9. **Recommend two brisk 10-15 minute daily walks.** Exercise is beneficial and increases the chance of success (see page 6-20).

10. **Examine and weigh the animal, ideally at least every 2 weeks.** The frequency of office visits for obese patients undergoing weight reduction has a direct impact on the success of the program. If there is little or no weight loss, the most common cause is consumption of more calories than prescribed. If the client insists the pet is receiving no more than the prescribed amount of low-calorie diet, reduce the amount prescribed by 20%. If the rate of loss is still slower than expected (Table 11, page 6-22), hospitalize the pet to confirm the amount of food consumed and adjust it accordingly. If the animal is not losing weight at home and the owner claims the pet is eating the prescribed number of calories, never

indicate that you do not believe the owner. Instead request hospitalization of the pet for 5-10 days so that you can determine why the animal is not losing weight.

11. **Make a graph of the animal's body weight versus time.** Instruct the owner to record the animal's weight at least weekly and bring the record to each office visit. In conjunction with frequent office visits, a weight record (in the form of a graph as shown on page 6-35) is helpful in reinforcing the client's resolve to see the pet reach the established weight goal, which should be marked on the graph.

The animal should be weighed the first thing in the morning before eating. Instruct clients to weigh themselves with and without the animal and to subtract the difference to obtain the animal's weight. This procedure lacks precision, however, for cats or small dogs and is unnecessary; most small pets will sit on a scale long enough to be weighed. If the dog is too large to be weighed by the client, a girth measurement at the level of the xiphoid may be used instead.

12. **Once the weight goal has been reached, feed the amount necessary to maintain optimum weight.** Some animals' diets may

FIGURE 4

CANINE WEIGHT REDUCTION: STARVATION vs. CALORIC RESTRICTION

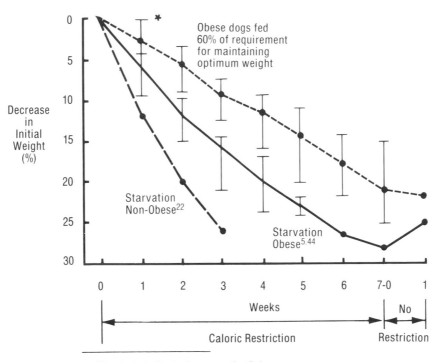

*Brackets indicate the range for 6 dogs.

be changed from the reducing diet to a re-stricted-calorie maintenance diet (such as Pre-scription Diet w/d, Hill's). However, many clients find it necessary and easier to continue feeding a larger amount of the reducing diet. Often, in these instances, the amount offered need not be restricted; whereas, the amount of a regular maintenance diet must be restricted to prevent recurrence of obesity.

13. **Instruct the client to continue weighing the animal weekly and record the weight,** preferably on the graph of the animal's body weight versus time (see page 6-35). If the animal begins to regain weight, lessen the amount fed by 10% or return to the reducing diet if it is not being fed. The reducing diets (Prescription Diets r/d, Hill's, or Recipes 4 or 10-Appendix Table 3), are nutritionally ade-quate for long-term maintenance of a dog or cat and are often used for maintenance of obese-prone dogs and cats.

14. **Reexamine the pet,** ideally one month and again three months after completion of the weight-reduction program. Follow-up exams are important in preventing recurrence. If clients know they will be bringing their pet

back, they will try harder to prevent the animal from regaining weight. In doing so they find weekly weighing of the pet and adjustment of the amount of diet fed are not difficult. These procedures soon become habit, thus greatly assisting in preventing recurrence of obesity.

STARVATION FOR WEIGHT REDUCTION

Weight reduction of obese subjects by starvation or total fasting has been used successfully both in human subjects[27,90] and dogs,[5,46,110] but not in cats. However, in human medicine fasting is rarely prescribed even during hospitalization.[27] It offers few advantages and many potential disadvantages, risks, and problems.

As shown in Figure 4, two phases of weight loss occur with starvation of either obese or non-obese dogs. First is a rapid loss of fluid as the body adjusts to using stored fat.[5,27] This occurs because of natruresis and reduction in renal-concentrating ability that characteristically accompany early star-vation or semistarvation.[177] Thus, much of the weight loss occurring during this initial period of starvation is water which is regained when feeding is

reinstituted.[5] These changes in fluid balance do not occur when a low-calorie reducing diet is fed in the amounts recommended (Figure 4). In addition, with starvation in people anxiety and depression are greatest, and satiety, interpersonal sensitivity, depression, diet-attitude, and self-esteem are lowest during this initial period.[154] After the first one to three weeks of starvation, weight loss is due primarily to utilization of adipose tissue which is relatively anhydrous; as a result the rate of loss slows. Thus, as has been reported for people[157] and as shown in Figure 4 for the dog, when this initial fluid loss is deleted, true weight loss as adipose tissue occurs at about the same rate with starvation as it does when a high-fiber low-calorie diet is consumed at 60% of caloric requirement for maintenance of optimum body weight.

Although the rate of weight loss with starvation of either obese or non-obese animals occurs in a hyperbolic fashion, becoming slower with time,[5,16,61] this is not the case when a low-calorie reducing diet is consumed (Figure 4). When a low-calorie reducing diet is consumed, body weight decreases at a rate of 3% per week for at least the first seven weeks. This same rate of loss occurs with starvation after the first one to three weeks of excess fluid losses (Table 16). After seven weeks the dog's body weight is 8% less with starvation than when the low-calorie reducing diet is fed (Table 16). However, when the starved dog begins eating again, fluid losses are regained, increasing the dog's body weight by about 4%.[5] Thus, the dog's non-dedehydrated body

weight is only about 4% less after seven weeks of starvation than it is when a low calorie reducing diet is consumed (Table 16).

Starvation not only produces about the same rate of weight loss as occurs when a low-calorie reducing diet is fed; it also creates a much greater loss of body protein.[157] With fasting by obese people, one-half the weight loss in the first month and one-fourth thereafter is due to protein catabolism.[18] In one study in people, although fat loss was 47% greater in fasting subjects than it was in subjects fed either a low-or a high-carbohydrate restricted-calorie diet, protein loss was 250 to 500% more.[61] This protein loss may be lessened by a high-protein diet,[157] but these diets significantly multiply the risk of precipitating health problems (see page 6-24).[59,152,166]

Fasting, in addition to increasing protein loss, causes magnesium depletion,[29] increases the risk of hypotension,[27] and causes alterations in intestinal villi, which decrease intestinal absorption.[157] In obese people, fasting has also been shown to decrease renal function and cause hepatocellular degeneration and focal hepatic necrosis, although these pathologic changes are reversible and return to normal when eating is resumed.[18]

In the fasted obese dog, although plasma ALT (formerly called SGPT) activity increases, results of liver function tests remain normal, and liver biopsies show no histologic abnormalities.[5,46,47] As shown in Table 17, many of the alterations that occur with fasting in obese people and rats, do not occur in obese dogs. The plasma ketone body

TABLE 16

RATE OF DECREASE IN OBESE DOG'S WEIGHT WITH CALORIC RESTRICTION

Feeding Regimen	% Over-Weight Initially	% Below Initial Weight at End of Each Week							No Restriction 1
		Caloric Restriction							
		1	2	3	4	5	6	7	
60% of Requirement at Optimum Wt.	28.3 (16–43)	2.7[a] (0.4–4.3)	5.5 (3.2–8)	9.5 (7.4–12)	11.9 (10–13)	14.5 (12–20)	17 (14–22)	21 (18–25)	22[c]
Starvation[5,46,47,101]	>30	7[b] (4–9)	12 (9–15)	17 (15–22)	20 (17–24)	23 (22–24)	27	29	25[c]

[a]Mean and (range) of 6 dogs.

[b]With starvation the rapid weight loss that occurs initially is due primarily to fluid loss. Weight loss as adipose tissue (which is relatively anhydrous) occurs at nearly the same rate with the degree of caloric restriction shown as it does with total starvation.

[c]End of the first week after caloric restriction. The amount of food fed during this week was just adequate to meet requirements for maintenance. The 4% increase in body weight after starvation is due to the regain of excess fluid loss that occurred during the first 1–3 weeks of starvation. These fluid losses and, therefore, regain do not occur when a high-fiber low-calorie diet is fed at 60% of caloric requirement.

TABLE 17

EFFECTS OF FASTING IN OBESE DOGS, PEOPLE, AND RATS[47]

Plasma Concentration	Dogs	People & Rats
Glucose	NC*	decreased
Insulin	NC	decreased
Glucagon	NC	increased
Growth Hormone	NC	---
Thyroxine	NC	---
Active T3	decreased	decreased
Inactive T3	NC	increased
Ketone Bodies	NC	increased
Ketone Bodies—mM/L	0.26	6–8

*NC = no change

concentration with fasting remains the same in the obese dog (0.23 to 0.26 mM/L); it increases from 0.06 to 0.28 mM/L in the fasting non-obese dog, and increases to 6-8 mM/L in fasting obese people and rats.[47] The low ketonemia in dogs is due to efficient peripheral use of ketone bodies and not due to reduced hepatic production. Use of glucose by the dog during fasting decreases by one-third[22] and is less than it is in fasting people or rats.[47] The fasting obese dog loses about 1g of body protein/kg body wt/day.[156] As a result, plasma protein and albumin concentrations decrease; in one study they dropped from 7.3 to 6.0 g/dl and from 3.8 to 3.0 g/dl, respectively, after a five week fast.[47] No other clinical or biochemical alterations were noted. Urine excretion of the primarily extracellular ions, sodium and calcium, decreased. In contrast, urine excretion of the primarily intracellular ions, potassium and magnesium, increased and remained high throughout fasting. Polyuria and polydipsia may[5] or may not occur.[47]

Regardless of the degree of caloric deficit, obese dogs lose body weight much more slowly than the dogs of normal weight[22,47] (Figure 4, page 6-27). The obese animals lose weight more slowly because primarily adipose tissue, which contains 10-15% water and has a caloric density of 8 kcal/g, is being utilized; in the non-obese animal more lean body tissue, which contains about 75% water and has a caloric density of about 1 kcal/g, is being utilized.

Total starvation of obese dogs has no detrimental effects and may be used as a means of weight reduction.[5,47,110] There are, however, major disadvantages and few advantages to its use.

1. Weight loss as adipose tissue is only 3-5% greater after seven weeks of fasting than it is

when a low-calorie reducing diet is fed (Table 16),

2. Many people view fasting as inhumane and therefore will not use it.

3. Hospitalization is required, which is more costly (generally at least twice the cost of weight reduction by the in-home caloric-restriction method described).

4. Because the client is not involved in the weight-reduction program, obesity recurrence can be expected to be greater than it is with the in-home program in which the pet owner is an integral part.

Total starvation of obese cats is not recommended. No studies on its safety and efficacy have been reported. It may result in severe hepatic lipidosis and death. Both obesity and fasting, particularly by obese cats, increase hepatic fat deposition, thus **obese cats should not be allowed to fast for more than a few days.** This is extremely important and can't be overemphasized! The greater the obesity, the greater the risk.

DRUG USE FOR WEIGHT REDUCTION

Many drugs have been used to treat obesity. However, as concluded by Bray,[27] **"There is no acceptably safe and effective pharmacologic treatment for obesity."** In one study there were no differences in weight loss between human patients treated with drugs (mazindol or diethyl-propion), placebo, or behavioral therapy.[41] Drugs that have been used include those which:

1. Decrease appetite, such as cholecystokinin, glucagon, mazindol, fluoxetine and numerous phenethylamines including amphetamines, phenmetrazine, phentermine, diethylpropion, fenfluramine and phenylpropanolamine

2. Cause nausea

3. Decrease digestion or absorption, such as starch or amylase blockers

4. Increase metabolic rate, such as thyroid hormone, growth hormone, and human chorionic gonadotropin (HCG)

5. Tranquilize

6. Induce diuresis

7. Decrease diet caloric density, such as the fat substitute, sucrose polyester

In evaluating any drugs or methods of treatment for any condition, especially weight loss, it is important to use placebos with neither the patient nor the clinician knowing which is the placebo and which is the drug being tested. Obese human

patients receiving placebos lose more weight than those subjected to behavioral, dietary or pharmacological techniques.[75,189]

Although some reports state that **amphetamines** hasten the rate of weight loss,[68] in 160 controlled studies evaluated by the U.S.A. Food and Drug Administration (FDA), 4543 human subjects given amphetamines lost only 0.08 lb more per day than 3182 given placebos.[42] Another series of double-blind studies of the efficacy of both **phenethylamine** and **nonphenethylamine** in reducing weight in more than 5000 people showed that these drugs had comparable efficacy and increased the rate of weight loss an average of only 0.6 lb/week more than placebos.[169] Both amphetamines and **fenfluramine** have been found to be ineffective in increasing the rate of weight loss in dogs.[20,46] When administration of any of these drugs is discontinued, rebound hyperphagia and rapid weight regain occur.[170] In addition, all of the phenethylamine drugs induce a variety of undesirable side effects such as dry mouth, restlessness, insomnia, irritability and increased heart rate and blood pressure.[27,121,170]

Administration of **cholecystokinin** reduces food intake by monkeys, rats, and lean and obese human beings, [69,164] but not by wolves.[129] Opiate antagonists, **naloxone** and **naltrexone,** prevented overeating by genetically obese mice, decreased feeding in rats after acute food deprivation and suppressed food intake in obese people.[195] However, in other studies naloxone in human subjects produced no change in hunger drive.[195] The effects of these drugs presumably occur because they block the appetite-stimulating effects of endogenous opioids.

Fluoxetine, a selective inhibitor of serotonin uptake, has been shown to suppress food intake in a dose-dependent manner and to reduce body weight in both normal and obese mice.[190] However, fluoxetine, opiate antagonists and cholecystokinin are ineffective when taken orally. With the exception of fluoxetine, none of these drugs has been shown to be effective for increasing weight loss. The efficacies of all of these drugs in dogs and cats are unknown, as are toxic effects of chronic administration.[164,195] In addition, at certain dosages and in certain conditions, opiate antagonists stimulate rather than suppress food intake.[195]

Thyroid hormone increases the rate of weight loss,[68] but more than two-thirds of this effect is due to the breakdown of lean body mass rather than adipose tissue.[25] In addition, chronotropic and inotropic properties of cardiac muscle and cardiac workload are increased, which could be detri-

mental.[27] Because it increases metabolic rate, growth hormone has been used to treat obesity. However, in controlled studies, it was no more effective than placebos.[75]

It has been claimed that **human chorionic gonadotropin (HCG)** is beneficial for weight loss because it renders "abnormal" fat deposits readily available, enabling the obese subject to adhere to and live comfortably on a restricted-calorie diet.[42] However, it was found ineffective in two clinical trials.[4] The American Medical Association and FDA both found no convincing scientific evidence that HCG was beneficial for inducing weight loss and consider it unphysiologic and unsafe.[42]

Because metabolic rate is increased by norepinephrine, which is mediated via primarily **beta-adrenoceptors,** drugs that stimulate these receptors have been used to increase energy utilization and, as a result, weight loss. These drugs have been shown to reduce weight gain and body weight with no change in food intake in either obese or non-obese mice.[8] They have not been reported effective in other species.

Starch blockers, which are inhibitors of alpha-amylase, supposedly decrease starch digestion and thus decrease use of energy from starch. All controlled studies in both human subjects[82] and dogs[163] have demonstrated no efficacy. They have no effect on decreasing starch or total carbohydrate digestion, postprandial plasma glucose or insulin concentrations, or on increasing fecal caloric content.[82,163] They are ineffective because starch continues to be digested by intestinal brush-border enzymes and is converted by bacteria in the large intestine to volatile fatty acids which are absorbed and utilized for energy. Ingestion of starch blockers may result in excessive production of intestinal gas. This may cause vomiting, diarrhea, abdominal cramps and flatulence.[82] However, in one study in dogs, starch blockers had no effect on gastrointestinal function.[163]

Chlorocitrate, a drug that reduces the rate of gastric emptying, has been shown in both dogs and rats to decrease food intake.[170] Rebound hyperphagia did not occur when the drug was discontinued. It reduced body weight in both lean and obese rats by a selective reduction in body fat.[170] However, it is not effective orally, its toxic effects are unknown and it is currently not available for clinical use.

Substances that appear to hold promise of benefit without undue risk or side effects in the treatment of obesity are the **synthetic fat substitutes.** Some are being considered by FDA for approval for inclusion in human foods. The synthetic fat

substitutes under consideration have physical and organoleptic properties almost identical to those of dietary fats but are indigestible. They may, therefore, be substituted for fat without changing the taste or physical properties of the diet, but they decrease caloric density. When the fat substitute, sucrose polyester, replaced one-half the dietary fat (resulting in an intake of 60 g of sucrose polyester/day) in the diet of obese people, it had no effect on the amount of food eaten or stool characteristics, but it decreased caloric density 21% and caloric intake 23% (540 kcal/day).[72] Patients could not tell the difference between the diets with and without sucrose polyester. An added benefit of some of the fat substitutes in people is that they decrease cholesterol absorption, which results in a decreased plasma low-density lipoprotein cholesterol concentration[72,124] and therefore, may decrease atherosclerosis.

SURGERY FOR WEIGHT REDUCTION

Surgery as a means of treating obesity is rarely used in either veterinary or human medicine. Because of numerous and common complications and risks it appears to be rarely indicated for either human beings or animals. In contrast to the extensive studies of surgical treatment of obesity conducted in human medicine, there appear to be none in veterinary medicine. This is probably because veterinarians have not had to rely on these procedures to attain weight loss in their patients and have had the good sense not to use them.

Surgical procedures used in human medicine for treating obesity include: 1) jejunoileal bypass, 2) many procedures to decrease stomach size, and 3) jaw-wiring. Wiring the jaws results in aspiration and death if the patient vomits or regurgitates. The procedure is unsuccessful because large quantities of food in liquid form can be ingested.[27] If weight loss occurs, it is rapidly regained after the wires are removed. In human medicine, the two other procedures result in a surgical mortality of 2.8% and are considered appropriate only when all three of the following requirements are met: 1) all other methods have failed repeatedly, 2) risk from obesity is greater than the risk of surgery and the extensive common complications, and 3) the surgery is conducted and monitored by an experienced team of surgeons, internists, and psychiatrists.[27]

Although both surgical procedures commonly cause many surgical and long-term postsurgical complications, these complications and the weight regained are greater with jejunoileal bypass.[76,81] As a result, most surgeons knowledgeable on this subject

no longer consider jejunoileal bypass surgery justified in treating obesity.[81]

Removing the distal 50-70% of the dog's small intestine results in 80-90% of ingested fat (from either a high or a low-fat diet) being excreted in the feces and a decrease in protein absorption; the result is a 20% weight loss.[101] Removing more of the dog's intestinal tract or bypassing the ileocecal valve leads to malnutrition, hepatic damage, electrolyte imbalances, and progressive weight loss terminating in death.[162] Removal of the proximal 50-70% of the dog's small intestine results in only a small decrease in body weight and a 10% decrease in fat absorption.[101,162]

The effects of procedures to reduce gastric size in the dog and cat have not been reported, but the procedures have been well studied in human subjects. Reducing gastric volume results in gastric distention, with less food intake. Gastric distention stimulates satiety.[49] A new method of decreasing gastric volume undergoing clinical trials in human medicine is a capsule that after its ingestion inflates in the stomach. It deflates with time, however, and currently must be replaced one to three times a year. Surgical procedures for decreasing gastric volume result in fewer long-term complications than those for jejunoileal bypass. However, surgical problems still occur in 62.5% of the cases.[27] In addition, 87% of cases develop either or both an iron and/or vitamin B-12 deficiency anemia; 50% of cases show musculoskeletal symptoms such as osteoporosis resulting from decreased calcium absorption.[37] Severe persistent vomiting, dumping syndrome, hair loss, kidney stones and unexplained neurologic disorders also occur.[1,27] After gastric reduction, marked alterations in eating behavior are necessary to achieve weight loss.[1] In addition, the remaining stomach pouch may gradually enlarge; and with small meals there is no decrease in food intake and, therefore, no weight loss.[27]

PREVENTION

Prevention of obesity has two aspects: 1) prevention of occurrence and 2) prevention of recurrence after a successful weight loss program. As with any disease, the best means of prevention is to eliminate causative factors. One of the causes of obesity is the development of too many fat cells during growth. Once formed, the number of fat cells cannot be decreased, and their size cannot be reduced to less than a certain limit.[16,17] Thus, the only way an animal with too many fat cells can maintain optimum body weight is by losing lean body mass.[182] However, loss of lean body mass is detrimental and is quite difficult to achieve and maintain because of

the body's many mechanisms to prevent it. The greater the number of fat cells that develop during growth, the more difficult it is to lose weight and to maintain a lower body weight.[153] More than 80% of overweight children become overweight adults. The more overweight the child, the more likely the child is to become an obese adult.[25,27,151] Although comparable information has not been determined for the dog or cat, it is available for a number of other animal species and extrapolation to the dog and cat appears logical. Thus, **one of the most important means of preventing obesity in the adult is to prevent obesity during growth.** This can be accomplished by feeding the puppy and kitten properly as described beginning on pages 3-12 and 4-10.

The most important aspect in preventing obesity during growth is to encourage exercise and play, and to avoid having food always available so that the puppy can eat as much as it wants, whenever it wants. This was well demonstrated in a study in which Labrador and Beagle puppies were allowed free access to a commercial puppy food. The pups allowed free access were 22-25% heavier at one year of age than were those fed 20% less, but were the same height and length and had the same muscle and skeletal development.[93] As these authors concluded, "free-choice feeding during growth, even of only a moderately palatable dry dog food, can produce a marked degree of obesity."

In addition to preventing obesity during growth, feeding the proper amount and allowing and encouraging exercise throughout life greatly assists in preventing obesity. As discussed previously (page 6-14) excess consumption of fat is more likely to induce obesity than is a similar number of calories derived from carbohydrate or protein. However, chronic intake of excess protein may predispose to renal failure (see page 8-10). Thus, to prevent obesity and possibly renal failure, calories for energy should come primarily from carbohydrates. In affluent societies where high calorie intake is common,[45] increasing the carbohydrate/fat ratio in the diet helps overcome the tendency to become obese and therefore, reduces the high prevalence of obesity.

Exercise helps prevent obesity because normal internal mechanisms that regulate appetite and satiety do not operate properly at low levels of physical exertion.[131] At one year of age sedentary rats given all they wanted to eat after weaning weighed 700-1000g; those forced to exercise moderately for one to two hours per day weighed 400g.[83] Maintenance of physical activity also lessens the increase in body fat and decrease in lean body mass that normally occurs with increasing age after puberty.[27]

Preventing an increase in the number of fat cells by preventing obesity during growth is important, not only in preventing occurrence of obesity later in life, but also in preventing recurrence of obesity after weight loss. The more fat cells in the body, the more difficult it is to lose weight and to maintain that loss.[16] The duration of maintenance of reduced body weight is inversely proportional to the number of fat cells in the body.[16,102] Hypertrophic obese people remain at a reduced weight more than four times longer than hyperplastic obese subjects who generally start to relapse within three to four months.[16]

Even without an increased number of fat cells, continual care must be taken to prevent recurrence of obesity. This is necessary, both to prevent recurrence of the environmental factors responsible for causing the obesity initially and because after weight loss, caloric requirements are less. After weight loss in human beings, caloric intake must be reduced by 40 kcal for each 1 lb of weight reduction to maintain the new weight.[13] This decrease in caloric requirement after weight loss is due to: 1) a decrease in lean body mass, 2) a decrease in energy cost of physical activity for the same level of activity, and 3) a decrease in meal-induced heat production. In obesity, both body fat and lean body mass increase; both decrease with weight loss. The decrease in lean body mass lowers resting metabolic rate or energy expenditure for maintenance. Energy cost for physical activity is also reduced after weight loss because there is less body mass to move. Additionally, meal-induced heat production is less in obese animals than in non-obese animals[13,88] and is further reduced after weight loss.[161] The lower amount of meal-induced heat produced contributes to obesity, and its further reduction with weight loss is often a cause of recurring obesity after weight loss.[161]

The high incidence of recurrent obesity is also explained by a study which demonstrated that adipocyte metabolism is similar: 1) for weight-stable never-obese people and obese people; 2) for fasted never-obese people, and weight-stable reduced obese people, but differs greatly between these two groups.[105] Thus, the reduced obese individual's adipocytes, like those of the fasted individual, perceives the reduced body weight as abnormally low. This suggests that, like fasted never-obese individuals, the reduced-obese individual has a homeostatic tendency for body weight to return to what is perceived as a non-fasted state, i.e. the previously obese weight. This would be expected if the obesity is caused by a metabolic abnormality that remains after weight reduction.

In most people, a reduced weight is maintained for only one to one and one/half years.[90] Subsequently a steady weight gain begins so that 50% of people regain their lost weight within two to three years.[16] More than 90% of people regain or exceed their original weight within nine years; only 3 to 4% remain at a reduced weight.[90] The rate at which lost weight is regained is uniform regardless of original weight, degree of weight loss, or duration of obesity.[16] These statistics make the treatment of obesity extremely discouraging and further emphasize the importance of doing everything possible to prevent its occurrence. Fortunately, the incidence of recurrence in dogs and cats need not be nearly this high if the detrimental effects of obesity are adequately explained and emphasized to the client, and if the procedures for weight reduction by dietary caloric restriction are followed as described, particularly steps 12-14 (pages 6-26 and 27).

CONCLUSIONS

On the basis of clinical examination, 23-32% of dogs and many cats are more than 15% overweight (Tables 2 and 3, pages 6-3 and 4). Health and longevity are impaired because of locomotion and respiratory difficulties, heart disease, neoplastic diseases, hypertension, impaired hepatic function, reduced reproductive ability, less heat tolerance, decreased resistance to both viral and bacterial diseases, increased dystocia, irritability, dermatosis, surgical risk and difficulty, bone disease, and diabetes mellitus (Tables 1 and 7, pages 6-3 and 7 and Figure 1, page 6-9).

There are two stages of obesity: initial and static. During the initial stage, when obesity is developing, caloric intake exceeds expenditure of energy. During the static stage caloric intake equals expenditure of energy, and excess body weight is maintained. Excess caloric intake is caused by or predisposed to by factors that interfere with either internal (physiologic) or external (environmental) signals that induce satiety (Figure 1, page 6-9).

Factors that interfere with internal satiety signals are thought to be less common than those that interfere with external satiety signals. The factors most commonly interfering with external satiety signals include constant and easy access to excessive amounts of highly palatable energy-dense foods. Coupled with inactivity, these appear to be the most common causes of obesity. Other obesity-inducing factors include:

1. Increased efficiency of energy utilization due to a decrease in meal-induced heat production
2. Alterations in hypothalamic satiety or hunger centers

3. Alterations in signals to these centers or their response
4. Decreased energy expenditure due to a decrease in metabolic rate

Although these factors are known to induce obesity their prevalence among obese dogs and cats is unknown. These obesity-inducing factors may be due to alterations in the sympathetic nervous system or thyroid hormone secretion, or to response of brown adipose tissue in using energy for heat production. These alterations, and/or an increased number of fat cells may be inherited. An increased number of fat cells, which greatly predisposes to obesity, may also be induced by excess fat deposition during growth. The majority of animals that have obese parents or that have excess fat deposition during growth have a problem with obesity throughout life. Therefore, preventing obesity during growth is very important in preventing obesity in the adult.

A weight reduction program should be instituted for all dogs and cats that are more than 15% above their optimum weight so as to: 1) minimize health problems, 2) reduce future health-care costs, 3) improve appearance, and 4) increase the animal's longevity and enjoyment of life. There are five possible methods for managing obesity: psychological, exercise, dietary, pharmacological, and surgical. Surgery and currently available drugs are of no value. The psychological aspect of weight reduction includes the essential task of convincing everyone associated with the animal of the importance of weight reduction and maintaining a lower body weight. Exercise is quite helpful, not only in increasing energy expenditure (Table 10, page 6-20), but also because an increase in exercise from sedentary activity lessens appetite and food intake.

Success in treating obesity and preventing its recurrence is greatest when caloric intake is reduced by feeding a nutritionally balanced, high-fiber low-calorie reducing diet which is 35-45% lower for dogs, and 20-30% lower for cats, in caloric density than average commercial pet foods (Table 15, page 6-26). A diet of this type reduces intake of energy and induces satiety, thereby increasing diet compliance and weight loss. Depending on the individual case, the actual amount of food fed may or may not require limitation (Table 14, page 6-25). In contrast to reducing the amount fed of a higher calorie-dense diet, or feeding a high-protein or low-carbohydrate diet, a nutritionally balanced high-fiber low-fat low-calorie-dense diet has no detrimental effects. If necessary, it may be and, in some cases, should be fed indefinitely to prevent recurrence of obesity.

CLIENT INFORMATION ON CANINE AND FELINE OBESITY

Obesity is the most common nutritional disease of dogs and cats. It is an excess of body fat and is associated with many health problems. Obesity occurs in 20-30% of pet dogs and cats. It is most common in older animals and females.

WHY IS OBESITY DANGEROUS?

Overweight pets suffer more physical ailments and don't live as long as animals of average weight. Obesity often reduces a pet's enjoyment of life, its performance, and the owner's enjoyment of the pet.

Obesity can cause, worsen or increase:
1. Cancer
2. Arthritis, hip dysplasia, back or spinal disk problems, and ligament rupture
3. Lung disease
4. Heart disease
5. Liver disease
6. Diabetes
7. Constipation, excessive gas and pancreatitis
8. Risk with surgery and anesthesia
9. Heat intolerance
10. Skin disease
11. Mental irritability (related to discomfort)
12. Susceptibility to infectious diseases
13. Exercise intolerance

Weight reduction will lessen the chances of these problems. Strict adherence to a weight control program will improve your pet's appearance, health and enjoyment of life, your enjoyment of the animal, and your future health-care costs for the pet.

WHAT CAUSES OBESITY?

Obesity is caused by consumption of more calories than needed: too much food, too little exercise, or both.

Pets fed table scraps, treats or snacks are more likely to be obese than those fed only commercially prepared rations. Overfeeding puppies predisposes them to obesity as adults by increasing their number of fat cells. After an animal matures, its number of fat cells do not multiply as readily. Instead, the size of the fat cells can increase. The primary effect of weight reduction, is to make the fat cells smaller but not fewer. Thus, puppies and kittens that become obese during growth will often be plagued by obesity throughout life.

Some diseases can cause obesity, but they are uncommon. The most common causes of obesity are overfeeding and inadequate exercise.

IS MY PET OVERWEIGHT?

If your pet weighs over 15% more than it did as a young, healthy adult it is overweight. If you do not know your pet's optimum weight, the amount of tissue overlying the rib cage is the most practical way to evaluate your pet. Your pet is thin or normal if its ribs are easy to feel, overweight if its ribs are difficult to feel, and dangerously obese if its ribs cannot be felt at all. Some overweight pets, may have a pendulous abdomen.

Before beginning a weight-reduction program for your pet, a veterinary examination is recommended. This will rule out the presence of conditions that resemble obesity, such as excessive fluid in the body. It is important to confirm that your pet is really overweight and not showing symptoms of heart, kidney or other diseases, or that other diseases if also present, are treated.

HOW IS OBESITY MANAGED?

The most important aspect of a successful weight-reduction program is to convince yourself and everyone associated with your pet that the program is essential. Anything short of your total commitment will result in frustration and wasted time, effort and money. Management requires that your pet use more calories than it eats. This means that the intake of calories must be reduced, and, if possible, the amount of exercise increased.

Drugs and hormones are not beneficial for achieving weight loss unless your pet has a confirmed disease in addition to obesity.

Together with your veterinarian, set a specific goal for weight reduction and estimate the time required to reach that goal. Your pet's weight should decrease by 3% per week. From 8–12 weeks are required for most obese pets to reach their ideal weight. Your veterinarian will want to see and weigh your pet at regular intervals during and after the weight-reduction program.

Management of an overweight pet should include:
1. Reduce your pet's caloric intake by feeding it a low-calorie, high-fiber dietary food specifically formulated for reducing weight.
2. Keep your pet out of the room when food is being prepared or eaten.
3. Do not feed obese pets with other pets.
4. Do not feed anything other than the amount of food prescribed by your veterinarian. Withholding food shows much more care and concern for your pet than allowing it to suffer the effects of

obesity. Don't make your pet suffer these effects because you can't resist its demands for food.

5. Exercise your pet regularly as directed.

6. At least once weekly weigh your pet and record its weight on the graph below.

If you cannot successfully reduce your pet at home, hospitalization may be recommended. This allows your veterinarian to determine why your pet is not losing weight, to implement a successful weight-reduction program, and to spare you the difficulties involved.

DIETARY MANAGEMENT

Successful weight-reduction is rare if your pet is fed its regular diet. If any snacks are fed it is virtually impossible to reduce the pet. Decreasing the amount of regular food enough to produce weight loss may cause nutritional deficiencies and begging. Feed your pet a diet specifically formulated for weight reduction. These are available from most veterinarians. The greater your concern for your pet's health, the greater your resolve should be to help your pet reach and maintain ideal weight.

VETERINARY INSTRUCTIONS

For Weight Reduction of_____

1. Diet Prescribed: _____

Total amount to feed daily:_____

Divide total amount into_____ feedings/day.

All right to feed _____ amount

daily of celery, lettuce, green beans, unbuttered

popcorn or _____ .

2. Exercise: ____minutes____times/day

3. Estimated time to reach goal **IF** all

instructions are followed: ____ weeks

4. Return with pet and graph on:

_____

_____

WEIGHT LOSS PERFORMANCE CHART:

1) Enter optimum weight or goal weight on the vertical axis near the bottom of the scale.

2) Enter obese weight at appropriate distance on the vertical axis near the top of the scale.

3) Plot weight weekly.

W E I G H T

(   )

< - - GOAL - - > --- --- --- --- --- --- --- --- --- --- --- ---

1   2   3   4   5   6   7   8   9   10   11   12   13   14   15

TIME (Weeks)

Date:_____

REFERENCES

1. Alpers DH: Surgical therapy for obesity. New Engl J Med 308:1026-1027 (1983).

2. Anand BK: Central chemosensitive mechanism related to feeding. In Handbook of Physiology Sec 6 Alimentary Canal Vol 1, Editor CF Code, American Physiological Society, Washington DC, pp 249-263 (1967).

3. Anderson JW: Physiological and metabolic effects of dietary fiber. Federation Proc 44:2902-2906 (1985).

4. Anderson RS: Obesity in the dog and cat. The Vet Ann 186 (1973).

5. Anderson GL, Lewis LD: Obesity. In Current Vet Therapy VII, Editor RW Kirk, WB Saunders Co. Philadelphia, PA, pp 1034-1039 (1980).

6. Anonymous: Breed requirements as recognized by AKC. In the New Dog Encyclopedia, Stackpole Books, Harrisburg, PA pp 447-702 (1970).

7. Applegate EA, Upton DE, Stern JS: Exercise and detraining effect on food intake, adiposity and lipogenesis in Osborne-Mendel rats made obese by a high fat diet. J Nutr 114:447-459 (1984).

8. Arch JRS, DePhil MA, Ainsworth AT: Thermogenic and anti-obesity activity of a novel beta-adrenoceptor agonist (BRL 26830A) in mice and rats. Amer J Clin Nutr 38:549-558 (1983).

9. Baecke JAH, van Staveren WA, Burema J: Food consumption, habitual physical activity and body fatness in young Dutch adults. Amer J Clin Nutr 37:278-286 (1983).

10. Bartoshuk LM, Harned MA, Parks LTL: Taste of water in the cat:Effect of sucrose preference. Science 171:699-701 (1971).

11. Beauchamp GK, Maller O, Roberts JG Jr: Flavor preferences in cats(Felis catus and Panthera species). J Comp Physiol Psychol 91:1118-1127 (1977).

12. Bertrand HA, Stacy C, Masoro EJ, et al: Plasticity of fat cell numbers. J Nutr 114:127-131 (1984).

13. Bessard T, Schutz Y, Jequier E: Energy expenditure and postprandial thermogenesis in obese women before and after weight loss. Amer J Clin Nutr 38:680-693 (1983).

14. Bistrain BR: Prevalence, causes and therapy of obesity. In Obesity—A Comprehensive Approach, Ross Laboratories publication, Columbus, Ohio, pp 2-7 (1980).

15. Bistrain BR, Blackburn GL, Flatt JP, et al: Nitrogen metabolism and insulin requirements in obese diabetic adults on a protein-sparing modified fast. Diabetes 25:494-504 (1976).

16. Bjorntorp P: Results of conservative therapy of obesity: correlation with adipose tissue morphology. Amer J Clin Nutr 33:370-375 (1980).

17. Bjorntorp P, Carlgren G, Isaksson, et al: The effect of energy reducing dietary regime in relation to adipose tissue cellularity in obese women. Amer J Clin Nutr 28:445-452 (1975).

18. Bloom WL: Fasting as an introduction to the treatment of obesity. Metabolism 8:214-220 (1959).

19. Bolton RP, Heaton KW, Burroughs LF: The role of dietary fiber on satiety, glucose and insulin: studies with fruit and fruit juice. Amer J Clin Nutr 34:211-217 (1981).

20. Bomson L, Parket CHL: Effect of fenfluramine on overweight spayed bitches. Vet Rec 96:202-203 (1975).

21. Bonde AA, Hendler R, Felig P: Impaired glucose tolerance and insulin resistance following extended cafeteria feeding in female rats. Abstr 2998 Fed Proc 43:798 (1984).

22. Brady LJ, Armstrong MK, Muiruri KL, et al: Influence of prolonged fasting in the dog on glucose turnover and blood metabolites. J Nutr 107:1053 (1977).

23. Bray GA: Clinical management of the obese adult, Postgrad Med 51:125 (1972).

24. Bray GA: Obesity in perspective. In NIH Fogarty Inst Series on Preventive Med, Vol II, Part 2, DHEW Publication No (NIH) 75-708, Washington DC (1975).

25. Bray GA: The obese patient. In Major Problems in Internal Medicine, Editor LH Smith Jr, WB Saunders, Philadelphia, Vol 9 (1976).

26. Bray GA: The inheritance of corpulence. In Body Weight Regulatory System: Basic Mechanisms and Clinical Implications, Editors WPT James, L Cioffi, TB Van Itallie, Raven Press, NY (1981).

27. Bray GA: Obesity. In Current Concepts, Scope Publication by UpJohn, Kalamazoo, MI, pp 1-52 (1982).

28. Bray GA, York DA: Hypothalamic and genetic obesity in experimental animals: An autonomic and endocrine hypothesis. Physiol Rev 59:719-809 (1979).

29. Brown MR, Klish WJ, Hollander J, et al: A high protein, low calorie liquid diet in the treatment of very obese adolescents: long-term effects on lean body mass. Amer J Clin Nutr 38:20-31 (1983).

30. Burrows CF, Kronfeld DL, Banta CA, Merritt AM: Effects of fiber on digestibility and transit time in dogs. J Nutr 112:1726-1732 (1982).

31. Chandra RK: Cell-mediated immunity in genetically obese mice. Amer J Clin Nutr 33:13-16 (1980).

32. Chumlea WC, Roche AF, Siervogal RM, et al: Adipocytes and adiposity in adults. Amer J Clin Nutr 34:1798-1803 (1981).

33. Cianzio DS, Topel DG Whitehurst GB, et al: Adipose tissue growth and cellularity: Changes in bovine adipocyte size and number. J Amer Sci 60:970-976 (1985).

34. Colliver JA, Frank S, Frank A: Similarity of obesity indices in clinical studies of obese adults: a factor analysis study. Amer J Clin Nutr 38:640-647 (1983).

35. Compston JE, Vedi S, Ledger JE, et al : Vitamin D status and bone histomorphometry in gross obesity. Amer J Clin Nutr 34:2359-2363 (1981).

36. Conway JM, Bulman SD, Collins JS, et al: A comparison of new methods for estimating body composition: whole body impedance and near infrared interactance. Amer J Clin Nutr 41:839 (1985).

37. Crowley L, Seay J, Mullin G: Late effects of gastric bypass for obesity. Fed Proc 43:Abstr 676:400 (1984).

38. Cummings JH: Nutritional implications of dietary fiber. Amer J Clin Nutr 31:21-29 (1978).

39. Cunningham J, Calles-Escandon J, Zawalich W, Felig P: Exercise and appetite: evidence for an anorexigenic effect of exercise in hyperphagic rats and a hyperphagic effect in normal rats. Amer J Clin Nutr 39, Abstr 686 (1984).

40. Czaja JA, Gay RW: Ovarian hormones and food intake in female guinea pigs and rhesus monkeys. Horm Behav 6:329-349 (1975).

41. Daham WT, Molitch ME, Bray GA, et al: Treatment of obesity: cost-benefit assessment of behavioral therapy, placebo, and two anorectic drugs. Amer J Clin Nutr 31:774-778 (1978).

42. Dairy Council Digest: What's new in weight control? National Dairy Council, 6300 N River Rd, Rosemont IL publication 49 (No. 2) (1978).

43. Dairy Council Digest: Dietary factors and blood pressure. National Dairy Council, 6300 N River Rd, Rosemont IL (No. 5) (Sept-Oct 1981).

44. Danforth E Jr: The role of thyroid hormones and insulin in the regulation of energy metabolism Amer J Clin Nutr 38:1006-1017 (1983).

45. Danforth E Jr: Diet and obesity. Amer J Clin Nutr 41:1132-1145 (1985).

46. de Bruijne J J, Lubberink AMME: Obesity. In Current Veterinary Therapy VI, Editor RW Kirk, Philadelphia, WB Saunders, pp 1068-1070 (1977).

47. de Bruijne JJ: Ketone-body metabolism in fasting dogs. PhD Thesis, State University of Utrecht, The Netherlands, pp 1-104 (1982).

48. Delorne CB, Wojcik J: Interaction of dietary protein with cellulose in the adaptation to caloric dilution by weanling rats. J Nutr 112:21-28 (1982).

49. Deutsch JA, Phil D: The role of the stomach in eating. Amer J Clin Nutr:1040-1043 (1985).

50. Diamond PR, Brondel L, DeBlanc J: Palatability and postprandial thermogenesis in dogs. Abstr 42, Fed Proc 43:291 (1984).

51. Duch DS, Chow FHC, Hamar DW, Lewis LD: The effect of castration and body weight on the occurrence of the feline urological syndrome. Feline Pract 8:35-40 (1978).

52. Duncan KH, Bacon JA, Weinsier RL: The effects of high and low energy density diets on satiety, energy intake, and eating time of obese and nonobese subjects. Amer J Clin Nutr 37:763-767 (1983).

53. Edney ATB: Current trends in small animal nutrition. The Vet Ann 195:195 (1972).

54. Edney ATB: Management of obesity in the dog. VM/SAC 69:46 (1974).

54a. Edney ATB, Smith PM: Study of obesity in dogs visiting veterinary practices in the United Kingdom. Vet Rec 118:391-396 (1986).

55. Elahi D, Nagulesparan M, Hershcopf RJ, et al: Feedback inhibition of insulin secretion by insulin: relation to the hyperinsulinemia of obesity. New Engl J Med 306:1196-1202 (1982).

56. Etherton TD, Wangsness PJ, Hammers VM, Ziegler JH: Effect of dietary restriction on carcass composition and adipocyte cellularity of swine with different propensities for obesity. J Nutr 112:2314-2323 (1982).

57. Fabry P, Tepperman J: Meal frequency—A possible factor in human pathology. Amer J Clin Nutr 23:1059 (1970).

58. Faust IM, Johnson PR, Hirsch J: Long-term effects of early nutritional experience on the development of obesity in the rat. J Nutr 110:2027-2034 (1980).

59. Felig P: Very low calorie protein diets. New Engl J Med 310:589-591 (1984).

60. Fernandez R, Phillips SF: Components of fiber impair iron absorption in the dog. Amer J Clin Nutr 35:107-112 (1982).

61. Fidanza F: Effects of starvation on body composition. Amer J Clin Nutr 33:1562-1566 (1980).

62. Flatt JP: Role of the increased adipose tissue mass in the apparent insulin insensitivity of obesity. Amer J Clin Nutr 25:1189 (1972).

63. Food and Drug Administration Consumer Update: Weight reduction diets. Washington DC (July 1982).

64. Forbes GB: Energy intake and body weight a reexamination of two "classic" studies. Amer J Clin Res 39:349-350 (1984).

65. Forman LP, Schneeman BO: Effects of dietary pectin and fat on the small intestinal contents and exocrine pancreas of rats. J Nutr 110:1992-1999 (1980).

66. Friedman GJ: Diet in the treatment of diabetes mellitus. In Modern Nutrition in Health and Disease, Editors Goodhart RS and ME Shils, Lea & Febiger, Philadelphia, pg 977 (1980).

67. Garn SM, Hawthorne VM, Pelkington JJ, Pesick SO: Fatness and mortality in west Scotland. Amer J Clin Nutr 38:313-319 (1983).

68. Gershberg H: Use of drugs in the treatment of obesity. Postgrad Med 51:135 (1972).

69. Gibbs J, Smith GP: Cholecystokinin and satiety in rats and rhesus monkeys. Amer J Clin Nutr 30:758-761 (1977).

70. Glick Z, Bray A, Teague RJ: Effect of prandial glucose on brown fat thermogenesis in rats: Possible implications for dietary obesity. J Nutr 114:286-291 (1984).

71. Glick Z, Wickler SJ, Stern JS, Horwitz BA: Blood flow into brown fat of rats is greater after a high carbohydrate than after a high fat meal. J Nutr 114:1934-1939 (1984).

72. Glueck CJ, Hastings MM, Allen C, et al: Sucrose polyester and covert calories dilution. Amer J Clin Nutr 35:1352-1359 (1982).

73. Gordon DT, Besch-Willford C, Ellersieck MR: The action of cellulose on the intestinal mucosa and element absorption by the rat. J Nutr 113:2545-2556 (1983).

74. Grace J, Russek M: The influence of previous experience on the behavior of dogs toward sucrose and saccharin. Physiol Behav 4:553-558 (1969).

75. Greenway FL, Bray GA: Human chorionic gonadotropin (HCG) in the treatment of obesity: A critical assessment of the Simeons Method. West J Med 127:461-463 (1977).

76. Halverson JD, Scheff RJ, Gentry K, Alpers DH: Long-term follow-ups of jejunoileal bypass patients. Amer J Clin Nutr 33:472-475 (1980).

77. Hart BL, Barrett RE: Effects of castration on fighting, roaming, and urine spraying in adult male cats. J Amer Vet Med Assoc 163:290 (1963).

78. Haymes EM, Lundegren HM, Loomis JL, Buskirk ER: Validity of the ultrasonic technique as a method of measuring subcataneous adipose tissue. Ann Human Biol 3:245-251 (1976).

79. Himms-Hagen J, Phil D: Thermogenesis in brown adipose tissue as an energy buffer. Implications for obesity. New Engl J Med 311:1549-1558 (1984).

80. Hirsch J: Can we modify the number of adipose cells? Postgrad Med 51:83 (1972).

81. Hocking MP, Duerson MC, O'Leary JP, Woodward ER: Jejunoileal bypass for morbid obesity. New Engl J Med 308:995-999 (1983).

82. Hollenbeck CB, Coulston AM, Orlan R, et al: Effects of a common starch blocker preparation on carbohydrate digestion and absorption: in vivo and in vitro studies Amer J Clin Nutr 38:498-503 (1983).

83. Holloszy JO: Reaction: Effectiveness of exercise in weight loss. In Obesity—A Comprehensive Approach, Ross Laboratories publication, Columbus Ohio, pp 27-29 (1980).

84. Hoover-Plow J, Nelson B: Oxygen consumption in mice (I strain) after feeding. J Nutr 115:303-310 (1985).

85. Hopkins GS, Schubert TA, Hart BL: Castration of adult male dogs: Effects on roaming, aggression, urine marking, and mounting. J Amer Vet Med Assoc 168:1108 (1976).

86. Horton ES: An overview of the assessment and regulation of energy balance in humans. Amer J Clin Nutr 38:972-977 (1983).

87. Houpt KA, Coren B, Hintz HF, Hilderbrandt JE: Effect of sex and reproductive status on sucrose preference, food intake and body weight of dogs. J Amer Vet Med Assoc 174:1083-1085 (1979).

88. Houpt KA, Smith SL: Taste preference and their relation to obesity in dogs and cats. Canad Vet J 22:77-81 (1981).

89. Jequier E, Schutz Y: Long-term measurements of energy expenditure in humans using a respiration chamber. Amer J Clin Nutr 38:989-998 (1983).

90. Johnson D, Drenick EJ: Therapeutic fasting in morbid obesity. Long-term follow-up. Arch Intern Med 137:1381-1382 (1977).

91. Johnston JL, Warsh JJ, Anderson GH: Obesity and precursor availability affect urinary catecholamine metabolite production in women. Amer J Clin Nutr 38:356-368 (1983).

92. Kane E, Morris JG, Rogers QR: Acceptability and digestibility by adult cats of diets made with various sources and levels of fat. J Anim Sci 53:1516-1523 (1981).

93. Kendall PT, Burger IH: The effect of controlled and appetite feeding on growth and development in dogs. Proc 3rd Kal Kan Symp, pp 60-63 (1979).

94. Kinsell LW, Gunning B, Michaels GD: Calories do count. Metabolism 13:195 (1964).

95. Knehans AW, Romsos DR: Effects of diet on norepinephrine turnover in obese mice. J Nutr 114:2080-2088 (1984).

96. Kleerekoper M, Tolia K, Parfitt AM: Nutritional, endocrine and demographic aspects of osteoporosis. Orthop Clin N Amer 12:547-558 (1981).

97. Knittle JL, Hirsch J: Effect of early nutrition on the development of rat epididymal fat pad: cellularity and metabolism. J Clin Invest 47:2091-2098 (1968).

98. Kolterman OG, Insel J, Saekow M, Olefsky JM: Mechanisms of insulin resistance in human obesity: Evidence for receptor and postreceptor defects. J Clin Invest 65:1272-1284 (1980).

99. Koong LJ, Nienaber JA, Mersmann HJ: Effect of phase of nutrition on organ size and fasting heat production in genetically obese and lean pigs. J Nutr 113:1626-1631 (1983).

100. Krehans AW, Romsos DR: Reduced norepinephrine turnover in brown adipose tissue of ob/ob mice. Amer J Physiol 242, E253-E261 (1982).

101. Kremen AJ, Lanner JH, Nelson CH: An experimental evaluation of the nutritional importance of the proximal and distal small intestine. Ann of Surg 140:439-448 (1954).

102. Krotkiewski M, Sjostrom L, Bjorntorp P, et al: Adipose tissue cellularity in relation to prognosis for weight reduction. Int J Obesity 1:395-416 (1977).

103. Kuffert AM, Curry DL, Stern JS: Pancreatic hypersensitivity to glucose by obese Zucker rats. Fed Proc 44:1104 (1985).

104. LeBlanc J, Diamond P: The effect of meal frequency on postprandial thermogenesis in dog. Fed Proc 44:1678 (1985).

105. Leibel RL, Hirsch J, Berry EM, Gruen RK: Alterations in adipocyte free fatty acid re-esterification associated with obesity and weight reduction in man. Amer J Clin Nutr 42:198-206 (1985).

106. Lennon D, Nagle F, Stratman, F, Dennis S: Diet and exercise training effects on resting metabolic rate. Fed Proc 43, Abstr 3018:801 (1984).

107. Levine AS, Morley JE, Sievert CE, et al: Peptidergic regulation of feeding in the dog. Fed Proc 43, Abstr 672:399 (1984).

108. Lewis BA: Effect of diet caloric density on amount of food and calories consumed and body weight of the cat. Unpublished data (1984).

109. Lewis DS, Bertrand HA, Masoro EJ, et al: Preweaning nutrition on fat development in baboons. J Nutr 113:2253-2259 (1983).

110. Lewis LD: Obesity in the dog. J Amer Anim Hosp Assoc 14:402-409 (1978).

111. Lukaski HC, Bolonchuk WW, Johnson PE, et al: Assessment of fat-free mass using bioelectrical impedance measurements of the human body. Amer J Clin Nutr 39:Abstr 657 (1984).

112. Lukaski HC, Johnson PE, Bolonchuk MSc, Lykken GI: Assessment of fat-free mass using bioelectrical impedance measurements of the human body. Am J Clin Nutr 41:810-817 (1985).

113. Lyons MJ, Faust IM, Hemmes RB, et al: A virally induced obesity syndrome in mice. Science 216:82-85 (1982).

114. MacMahon SW, Wilcken EL, Macdonald GJ: The effect of weight reduction on left ventricular mass. A randomized controlled trial in young, overweight hypertensive patients. New Engl J Med 314:334-339 (1986).

115. Mann GV: New Engl J Med 291:178&226 (1974).

116. Marchington D, Rothwell NJ, Stock MJ, York DA: Diet induced thermogenesis and brown adipose tissue in lean and obese,(fa/fa)Zucker rats after adrenolectomy. J Nutr 113:1395-1402 (1983).

117. Mason E: Obesity in pet dogs. Vet Rec 86:612 (1970).

118. Mattheeuws D, Rottiers R, Kaneko JJ, Vermeulen A: Diabetes mellitus in dogs: relationship of obesity to glucose tolerance and insulin response. Amer J Vet Res 45:98-103 (1984).

119. Mattheeuws D, Rottiers R, Baeyens D, Vermeulen A: Glucose tolerance and insulin response in obese dogs. J Amer Anim Hosp Assoc 20:287-293(1984).

120. Mayer J: Obesity. Postgrad Med 51:67 (1972).

121. Mayer J: Obesity. In Modern Nutrition in Health and Disease, ed 5, Editors RS Goodhart and ME Shils, Lea & Febiger, Philadelphia, p 639 (1973).

122. Mayer J, Marshall NB, Vitale JJ, et al : Exercise, food intake and body weight in normal rats and genetically obese adult mice. Amer J Physiol 177:544-548 (1954).

123. McLaughlin CL: Role of peptides from gastrointestinal cells in food intake regulation. J.Anim Sci 55:1515-1527 (1982).

124. Mellies MJ, Vitale C, Jandacek RJ, et al: The substitution of sucrose polyester for dietary fat in obese, hypercholesterolemic outpatients. Amer J Clin Nutr 41:1-12 (1985).

125. Mendex J, Lukaski HC, Buskirk ER: Fat-free mass as a function of maximal oxygen consumption and 24-hour urinary creatinine, and 3-methylhistidine excretion. Amer J Clin Nutr 39:710-715 (1984).

126. Mersmann JH, Pond WG, Yen JT: Use of carbohydrate and fat as energy source by obese and lean swine. J Anim Sci 58:894-902 (1984).

127. Meserole VK, Etherton TD: Insulin binding to liver microsomes from lean and obese swine during growth to market weight. J Anim Sci 59:650-657 (1984).

128. Meyer H, Drochner W, Weidenhaupt C: Contribution to incidence and treatment of obesity in dogs. Dtsch Tierarztl Wschr 85:113-152 (1978).

129. Morley JE, Levine AS, Plotka ED, Seal US: The effect of naloxone on feeding and spontaneous eating locomotion in the wolf. Physiol Behav 30:331-334 (1983).

130. Morris ML Jr: Index of Dietetic Management. In Current Veterinary Therapy VI, Editor RW Kirk, WB Saunders Co. Philadelphia, pp 59-73 (1977).

131. National Institutes of Health: Facts About Obesity. Washington DC (1976).

132. Nesbitt GH, Izzo J, Peterson L, Wilkins RJ: Canine hypothyroidism: A retrospective study of 108 cases. J Amer Vet Med Assoc 177:1117-1122 (1980).

133. Newberne PM: Overnutrition and resistance of dogs to distemper virus. Fed Proc 25, 1701 (1966).

134. Nisbett RE: Eating Behavior and Obesity in Men and Animals. In Advances of Psychosomatic Medicine 7:175 Basel-Karger (1972).

135. Nutrition Notes: Consumers union analyzes the Pritikin Program. pp 7-8 (Dec 1982).

136. Obarzanek E, Levitsky DA: Weight gain through overeating and return to normal without undereating. Abstr 4518, Fed Proc 43, 1057 (1984).

137. Orosco M, Jacquot C, Cohen Y: Brain catecholamine levels and turnover in various models of obese animals. Gen Pharmacol 12:267-271 (1981).

138. Pacy PJ, Barton N, Webster JD, Garrow JS: The energy cost of aerobic exercise in fed and fasted normal subjects. Amer J Clin Nutr 42:764-768 (1985).

139. Padwee HS: The Live-Longer Diet for Dogs and Cats. St. Martin's Press, NY, NY pp 1-134 (1980).

140. Parizkova J: Body composition and body build of champion athletes in relation to fitness and performance. In Body Fat and Physical Fitness, Editors Parizkova J, Martinus BU, The Hague, The Netherlands, pp 197-208 (1977).

141. Peterson ME: Canine and feline endocrinology. Proc Amer Anim Hosp Assoc 50th Ann Meeting, pp 151-158 (1983).

142. Pettitt DJ, Baird HR, Alleck KA, et al: Excessive obesity in offspring of Pima Indian women with diabetes during pregnancy. New Engl J Med 308:242-245 (1983).

143. Pilkington TR, Rosenoer VM, Gainsborough H: Diet and weight reduction in the obese Lancet I:856 (1960).

144. Pi-Sunyer FX, Woo R: Effect of exercise on food intake in human subjects. Amer J Clin Nutr 42:983-990 (1985).

145. Presta E, Wang J, Harrison, et al: Measurement of total body electrical conductivity: a new method for estimation of body composition. Amer J Clin Nutr 37:735-739 (1983).

146. Presta E, Yang MU, Segal KR, Bjorntorp P: Energy depot replenishment in rats during refeeding after fasting: effect of exercise. Amer J Clin Nutr 40:1011-1016 (1984).

147. Ravussin E, Burnand B, Schuta Y, Jequier E: Twenty-four hour energy expenditure and resting metabolic rate in obese, moderately obese and control subjects. Amer J Clin Nutr 35:566-573 (1982).

148. Reisin E, Abel R, Modan M, et al: Effect of weight loss without salt restriction on the reduction of blood pressure in overweight hypertensive patients. New Engl J Med 298:1-6 (1978).

149. Richard D, Labrie A, Lupien D, et al: Role of exercise-training in the prevention of hyperinsulinemia caused by high energy diet. J Nutr 112:1756-1762 (1982).

150. Rijnberk A: Clinical endocrinology. Proc Delaware Valley Forum, April 16 (1975).

151. Rimm IJ, Rimm AA: Association between juvenile onset obesity and severe adult obesity in 73,332 women. Amer J Public Health 6:479-481 (1976).

152. Roberts HJ: Thrombophlebitis complicating liquid protein diets. New Engl J Med 298:165 (1978).

153. Rolland-Cachera MF, Deheeger M, Bellisle F, et al: Adiposity rebound in children: a simple indicator for predicting obesity. Amer J Clin Nutr 39:129-135 (1984).

154. Rosen JC, Gross J, Loew D, Sims EAH: Mood and appetite during minimal-carbohydrate and carbohydrate-supplemented hypocaloric diets. Amer J Clin Nutr 42:371-379 (1985).

155. Rosenbaum MS, Faris AW, Shriner JF, Suskind RM: Weight reduction and physical fitness in overweight. Abstr Amer J Clin Nutr 84:646 (1981).

156. Rule DE, Beitz DC: Evidence of fat cell hyperplasia in obese cattle. Fed Proc 43, Abstr 2949 (1984).

157. Schemmel RA, Stone M, Warren MJ, Stoddart KA: Nitrogen and protein losses in rats during weight reduction with a high protein, very low energy diet or fasting. J Nutr 113:727-734 (1983).

158. Schneeman BO, Gallaher D: Changes in small intestinal digestive enzyme activity and bile acids with dietary cellulose in rats. J Nutr 110:584-590 (1980).

159. Schneider MU, Domschke S, Domschke W: Effect of dietary fiber on exocrine pancreatic enzyme activity in vitro and in vivo. Digestion 25:Abstr 67 (1982).

160. Schutz Y, Bessard T, Jequier E: Diet-induced thermogenesis measured over a whole day in obese and nonobese women. Amer J Clin Nutr 40:542-552 (1984).

161. Schutz Y, Golay A, Felber JP, Jequier D: Decreased glucose-induced thermogenesis after weight loss in obese subjects: predisposing factor for relapse of obesity. Amer J Clin Nutr 39:380-387 (1984).

162. Sclefani A: Animal models for the intestinal bypass approach to morbid obesity. Amer J Clin Nutr 33:360-370 (1980).

163. Sheffy BE: Annual report James A Baker Institute for Animal Health, Cornell Univ, Ithaca, NY 33:13 (1983).

164. Smith GP, Gibbs J: Gut peptides and postprandial satiety. Fed Proc 43:2889-2892 (1984).

165. Smith RR, Rumsey GL, Scott ML: Heat increment associated with dietary protein, fat, carbohydrate and complete diets in salmonids: comparative energetic efficiency. J Nutr 108:1025-1032 (1978).

166. Sours HE, Frattali VP, Brand CD, et al: Sudden death associated with very low calorie weight reduction regimens Amer J Clin Nutr 34:453-461 (1981).

167. Stasse-Wolthuis M, Albers HFF, Van Jeveren JGC, et al: Influence of dietary fiber from vegetables and fruits, bran or citrus pectin on serum lipid, fecal lipids, and colonic function. Amer J Clin Nutr 33:1745-1756 (1980).

168. Stock-Damge C, Bouchet P, Dentinger A, et al: Effect of dietary fiber supplementation on the secretory function of the exocrine pancreas in the dog. Amer J Clin Nutr 38:843-848 (1983).

169. Sullivan AC, Comai K: Pharmacological treatment of obesity. Int J Obes 2:167-189 (1978).

170. Sullivan AC, Gruen RK: Mechanisms of appetite modulation by drugs. Feder Proc 44:139-144 (1985).

171. Swaminathan R, King RFGJ, Holmfield J, et al: Thermic effect of feeding carbohydrate, fat, protein and mixed meal in lean and obese subjects. Amer J Clin Nutr 42:177-181 (1985).

172. Tarttelin MF, Gorski RA: Variations in food and water intake in normal and acyclic female rats. Physiol Behav 8:847-852 (1971).

173. Thompson JK, Jarvie GJ, Lahey BB, Cureton KJ: Exercise and obesity: etilogy, physiology and intervention. Psychol Bull 91:55-79 (1982).

174. Thurlby PL, Trayhurn P: The role of thermoregulatory thermogenesis in the development of obesity in genetically obese (ob/ob) mice pair-fed with lean siblings. Brit J Nutr 42:377-385 (1979).

175. Tuck ML, Sowers J, Dornfeld L, et al: The effect of weight reduction on blood pressure, plasma renin activity, and plasma aldosterone levels in obese patients. New Engl J Med 304:930-933 (1981).

176. Tulp OL, Frink R, Danforth E Jr: Effect of cafeteria feeding on brown adipose tissue cellularity, thermogenesis and body composition in rats. J Nutr 112:2250-2260 (1982).

177. Van Itallie TB, Yang MU: Diet and weight loss. New Engl J Med 297:1158-1161 (1977).

178. Van Itallie TB: "Morbid" obesity: a hazardous disorder that resists conservative treatment. Amer J Clin Nutr 33:358-363 (1980).

179. Van Itallie TB, Kissileff HR: The physiologic control of energy intake an econometric perspective. Amer J Clin Nutr 38:978-988 (1983).

180. Van Itallie TB, Yang MU: Cardiac dysfunction in obese dieters: a potentially lethal complication of rapid, massive weight loss. Amer J Clin Nutr 39:695-702 (1984).

181. Vaughan RW, Conahan RJ: Cardiopulmonary consequences of morbid obesity. Life Sciences 26:2119-2127 (1980).

182. Walks D, Lavau M, Presta E, Bjorntorp P: Refeeding after fasting in the rat: effects of dietary-induced obesity on energy balance regulation. Amer J Clin Nutr 37:387-395 (1983).

183. Ward A: The fat-dog problem: how to solve it. VM/SAC 79:781-786 (1984).

184. Weinsier RL, Wadden TA, Ritenbaugh C, et al: Recommended therapeutic guidelines for professionsl weight control programs. Amer J Clin Nutr 40:865-872 (1984).

185. Welle S: Metabolic responses to a meal during rest and low-intensity exercise. Amer J Clin Nutr 40:990-994 (1984).

186. Williams GD, Newberne PM: Decreased resistance to Salmonella infection in obese dogs. Fed Proc 30:572 (1971).

187. Williams T, Berelowitz M, Joffe SN, et al: Impaired growth hormone responses to growth hormone-releasing factor in obesity; a pituitary defect reversed with weight loss. N Engl J Med 311:1403-1407 (1984).

188. Wilmore JH: Body composistion in sport and exercise: Directions for future research. Med Sci Sports Exerc 15:21-31 (1983).

189. Wing RR, Jeffery RW: Outpatient treatments of obesity: A comparison of methodology and clinical results. Int J Obesity 3:261-279 (1979).

190. Wong DT, Yen TT: Suppression of appetite and reduction of body weight in normal and obese mice by fluoxetine, a selective inhibitor of serotonin uptake. Fed Proc 44:1162 (1985).

191. Woods SC, Porte D Jr, Bobbioni E, et al: Insulin: its relationship to the central nervous system and to the control of food intake and body weight. Amer J Clin Nutr 42:1063-1071 (1985).

192. Wov R, Garrow JS, Pi-Sunyer FX: Effect of exercise on spontaneous caloric intake in obesity; and voluntary food intake during prolonged exercise in obese women. Amer J Clin Nutr 36:470-484 (1982).

193. Wurtman JJ, Moses PL, Wurtman RJ: Prior carbohydrate consumption affects the amount of carbohydrate rats choose to eat. J Nutr 113:70-78 (1983).

194. Yang M-U, Van Itallie TB: Composistion of weight loss during short-term weight reduction. J Clin Invest 58:722-730 (1976).

195. Yim GKW, Lowy MT: Opioids, feeding and anorexias. Fed Proc 43:2893-2897 (1984).

196. Yen JT, Pond WG: Plasma thyroid hormones, growth and carcass measurements of genetically obese and lean pigs as influenced by thyroprotein supplementation. J Anim Sci 61:566-572 (1985).

197. Young CM, Scanlan SS, Im HS: Effect on body composition and other parameters in obese young men of carbohydrate level of reduction diet. Amer J Clin Nutr 24:290 (1971).

198. Young JB, Saville E, Rothwell NJ, et al: Effect of diet and cold exposure on norepinephrine turnover in brown adipose tissue of the rat. J Clin Invest 69:1061-1071 (1982).

199. Young JB, Landsberg L: Diet-induced changes in sympathetic nervous system activity: possible implications for obesity and hypertension. J Chronic Dis 35:879-885 (1982).

CHAPTER 7

Gastrointestinal, Pancreatic and Hepatic Diseases

CONTENTS

SUMMARY OF MANAGEMENT RECOMMENDATIONS

REGURGITATION

1. **Reflux esophagitis:**
   a. Administer cimetidine, metoclopramide, and an antibiotic for at least 5-7 days (Table 1).
   b. Withhold food for 3-4 days then offer small amounts of a food slurry 3-6 times daily for several days. If this is well tolerated, feed a canned food for several more days; thereafter, gradually return to the normal diet.

2. **Cricopharyngeal achalasia, vascular ring anomalies, strictures, tumors, and *Spirocerca lupi* granulomas** are usually amenable to surgery or bougienage and treatment of esophagitis.

3. **Foreign bodies**—remove and treat for esophagitis.

4. **Megaesophagus**
   a. Feed the animal on stairs or from an elevated platform.

b. Different forms of food (dry, soft-moist, or gruel) and feeding regimens should be tried to find those best tolerated.

c. Observe closely for aspiration pneumonia and give an antibiotic at first sign.

5. **Achalasia**

a. Esophagomyotomy may be helpful.

b. Manage the same as megaesophagus from other causes.

VOMITING

1. If dehydration is present, give parenterally an isotonic saline solution with 10-30 mEq/L of potassium choloride added. Enough should be given to correct the fluid deficit. Clinical signs of mild, moderate or severe dehydration indicate a fluid deficit of about 60, 80 or 100 ml/kg, respectively. If given intravenously one-half the fluid deficit may be given during the first 1-3 hours, and the remainder over the following 8-24 hours.

2. Withhold all food for 24-48 hours and water for 24 hours.

3. If the cause of vomiting is detected from the history and initial examination, specific therapy as indicated should be instituted.

4. If vomiting has stopped, over the next 3-5 days gradually return the patient to full feed and water. Feed small amounts frequently (3-6 times daily) of a highly-digestible low-fiber diet (Prescription Diets Canine i/d for dogs and Feline c/d for cats, Hill's, or Recipes 1 or 8, Appendix Table 3).

5. If vomiting persists, do a complete evaluation to determine the cause (Figure 3, page 7-14) and appropriate therapy, and give metoclopramide (Table 1).

6. For vomiting caused by stimulation of the chemorecptor trigger zone (such as that due to drugs, uremia, bacterial toxins and other metabolic disorders) phenothiazine tranquilizers, pimozide, and, in dogs only, trimethobenzamide (Table 1) may help.

7. For motion sickness or vestibulitis, give antihistamines (Table 1).

8. For hematemesis, ulcers, gastritis, uremia, bloat or acute pancreatitis give cimetidine (Table 1). Staggered administration of sucralfate (Table 1) and cimetidine may be helpful for ulcer therapy.

9. **Acute Pancreatitis**

a. Give rapidly large volumes of Ringer's lactate intravenously to treat hypotension and shock.

b. Give antibiotics daily.

c. Give meperidine at 5-10 mg/kg 2-3 times daily to relieve pain.

d. Give nothing orally for 2-5 days, only water for the next 3 days, then over the next 3-5 days gradually return to full feed. Feed small amounts frequently (3-5 times daily) of a highly-digestible, moderate fat-restricted diet (Prescription Diet i/d, Hill's). This diet and feeding regimen should be continued thereafter to prevent recurrence and eventual development of either, or both, exocrine or endocrine insufficiency.

10. **Eosinophilic Gastroenteritis**

a. Feed a hypoallergenic diet (Prescription Diet d/d, Hill's or Recipe 6, Appendix Table 3).

b. Give 20 mg/cat of methylprednisolone acetate (Depo-Medrol, Upjohn) subcutaneously 2-3 times yearly.

c. Give the dog prednisolone (Table 1).

GASTRIC DILATATION WITH VOLVULUS

1. Decompress the stomach by passing a tube, if possible; if not by taping the stomach through the abdominal wall with a needle.

2. If poor tissue perfusion is present, give oxygen and administer intravenously large volumes (90 ml/kg in the first hour) of Ringer's lactate containing corticosteroids and antibiotics.

3. If cardiac arrythmia is present, give intravenously a 2-4 mg/kg bolus of lidocaine hydrochloride without epinephrine.

4. If the stomach or pylorus is displaced, correct surgically and do a circumcostal gastropexy to prevent recurrence.

5. Withhold food and water for the first 24 hours, then feed small amounts of water frequently.

6. When vomiting has not occurred for 24 hours, feed one-third of the daily requirement of a highly digestible diet (Prescription Diet i/d, Hill's, or Recipe 1, Appendix Table 3) divided into 3-6 small meals. Over the next several days gradually increase the amount fed back to normal.

DIARRHEA

1. If dehydration is present, give Ringer's lactate with 40-70 mEq/L of sodium bicarbonate added. It should be given in the same amount and at the same rate as described for vomiting (step 1).

TABLE 1

DRUGS AND NUTRIENTS USEFUL IN DIAGNOSIS OR MANAGEMENT OF GASTROINTESTINAL, PANCREATIC, AND HEPATIC DISEASES

Chemical Name	Product Name	Source	Dosage*	Mode of Action	Reasons for Administration	Contraindications	Complications
Ampicillin	Many	Many	5–10 mg/kg 3–4x/day parenterally	Antibiotic	Hemorrhagic diarrhea, fever, leukocytosis or degen. left shift of hemogram		May induce or prolong diarrhea
Amphotericin B	Fungizone	Squibb	0.5–1 mg/kg/day in fluids IV for 3–6 days	Fungicidal and fungistatic	Histoplasmosis blastomycosis		Anorexia, emesis, cardiac depression, renal damage, hypokalemia, particularly in cats
Aspirin	Many	Many	10 mg/kg for dogs 2x/day & cats every other day	Antiprostaglandin which decreases intestinal secretion	Bacterial toxin-induced diarrhea	Use for more than 1–2 days	Gastric ulcers and bleeding
Azathioprine	Imuran	Burroughs Wellcome	2 mg/kg/day	Immunosuppressive	Chronic active hepatitis		Diarrhea, leukopenia, thrombocytopenia
Balneol	Balneol	Rowell	3–4x daily	Perianal cleansing lotion & emollient	Perianal sores, colitis, proctitis		
Bethanechol	Urecholine	Merck, Sharpe & Dohme	2.5–10 mg/animal orally 4x/day & titrate to effect	Increase gastroesophageal sphincter pressure, improve gastric emptying	Reflux esophagitis	Hypotension, epilepsy, pregnancy, GI-obstruction or surgery	Colic, diarrhea, hypotension
Bisacodyl	Ex-Lax or Dulcolax	Boehringer Ingelheim	5–20 mg/dog, 2–5 mg/cat 1–2x/day orally	Stimulant laxative	Chronic intractable constipation		
Bismuth subsalicylate	Pepto-Bismol	Norwich-Eaton	1–2 ml/kg 4–6x/day	Antiprostaglandin which decreases int. sec.	Bacterial toxin-induced diarrhea	Use for more than 1–2 days	Gastric ulcers and bleeding
Chlordiazepoxide and clidinium	Librax	Roche	1/4 cap/5 kg to max of 1 cap 2–3x/day	Antianxiety and anticholinergic	Spastic or irritable colon	Glaucoma	Uncommon
Cimetidine	Tagamet	Smith Kline & French	5 mg/kg orally 2–4x/day or 10 mg/kg IV 2x/day before meal	Decreases gastric acid and increases gastroesophageal sphincter pressure	Reflux esophagitis, gastritis, pancreatic exocrine insufficiency, ulcers	None	None in dogs
Colchicine	Colchicine	Lilly, Danbury, Merck	0.3 mg/kg orally once daily	Fibrinolytic	Chronic active hepatitis and fibrosis		In people malaise, vomiting, diarrhea, abdominal pain, agranulocytosis, anemia, myopathy, alopecia[174]
Corticosteroid enemas	Cortenemas	Rowell	1 tube (60 ml & 100 mg hydrocortisone)/>20 kg, 1/2 tube/5–20 kg, 1/4 tube/<5 kg & cats, 3x/day	Anti-inflammatory	Tenesmus & dyschezia		Uncommon
Dimenhydrinate	Dramamine	Searle	dogs 4 mg/kg 30 min before travel & 3x/day	Antihistamine, decreases hyperstimulated labyrinth	Nausea due to motion sickness or vestibulitis	None known	Sedation
Dioctyl sodium sulfosuccinate	Many	Many	As needed	Enema or orally to soften stool	Constipation or impaction		
Diphenoxylate	Lomotile	Searle & Co.	0.1–0.2 mg/kg 3–4x/day for dogs	See opium	Diarrhea	See opium	See opium
D-penicillamine	Cuprimine	Merck, Sharp & Dohme	10 mg/kg orally 2x/day at least 30 min before or more than 2 hrs after a meal	Increases urinary copper excretion	Copper – storage disease	Within 3 weeks of surgery or trauma. Chronic liver disease	Vomiting. Copper deficiency after 1-2 years? Pyridoxine deficiency. Decreases wound healing, cytopenia, anorexia, dysgeusia, proteinuria, skin rash & death
Erythromycin	Many	Many	10 mg/kg 3x/day parenterally	Antibiotic	ntestinal bacterial overgrowth, hepatic encephalopathy		May induce or prolong diarrhea

Chemical Name	Product Name	Source	Dosage*	Mode of Action	Reasons for Administration	Contraindications	Complications
Fenbendazole	Panacur	American Hoechst	25 mg/kg (1 tsp/20 kg) 2x/day for 3 days (10 days for larval migrans)	Anthelmintic & Toxocara canis visceral larval migrans	Gastroenteritis or trichuriasis		Vomiting
Flunixin meglumine	Banamine	Schering	1 mg/kg once/day	Antiprostaglandin, decreases int. sec.	Bacterial toxin-induced diarrhea	Use for more than 1–2 days	Gastric ulcers and bleeding
Furazolidone	Furoxone	Norden	4 mg/kg 2x/day for 5 days	Antiprotozoal	Giardiasis		
Furosemide	Lasix	Hoechst-Roussel	0.25–0.5 mg/kg twice daily, if no response in 7 days, double dose	Diuretic	Edema, ascites or pleural effusions with hepatic disease	Dehydration, hypotension, encephalopathy	Increased potassium and calcium excretion
Glycerine	Many	Many	As needed	Enema to soften stool	Constipation or impaction		
Hypertonic phosphate enemas	Fleet PVL	CB Fleet Prof. Vet Lab	As needed	Draws fluid into gut & softens stools	Constipation	Cats and toy breed dogs	Fatal alterations in plasma electrolyte concentrations
Ipropan	Ipropan	Roche	126 mg/L of drinking water	Antiprotozoal	Giardiasis		
Kaolin, pectin, antacids, activated charcoal	Many	Many	Generally higher than recommended by mfg.	Intestinal protectants, little proof of benefit	Absorb bacteria, toxins & bile acids, protect mucosa		Interfere with absorption of many drugs
Ketoconazole	Nizoral	Janssen	dogs 3–10 mg/kg/day, cats 5–20 on alternate days orally	Antifungal	Histoplasmosis		Vomiting, colic
Lactulose	Cephulac Chronulac Duphalac	Merrell Dow Merrell Dow Philips Roxane	5–15 ml/dog 3x/day and adjusted to produce 2–3 soft stools daily	Acidifies luminal contents	Hepatic encephalopathy		Diarrhea
Lidocaine HCl	Xylocaine without epinephrine	Astra	2–4 mg bolus IV	Increase electrical stimulation threshold	Control arrythmias in dogs with bloat & volvulus	Intraventricular block	Uncommon
Loperamide	Imodium	Janssen Pharmaceutical	0.1–0.3 mg/kg 2x/day	See opium	Diarrhea	See opium	See opium
Medium Chain Triglycerides	MCT oil and Portagen Powder	Mead Johnson	Gradually increase up to 2 ml oil or 4 g powder/kg/day	If fully utilized, provides 8.3 kcal/ml & 4 kcal/g powder	To increase wt gain or maintain condition	Cats, ketosis, acidosis, severe hepatocellular damage	Hepatic lipidosis, abdominal cramps, diarrhea, poor palatability
Metoclopramide	Reglan	AH Robins	0.2–0.4 mg/kg orally or SC into fat pads 2–4x/day	Increase gastroesophageal sphincter pressure, improve gastric emptying	Reflux esophagitis, gastritis, vomiting, gastric paresis, bloat, constipation, pyloric stenosis	Gastric outlet obstructions,[37] epilepsy, & with phenothiazines[202]	Restlessness and hyperactivity or 4–5 hrs of depression
Metronidazole	Flagyl	Searle	25 mg/kg twice daily / 7.5 mg/kg 3x/day / 25 mg/kg for dogs or 10 for cats 2x/day for 5 days	Antibiotic / Antibiotic / Antiprotozoal & Colitis	Suppurative cholangiohepatitis in cats. Control bacterial overgrowth with lymphocytic-plasmocytic enteritis. Giardiasis or trichomoniasis	Pregnancy	
Naloxone	Narcan	Endo Pharm.	To effect parenterally, start with 0.01 mg/kg, may repeat every few min	Narcotic antagonist	Reverse effects of opiates		Vomiting
Neomycin	Many	Many	20 mg/kg 3x/day orally	Antibiotic	Intestinal bacterial overgrowth, hepatic encephalopathy		May induce or prolong diarrhea
Opium tincture	Paregoric	Roxane Labs	0.01–0.02 mg/kg 2x/day	Paralyzes intestinal motility, increases absorption and decreases secretion	Diarrhea	Use for greater than a few days, toxigenic bacterial intestinal infections or pseudomembranous colitis	CNS depression, constipation
Opium tincture & bismuth subsalicylate	Corrective mixture	Beecham	1–2 ml/kg orally 4–6x/day	Opium + antiprostaglandin	Diarrhea	See opium	See opium
Oxytetracycline	Many	Many	10–20 mg/kg 2x/day orally	Antibiotic	Intestinal bacterial overgrowth, hemobartonellosis		May induce or prolong diarrhea

TABLE 1—Continued

DRUGS AND NUTRIENTS USEFUL IN DIAGNOSIS OR MANAGEMENT OF GASTROINTESTINAL, PANCREATIC, AND HEPATIC DISEASES

Chemical Name	Product Name	Source	Dosage*	Mode of Action	Reasons for Administration	Contraindications	Complications
Pancreatic enzymes	Viokase-V	AH Robins	Begin with 1 tsp/10 kg/meal then decrease to minimum needed for favorable response	Digests dietary fat, carbohydrate, and protein	Pancreatic exocrine insufficiency	None	Less effective than a highly digestible diet
Phenothiazines	Many	Many	According to mfg.	Tranquilizer, & blocks vomiting center CTZ	Vomiting due to uremia, toxins, drugs, metabolic disorders, and colitis	Hypotension	Sedation
Pimozide	Orap	McNeil Pharm.	0.025-0.1 mg/kg	See phenothiazine	Same as phenothiazines with longer duration of action		
Prednisolone	Prednisolone	Many	1-4 mg/kg 2x/day until 1-2 weeks after response, then taper off over next 2-3 weeks or alternate day therapy	Anti-inflammatory, immunosuppressive, antifibrotic	Lymphocytic-plasmacytic enteritis & colitis, eosinophilic colitis & gastroenteritis, chronic active hepatitis or fibrosis[44]	Supportive cholangio-hepatitis	Gastritis, ulcers, hepatopathy
Quinacrine	Atabrine	Winthrop	6 mg/kg 2x/day for 5 days	Antiprotozoal	Giardiasis	Pregnancy	Anorexia, fever & lethargy are common, & vomiting
Ranitidine	Zantac	Glaxol	0.5 mg/kg orally 2x/day	Same as cimetidine but more potent	Same as cimetidine	Don't give other drugs for at least 2 hours after it	Decreases absorption of other drugs
Spironolactone	Aldactone	Searle	1-2 mg/kg twice daily, if no response in 4 days, double dose	Potassium sparing diuretic	Edema, ascites, or pleural effusions with hepatic disease	Dehydration, hypotension, encephalopathy	Hyperkalemia, gynecomastia
Sucralfate	Carafate	Marion Labs	1 tab/25 kg orally 3x/day	Protective barrier, inactivates pepsin and bile	Ulcers, gastritis, stomatitis		Uncommon
Sulfasalazine	Azulfidine	Pharmacia Labs	For 3-4 weeks orally: dogs 25 mg/kg 3x/day,[34] cats 250 mg 3x first day then once daily[129]	Prostaglandin inhibitor and antibiotic	Colitis-drug of choice	None known	Keratoconjunctivitis, allergic response, salicylate toxity, stomatitis
Thiabendazole	Thiabendazole	Merck, Sharp & Dohme	25 mg/kg 2x/day for 10 days orally	Toxocara canis visceral larval migrans	Eosinophilic gastroenteritis		
Tinidazole	Fasigyn	Pfizer	44 mg/kg 1x/day for 3 days	Antiprotozoal	Giarciasis and trichomoniasis		
Tylosin	Tylan plus Vitamins	Elanco	10 mg/kg 2-3x/day (440 mg/tsp) for at least 1-2 weeks	Antibiotic	One of most effective for control of bacterial over-growth & inflam bowel disease. Colitis		
Trimethobenzamide	Tigan	Beecham	For dogs only at mfg. recommendation	Same as phenothiazines	Same as phenothiazines	Cats	Sedation
Vitamin K-1	Aqua MEPHYTON	Merck, Sharp & Dohme	1-3 mg/kg parenterally or 5 mg/kg orally	Correct deficiency	Prolonged prothrombin time		Parenteral administration may cause Heinz body anemia
Xylazine	Rompun	Haver Lockhart	1-2 mg/kg SC	Stimulates vomiting center	Induce vomiting of hairballs	With tranquilizers	Sedation
Zinc	Many	Many	2-3 mg elemental zinc/kg/day	Decreases copper absorption	Copper – storage disease		In people malaise, vomiting, diarrhea, abdominal pain, agranulocytosis, anemia, myopathy, alopecia[174]

*Unless specified, dosage is for both dogs and cats; SC means subcutaneous, IM intramuscular, and IV intravenous.

2. Withhold all food, but not water, for 1-4 days (longer the more severe the intestinal disturbance).

3. If the cause of diarrhea is detected from history and initial examination, specific therapy as indicated should be instituted.

4. Over the next 3-5 days gradually return the patient to full feed. Feed small amounts frequently (3-6 times daily).

5. Except for animals with lymphangiectasia or colonic dysfunctions, feed a highly-digestible, low-fiber diet (Prescription Diets Canine i/d for dogs and Feline c/d for cats, Hill's, or Recipes 1 or 8, Appendix Table 3).

6. For dogs or cats with **lymphangiectasia** or **colonic dysfunctions** (see Table 3, page 7-27) feed a high-fiber, severely-restricted fat diet (Prescription Diets r/d, or instead for dogs w/d, Hill's, or Recipes 4 or 10, Appendix Table 3).

7. If diarrhea has been a chronic problem, or intestinal parasites or giardiasis are suspected, administer an anthelmenic and metronidazole (Table 1).

8. If **colitis** is present, feed as described in steps 4 and 6 and give sulfasalazine (Table 1). If a satisfactory response does not occur within 1-2 weeks, change to one of the highly-digestible diets given in step 5.

   a. If whipworms are suspected, or are common in that area, give fenbendazole or fenbantel (Table 1).

   b. Giving tylosin (Table 1) may be beneficial, particularly if bacterial overgrowth is present.

   c. If eosinophilic colitis is present, give corticosteroids (Table 1).

   d. If tenesmus and dyschezia due to severe colitis are present, give corticosteroid retention enemas (Table 1).

9. If diarrhea persists, do a complete evaluation to determine the cause (Figure 4, page 7-29) and appropriate therapy.

STEATORRHEA

1. Determine cause (Figure 5, page 7-39) and manage accordingly.

2. If due to **pancreatic exocrine insufficiency,** see page 7-45).

CONSTIPATION OR TENESMUS

1. Give 2-3 enemas daily until constipation is relieved (Table 1).

2. To assist in preventing recurrence

   a. Feed as described in steps 4 and 6 for diarrhea.

   b. Exercise the animal frequently to encourage defecation.

   c. Do not feed bones.

FLATULENCE

1. Feed the animal free-choice, or several times daily, in a quiet location by itself.

2. Feed a highly-digestible, low-fiber, moderately low-protein, soy-free, wheat-free diet (Prescription Diets Canine i/d or Canine k/d for dogs and Feline c/d for cats, Hill's, or Recipes 1, 2 or 8, Appendix Table 3).

3. Do not feed any vegetables, milk, table scraps or vitamin-mineral supplements.

HEPATIC DISEASE

1. If **dehydration** and neither ascites nor edema is present, give isotonic saline solution. It should be given in the same amount and at the same rate as described for vomiting (step 1).

2. If **ascites** or **edema** is present, correct dehydration using half-strength saline solution with 2.5% glucose (a mixture of equal parts isotonic saline and isotonic glucose solutions). If encephalopathy is not present, give spironolactone (Table 1). If after 3-4 days ascites or edema is still present, also give furosemide. If necessary, give additional quantities of fluid to prevent hypovolemia. Ascitic fluid should not be removed unless necessary to relieve dyspnea and patient discomfort.

3. Provide cage rest and frequently feed small amounts of a highly-digestible diet that is moderately restricted in salt, fat and high-quality protein, and high in B-vitamins (Prescription Diets k/d, Hill's, or Recipes 2 or 9, Appendix Table 3). Ensure sufficient food intake to meet caloric needs. If necessary, force-feed or tube-feed (see Chapter 5).

4. If **encephalopathy** is present:

   a. If feeding the previously recommended diets doesn't alleviate signs, change the dog to a lower-protein diet (Prescription Diet u/d, Hill's, or Recipe 2, Appendix Table 3,

substituting 1/4 cup of non-creamed cottage cheese for the egg), and give lactulose (Table 1).

   b. If signs are still not alleviated, give poorly absorbed antibiotics orally, and enemas containing 1% neomycin and 10% vinegar.

   c. Control gastrointestinal bleeding if present (pages 7-21 & 58).

   d. Don't give diuretics or lipotrophic agents (e.g. methionine and choline).

   e. If a portasystemic shunt is present, it should be corrected surgically, if possible, and the dietary management described followed.

5. If blood coagulation is impaired, give vitamin K-1 (Table 1).

6. If **fever, cholangitis** or **cirrhosis** is present, give systemic antibiotics (e.g. ampicillin, cephalosporins, streptomycin, gentamicin or kanamycin).

7. If **chronic active hepatitis** or **fibrosis** is present, give prednisolone (Table 1).

INTRODUCTION

Problems that interfere with use of nutrients are common in veterinary practice. Interference with nutrient utilization can arise from oral, esophageal, gastric, intestinal, pancreatic, or hepatic dysfunctions. These dysfunctions are often empirically pursued or symptomatically treated with little or no improvement in the initial problem or complaint. Rational therapeutic plans are directly related to, and should follow, good diagnostic plans. This chapter is a problem-oriented approach to the diagnosis and management of disorders of organs involved with nutrient assimilation. The drugs and nutrients useful in the diagnosis and management of gastrointestinal, pancreatic and hepatic diseases are given in Table 1.

Most gastrointestinal, pancreatic, and hepatic disorders result from some alteration in the physiologic function of these organs. Dietary management of these disorders should be directed at compensating for these altered physiologic functions. For example, dietary management of diarrhea is the same, whether its etiology is infectious, caustic, toxic, or mechanical, and whether its origin is central or peripheral.

Major problems related to the gastrointestinal tract that can be identified easily include regurgitation, vomiting, bloat, abnormal stools, and flatulence. Abnormal stools include feces that have an altered consistency, color, or shape. Diarrhea is the main problem in this category. Constipation and steatorrhea are also common problems.

Major problems related to the pancreas include acute pancreatitis and exocrine and endocrine insufficiencies. Pancreatic exocrine insufficiency impairs food digestion, resulting in malassimilation of nutrients. Malassimilation may also be caused by hepatic, intestinal, or lymphatic dysfunctions. Hepatic dysfunctions may also result in anorexia, weight loss, and either ascites, or encephalopathy, or both.

REGURGITATION

Regurgitation is the reflux of undigested food from the mouth or esophagus before it has reached the stomach. Food that has been chewed is expelled from the mouth, usually during or immediately after deglutition, although occasionally it may not occur for several hours after prehension. The occurrence of regurgitation indicates that the problem is in the posterior pharynx or esophagus. In certain cases, the subjective data or history may not allow the clinician to determine whether the patient is actually regurgitating or is vomiting. In this situation, feeding, followed by observation, can provide information for differentiation of these two problems. The major factors useful in differentiating between regurgitation and vomiting are given in Table 2.

Animals with chronic regurgitation may exhibit other clinical signs. These include dehydration (degree variable depending on the patient's ability to retain water), emaciation, malnutrition, and aspiration pneumonia, which is the usual cause of death of affected animals.

DIAGNOSIS OF CAUSES OF REGURGITATION

The diagnostic procedures are similar for each of the conditions that result in regurgitation. Listed in order of their ease and availability, these procedures are:

1. Direct visual examination of the pharynx

2. Digital palpation of the throat and neck and observe for pain or enlargement of the esophagus

3. Survey radiographs of the neck and chest

4. Barium swallow for dogs. Esophotrast (Barnes-Hind) is better for cats because it passes through the esophagus more slowly.[194] When

TABLE 2

DIFFERENTIATION BETWEEN REGURGITATION AND VOMITION

Clinical Signs*	Regurgitation from		Vomition from Stomach
	Pharynx	Esophagus	
Time of food ejection following eating	Immediate	Delayed a few seconds	Delayed a few minutes to hrs.
Character of food ejected	Undigested Neutral pH	Undigested Neutral pH, may be covered with mucous and tubular shaped	Partially digested, ± bile stain, pH less than 5
Number of swallowing attempts	Multiple	Multiple	Single
Bolus in cervical esophagus	Absent	Present, may be prolonged	Absent
Ability to drink	Poor	Normal to poor	Normal
Dysphagia	Present	Present	Absent
Associated signs	± Dyspnea, cough, abdominal pressure absent	± Dyspnea, cough, abdominal pressure absent	Hypersalivation, repeated swallowing, abdominal pressure present
Aggravating or alleviating factors	Food consistency	Exercise, food consistency	None

*Clinical signs by themselves are not conclusive but are helpful, particularly when several are present. Occasionally food may be retained in the pharynx or esophagus and regurgitation may not occur for hours. Food vomited quickly after eating will have undergone minimal digestion and lowering of the pH. In addition it may be difficult to distinguish between partially digested food and macerated food. Some animals that regurgitate, such as puppies with congenital megaesophagus, do not have dysphagia and therefore do not exhibit multiple swallowing attempts or difficulty in drinking.

barium is used, a pastelike suspension is best for evaluating the esophagus; whereas, some radiologists prefer a dilute solution for evaluating the gastrointestinal tract.[228] If esophageal perforation is suspected, use a water-soluble organic iodide contrast preparation (e.g. Gastrografin, E. R. Squibb & Sons) instead of barium sulfate.[228]

5. Esophagoscopy

6. Measurements of pharyngoesophageal and gastroesophageal pressures. In the normal, untreated dog, the pharyngoesophageal pressure measured during continuous perfusion at a rate of 0.6 ml/min, was 18 mmHg.[178] Using the same technique, pressure in the gastroesophageal sphincter was found to be 47.9 ± 1.2 mmHg in one study[130] and in another, 38.5 ± 1.3 (mean ± SE) after fasting and 55.5 ± 2.0 after eating.[199] Giving tranquilizers, (e.g. acepromazine or xylazine), narcotics (e.g., meperidine) or atropine, greatly reduces sphincter pressure.[130,199]

The results of these procedures should provide the information needed for diagnosing the cause of regurgitation (also see Figure 1).

The following are considerations for the various disorders that result in regurgitation and should be ruled out systematically as data and judgement permit.

Regurgitation—Acute

Rule out:

1. Esophageal or pharyngeal **foreign body**

   These are a common cause of regurgitation in dogs, particularly young dogs. One in every 200 canine patients has been reported to have a foreign body in the digestive tract.[64] In contrast, foreign bodies are uncommon in cats, primarily because of their fastidious eating habits. Clinical signs include frequent gulping, and often drooling, and regurgitation which occur shortly after eating. Often, liquids can be swallowed. The animal may stop attempting to eat, appear to have a stiff neck, and object to being picked up. Cervical esophageal foreign bodies can usually be palpated. Radiographs or esophagoscopy are necessary to confirm the presence of those further down the esophagus. Bone is the most common esophageal foreign body in dogs, and is located:

   a. At the thoracic inlet

   b. Heart base or

   c. Just proximal to the gastroesophageal sphincter.

FIGURE 1

DETERMINING CAUSE FOR WEIGHT LOSS, POOR GROWTH, OR REGURGITATION

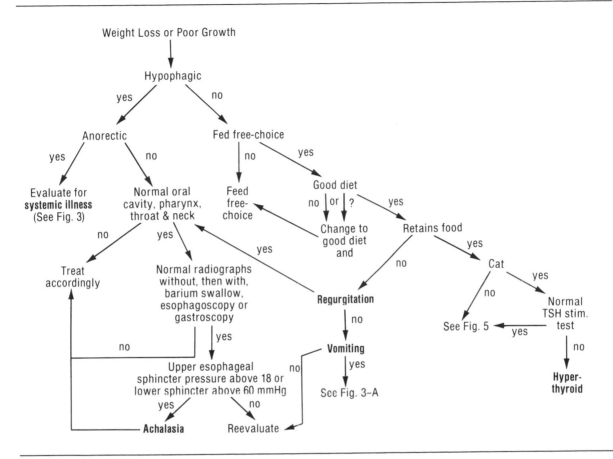

2. **Esophagitis** or **pharyngitis**

   May cause dysphagia, salivation, or pain upon swallowing.

   Causes include:

   a. Trauma from a foreign body or efforts to extract it

   b. Toxicity

   c. Infectious, e.g. calicivirus in cats

3. **Gastroesophageal intussusception** (rare)

   This should be considered when regurgitating puppies become acutely and severely ill. The disease is quite different from hiatal hernia (see page 7-11). Gastroesophageal intussusception results in regurgitation and vomiting in 80% of affected dogs, dyspnea in 40%, hematemesis in 30%, and abdominal discomfort in 30%.[126] In 21 cases, 20 occurred in dogs less than 1 year old, 17 in dogs under 3 months of age, 14 in German Shepherds; 20 died or were euthanized.[126] All deaths occurred within 1-3 days after

signs first appeared. The presence of a dilated or abnormal esophagus, or incompetent gastroesophageal sphincter may be needed for intussusception to occur. Of the 21 cases, only 3 had a normal esophagus. Diagnosis is based on history, physical examination and radiographs. Successful treatment requires early diagnosis, immediate surgical correction, and circumcostal gastropexy to prevent recurrence.

Regurgitation—Chronic

1. **Immature** dogs or cats

   Rule out:

   a. **Congenital megaesophagus**

      Occurs in all breeds of dogs with highest incidence in Great Danes and Irish Setters, followed by German Shepherds, Labrador Retrievers, Miniature Schnauzers, and Wirehaired Fox Terriers.[127] In the last two breeds it is reported to be heritable.[22] It may involve one to all puppies in a litter. Its occurrence

in cats, primarily Siamese, also has been reported.[53,73] It appears to be due to impaired motor neuron function and not an increase in gastroesophageal sphincter pressure, i.e. achalasia. Clinical signs usually become apparent when young are started on solid food at weaning. However, clinical signs may not be observed until maturity. Regurgitation can occur immediately after eating to many hours later, and as frequently as 20 times per day to once every several days.[127] Water is often regurgitated shortly after drinking. Unless a secondary aspiration pneumonia occurs, as it does in most, affected animals usually maintain a good appetite and dogs often eat regurgitated food immediately after regurgitating. Occasionally respiratory signs may be present without evidence of regurgitation. Affected animals are usually smaller than is considered normal; they may be thin and have dull coats. Radiographs after a barium swallow reveal a dilated esophagus.

b. **Cricopharyngeal achalasia**
This term implies that the cricopharyngeal muscle fails to relax when food enters the pharynx, which increases pharyngoesophageal sphincter pressure and prevents food from entering the esophagus. Therefore, this form of achalasia should be amenable to cricopharyngeal myotomy. However, achalasia is used to indicate a swallowing dysfunction resulting in dysphagia that occurs as a result of a variety of neuromuscular disorders involving a number of nerves.[219] Dogs affected by these disorders usually present with dysphagia.[127] There may be frequent attempts to swallow, followed by regurgitation of a large bolus. Liquids are better tolerated.

c. **Vascular ring anomalies**
These are anomalies of the right aortic arch that cause esophageal stenosis near the base of the heart. Persistent regurgitation occurs and is usually present from the time of weaning. Occasionally respiratory signs due to aspiration pneumonia may develop. Radiographs reveal esophageal dilation proximal to the vascular malformation only.

d. **Esophageal diverticula**

e. **Esophageal strictures** (See 2. e.)

2. **Adult** dogs and cats.
Rule out:

a. **Acquired megaesophagus**
Clinical signs usually resemble those in pup-

pies with congenital megaesophagus. Weight loss usually occurs. Some animals present with respiratory signs from a secondary aspiration pneumonia without signs of regurgitation.[127] Megaesophagus associated with myasthenia gravis, systemic lupus erythematosus, polyneuropathy, or other neuromuscular diseases may occur.[127]

b. **Reflux esophagitis**
Esophagitis due to reflux of gastric contents causes a burning sensation beneath the sternu, called "heartburn" in people. It is caused by decreased gastroesophageal sphincter pressure. Although common in people, it is rare in dogs and cats. However, it may occur after the administration of such drugs, as atropine, acepromazine and xylazine. These drugs reduce gastroesophageal sphincter pressure (in one study to 23-39% of normal[198]). Anesthetic-induced relaxation of the gastroesophageal sphincter and positioning the animal with its head lower than its stomach may result in reflux esophagitis. To prevent this, the animal should not be put in this position during surgery.

c. **Hiatal hernia**
This occurs when a part of the stomach passes into the thorax through the esophageal hiatus of the diaphragm. Hiatal hernias result in chronic, recurring intermittent regurgitation, vomiting, dysphagia and frequently, reflux esophagitis. It occurs primarily in adults.[58] Diagnosis is usually made by radiography.

d. **Esophageal neoplasia** (rare)

e. **Esophageal strictures**
These frequently are a sequel to severe esophagitis or esophageal damage from foreign bodies or reflux esophagitis, but may also be caused by periesophageal masses (e.g. tumors, hilar lymphadenopathy, abscesses, etc.).

f. **Mediastinal lymphosarcoma**
This disease may cause compression of the esophagus. Radiographs will reveal a mediastinal mass, and an aspiration cytological study can confirm the diagnosis of lymphosarcoma. It is more common in cats.

g. *Spirocerca lupi* **granuloma**

h. **Systemic mycoses** (histophasmosis, blastomycosis) (see page 7-37)

i. **Polymyopathy** and **polyneuropathy** causing a myasthenia-like syndrome

j. **Esophageal diverticulum** (rare)

MANAGEMENT OF REGURGITATION

For **reflux esophagitis** administer cimetidine for at least 5-7 days (Table 1). Cimetidine decreases gastric acid secretion and increases gastroesophageal sphincter pressure.[83] Administration of metoclopramide or bethanechol (Table 1) to further increase gastroesophageal sphincter tone and improve gastric emptying has also been recommended.[58,106]

With **esophagitis** in either dogs or cats from any cause there is: 1) a decrease in gastroesophageal sphincter tone, 2) decreased ability of the sphincter to relax in response to swallowing and 3) severely disordered esophageal motor activity.[69,90] These defects result in reflux of gastric contents into the esophagus, exacerbating esophagitis and establishing a vicious cycle of further inflammation that may continue indefinitely.[239] Such a cycle would result in formation of an esophageal stricture or perforation of the esophagus. To break the cycle, the treatment for reflux esophagitis described above should be initiated. In addition, an antibiotic such as ampicillin should be given.[239] The damaged esophagus is susceptible to secondary bacterial infection. Unless the animal is in a poor nutritional state, food should be withheld for 3-4 days to minimize trauma to the esophagus. Afterwards, initiate food intake with small volumes of food slurries offered at frequent intervals (3-6 times daily). If the animal does well clinically, offer a canned food for several days; thereafter, gradually return to the normal diet.

Cricopharyngeal achalasia, vascular ring anomalies, strictures, tumors, _Spirocerca lupi_ granulomas and **foreign bodies** are usually amenable to surgery, bougienage or removal, and the treatment for esophagitis described above. Esophageal foreign bodies rarely pass and the risk of serious complications increases with time. First choice for removal is oral extraction, second is propulsion into the stomach with or without removal by gastrotomy, and third is esophagotomy. Bones left in the stomach will usually dissolve within a few weeks.[239] After removal of a foreign body by any of these means, esophagitis can persist or progress.[239] Damaged esophageal tissue heals slowly. An esophageal incision reaches its maximum tensile strength 6-8 days after surgery. Many complications can follow esophageal surgery; therefore, it is recommended only after all other approaches to alleviate the problem have failed. Recovery from any cause of regurgitation, and its correction relates directly to the dietary and medical management employed.[239]

After esophageal surgery, some veterinarians recommend inserting a gastrotomy or nasogastric tube in all dogs. Others feel tube feeding is unnecessary and may result in greater constriction at the surgical site, and that the dietary management described earlier (slurry feeding), is preferable. If a feeding tube is inserted, daily requirements of food and water should be supplied through this tube for one week after surgery. The daily amount of food and water can be blended into a thin gruel and given through the tube (see Chapter 5). One week after surgery, the gastrotomy or nasogastric tube should be removed and the patient started on canned food and water.

Megaesophagus management is controversial. True esophageal achalasia in people is best managed with cardiomyotomy. However, dogs with megaesophagus usually do not have achalasia,[127] therefore, surgical manipulation of the esophagus or cardia seldom benefits a canine patient with a dilated esophagus. In one study of 79 cases, it was concluded that dietary management was superior to surgical treatment.[87] Thus, dietary management is the therapy of choice for the majority of dogs or cats with megaesophagus (congenital or acquired). However if true achalasia is present, as indicated by an elevated gastroesophageal sphincter pressure (determined by manometry), or there is little or no improvement using dietary management, surgery may be effective. Surgical correction of achalasia using a modified Heller esophagomyotomy procedure has been recommended for dogs.[95] In most instances dietary management must be continued even after surgery.[127] Management is aimed at controlling regurgitation and secondary pneumonia in the hope that the animal can be maintained and/or that esophageal motility will improve with time.

Feeding dogs or cats on stairs or teaching them to eat from an elevated platform is beneficial in managing megaesophagus (Figure 2). This places the esophagus in a vertical position and lets gravity help the passage of food through the dilated esophagus. Maintaining the dog in this positon for 15-20 minutes after it has eaten also helps.[127] With this technique, dry expanded food can be fed successfully to most affected dogs or cats. Dry foods serve as a better bolus stimulator of esophageal motility than do liquids, and tend to reduce esophageal overloading.[85] Allow the animal 4-7 days to adjust to the diet.

If problems occur, feed only soft-moist or a ration-type canned food containing at least 4% fat. Gruel diets usually are not necessary, and the incidence of aspiration pneumonia may be

FIGURE 2

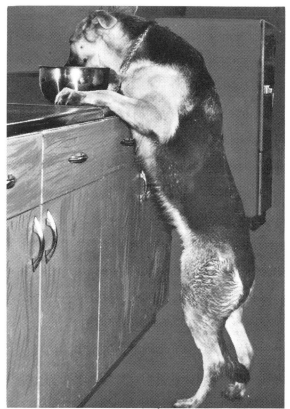

FIGURE 2: Feeding so gravity helps move food through the esophagus is beneficial in managing megaesophagus.

greater in patients fed gruel. However, if the entire esophagus is involved, liquid or gruel diets may be required. Each animal differs in its ability to tolerate a given form of food or feeding regimen. Different forms of food and feeding regimens should be tried to find those best tolerated. Regardless of the diet fed, the patient's daily caloric intake should be divided into three or more equal feedings. Broad-spectrum antibiotics should be given at the first sign of a respiratory problem, as aspiration pneumonia commonly occurs in regurgitating animals.

Although significant improvement or complete remission of clinical signs may occur, prognosis is poor. In some cases, the congenital form has been reported to improve as the animal matures,[55] and the acquired form to improve with treatment of the primary disease process.[22] However, in most cases of acquired megaesophagus the cause cannot be determined.[22] Few, if any, dogs with megaesophagus actually recover.[127] The clinical course varies tremendously. Clinical signs may repeatedly abate, then reappear. Affected dogs may do well

for a long time, then deteriorate rapidly and die.[127]

In two studies involving a total of 145 dogs, overall mortality directly related to megaesophagus was 63% and 75% within 18 months of diagnosis.[87,127] Most (94%-98%) had recurrent regurgitation. In another report, none of 18 young dogs with congenital megaesophagus showed clinical improvement, and only 3 were alive 3 months after diagnosis.[22] Of 32 adult dogs with acquired megaesophagus, 10 had an extra-esophageal disorder. Among these 10 dogs 3 of 4 responded to therapy for that disorder and became asymptomatic.[22] Only 4 of the 32 other dogs improved with time but they remained symptomatic. Pneumonia occurred in 60% of all 50 of these dogs and was the most common cause of death.[22]

VOMITING

Vomiting is the forceful ejection of the contents of the stomach and, in most cases, the contents of the proximal small intestine, through the mouth following a coordinated effort of the digestive, respiratory, musculoskeletal, and nervous systems. Many healthy dogs and cats vomit occasionally; however, frequent or persistent vomiting is abnormal. Regardless of the cause of vomiting, the emetic center, located in the caudal brain stem, mediates this complex reflex. Three broad categories that usually contain the cause of vomiting are: 1) functional disorders of the gastrointestinal tract (obstruction, stenosis, achlorhydria), 2) generalized or metabolic disease affecting the tract or emetic center, and 3) intrinsic disease of the gastrointestinal tract wall (gastric, small-bowel or large-bowel distention or irritation).

Vomiting may create life-threatening problems in the patient through disturbances in fluid, electrolyte, and acid-base balances. Dehydration develops because of inadequate water absorption and excessive losses of gastrointestinal secretions. Sporadic vomiting (several times per week) will not result in abnormalities in a patient if water and nutrients are absorbed between vomiting episodes. With persistent vomiting, dehydration may be severe and is usually accompanied by clinical signs of weakness, lethargy, and depression. Large quantities of sodium, potassium, and chloride are lost in vomitus. Hypokalemia and hyponatremia contribute to muscle weakness, depression, lethargy and anorexia commonly present in the chronically vomiting animal. Hypokalemia is the most frequent electrolyte disturbance observed. In some cases, the fluid and electrolyte alterations may be more severe than the disease that initiated the vomiting.

FIGURE 3-A

DETERMINING CAUSE OF VOMITING

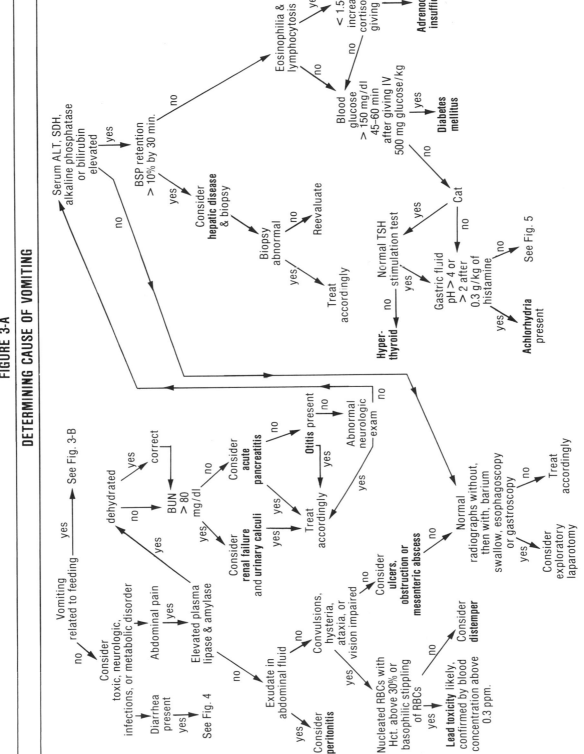

FIGURE 3-B

DETERMINING CAUSE OF VOMITING

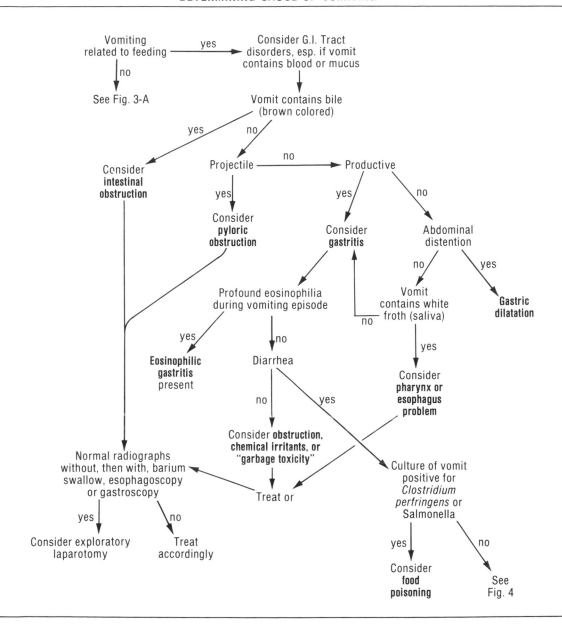

Loss of sufficient gastric contents, which contain a large amount of hydrogen ions, results in metabolic alkalosis. In contrast, loss of sufficient small intestinal contents, which contain a large amount of bicarbonate, results in metabolic acidosis. Historically, it has been assumed that alkalosis occurs with vomiting, and acidosis with diarrhea. However, measurement of the acid-base status in vomiting dogs has shown that, unless pyloric obstruction is present, or there is frequent profuse vomiting, gastric and duodenal losses are sufficiently balanced so that often no alteration in acid-base balance occurs.[235] If a sodium and potassium deficit occurs with vomiting, the kidneys retain these ions in exchange for hydrogen ions, resulting in an acid urine regardless of the animal's acid-base balance. If alkalosis is present, this is called "paradoxical aciduria."

DIAGNOSIS OF CAUSES OF VOMITING

Vomiting can be classified as short-term or chronic. Regardless of the duration, the clinician should obtain a history designed to reveal or localize the cause of the problem. The time of vomiting in relation to the time of eating is valuable information for localizing the cause of vomiting. See Table 2 (page 7-9) for factors useful in differentiating between regurgitation and vomiting, and Figure 3 for a systematic approach to determining the cause of vomiting. In general, as the interval between eating and vomiting lengthens, the lesion will be found more distally in the gastrointestinal tract. Normally, the stomach is completely emptied within 6-8 hours after a meal. Vomiting of food when the stomach should be empty suggests a gastric outlet obstruction or motility disorder. Sudden projectile vomiting may occur with pyloric obstruction. Acute onset of frequent attempts to vomit, with nonproductive retching and abdominal distention, is associated with gastric dilatation. Typically, acute gastritis will produce frequent vomiting episodes shortly after the animal has ingested food or water; whereas, with chronic gastritis, vomiting may occur as seldom as once every few days. If vomiting is unrelated to eating, a toxic, metabolic or neurologic disorder should be suspected. A history of the animal's habits and environment may be helpful in suggesting possible access to toxins. If food poisoning is suspected, vomitus should be cultured specifically for staphylococcus, *Clostridium perfringens* or salmonella.

The clinician should determine the physical characteristics of the vomitus. Intrinsic disease of the gastrointestinal wall may cause vomitus that contains blood or excessive mucus. Blood in vomitus may look like coffee grounds. Animals that vomit bile or bile-tinged fluid usually have an intestinal obstruction. The presence of bile may be differentiated from blood turned brown due to gastric acid, by diluting the vomitus with water. Under these conditions, bile appears greenish. Brown vomitus due to the presence of bile suggests intestinal obstruction. Yellow vomitus is usually gastric in origin. Vomitus containing an excessive amount of white froth usually indicates the presence of saliva and suggests problems of the pharynx or esophagus.[165]

An improper immunization program may suggest an infectious cause of vomiting, especially in young patients. Feline and canine distemper, and obstructions are common causes of vomiting. If diarrhea also is present, obstructions or chemical irritants are unlikely. General questions designed to review other body systems may reveal information suggesting metabolic disease secondarily involving the gastrointestinal tract and manifested primarily through vomiting (e.g. renal or adrenal insufficiency).

In addition to a good history, the minimum data for all vomiting patients should include a complete physical examination. Thorough examination of the pharynx, and abdominal palpation for an obstruction is a must, and may reveal the cause of vomiting. Abdominal pain suggests acute pancreatitis as a cause of vomiting but may also be due to gastrointestinal obstruction, mesenteric abscess, peritonitis, or lead toxicity. If not contraindicated, tranquilization of the patient is helpful in relaxing a tense or painful abdomen to facilitate examination. Contents of the cranial abdomen are best palpated by raising the patient by its front legs into a vertical position. Gently shake the patient to allow the viscera in the cranial abdomen to fall caudal to the sternum where they are easier to palpate. Even when this procedure is used, the cat's stomach cannot usually be palpated. When it can be, the presence of a foreign body or tumor—most commonly a lymphoma—is suggested.[194]

A complete blood count and urinalysis are tests that screen many body systems and may quickly reveal clues to systemic diseases. These two tests should be considered an extension of the physical examination. The common association of vomiting with internal parasites, in many geographic areas, requires the addition of a fecal flotation to the minimum data base for vomiting.

Short-Term Vomiting

Rule out:

1. Life-threatening causes
   a. **Gastrointestinal obstruction**
      such as foreign bodies or intussusception
   b. **Systemic diseases**
      such as hepatic disease, peritonitis, uremia and septicemia
   c. **Toxin** ingestion
   d. **Colonic perforation**
      The most frequent clinical signs are depression, anorexia, emesis, and, less commonly, abdominal pain and constipation. Death usually occurs within 24 hours. Treatment appears to be of little benefit. Perforation occurs at the antimesenteric border, most often at or near the left colic flexure.[209] It almost always occurs in dogs treated with corticosteroids (especially dexamethasone).

These dogs most commonly have paresis or paralysis secondary to intervertebral disc disease or after major surgical stress; however, perforation can occur in dogs given corticosteroids for other reasons. Dexamethasone given at any dosage for longer than 2-3 days increases the prevalence of gastrointestinal complications in dogs.[151]

2. **Acute gastroenteritis**
This is confirmed by endoscopic observation of the gastric mucosa or an exclusion diagnosis when the minimum data base is normal. Hemorrhagic gastroenteritis, which is a potentially fatal syndrome characterized by peracute onset of hemorrhagic diarrhea, often begins with hematemesis. Hematocrit usually exceeds 50-60%. Hemorrhagic-erosive gastritis and ulcers may result from corticosteroid[192] or antiprostaglandin administration. Corticosteroids reduce production of gastric mucus and mucosal cell removal, and thus protection from gastric acid.

3. **Intestinal parasites** (see page 7-31)

4. **Hairballs**
Hairballs may cause cats to vomit but are not the main cause of vomiting in this species, contrary to popular belief.[194] Vomiting of hairballs may be induced in most cats by administering xylazine (Table 1).[194]

5. **Gastroesophageal intususception** (See page 7-9)

6. **Acute pancreatitis**
This disease occurs most often in middle-aged, obese, and sedentary dogs; least often in dogs in good physical condition. It occurs less commonly in cats.[23] Acute pancreatitis often follows a large meal. It also occurs postoperatively. Glucocorticoid administration or stimulation of endogenous secretion, and many drugs (including salicylazosulfapyridine, chloropromazine, diuretics, chemotherapeutics and estrogen) have been incriminated as a cause. Chronic feeding of high-fat diets has also been thought to predispose to acute pancreatitis; however, there are substantial data to refute this, at least at fat levels up to the amount in pet foods (see page 1-18). Abdominal trauma is a cause in some cases. A number of viruses have also been incriminated. Vascular impairment from any cause may induce pancreatitis.[67]

In dogs the disease generally manifests as sudden severe vomiting and abdominal pain. Affected dogs may vomit many times per hour for extended periods. The abdominal pain may be severe and particularly evident in the cranial right abdomen. Affected animals may be extremely sensitive to handling, walk with an arched back and a stiff, saw-horse gait, or take a praying stance (down in front, standing in back). Fever, shock, ileus, anorexia and depression often occur. Anorexia, depression, dehydration and generalized abdominal pain occurred in all dogs with experimentally induced acute-necrotizing pancreatitis; vomiting occurred in 92%, diarrhea in 54%, fever in 46%, abdominal distention in 38%, and cardiac complications in 23% of the dogs.[155] Attacks usually last 3-7 days. Recurrent bouts later in life are not uncommon.

Laboratory findings in affected dogs include elevated plasma cholesterol, amylase, lipase, and glucose, as well as glucosuria, hypocalcemia, and leukocytosis due to a neutrophilia with a left shift. Icterus may be present due to compression of the bile duct by inflamed pancreatic tissue. An increase in amylase in peritoneal fluid correlates highly with acute pancreatitis in dogs.[115] In addition, more than 1000 white blood cells/ml of peritoneal fluid and the presence of bacteria or toxic neutrophils indicate septic pancreatic necrosis. This condition requires exploratory celiotomy and usually indicates pancreatic abscessation.[115] An elevated plasma lipase is considered the most reliable indication of acute pancreatitis in both dogs and cats.[119] An increase in peak 3 isoamylase activity may also be a useful diagnostic indicator of acute pancreatitis.[156]

A diagnosis of acute pancreatitis is seldom made in cats, probably because clinical signs of the disease and laboratory tests are subtle and nonspecific. In experimentally induced acute pancreatitis in cats, the only change that would lead to suspicion of the disease was an increase in plasma lipase for the first 4 days after the disease was induced.[119] Only 2 of 7 cats vomited, and then only once. Diarrhea, depression, anorexia, and hematologic changes did not develop. All cats showed variable degrees of abdominal discomfort during palpation. Plasma calcium and phosphorus were reduced by the fourth day. In contrast to the plasma amylase in dogs, it is of no diagnostic value in cats with acute pancreatitis because: 1) it is reduced rather than elevated during the acute phase of the disease[119] and 2) it is usually increased to 1500-3000 Harleco units in vomiting cats regardless of the cause of vomiting.[194]

Chronic Vomiting

Rule out:

1. **Foreign body**
   Survey abdominal radiographs, gastroscopy, and a complete barium series are examinations designed to localize foreign bodies that cannot be palpated.

2. **Intestinal intussusception**
   Most can be palpated; however, the decision to operate may depend upon characteristic findings of intussusception in a barium series or barium enema.

3. **Renal Failure**
   Blood urea nitrogen and creatinine are elevated. A non-regenerative anemia, fixed urine specific gravity, and significant proteinuria often are present (see Chapter 8).

4. **Hepatic dysfunction**
   May result in gastric ulcers and chronic vomiting. See page 7-52 for other clinical signs, diagnosis, and management of liver disease.

5. **Pyometra**
   Information from the minimum data base usually provides sufficient information to allow diagnosis of this condition. In some cases, survey abdominal radiographs are helpful.

6. **Infectious diseases**
   a. Canine distemper (see page 7-28)
   b. Canine infectious hepatitis
   c. Canine parvovirus (see page 7-30)
   d. Leptospirosis
   e. Feline enteritis (see page 7-30)
      In addition to vomiting, diarrhea and a neutrophil:lymphocyte ratio of less than 1:2 are usually present.
   f. Feline infectious peritonitis
   g. Feline leukemia

7. **Adrenocortical insufficiency**
   Eosinophilia with lymphocytosis, in the face of stress, may be evident. A decreased sodium/potassium ratio is present in most cases. An ACTH stimulation test is diagnostic (see page 6-5).

8. **Diabetes mellitus**
   A fasting blood glucose concentration greater than 150 mg/dl is present in dogs with Type I or II diabetes, but may be normal in what some refer to as Type III diabetes. However, the presence of a blood glucose concentration above 150 mg/dl 45-60 minutes after intravenous administration of 500 mg of glucose/kg body weight confirms the presence of all types of diabetes.[142] See page 6-4 for description of types of diabetes.

9. **Hyperthyroidism**
   Occurs primarily in cats and is characterized by a normal to increased appetite accompanied by weight loss. Mild diarrhea or steatorrhea may also occur.

10. **Gastric neoplasia**
    Accounts for less than 1% of all neoplasms in dogs and cats.[107] Adenocarcinomas are the most common gastric tumor in dogs, followed by benign neoplasms (such as polyps), sarcomas, and leiomyomas; whereas, lymposarcomas are the major gastric tumor in cats.[107] Gastroscopy with cytologic exam of tissue or secretions provides the easiest means of documenting the presence of gastric neoplasia. An upper gastrointestinal series may provide localizing information. Exploratory laparotomy should be considered early in the diagnostic workup if a gastroscope is unavailable.

11. **Intestinal neoplasia**
    A complete gastrointestinal barium series will usually show the site of the lesion. A definitive diagnosis and prognosis are made through exploratory laparotomy. The presence of immature lymphocytes suggests the presence of lymphosarcoma.

12. **Phycomycosis**
    In addition to, or instead of, chronic vomiting, phycomycosis may cause abdominal masses, granulomas, draining fistulous tracts, and subcutaneous nodules. Diagnosis is made by culture of biopsies or exudates. Treatment is surgery and amphotericin B (Table 1).

13. **Central nervous system or vestibular diseases**
    A complete neurological examination is indicated if these problems are suspected. Basophilic stippling and many nucleated red blood cells, with a hematocrit above 30%, may indicate lead intoxication as the cause.

14. **Chronic gastroenteritis**
    Exclude other causes of vomiting and eosinophilic gastroenteritis. An endoscopic examination, or gastric mucosal biopsy, may be needed to confirm the diagnosis. In most cases a definitive diagnosis is not determined. Some people feel that some cases may be due to an autoimmunity against gastric secretions or the gastric wall. It may also be caused by a food allergy or reflux of bile into the stomach. **Reflux gastritis** is characterized by chronic vomiting of bile-stained material and mucus

after a prolonged fast—often early in the morning. The gastric nematode *Ollulanus tricuspis* may cause gastritis and chronic vomiting and weight loss in cats. Diagnosis of this parasite is difficult because larvae rarely, if ever, are passed in the feces. The prevalence and treatment of this parasite are unknown.

15. **Eosinophilic gastroenteritis**
A rare condition affecting both dogs and cats characterized by diffuse eosinophilic and fibrous tissue infiltration involving many layers of the stomach and/or intestinal wall. In cats the chief clinical sign is vomiting generally occurring about 30 minutes after a meal for several days followed by a period of several days with no vomiting. This pattern then repeats itself.[194] Treat by giving 20 mg/cat of methylprednisolone acetate (Depo-Medrol, Upjohn) subcutaneously 2-3 times yearly[194] and feed a hypoallergenic diet[212] (Prescription Diet d/d, Hill's). In dogs the chief clinical sign is diarrhea (see page 7-36).

16. **Pylorospasm, pyloric stenosis or obstruction**
Pyloric stenosis is particularly prevalent in Siamese cats and brachycephalic breeds of dogs, especially Boston Terriers and Boxers.[213] Pyloric spasms or stenosis may be acquired or present at birth and result in persistent vomiting when the animal begins eating solid food. The vomiting frequently worsens with age.[66] These dysfunctions are characterized by persistent postprandial vomiting, often with food remaining in the vomitus for up to 24 hours after a meal. Vomiting of undigested food may be projectile, or vomiting may occur 4-8 hours after eating and may be non-productive. Bloating may develop 1-4 hours after eating. Retention of barium in the stomach for 8-10 hours confirms the presence of pyloric obstruction. However, in some affected animals the barium passes in a normal period of time (2-3 hrs). Treatment for pyloric stenosis is surgery. For pylorospasms, frequent feeding of a canned or pureed food or, if necessary, administration of an anticholinergic drug or tranquilizer may alleviate signs.

17. **Chronic hypertrophic pyloric gastropathy** (CHPG) with or without gastritis
CHPG causes obstruction of gastric outflow and is secondary to pyloric muscular hypertrophy, with or without mucosal hyperplasia. This condition has been called hypertrophic gastritis, aquired pyloric hypertrophy and gastric polyps. The cause is thought to be exces-

sive gastrin secretion induced by chronic overdistention of the gastric antrum, or other causes. Gastrin is trophic to pyloric smooth muscle and mucosa. With CHPG a generalized hypertrophic gastritis may or may not be present.

CHPG affects primarily middle-aged to older dogs of small breeds that present with chronic intermittent vomiting of several weeks to months duration.[143,188] Vomiting usually occurs at various intervals after eating. Infrequently there is postprandial projectile vomiting or an acute episode of vomiting. A few cases are presented because of abdominal distention after eating. Anorexia and weight loss are features in about one-fourth of the cases.[143] There are no consistent findings on physical examination, and no hematologic or biochemical abnormalities.

Diagnosis is based on abdominal radiographs and positive-contrast studies demonstrating delayed gastric emptying, filling defects, or thickening of the pyloric wall and/or marked gastric distention.

Treatment is pyloroplasty except in patients with significant mucosal hyperplasia. In these cases, or those that do not respond to pyloroplasty, pyloric and antral resection and anastamosis are recommended.[143,222] This treatment provided good to excellent results in 33 of 39 dogs in one study[143] and 16 of 19 in another.[222]

18. **Achlorhydria** (rare)
Gastric contents should have a pH of 0.5-3.5 postprandial or fasted[243] and a pH of 2, or less, one hour after subcutaneous administration of 0.3 g/kg of histamine.[17] A gastric pH above these values is diagnostic for achlorhydria.

19. **Gastric or duodenal ulcers**
These result in any or all of the following: chronic intermittent vomiting, and occasionally diarrhea, hematemesis, anorexia, weight loss, abdominal pain, anemia, and, if perforation occurs, sudden collapse. A generalized erosive gastritis is usually present. Vomitus often resembles coffee grounds due to partially digested blood. Diagnosis is made from clinical signs, contrast radiography, and endoscopic examination or exploratory surgery with biopsy. It is important to differentiate between benign peptic ulcer and a gastric ulcer associated with neoplasia and, if possible, to determine the cause of the ulcers. Gastric or duodenal ulcers may be caused by:

a. Excessive gastric acid secretion stimulated by:
   1) Stress
      For example, ulcers and erosive gastritis occur in animals in intensive care units.
   2) Mastocytoma
      Neoplastic cells release histamine, which stimulates gastric acid secretion.[4] This tumor is most common in Boxers and Boston Terriers.
   3) High plasma gastrin concentration* due to:
      i) Excessive gastrin secretion from a pancreatic tumor (gastrinoma or Zollinger-Ellison syndrome). Although this condition occurs, it is uncommon in dogs and cats. Affected animals tend to be middle-aged or older and exhibit chronic vomiting, weight loss, and diarrhea.[216] Usually the tumor is small and can be removed surgically.
      ii) Decreased gastrin excretion due to renal failure.
b. Reduced gastric mucosal defense to gastric acid due to any of the following: uremic toxins, bile reflux, calorie-protein malnutrition, caffeine, alcohol, indomethacin, corticosteroids, acetylsalicylic acid (aspirin), flunixin meglumine (Banamine, Schering), or phenylbutazone. Corticosteroids and Banamine decrease mucosal cell turnover and mucus production, and stimulate gastrin secretion. Several days of Banamine administration results in severe ulcers.[38]
c. Inadequate mucosal circulation from any cause.
d. Liver disease. In one study, 16 of 22 dogs with fatty and degenerative hepatic changes had peptic ulcers.[107]

20. **Colitis** (see page 7-47)
    About 30% of dogs with colitis vomit.[34]

21. **Gastric paresis**
    Absence of gastric contractions due to a defect in the enteric nervous system. The cause is generally unknown. Gastric emptying is delayed, vomiting (usually of undigested or only partially digested food 6-12 hours after eating) and frequent bloating may occur, but without the gastric torsion that accompanies acute gastric dilatation. Pyloric stenosis and chronic hypertrophic pyloric gastropathy should be ruled out in such cases (see #16 and #17 page 7-19). After a meal, the normal stomach should be empty within 6-8 hours.

22. **Ineffective intestinal propulsion**
    This results in signs of obstruction without luminal occlusion. The acute form may be called ileus, spastic ileus or paralytic ileus. It may develop after surgery, be associated with pancreatitis or trauma, or present as an idiopathic entity. Chronic or recurrent intestinal pseudo-obstruction may result from disorders involving the smooth muscle, myenteric plexus or endocrine controls of gastrointestinal motility. The dysfunction is characterized by chronic intractable vomiting, diarrhea and weight loss of several weeks to months duration, and radiographic evidence of obstruction without occlusion of the lumen.[150] Cholinergics, metoclopramide, and prednisone may be of little benefit. Oral administration of antibiotics may help suppress intestinal bacterial overgrowth. The diet should be lactose-free and contain lowered amounts of highly digestible fat to avoid the potential for bacteria to metabolize these substances into products that enhance intestinal secretion.[150] Dietary fiber content should be low because of the potential to form bezoars.[150] Thus, a highly digestible, low fat, low fiber diet (Prescription Diet i/d, Hill's, or Recipe 1 or 10, Appendix Table 3) should be fed in small smounts at frequent intervals.

23. **Iatrogenic**
    Overdosage or prolonged administration of anticholinergic drugs or narcotic analgesics may cause severe gastric atony and gastric retention, resulting in persistent vomiting.[213] Withdrawal of these medications resolves the problem.

24. **Hiatal hernia** (see page 7-11)

MANAGEMENT OF VOMITING

The objective of the management of vomiting is to enable the patient to tolerate the disease while logical diagnostic plans and an indepth study of the patient are carried out (if necessary). Treatment steps 1 and 2 (p. 7-21) will resolve many cases of vomiting due to acute gastroenteritis or dietary indiscretion. If the cause of vomiting is detected from the history and initial examination, specific therapy, as indicated, should be instituted. If the cause of vomiting is not determined and vomiting persists for longer than 24 hours, an indepth evaluation should be conducted to determine the

---

*Normal is less than 100 pg/ml in fasted dogs and less than 200 after a meal (peak at 15-30 minutes).[77] The gastrin RIA kit for humans (Becton, Dickinson & Co) is accurate for the dog.[77]

specific cause, and appropriate therapy to alleviate that cause should be instituted.

1. For all vomiting patients, if dehydration is present, give parenterally an isotonic saline solution with 10-30 mEq/L of potassium chloride added. See Chapter 5 for specifics of fluid and electrolyte therapy.

2. Withhold all food for 24-48 hours and water for 24 hours. This helps break the drink/vomit cycle that develops in cases of simple emesis. If no vomiting occurs during the initial period of management, over the next 3-5 days gradually return the patient to full feed and water. Until vomiting is well controlled, feed small amounts frequently (3-6 times daily) of a highly-digestible, low-fiber diet (e.g. Prescription Diets i/d for dogs and Feline c/d for cats, Hill's, or Recipes 1 or 8 respectively, Appendix Table 3). Almost 90% of vomiting dogs and cats respond to this management.[38]

3. If vomiting persists, the following treatments should be considered:

   a. Give metoclopramide (Table 1). It has both a central and peripheral antiemetic effect, and may be beneficial for either initial therapy or long-term management of vomiting.[202] It is indicated as an antiemetic, particularly for **gastric paresis, bloat, reflux esophagitis or gastritis,** and **constipation.** The drug stimulates and coordinates gastrointestinal motility and increases gastroesophageal sphincter pressure (from 49 to 76 mmHg in dogs in one study).[199] It may be effective as an antiemetic agent in dogs with **parvovirus** when it is given by continuous intravenous drip with fluids at a dosage of 1 mg/kg/24 hours.[106] A single dose at bedtime often alleviates **early morning nausea and vomiting** in dogs that exhibit this as a chronic problem of unknown cause.[202] It is also useful in managing **pyloric stenosis** as an aid in diagnosis (good response to therapy) or treatment when there is a desire to avoid surgery.[202]

   b. Administration of **anticholinergics** to block afferent vagal impulses to the vomiting center **are not effective** in most cases. They are contraindicated in pyloric or intestinal obstruction, ileus, urinary retention, or glaucoma.[234]

   c. Phenothiazine tranquilizers and, in dogs only, trimethobenzamide (Tigan-Beecham) block the vomiting center chemoreceptor trigger zone. Therefore, they are useful when vomiting is caused by stimulation of this zone (e.g. **drugs, uremia, bacterial toxins,** and other **metabolic disorders).** These tranquilizers are effective as antiemetics at doses less than that which causes sedation. They should not be given until after body fluid deficits have been corrected, as they potentiate hypotension.

   d. Pimozide (Table 1) blocks the vomiting center chemoreceptor trigger zone and given once protects dogs from **drug**-induced emesis for up to 6 days.[231]

   e. Antihistamines (e.g. Dramamine, Searle) are useful in preventing nausea and vomiting caused by **motion sickness** or **vestibulitis**.[37]

   f. Oral administered protectants such as kaolin, pectin, aluminum silicate, or bismuth preparations, although often prescribed, are usually not useful in therapy for the vomiting patient.[235]

   g. Oral administered antibiotics should be used only if a bacterial infection is present. They may promote vomiting and do more harm than good by altering the normal gastrointestinal flora.

4. If **hematemesis** is occurring, or **ulcers, gastritis, esophagitis, uremia, bloat, or acute pancreatitis** are present, give cimetidine orally or intravenously (Table 1). If hematemesis is severe, intragastric lavage using ice water with 16 mg of norepinephrine/L will help stop gastric hemorrhage.[107] If the hematocrit is less than 25%, consider intravenous administration of whole blood. A number of other drugs have also been effective in promoting ulcer healing.

   Ranitidine (Zantac, Glaxol) as compared to cimetidine is (on a molar basis) 5-12 times more potent, causes 30-50% greater reduction in gastric acid secretion and is a more specific parietal cell histamine H_2-receptor blocker.[238] This increased specificity results in fewer adverse side effects such as confusion, depression, thrombocytopenia and agranulocytosis that occasionally occur in people given cimetidine.[238] However, cimetidine is not known to cause any untoward effects in dogs. The main advantage of ranitidine is that it requires only twice-daily administration (Table 1). Currently, ranitidine is more expensive than cimetidine.[37]

   Omeprazole, a drug being used in clinical studies, recently has been shown in people to be more effective than cimetidine for ulcer therapy[124] and more effective than ranitidine for reflux esophagitis.[19] However, after 2 years

of high doses of omeprazole to rats, gastric carcinoid tumors developed, therefore it may not become available commercially. It is a long-acting inhibitor of gastric ATPase, the enzyme needed for secretion of hydrogen ions by parietal cells.

Antacids, in contrast to gastric acid secretion inhibitors, are not usually beneficial. In people, and quite likely dogs and cats, antacids must be given every 2 hours for adequate buffering. It has been stated that in contrast to people, dogs secrete gastric acid only when food is ingested. However, radiotelemetric studies conducted in dogs refute this and have shown that even after a 24-hour fast gastric pH is 0.9-2.5 (mean 1.5) and duodenal pH is 4.5-7.5 (mean 6.1).[243]

Sucralfate may be beneficial for ulcer therapy (Table 1). It acts as a protective barrier, promotes mucous production and inactivates pepsin and bile. It should not be given within 2 hours of other drugs as it may decrease their absorption or bind them, as it does cimetidine and ranitidine. If sulcrafate is given with gastric acid secretion inhibitors, their administration should be staggered.

Fat, carbohydrate and fiber stimulate the least, and protein the greatest amount of gastric acid secretion.[27] The amount of acid secreted also increases with meal size.[27] Thus, the animal with ulcers should be fed small amounts frequently of a low-protein diet.

5. If **acute pancreatitis** is suspected, large volumes of an extracellular replacement fluid, such as Ringer's lactate solution, should be given rapidly to treat the hypotension and shock which are often present. Failure to give adequate amounts of fluid rapidly is the primary cause of death of patients with acute pancreatitis.[155] In dogs with experimentally induced acute hemorrhagic pancreatitis, it has been shown that, in contrast to what has been suggested, Ringer's lactate solution is better than colloid-containing fluids.[138] This study also demonstrated that large volumes of fluid may be safely given (2675 ± 131 ml in 4 hours). It may be beneficial to add 10 ml of 23% calcium gluconate per liter of fluid administered. This will help correct the hypocalcemia often present but is not harmful if hypocalcemia is not present.

Antibiotics, such as procaine penicillin G (20,000 IU/kg) for anerobes and kanamycin (5 mg/kg) for Gram-negative bacteria, given twice daily, have been recommended.[67,155] Anal-

gesics should be administered to relieve pain. Meperidine (at 5-10 mg/kg 2-3 times daily) is reported to be the analgesic of choice for dogs with acute pancreatitis.[155] Atropine or other anticholinergic drugs have been recommended to reduce pancreatic secretion. However, these drugs reduce motility of an already atonic intestine and are reported to be of questionable value.[67,115] Corticosteroids are not recommended.

Nothing should be given orally for 2-5 days, then only water for the next 3 days.[155] After recovery from the acute episode there may be recurrences and eventual development of either, or both, exocrine or endocrine insufficiency. The most important means of preventing this is strict adherence to feeding a highly digestible, moderate fat-restricted diet (Prescription Diet i/d, Hill's).[67] Small amounts should be fed several times daily.

A pancreatic pseudocyst or abscess rarely may occur after a severe episode of acute pancreatitis. If this occurs (as can be detected ultrasonographically or radiographically usually 1-3 weeks after the acute episode), surgical drainage may be necessary.[182]

6. **Achlorhydria** may respond to the feeding of a highly digestible diet (Prescription Diets i/d for the dog or Feline c/d for the cat, Hill's, or Recipes 1 or 8, Appendix Table 3) and if diarrhea is present, the oral administration of an antimicrobial drug for 1-2 weeks.[173] Adding 1/8 to 1/4 teaspoonful of salt to the dog's food has also been reported to be helpful in some cases.

ACUTE GASTRIC DILATATION (BLOAT)

GASTRIC DILATATION WITHOUT VOLVULUS

Gastric dilatation may occur with or without volvulus. Gastric dilatation without volvulus most often occurs intermittently, usually in young dogs, particularly as a result of overeating. Clinical signs include nausea, belching, and vomiting. Conversely, there may be no effort to vomit, but instead lethargy, a reluctance to move, and grunting sounds with respiratory effort. Usually, gastric tympany is not detected by abdominal percussion, whereas it is in dogs with gastric dilatation with volvulus. Administration of metoclopramide (Table 1) has been reported to be beneficial in dogs repeatedly affected.[202]

GASTRIC DILATATION WITH VOLVULUS (GDV)

Gastric dilatation with volvulus occurs most commonly in middle-aged and older, deep-chested, large breeds of dogs, although it has occurred in Dachshunds, Pekingese, terriers, and cats.

Causes of GDV

Three things are necessary for the development of GDV. They are:

1. Laxity of the gastrohepatic ligament
2. Gastric dilatation with gas
3. Obstruction to eructation and passage of gas from the stomach

Laxity of the gastrohepatic ligament occurs as a result of the prolonged, repeated consumption of large amounts of food at a single feeding. It may be worsened if physical activity closely follows a large meal. A chronic feeding pattern of large amounts of food fed at one meal daily also results in an enlarged, heavy, muscular stomach, and increases gastrin secretion.[221] Gastrin secretion is also stimulated by excess calcium ingestion.[143,188,221] Chronic excessive calcium intake results in continuously elevated gastrin secretion.[221] Hypergastrinemia is present in dogs with acute GDV and persists after treatment and recovery, suggesting that dogs with GDV have a preexisting hypergastrinemia.[130] In turn, gastrin stimulates hyperplasia and hypertrophy of the gastroduodenal musculature and mucosa, delays gastric emptying, increases gastroesophageal sphincter pressure, and may increase aerophagia.[130,199,221] Hyperplasia and hypertrophy of the gastroduodenal musculature and mucosa are routinely present in dogs that bloat. These effects impair passage of gas from the stomach and lead to a pendulous atonic stomach susceptible to volvulus.

Gas in the stomach of dogs with GDV has been shown to be primarily air, which differs greatly in composition from the gas produced by bacterial fermentation.[43,214] Thus, aerophagia is the primary source of gas in dogs with GDV, not bacterial fermentation. Production of gas in the stomach from bacterial fermentation occurs following death and initially led to the belief that it was responsible for GDV. Aerophagia can be caused by spasms of the upper gastrointestinal tract, which may be induced by gastrin.[160] Aerophagia also increases as the rate of food consumption increases, and with excitement and stress.

As described above, the following factors appear to predispose to acute GDV:

1. Consumption of large amounts of food at a single feeding
2. Physical activity shortly after eating a large meal
3. Excessive dietary calcium
4. Rapid food consumption, which occurs to a greater extent when:
   a. Dogs are fed with others
   b. If they are excited when fed
   c. The less frequently they are fed

A number of other factors, including soy and dry expanded cereal based commercial dog foods, have been speculated, without any valid supportive data, to predispose to GDV. However, as has been reported,[214] GDV occurs in animals whether they are being fed 1) free-choice or meal-fed, 2) meat or cereal based diets, 3) soybean-containing or soybean-free foods, or 4) small or large quantities. Attempts to reproduce GDV by dietary manipulation have been unsuccessful. In one study, no difference was found in gastric motility or emptying in large-breed dogs fed either: 1) a canned meat-based, soybean meal-free, commercial dog food, 2) a dry, expanded cereal-based, soy-containing commercial dog food moistened with water before feeding or 3) the same food fed dry.[39] Thus, this study suggests that neither soybean meal nor a dry expanded dog food fed dry appear to be causative factors for GDV. As these investigators concluded, most large dogs are fed dry cereal-based food for reasons of cost and ease of use, and these diets may have been wrongly incriminated as a predisposing factor in GDV.[39]

Clinical Signs of GDV

Volvulus is characterized by sudden abdominal bloating, retching with an inability to vomit, increased respiratory effort, hyperpnea, open-mouthed panting, collapse, and death. This is an emergency. Prompt proper veterinary attention is required to relieve distention immediately, by any means necessary, and to treat hypovolemic shock. If gastric distention is not promptly relieved, absorption of endotoxins, acidosis, tissue hypoxia, strangulation of the spleen, and hypovolemic or hypotensive shock may occur. Any combination of these conditions may result in death.

Treatment of GDV

Therapy for shock and gastric decompression are necessary. Decompression by any means should be accomplished as quickly as possible. In some cases a stomach tube may be passed. This is best accomplished with a large-bore, firm, flexible,

well-lubricated tube. It should be passed to a premeasured distance from the nose to the 11th rib (third from the last). If a stomach tube cannot be passed, large-bore needles should be used to tap the stomach through the abdominal wall. If poor tissue perfusion is present, give oxygen and rapidly administer intravenously, large volumes (90ml/kg in the first hour) of an extracellular replacement fluid, such as Ringer's lactate, containing corticosteroids, and antibiotics. Sodium bicarbonate should not be given unless acidosis has been confirmed. In contrast to experimentally induced GDV, most clinically affected dogs have normal acid-base parameters[236] or rarely may be alkalotic.[111] If cardiac arrhythmia is present, as it is in 30-50% of affected dogs, the intravenous administration of a 2-4 mg/kg bolus of lidocaine hydrochloride without epinephrine (Table 1), may be of benefit.[153] If the stomach or pylorus is displaced, surgical correction is indicated.

Intravenous administration of fluid, with 15-25 mEq/L of potassium chloride added, should be continued, and food and water withheld for the first 24 hours. After either surgery or radiographic evidence that the stomach has returned to its proper position, gradually feed ice cubes and small amounts of water. Withhold food until the dog has not vomited for 24 hours, then feed one-third of the daily requirement of a highly digestible diet (Prescription Diet i/d, Hill's, or Recipe 1, Appendix Table 3) divided into 3-6 small meals. Over the next 3-4 days, gradually increase the amount fed back to normal.

Prevention of GDV

1. During growth meal-feed a good-quality, low-fiber, highly-digestible, nutritionally balanced diet. Avoid high calcium diets (greater than 2.0% of dry matter) and do not give calcium supplements of any type.
2. Feed the puppy as described beginning on page 3-12.
3. Feed all dogs throughout their lives at least twice daily or free-choice. In a dog previously affected with GDV, feed a highly digestible diet (Prescription Diet i/d, Hill's, or Recipe 1, Appendix Table 3) at least 3 times daily.
4. Minimize excitement and physical activity before, during and for 1 hour after feeding. Feed the dog by itself and in a quiet location.
5. If the above procedures are unsuccessful or if surgery is necessary in treatment, permanent gastropexy to prevent volvulus will prevent recurrence in most cases. A circumcostal gastropexy appears to be the most successful procedure for preventing recurrence[128] and has a higher adhesion strength than permanent or tube gastrotomy techniques.[75]

DIARRHEA

Diarrhea is the passage of loose or liquid stools at an increased frequency. It is the primary clinical sign of intestinal disease and occurs secondary to many non-intestinal diseases. The intestinal tract has four main functions:

1. Transport of luminal contents (motility)
2. Secretion of enzymes, hormones, fluids, and electrolytes
3. Digestion and absorption of ingested materials and reabsorption of much of the secreted fluid and electrolytes
4. Immune responses

PATHOPHYSIOLOGY AND CAUSES OF DIARRHEA

Diarrhea may result from nearly any intestinal dysfunction, resulting in the following types of diarrhea:

1. Motility
2. Active secretory
3. Passive secretory or osmotic
4. Increased permeability or exudative
5. Mixed

The small intestine may initiate diarrhea by exposing the colon to intestinal contents at a rate or volume that exceeds the absorptive capacity of the colon (simple volume overload), or by allowing the entry of substances into the colon (such as excessive bile salts and fatty acids) that stimulate colonic secretion and rapid colonic emptying of the colon. Colonic absorptive reserve capacity is low in dogs and cats because they have a relatively small colon. Extra fluid delivered from the small intestine will therefore rapidly overwhelm colonic capacity.

Disturbed motor function may manifest as abdominal pain or alteration in transit time, resulting in either constipation or motility-induced diarrhea. In contrast to historic beliefs, a decrease in intestinal motility is present in most patients with diarrhea. Generalized absence of intestinal motility is called "ileus." The lack of resistance to peristalsis, and reduced rhythmic segmentation and sphincter tone, result in rapid movement of fluid through the intestinal tract (peristaltic rush), causing diarrhea.

Increased intestinal secretion and/or decreased absorption of fluid and electrolytes are primary

causes of diarrhea. Increased secretion may be either active or passive. Toxins secreted by some **bacteria** (e.g., toxigenic *Escherichia coli*, *Vibrio cholera*, Corynebacterium spp, *Colostridium perfringens*, Salmonella spp and Klebsiella spp) cause an increase in active intestinal secretion. These toxins attach to intestinal epithelial cells and activate the membrane enzyme, adenyl cyclase, which converts intracellular ATP to cyclic AMP. The cyclic AMP accumulates in the intestinal epithelial cells and stimulates an active secretion of water and electrolytes. This may also be induced by a number of **hormone-secreting neoplasms**, including non-beta cell, non-gastrin secreting tumors of the pancreatic islet cells (resulting in what is called pancreatic cholera), malignant carcinoids, medullary carcinoma of the thyroid, mast-cell tumors, bronchogenic carcinoma, and neural-crest tumors.[50] Prostaglandins appear to play a role in causing the secretory diarrhea that occurs as a result of these bacterial toxins or the hormones produced by these tumors. As a result, prostaglandin inhibitors, such as indomethacin and salicylates (e.g. aspirin; Corrective Mixture, Beecham; and Pepto-Bismol, Norwich-Eaton), may be beneficial.[100] However, these causes of active secretory diarrhea are uncommon in dogs and cats.[38]

Hydroxy fatty acids are a more common cause of active secretory diarrhea. They are produced by enteric bacteria from unabsorbed dietary fatty acids, but not triglycerides.[38] Because dietary fats are triglycerides (see Figure 1, page 1-3), they must be digested by pancreatic lipase to release their fatty acids in order for dietary fats to induce diarrhea. Thus, hydroxy fatty acid-induced secretory diarrhea occurs only if there is: 1) sufficient pancreatic lipase, 2) sufficient fat ingested and 3) insufficient fatty acid absorption as may occur with small intestinal, hepatic, or lymphatic dysfunction. This is one reason a diet containing a low or only moderate amount of a highly digestible fat is indicated for animals with these dysfunctions.

Increased intestinal secretion is often accompanied by a compensatory increase in absorption. However, if absorptive capacity is overwhelmed (simple volume overload), diarrhea occurs. A passive (rather than an active) increase in intestinal secretion exceeding that absorbed may result from: 1) an increased osmolality of intestinal contents brought about by the presence of poorly absorbed substances resulting in an **osmotic diarrhea** or 2) **increase in intestinal permeability.** Poor absorption of ingested carbohydrates, fats, and proteins may occur because they are constituents of

poorly digestible foods or because of **maldigestion** due to a lack of sufficient:

1. Pancreatic enzymes for digestion of all three nutrients
2. Bile salts for fat digestion and absorption
3. Intestinal brush border dissacharidase enzymes for soluble carbohydrate digestion.

These are the reasons a highly digestible diet is indicated for animals with pancreatic insufficiency, intra- or extra-hepatic obstructive diseases, or enteritis.

A passive increase in intestinal secretion due to an increase in intestinal permeability may result from: 1)intestinal damage from any cause or 2) increased hydraulic pressure in the mucosa because of **lymphatic obstruction,** or increased mesenteric venous pressure due to **congestive heart failure** or **hepatic congestion.** In addition to increasing intestinal permeability, damage to the intestinal mucosa may decrease absorption.

Because absorption occurs from the tips of the intestinal villi, any condition that blunts the villi reduces absorption and may lead to diarrhea (malabsorption diarrhea). This mechanism is responsible for the diarrhea associated with many **viral** (e.g. parvovirus, rotavirus, and coronavirus), bacterial (e.g. invasive *E. coli*, Corynebacterium spp., Salmonella spp., and *Campylobacter jejuni*), nonbacterial **toxin**-induced diseases, and enteritis due to radiation. Although **bacteria** are an important cause of diarrhea in many species, they are an uncommon cause of diarrhea in dogs and cats. **Radiation enteritis**-induced diarrhea, frequently steatorrhea and often, as a result, malnutrition, are common sequela of radiotherapy for abdominal or pelvic malignancies.[123] Acute irradiation of the small intestine causes reversible destruction of the mucosal epithelium.[210] However, the delayed effects of intestinal radiation include progressive enteritis with chronic ulceration and/or fibroatrophy that may result in the development of diarrhea years later.[162,181]

Frequently, with enteritis from any cause, there is a loss of the intestinal brush border and, therefore, of the disaccharidase enzymes that it contains (lactase, sucrase, maltase, and alpha-dextrinase). These enzymes are essential for the digestion of disaccharides (lactose or milk sugar, sucrose or table sugar, and maltose and alpha-dextrins from starch) and subsequent absorption of their constituent monosaccharides. Unabsorbed disaccharides or other carbohydrates are converted by colonic bacteria to lactic acid and volatile fatty acids, which lower the pH and increase the osmolality of the luminal contents. The lowered pH and

osmotic effects of these acids produce watery diarrhea. Often 1-2 weeks are needed for restoration of intestinal brush border disaccharidase activity after correction of the cause for their loss. Diarrhea may, therefore occur during this period when carbohydrates requiring disaccharidase digestion are ingested. This would include all carbohydrates except the monosaccharides glucose, galactose, and fructose. For this reason, during and for at least 2-3 weeks after diarrhea, a highly digestible diet that does not contain lactose or sucrose (such as Prescription Diet i/d for dogs and Feline c/d for cats, Hill's, or Recipes 1 or 8, Appendix Table 3) should be fed in small amounts at frequent intervals (3-6 times daily).

Inadequate intestinal disaccharidase activity is also the mechanism responsible for causing diarrhea due to **excess milk consumption,** and diarrhea which may occur following a rapid change in diet. Puppies and kittens have small amounts of lactase. As in other animals, after weaning age, lactase falls to about 10% of its peak activity. The continued consumption of milk does not alter the decline in lactase activity.[122] Diarrhea will occur if more lactose is consumed than the animal can digest. Bitch's milk contains only 3.1% lactose, and queen's milk 4.2%, as compared to 4.5-5% in cow's and goat's milk, 7% in human milk, and none in sea lion or walrus milk (Table 4, page 3-18). This is why puppies and kittens commonly have diarrhea when given cow's or goat's milk.

Inadequate intestinal disaccharidase activity also is one of the factors responsible for diarrhea subsequent to a **rapid change in diet.** Several days are required for intestinal disaccharidase enzyme activity to respond to a change in dietary carbohydrates. Such a diet change may occur between different batches of the same brand of pet food since the ingredients used in most popular commercial pet foods vary, depending on their availability and cost. This is the reason diarrhea may occur when feeding is initiated from a new bag of the same or different brand of food. To prevent this type of diarrhea, a fixed-formula diet can be fed (see page 2-16).

Diarrhea may be caused not only by decreased digestion or absorption of disaccharides, but also by decreased absorption of fats, proteins, or other carbohydrates. Diarrhea of this type is commonly referred to as the **malabsorption syndrome.** However, it can be caused by either malabsorption or maldigestion; therefore, malassimilation is a more appropriate name for this syndrome. Malabsorption may be caused by intestinal dysfunctions, a lack of hepatic bile salts, or lymphatic obstruction. Maldigestion is due to a lack of pancreatic digestive enzymes. Because fat absorption requires all of these processes, steatorrhea occurs regardless of the cause of malassimilation. Steatorrhea may or may not be clinically evident. If maldigestion (pancreatic exocrine insufficiency) is not present, the steatorrhea is primarily from fatty acids not absorbed in the jejunum and ileum. These fatty acids may inhibit the absorption of water and electrolytes in the colon, creating a watery diarrhea. In addition, high concentrations of fatty acids in the colon may alter colonic motility to favor more rapid luminal transport of ingesta. In contrast, the steatorrhea from maldigestion is primarily composed of neutral fats that do not alter colonic function as significantly as free fatty acids. Therefore, rather than a profuse watery stool characteristic of malabsorption, maldigestion usually results in bulky malformed stools.

The colon stands guard against excessive water and electrolyte losses in the stool. The final common pathway resulting in frequent stools lies with an increase in the volume load, a decrease in the absorption capacity, or rapid transit through the colon. The most common mechanism of **altered colonic function** is simple volume overload due to inadequate absorption in the small intestine. Generalized inflammation may lessen the absorptive capacity of the colon. The motility alterations associated with diarrhea may produce a "quiet colon." A hypomotile colon does not effectively retard the movement of luminal contents, and diarrhea may develop. Hypomotile states may be present as a result of the irritable bowel syndrome and chronic inflammatory disease.

Fecal incontinence, with or without normal stool consistency, can occur as a result of decreased rectal sensation or impaired function of the external anal sphincter. These effects, as well as diarrhea, constipation, and impaired gastric emptying, may occur due to neurogenic dysfunctions of the gastrointestinal tract secondary to **diabetes mellitus.**[220]

EFFECTS OF DIARRHEA

The fluid and electrolyte losses and their effects are similar regardless of the alterations responsible for causing the diarrhea. The major losses are water, sodium, chloride, bicarbonate, and potassium. Losses of water, sodium and chloride result in dehydration; bicarbonate loss results in metabolic acidosis; and potassium loss results in weakness, lethargy, decreased appetite, and decreased muscle tone.[134]

Acidosis is an increase in the extracellular hydrogen ion concentration. This increase results in

increased movement of hydrogen ions into the cells, which is called "tissue buffering." The increased movement of positively-charged hydrogen ions into the cells results in an increased movement of positively charged potassium ions out of the cells in order to maintain electrical neutrality of both intracellular and extracellular fluids.[134] Depending on the rate of potassium loss from the cells and from the body, the plasma potassium concentration may be increased, decreased, or unchanged.

When extensive fluid losses occur rapidly, the losses are primarily from the extracellular space which results in hypovolemia; whereas, when they occur more slowly, there is a more nearly equal loss of fluids from all body compartments.[134] Hypovolemia results in less tissue perfusion and reduced hepatic and renal blood flow. The resulting tissue hypoxia increases lactic acid production. In addition, there is a decrease in hepatic uptake of lactic acid. As a result, lactic acidosis may occur which worsens the acidosis resulting from the intestinal loss of bicarbonate. Hyperkalemia may result from the decrease in renal blood flow and increase in potassium movement out of cells in response to tissue buffering. In contrast, when fluid losses occur more slowly, hypokalemia is more likely. However, regardless of the plasma potassium, sodium, or chloride concentrations, the diarrheic animal has a total body deficit of these electrolytes and of water.

DIAGNOSIS OF CAUSES OF DIARRHEA

Diarrhea is the most common problem related to intestinal disease. However, bulky or excessively firm stools also may be signs of intestinal disorders or dysfunction of associated organs of digestion (liver and pancreas). The client should be asked about weight loss, vomiting, stool quantity, duration of diarrhea, and whether the diarrhea is continuous or intermittent. Continuous diarrhea is usually associated with organic disease; whereas, periods of diarrhea interspersed with passage of normal feces suggests a functional disorder.[31] A history of exposure to other animals with diarrhea suggests parasitic, viral or, less commonly, bacteria-induced diarrhea. Working dogs, such as guide dogs, police dogs, or those subjected to obedience training, have a higher incidence of stress-induced diarrhea.[31] A stress-induced diarrhea is also suggested by a recent change in environment. Stress-induced diarrhea should be suspected if diarrhea is intermittent in a healthy dog and is mainly large-bowel in character.[31] The

presence of blood, melena, undigested fat or food, or mucus in the feces should be determined.

To determine the cause, prognosis, and therapy of abnormal stools, an effort should be made initially to localize the problem to either the small or large bowel. A good history plus physical examination and observation of feces usually provides ample information on which to base the decision of whether small or large bowel signs predominate. Table 3 compares the clinical signs associated with the origin of chronic diarrhea.

Abnormal stools of small bowel origin are characterized by a watery or mushy consistency. The amount of stool passed may be normal or

TABLE 3

DIFFERENTIATION OF SMALL INTESTINE FROM LARGE INTESTINE DIARRHEA[33,34]

Clinical Sign	Small Intestine	Large Intestine
Feces		
Volume	Increased > 3 times	Increased 1–3 times
Mucus	Rare	Common
Blood	When present— melena, except in acute hemorrhagic diarrhea	Red (fresh) blood common
Fat or undigested food	May be present	Absent
Defecation		
Urgency	Absent unless very severe	Usually present
Tenesmus (prolonged squatting)	Absent	Frequently present
Frequency (normal 1–2/day)	3–5 times daily	Usually > 5 times daily
Difficult or painful	No	Present with distal colonic or rectal disease
Ancillary signs		
Weight loss	Sometimes	Rare except in severe colitis, diffuse tumors or histoplasmosis
General malaise	Sometimes	Rare
Vomiting	May be present with inflammatory diseases Often associated with eating	Occurs in 30% of dogs with colitis but is unrelated to eating
Flatulence and Borborygmus	Sometimes	Absent
Halitosis with no oral disease	Sometimes	Absent

increased. Frequency of defecation may be moderately increased. Stools do not usually contain mucus or blood. Blood, if present, is usually digested, resulting in melena.

Acute severe malassimilation of nutrients causes rapid fluid loss, electrolyte loss, and metabolic acidosis. Dehydration and depression soon develop. Malassimilation caused by malabsorption may result from defects in the mucosa, submucosa, or lympatics of the intestinal wall. Regardless of the site, the net effect is similar: Nutrients are not absorbed, water absorption is inhibited, and watery feces develop. Malassimilation from maldigestion is caused by a relative or absolute lack of pancreatic enzymes or bile. The effect of maldigestion is similar to malabsorption, except that stools tend to be bulky.

In addition to determining if diarrhea is due to small or large intestinal dysfunction, categorizing diarrhea as acute or chronic is clinically useful. As described in Table 4, acute diarrhea due to either small or large intestine dysfunctions generally has an abrupt onset and a short clinical course that ranges from transient and self-limiting to fulminating and life-threatening. In acute diarrhea, the elaborate gastrointestinal function tests used for chronic diarrhea are usually not necessary.

Acute Small Bowel Diarrhea

The minimum data for determining the cause of acute small bowel diarrhea should include:

1. History
2. Physical examination
3. Fecal flotations and colonic smears (at least three)

4. Survey radiographs (reserved for cases where palpation is difficult and obstruction is a possibility)
5. Serum amylase or lipase (reserved for cases with tense abdomen and vomition)
6. Parameters needed for administering and monitoring fluid therapy, e.g. hematocrit, plasma protein, potassium, and bicarbonate or total carbon dioxide concentrations

The following conditions should be considered as causes of acute small-bowel diarrhea. Figure 4 may be helpful in determining the cause of diarrhea.

1. Viral enteritis.[7,171,189]
    a. **Canine distemper**
    Affected dogs usually present with respiratory or neurologic signs; however, severe enteritis is the principal or sole manifestation in a few. Severe bloody diarrhea, dehydration, depression, and rapid weight loss can be the only presenting signs, or these signs may accompany "classic" distemper, occurring together with ocular and respiratory discharges, coughing, dyspnea, and neurologic disorders. These latter signs help differentiate distemper from parvoviral enteritis, but in their absence, clinical differentiation may be impossible. Both diseases can cause leukopenia, and both are most likely to be encountered in puppies or in dogs with a history of inadequate vaccination.

    b. **Canine coronavirus**
    Affects dogs of any age after a 1-3 day incubation period, which is followed by

TABLE 4

CLASSIFICATION OF DIARRHEA[35]

SMALL INTESTINE	
Acute	Chronic
Usually less than 48 hours in duration. Variable volume; seldom contains mucus. Fresh or partly digested blood not uncommon. Patients are usually inappetent or anorexic so no steatorrhea. Feces brown or red. Defecation has sense of urgency and increased frequency. Tenesmus present. Dyschezia absent. **Symptomatic therapy usually effective.**	Usually 7–10 days or longer in duration. Large volume, little or no mucus, blood if present is melena. Steatorrhea in maldigestion or malabsorption. Feces brown, little urgency, no tenesmus. Frequency 2–3 times normal. Dyschezia absent; weight loss may occur. Can often be controlled by dietary manipulation. **Specific diagnosis and therapy essential.**

LARGE INTESTINE	
Acute	Chronic
Usually less than 48 hours in duration. Feces are small volume, mucus may be abundant and fresh blood frequent; no steatorrhea. Fecal leucocytes abundant. Much urgency; "accidents" in house are common. Tenesmus is frequent and severe. Marked increase in frequency of defecation. Dyschezia variable, may be severe. **Symptomatic therapy usually effective; may become chronic.**	Usually 7–10 days or longer in duration (may be months). Feces are small volume, usually with abundant mucus; blood usually but not invariably present. Defecation associated with sense of urgency; accidents in the house are common. Tenesmus is common, frequency of defecation markedly increased. Dyschezia present if rectum involved. **Biopsy and specific therapy essential.**

FIGURE 4

DETERMINING THE CAUSE OF DIARRHEA

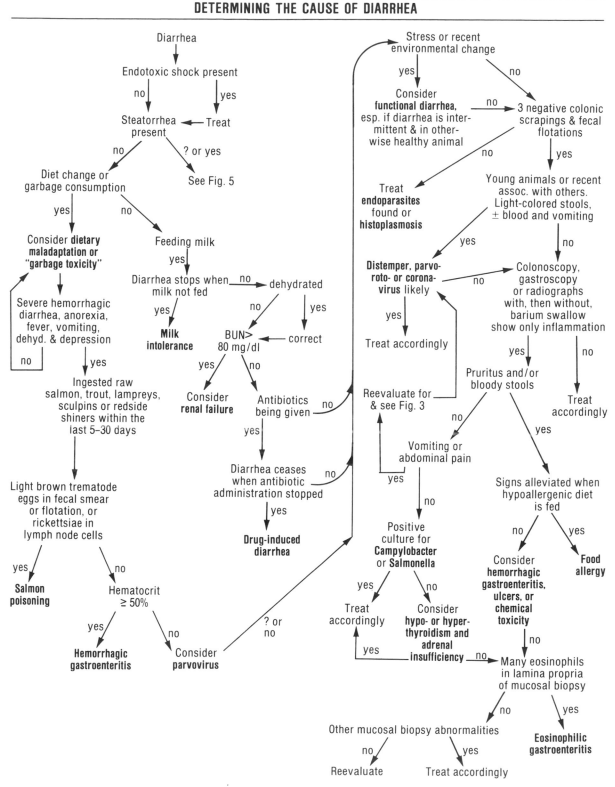

shedding of virus for several weeks. Usually there is a sudden onset of diarrhea, vomiting, depression, anorexia and weakness. Stools are loose, mucoid, usually orange, and foul smelling; infrequently, they contain blood. Recovery generally is complete within 7-10 days, but diarrhea may continue for 3-4 weeks. Occasionally, puppies die within two days. Leukopenia and fever usually are not present.

c. **Canine parvovirus**

As with coronavirus, dogs of all ages are susceptible, although clinical illness occurs primarily in puppies 6-20 weeks of age.[171] A higher incidence occurs in Doberman Pinschers and Rottweilers.[79] The disease may be subclinical to severe, depending on exposure, immunity, stress, nutritional status, and the presence or absence of intestinal parasites. However, there is usually a sudden onset of severe signs. In one study, the disease was fatal in 92% of 40 dogs which were all at least 8 months of age.[193]

Clinical signs are similar to those occuring with coronavirus except that with parvovirus: 1) vomiting is more severe and protracted; 2) stools are often hemorrhagic, darker colored, more watery, and less odorous; 3) diarrhea frequently is more acute; 4) fever, and in severe cases with concurrent infection or parasitism, severe leukopenia, especially lymphopenia, are present unless a secondary bacterial infection induces leukocytosis; and 5) in contrast to hemorrhagic gastroenteritis, the hematocrit is usually normal or reduced. The presence of leukopenia is associated with a poor prognosis and the need for aggressive treatment.[28] However, in one study any one of these signs or effects occurred in only 30-60% of dogs with parvovirus.[193]

Canine parvovirus may cause myocarditis and acute congestive heart failure in 4-12 week-old pups, although this is now rare because almost all dams are immune.[170] In contrast, many cases of myocarditis were reported when this disease was first identified in 1978.[170] Parvoviruses are a common cause of acute diarrhea in young dogs and cats.

d. **Feline panleukopenia or parvovirus**

This is one of the more common infectious diseases of cats. Its effects are similar to those of canine parvovirus.

e. **Feline coronavirus**

This virus is serologically different from feline infectious peritonitis (FIP), or canine coronavirus, and is shed in the feces by many asymptomatic cats. It causes a mild enteritis, diarrhea, and intermittent vomiting, particularly in 4-12 week-old kittens. Anorexia and dehydration are uncommon and occur only in severe cases.

2. **Bacterial enteritis**

Escherichia coli, clostridia, salmonellae and *Campylobacter jejuni* are common bacterial causes of diarrhea in many species but rarely cause diarrhea in dogs and cats.[7,189] All are commonly excreted in the feces of clinically normal dogs and cats.

Salmonella-induced diarrhea resembles that occurring with canine coronavirus and most commonly affects young, debilitated or stressed animals, or those being given antimicrobial drugs orally. Outbreaks thought to be caused by salmonellae resulting in anorexia, vomiting, diarrhea with mucus and blood, leukocytosis (but occasional severe leukopenia), and fever, have been reported to occur in mature cats.[185]

Campylobacter jejuni has been considered a rare cause of diarrhea in dogs and cats. However, in a survey of English small animal practices, the organism was recovered from 1.6% of dogs without diarrhea and 11.7% of dogs with diarrhea; in 72% the diarrhea was chronic.[71] It affects primarily the young, particularly in those kept under poor sanitary conditions in kennels or catteries.[7,150] However, it may also affect adults.[74] Compylobacter usually causes a peracute diarrhea, often accompanied by blood and mucus, depression, ataxia, emesis, and hypoglycemia—resembling that caused by parvovirus. Clinical signs can be precipitated by stress and usually last for 5-15 days, although they may persist for as long as 4 months.[71,74] Large numbers of organisms may be found in a direct smear of fresh feces from an affected animal.[74] Erythromycin given orally is effective in treating Campylobacter diarrhea.[150] *Campylobacter jejuni* may also affect people. Transmission from pets to family members, or the reverse, may occur.

Clostridia are rarely diagnosed as a cause of diarrhea in dogs or cats but have been suggested as a possible cause of hemorrhagic gastroenteritis (see #9, page 7-32).[189] An overgrowth of clostridia causing a pseudomem-

branous colitis may develop secondary to administration of antibiotics.

3. **Intestinal parasites**

At least three random fecal flotations or direct saline smears of feces, using the procedures given in Table 5, should be performed before any of the following parasites are ruled out.

a. **Strongyloides**

Associated with diarrhea which is often bloody, and also with pneumonia. Most often affects pet-store or humane-society puppies and kittens. Anorexia, depression, vomiting, dehydration, and weight loss may occur. Diagnosis is based on finding eggs or larvae in the stools.

b. **Ancylostoma (hookworms)** (see page 7-47)

May be associated with anemia and melena.

c. **Ascarids**

Heavy ascarid infestations resulting in clinical signs usually occur in young puppies and kittens. Clinical signs include abdominal discomfort, pot-bellied appearance, stunted growth, diarrhea and/or vomiting frequently with worms in the vomitus or stools. Finding the worms in vomitus or feces and/or identifying ascarid eggs from a fecal flotation is diagnostic.

4. **Coccidia**

Usually a problem in young puppies or kittens, resulting in a watery, mucoid feces, vomiting, depression and weight loss. Eosinophilia may occur. Diagnosis is based on identification of oocysts from a direct fecal smear.

5. **Giardiasis**

The protozoan parasite, Giardia, is a common cause of diarrhea in many species of animals, including humans, dogs, cats, and occasionally

horses and calves. Some species of Giardia are species-specific and some are not.[117] Giardia in dogs and cats may represent a threat to people, although this has not been proved.[117] Clinical signs may occur in animals of any age but usually in dogs and cats less than 1-3 years old.

Giardiasis is most commonly manifested by a sudden onset of a watery or cow-pie, light-colored, mucoid stool and steatorrhea. Abnormal stools may resolve spontaneously or be intermittent or chronic, persisting for weeks to years. For example, continuous and intermittent diarrhea over several years, particularly in the young but also in adults, in a cattery and in a kennel were found to be due to giardiasis.[116,179] Young dogs, and occasionally older dogs, would typically become diarrheic 2-6 weeks after entering the kennel.

Tenesmus, flatulence, borborygmus, and vomiting may occur.[29,169] Usually there is no blood in the stools. Relapses may occur several months after spontaneous or therapeutically induced recovery. Weight loss or retarded growth rate may or may not occur. A good appetite and adequate food intake are often maintained, although some animals may become hypophagic.[117] A fluid- and gas-filled intestine may be palpated. However, the animal may appear normal despite a history of diarrhea. Routine laboratory determined blood and plasma values are not altered.

Giardia spp. exist in two forms: motile trophozoites and nonmotile cysts. Both forms are transmitted by oral consumption and are passed intermittently in the feces by dogs and cats, fluctuating from undetectible to high concentrations.[118,240] As a result, trophozoites are observed in fresh fecal smears (the only way to observe them) in only 50% or less of infected animals.[20]

In one study trophozoites were found in 19% from 1, 43% from 3, and 49% from 6 fecal samples obtained on separate days.[240] Zinc sulfate concentration is the best procedure for finding cysts, but revealed their presence in only 50% of infected animals from 1 fecal sample and 94% from 3 fecal samples obtained on successive days.[240] Sugar and salt solutions render cysts unrecognizable. Use of a direct fecal smear* is recommended as a

TABLE 5

DIAGNOSIS OF INTESTINAL PARASITES[186]

Procedure	Diagnostic Finding
Fecal examinations	
Visual inspection	Tapeworm proglottids
Flotation (conventional)	Nematode and cestode ova
Flotation (zinc sulfate)	*Giardia* and coccidia cysts
Saline suspension	Protozoan trophozoites
Sedimentation/Baerman	*Strongyloides* larvae
Duodenal aspiration	*Giardia* trophozoites
Colonoscopy	Adult whipworms
Therapeutic trial	
Response to fenbendazole	Occult trichuriasis
Response to metronidazole	Occult giardiasis

*Suspend a sample of *fresh* feces in a drop of isotonic saline solution on a slide, apply a coverslip, examine at 100 and 400 magnification for Giardia trophozoites, which are pear-shaped with a posterior flagella and two nuclei which look like eyes. They dart around in an erratic circular pattern.

screening test. If the result is negative, do a zinc sulfate concentration* and look for cysts.[117,240] If it is negative, repeat this procedure two more times, using fecal samples taken on different days, or treat and assess the response. If results of all tests are negative or the animal does not respond to treatment, giardiasis is unlikely to be the cause of the diarrhea.[240]

Metronidazole (Table 1) has been considered the treatment of choice. This treatment eliminated cyst excretion in all 4 cats treated in one study,[118] but was only 67% effective in dogs.[241] Quinacrine (Table 1) was 100% effective in eliminating excretion of giardia by dogs.[241] However, 45% of these dogs when treated with quinacrine had some degree of anorexia, and 27% developed fever and lethargy. Because side effects are uncommon after metronidazole administration, and because it is 100% effective against **trichomoniasis,** it is recommended.[241] Trichomoniasis was found in 30% of dogs with giardiasis.[241] Although the pathogenicity of trichomonas in dogs has not been confirmed, anecdotal clinical experience suggests that they may cause diarrhea, especially in young animals, and therefore trichomoniasis warrants treatment.[241]

Dogs with giardiasis that do not respond to metronizabole should be treated with quinacrine.[241] Tinidazole (Table 1) has been shown to be as effective as metronidazole against both giardiasis and trichomoniasis and has the advantage of less frequent administration and a shorter course of therapy.[241] Furazolidone (Table 1) was also found equally effective to metronidazole in cats.[118] Ipronidazole added to the drinking water (126 mg/L) was effective in dogs.[1] A response to therapy may be noted in 12-24 hours and clinical signs alleviated in 2-3 days. Corticosteroid administration delays spontaneous recovery and partially inhibits the effects of these drugs.[118]

Reinfection with Giardia cysts was prevented in a cattery by cleaning all cages with detergent and thoroughly soaking them with a dilute bleach solution (sodium hypochlorite,

final concentration 1% by weight) twice during a 5-day treatment of all cats with furazolidone.[116] Giardia cysts are reported to be sensitive to sodium hypochlorite solutions.[103,112]

6. **Foreign body**
Partial intestinal obstruction may cause diarrhea but vomiting and abdominal distention are more common. Abdominal palpation and survey radiographs of the abdomen are indicated.

7. **Toxins**
Garbage, arsenic, lead, thallium and organophosphates can all cause diarrhea. History of exposure or concomitant systemic signs may provide clues to this diagnosis.

8. **Acute pancreatitis**
Usually associated with abdominal pain and acute vomiting (see page 7-17).

9. **Hemorrhagic gastroenteritis**
Affects all ages and breeds but especially young adults of small breeds. The cause is unknown. Clinical signs resemble those of parvovirus (page 7-30). They often begin suddenly in a previously healthy dog, with hematemesis followed by a severe bloody diarrhea with a fetid odor and jam-like stool consistency. If untreated, the animal will die within a few hours. The hematocrit is greater than 50% which, in conjunction with the clinical signs, is helpful in differentiating this disease from parvovirus.

10. **Drug induced**
a. Oral administration of chloramphenicol, neomycin, ampicillin, or tetracycline for 3-5 days in amounts used therapeutically have caused intestinal mucosal damage, and a malabsorption-induced diarrhea in calves.[176,177]

b. Antibacterial therapy may adversely affect normal intestinal flora, resulting in diarrhea.

c. Individual sensitivity or intolerance may occur, particularly to aspirin, indomethacin, digitalis, dithiazanine, anthelmintic drugs, and some anti-cancer drugs, such as cyclophosphamide.

11. **Food intolerance**
Overeating, rapid change in diet, or excessive lactose consumption can result in an acute diarrheal episode (for explanation of cause see pages 7-25 & 26). History is often helpful in confirming this diagnosis.

12. **Food allergy** [11,120,196]
Dietary hypersensitivity in dogs and cats results in a generalized pruritus usually without

---

*1) Mix 331 g of zinc sulfate in 1 liter of warm tap water. A specific gravity of 1.18 is wanted. 2) Mix 1 ml of feces (need not be fresh, but not frozen) in a 15 ml centrifuge tube one-half full of tap water. 3) Add water until tube is 2/3 full. 4) Centrifuge for 10 minutes at 400 times gravity. 5) Discard supernatant. 6) Resuspend sediment in the zinc sulfate solution. 7) Repeat step 4. 8) Remove a sample from the surface with a wire loop or capillary tube. 9) Put sample on a microscople slide and apply a coverslip. 10) Examine at 100 and 400 magnification for cysts. Giardia cysts are occasionally misdiagnosed as coccida oocysts as they are somewhat similar in appearance.

gastrointestinal signs. Gastrointestinal signs occur in only 10-15% of dogs with food-allergy induced pruritus.[154] In one report, 4 of 18 cats had gastrointestinal signs,[223] 0 of 4 cats in another,[12] and 2 of 30 dogs in another report.[230] In some cases, however, a voluminous, watery, often hemorrhagic diarrhea may occur. Less often the stools are just poorly formed and passed more often and in greater quantity. Vomiting, flatulence and borborygmus may occur with, or without, the presence of abnormal stools. If pruritus is present, these gastrointestinal signs are probably due to a food allergy. Uncommonly, a food allergy may result in chronic diarrhea without pruritus.[196,230] Food allergy may also result in superfical recurrent pyodermas, with or without pruritus and should be considered as a possible cause of these conditions.[230]

Other causes of pruritus, the most common being atopy (inhalant) and fleabite allergic dermatitis, are not associated with gastrointestinal signs. In addition, atopy begins with a mild pruritus that worsens with time; whereas, with food allergy, the onset of clinical signs is abrupt, and often explosive. The ensuing course is relatively static and is exacerbated by chronic self-trauma and secondary complications including pyodermas and seborrhea. Erythema, and papules, particularly on the face, neck, feet, back, and ventral abdomen, are the most predominant clinical signs.[230] Alopecia, hyperpigmentation, and seborrhea appear in repeatedly traumatized areas. Bilateral pruritic ceruminous otitis externa is usually present and occasionally may occur without generalized signs. Most affected animals are constantly pruritic, and no association with eating is observed. There is no predilection by breed, sex, age, or season.[230] Only one animal in a group is usually affected, although all may be fed the same diet.

Fleabite allergic dermatosis, in contrast to food allergy, is seasonal in some geographic areas. It affects particularly the dorsal lumbosacral region and may affect more than one animal in a group. Atopy is also seasonal and usually manifests before the animal is 3 years of age. The presence of greater than 10% eosinophils suggests an allergy,[120] but is not present in many cases.[125] Intradermal testing for fleabite allergic dermatitis should be done using a 1:1000 weight-to-volume dilution of flea antigen (Greer Labs). The reaction is read at 0.25, 24, 48, and 72 hours.

Other causes of pruritus include mange, dermatophytosis, pemphigus, irritant-contact dermatitis, hypersensitivity to intestinal parasites in young dogs, and drug allergies, including insulin.[230] Diagnosis of mange can be made from skin scrapings, and of dermatophytosis from Wood's lamp examination or fungal culture. Ninety-eight percent of all dermatophyte infections in cats are reportedly due to *Microsporum canis*. In a darkened room under a Wood's lamp, *Microsporum canis* infected hairs are blue-green.[159]

With food allergies, the offending food allergin is usually in the commercial pet food the animal has been consuming for an extended period of time. In one study, 68% of affected animals had been exposed to the offending antigen for 2 years or more before clinical manifestations became evident.[224] In one report hypersensitivities of dogs to various foodstuffs were: beef and/or milk 80%, cereals 5%, food additives 5%; and pork, horsemeat, chicken, egg, fish, and fungal contaminants in drinking water made-up the remainder.[11] Because the offending antigen is usually found in most commercial pet foods, changing brands rarely helps.[11,230] However, most cases are due to a single allergin. In one report, multiple sensitivities were observed only in 12 of 500 dogs and cats with dietary hypersensitivity.[224]

Skin testing and blood tests (radioallergosorbent test or RAST, and cytotoxic testing) are of minimal benefit in diagnosing food allergy.[125,230] False positive results are common with these tests.[125] Diagnosis and treatment are best accomplished in the following manner:[11]

a. If secondary skin complications are present, initially give antimicrobial therapy for 3 weeks, and weekly antiseborrheic and antibacterial shampoos with moisturizing rinses and otic preparations if necessary. On day 14 begin the following procedures.

b. Hospitalize.

c. Institute a 48-hour fast and give distilled drinking water.

d. Give 3 enemas at 12-hour intervals to remove residual antigens. Response to introduction of a hypoallergenic diet is slower if residual dietary antigens are not removed from the intestinal tract in this manner.

e. After the fast, feed a hypoallergenic diet (see Appendix Table 1) in at least 2 meals

TABLE 6

TESTS FOR DIAGNOSIS OF PANCREATIC EXOCRINE INSUFFICIENCY, MALABSORPTION, AND INTESTINAL BACTERIAL OVERGROWTH

Test	Normal	Pancreatic Insufficiency	Malabsorption
Stools			
Appearance	Normal	Bulky, cow-pie like	Profuse, watery
Fat droplets in acidified, warmed fecal emulsion	<2-3/low-power field[a]	Many, of large size	Absent to few in number. May be smaller in size. Severe cases—numerous
Fatty acid crystals[b]	Absent	Absent	May be present
Muscle fibers[b]	Occasional	Many	Occasional
Starch granules[b]	Absent to Occasional	Many	Absent to Occasional
Trypsin gel or x-ray film digestion[b]	Liquidification of gelatin or clearing of unexposed film	Absent	Present but 50% false negatives
Lipemia 1-3 hrs after oral administration of 3 ml/kg of cream or oil[c,d]			
pre-enzyme hydrolysis	Present	Absent	Absent
after-enzyme hydrolysis	Present	Present	Absent
Plasma trypsin activity[c,e]	5–35 μg/L	<2.5 μg/L	5–35 μg/L
PABA absorption[c,f] (give 50 mg in 5 ml of water/kg orally)	>400 μg/dl in plasma at 30 min & >600 at 60 min in dogs.[242] In cats >125 μg/dl at 60 or 90 min[88]	Less than normal	Normal or in dogs concentration at 60 min < concentration at 120 min
D-Xylose absorption[c] (give 0.5 g/kg orally)	9–12g/5 hr in urine or >45 mg/dl in plasma by 60–90 min in dogs[g]	Normal	Decreased in most dogs Decreased with bacterial overgrowth.[82,94] Increased in plasma and decreased in urine with reduced renal function.
Glucose absorption[c] (give 2g/kg orally)	Blood glucose increased by 30–35 mg/dl or more	Normal or greater and prolonged increase	Below normal increase which also occurs with bacterial overgrowth.[82,94] False normals may occur.
Intestinal biopsy	Normal histology	Normal histology	Clubbing and flattening of villi, thickening of mucosa and/or dilation of lymphatics
24-hr fat excretion[h]	dogs <5 g & cats <3.5 g	Increased up to 20–50 g	Increased
% dietary fat absorbed[h]	>90%	<85%	40–90%
Breath hydrogen (ppm)[c,i]		Increased with bacterial overgrowth[94] and decreased with intestinal ischemia[166]	
Fasting[226,227]	0.9 ± 0.1	3.6 ± 0.9	5.3 ± 1.3
2 hr after giving 0.5 g xylose/kg[226,227]	3.6 ± 0.4	19.0 ± 2.0	35.5 ± 7.2
Iodine 131 – Triolein[c]	8–15% absorption	Low absorption	Low absorption
Iodine 131 – Oleic acid[c]	10–15% absorption	Normal	Low absorption
Serum folate concentration[c,14-16]	<10 μg/L	Above normal if bacterial overgrowth is present	
Serum vit. B$_{12}$ concentration[c,14-16]	>200 ng/L	Below normal if bacterial overgrowth is present	
Nitrosonapthol[j]	Negative	Positive suggests presence of intestinal bacterial overgrowth	

[a]< Indicates less than and > greater than

[b]False negatives are common and, therefore, these tests are of little benefit.

[c]Should be measured, or test conducted, after a 12–24 hr fast. The development of a plasma xylose assay increases the clinical usefulness of this test.[145]

[d]If lipemia does not occur after cream or oil administration, wait several hours, mix pancreatic enzyme powder (Viokase-V, AH Robins) with the cream or oil, allow mixture to remain at room temperature for at least 30 minutes, then repeat test. This is the initial test recommended because it is simple and reliable. In one study, this test indicated the correct diagnosis in 93% of dogs tested.[242] Combined with clinical signs and physical exam, the test provides a sound basis for trial therapy with a highly digestible diet (see Appendix Table 1) and pancreatic enzymes (Table 1).

TABLE 6—Continued

[e]This is the most sensitive test for diagnosing pancreatic exocrine insufficiency.[14,232,233] Plasma trypsin activity is increased by renal insufficiency[140] and can be obtained by sending 1 ml of serum (does not need to be kept cold) to Box J-126JHMHC, University of Florida, Gainesville, FL 32610. Enzymatic assay kit (Trypsik Kit, Damon Diagnostics) for humans is not likely to be of benefit for other species as trypsin-like immunoreactivity exhibits a high degree of species specificity.

[f]Also called BT-PABA and bentiromide (Chymex, Adria Labs, Columbus, Ohio) which is cleaved by pancreatic chymotrypsin allowing passive absorption of PABA and subsequent excretion in the urine. In normal cats, peak plasma concentration is reached at 60–90 minutes and is 386 ± 134 $\mu g/dl$ (95% confidence interval 127–645).[88] Thus, a concentration below 125 is abnormal and may indicate presence of pancreatic exocrine insufficiency, although this has not been confirmed.

[g]Normal values for cats are about one-half those for dogs, are highly variable between individual cats, and are not significantly decreased with intestinal disease.[88]

[h]Meaningful **only** if animal is eating a sufficient amount of food containing at least 10% fat (dry matter basis) to meet its caloric need. When this is the case, the values given are valid, regardless of the diet consumer or size of the animal.[89,133]

[i]Fermentation of unabsorbed carbohydrate by intestinal bacteria results in the generation of hydrogen gas, a portion of which is absorbed and excreted by the lungs. There is a quantitative relationship between the amount of unabsorbed carbohydrate and pulmonary hydrogen excretion.[227] This test is a more sensitive indicator of decreased carbohydrate absorption than either glucose or xylose absorption tests,[226] but is not used clinically because few are equipped to measure breath hydrogen excretion.

[j]Excess bacteria in small intestine convert dietary tyrosine to 4-hydroxyphenylacetic acid which is absorbed, excreted in the urine, and can be detected by the nitrosonaphol test. Although this test is not specific for bacterial overgrowth in the small intestine, it gives an indication of which animals with chronic diarrhea might benefit from antibiotic therapy.[40] All reagents needed are inexpensive and stable. The test procedure is:[40] 1) put 1 ml of 2.63 N nitric acid in a test tube, 2) add 1 drop of sodium nitrite followed by 0.1 ml of 0.1% 1-nitroso-2 napthol (Eastman Organic Chemicals) made by dissolving 100 mg of this compound in 95% ethanol and diluting to 100 ml with 95% ethanol, 3) add 6 drops (about 0.15 ml) of urine to the test tube and mix, 4) the appearance of an orange-red color within 5 minutes is positive, whereas the maintenance of the original yellow color for at least 5 minutes is negative.

daily and **restricted** to the amount needed for maintenance. A hypoallergenic diet must contain ingredients not previously encountered by the patient and ideally as few ingredients as possible.

f. Send the patient home with instructions to the client to continue feeding the hypoallergenic diet and distilled water, and to avoid all other potential sources of dietary antigens, including rawhide chews, toys, table scraps, vitamin-mineral supplements, other sources of water, and access to the food and feces of other animals.

g. Response rarely occurs in the first week, but improvement will usually be apparent by the second or third week. When improvement does occur, reinstitute regular drinking water rather than distilled. If no change occurs within 7 days the client has the choice of: 1) confirming that a food allergy is present and trying to identify the offending food ingredient so that it can be avoided or 2) maintaining the animal on the hypoallergenic diet.

h. When clients make this choice they should know that food hypersensitivity is lifelong and that signs can be alleviated only by avoiding the offending food. No other

treatment is effective. Corticosteroids usually result in no more than a 50% reduction in signs.

i. If the client chooses to confirm the presence of a food allergy and wants to try to find the offending food ingredient, reintroduce the original diet. An exacerbation of signs usually follows within 12-72 hours but may take as long as 5 days. Exacerbation confirms the presence of a food allergy.

j. If signs recur, immediately return the dog to the hypoallergenic diet and give prednisolone (0.5 mg/lb each morning for 3-5 days). In most cases signs cease within 5-7 days.

k. Once signs cease, mix a small amount of one of the ingredients in the original diet, into the daily ration of the hypoallergenic diet. If there is no resumption of signs within 7 days, try a different ingredient until the offending ingredient is found. Life-long avoidance of that ingredient will be necessary to prevent recurrence.

Chronic Small-Bowel Diarrhea

If steatorrhea is grossly visible, the cause should be determined as described beginning on page 7-38

and as illustrated in Figure 5. If steatorrhea is not obvious, it has been recommended that since most dogs with chronic diarrhea but no steatorrhea respond to the initial management given on page 7-40 (steps 1-6), they be evaluated further only if they do not respond.[38] If the patient does not respond, the following data for diagnosis of chronic small-bowel diarrhea should be obtained.

1. History will usually indicate whether there is small or large intestinal dysfunction (Table 3, page 7-27).

2. Fecal smears and flotations on at least three random samples as described in Table 5, page 7-30.

3. Qualitative fecal-fat analysis
   The efficacy of this test is greatly increased by ensuring that the emulsion of equal parts feces and water is acidified and warmed to body temperature before a fat stain is added, and it is viewed for brightly stained spherical fat droplets.

4. Oral fat absorption test pre- and post-enzyme hydrolysis as described in Table 6. If the findings are not conclusive, have serum trypsin immunoreactivity measured or conduct the para-aminobenzoic acid (PABA) absorption test (Table 6). Glucose or xylose absorption tests can be conducted at the same time as fat or PABA absorption tests.

5. Complete blood counts and serum total protein and albumin concentrations for interpretation as described in Table 7.

6. Urinalysis

7. BUN

8. Colonic mucosal scraping

The following conditions should be considered as a cause of chronic diarrhea. Decreased fat digestion and absorption and, as a result, steatorrhea is not generally a prominent feature of these diseases, although occasionally steatorrhea as well as diarrhea may occur. In contrast, both chronic steatorrhea and diarrhea are generally a prominent aspect of the malassimilation syndrome (page 7-38). Determining the presence of a substantial decrease in fat digestion and absorption is, therefore, quite helpful in differentiating between the diseases described in this section and those that cause malassimilation. Causes of chronic diarrhea in which steatorrhea is not a prominent feature include the following:

1. **Intestinal parasites** (see page 7-31)

2. **Eosinophilic gastroenteritis**
   Most affected dogs and some cats have diarrhea, anorexia and, in some cases, progres-

TABLE 7

HEMATOLOGIC CHANGES WITH INTESTINAL DISEASE[186]

Hematologic Parameter	Clinical Associations
Neutrophils	
Increased	Inflammatory or Infectious diseases
Decreased	Parvovirus, Endotoxemia, or Overwhelming sepsis
Eosinophils	
Increased	Parasitism (e.g., hookworms, whipworms), Eosinophilic gastroenteritis, or Hypoadrenocorticism
Monocytes	
Increased	Chronic or granulomatous inflammation Systemic mycoses
Lymphocytes	
Decreased	Lymphangiectasia
Hematocrit	
Above 50%	Hemorrhagic gastroenteritis
Decreased	Enteric blood loss, or Anemia of malnutrition or chronic inflammation
Plasma proteins	
Increased	Basenji enteropathy
Decreased	Lymphangiectasia, Other protein-losing enteropathies, Blood loss

sive weight loss. These clinical signs may be chronic and persistent or cyclic, lasting for 2-3 days, then resolving for 6-30 days. Vomiting is often the major effect of this disease in cats (see page 7-19). In both dogs and cats eosinophilia, although associated with this condition, may occur only while clinical signs are occurring and is not specific for this disease. Two or three hemograms may be needed to detect eosinophilia. Large numbers of eosinophils in the lamina propria of a gastric or intestinal biopsy provide definitive proof of this disorder, although diagnosis is often made by exclusion or response to therapy. Eosinophil infiltration of the intestinal wall may be diffuse or segmental. The segmental or multifocal form has been reported to be induced by *Toxocara canis* visceral larval migrans and to respond to oral administration of either thiabendazole or fenbendazole (Table 1).[108,218] About the last day of treatment, or several days thereafter, diarrhea stops. If it does not stop, most dogs and cats respond to prednisolone administration (Table 1) and feeding a hypoallergenic diet[212] (Prescription Diet d/d, Hill's).

3. **Intestinal Neoplasia**

In most cases, intestinal neoplasia results in obstructive disorders of the intestinal lumen, which causes vomiting (see page 7-18). A barium series may demonstrate this obstruction. Nonobstructive adenocarcinomas and infiltrative neoplasia of the gut wall, such as lymphosarcoma, mast cell tumor, or adenocarcinoma, may result in chronic malabsorption, diarrhea, weight loss, protein-losing enteropathy, and a palpably thickened bowel. Steatorrhea may or may not occur. Although intestinal tumors occur predominantly in older dogs and cats, lymphosarcoma can occur in younger animals and is suggested by the presence of immature lymphocytes.

4. **Gastric or duodenal ulcers**

Ulcers may result in chronic diarrhea, often with melena and vomiting (see page 7-19).

5. **Functional or psychological diarrhea**

This is common and is suspected from the history and exclusion of organic disease. It may occur in conjunction with the spastic or irritable colon syndrome (page 7-46). It is most common in German Shepherd dogs, working dogs, and dogs subjected to excessive stress. Diarrhea is often intermittent, there is no loss of condition and results of intestinal function tests are normal.[33]

6. **Feline hyperthyroidism**

This is a common condition, particularly in older cats. It results in weight loss and poor condition, even though food intake is not reduced. It is confirmed by a TSH stimulation test (see page 6-5).

7. **Lymphocytic-plasmacytic enteritis and frequently colitis**

This disease occurs due to infiltration of the lamina propria by lymphocytes and plasma cells. A biopsy is necessary for diagnosis. It occurs in mature dogs and cats after many small intestinal insults. The cause is usually unknown. It results in malabsorption and, in most cases, intermittent vomiting (vomitus often contains bile), chronic diarrhea, often protein-loosing enthropathy, and occasionally lymphangiectasia. These effects result in steatorrhea and weight loss. Signs often occur intermittently. A thickened intestine may be palpated.

Generally there is response to feeding small amounts frequently of a highly digestible diet (Prescription Diets i/d for dogs and Feline c/d for cats,[158] Hills, or Recipes 1 or 8, Appendix Table 3) Some dogs and cats that do not respond to these diets within 2 weeks may instead respond to a hypoallergenic diet (Prescription Diet d/d, Hill's, or Recipe 6, Appendix Table 3). In one study clinical signs resolved in 5 of 6 affected cats within two weeks after dietary therapy began.[158] Diets containing different protein sources should be fed before dietary therapy is discarded. Failure to do so may result in reliance on chronic drug therapy.[158] The administration of corticosteroids and antibiotics, such as metronidazole or tylosine to control bacterial overgrowth (Table 1) may be beneficial in initial management and long-term when there is insufficient response to dietary management. Sulfasalazine (Table 1) administration may also be of benefit.[30,158]

8. **Immunoproliferative enteropathy of Basenjis**[24,25,26]

This condition is thought to be due to autosomal recessive inheritance, resulting in lymphoplasmocytic infiltration of the gastrointestinal lamina propria. Multiple other organ systems, including the skin, liver, adrenal, and thyroid, are also affected. A chronic, intermittent, progressivly worsening diarrhea and occasional vomiting may develop shortly after the dog is born, or not until it is several years old. Some affected dogs may have intermittent anorexia; others have excellent appetites but continue to lose weight. Affected dogs remain alert and active. Clinical signs are often initiated by stress. Hypergammaglobulinemia (greater than 1.2 g/dl) is an unusual feature of this disease which, in conjunction with hypoalbuminemia (less than 2.0 g/dl) and clinical signs, suggest this disease.

An intestinal biopsy is needed to confirm the diagnosis but is contraindicated if the plasma albumin is less than 2 g/dl, as such dogs are at risk of dehiscence of the biopsy site. Treatment is the same as for lymphocytic-plasmacytic enteritis described above. Survival time after first appearance of clinical signs is generally less than 2 years although a few live 5 years. Recovery is rare.

9. **Histoplasmosis**

In dogs this disease causes granulomatous lesions of either or both the lungs, or intestinal tract, lymph nodes, or colon. Although not contagious, other animals and people may be exposed to the same source of infection.[108] The most common signs of the disease are a chronic cough and an intractable, chronic diarrhea (often containing blood). Progressive weight loss, lassitude, anemia, ascites, hepato-

megaly, splenomegaly, and peripheral lymphadenopathy may occur. Diagnosis is made by
finding the organisms in macrophages obtained from colonic scrapings or in lymph
nodes or white blood cells. Treatment is keto-
conazole or amphotericin B (Table 1).[108] Relapses requiring retreatment may occur when
dosages lower than those given in Table 1 are
used.

10. **Campylobacter jejuni**
    This organism usually causes acute diarrhea,
    but diarrhea occasionally persists for several
    months (see page 7-30).

MALASSIMILATION SYNDROME

Although steatorrhea may occur with several of
the dysfunctions responsible for causing chronic,
small-bowel diarrhea, it is seldom a prominent
feature of the disease. In contrast, steatorrhea is
the hallmark of the condition commonly called the
"malabsorption or malassimilation syndrome." It
is so named because there is malassimilation of
fat, and, with some causes, also carbohydrates and
proteins. To compensate for the malassimilation
of energy-providing nutrients, more food is consumed unless the animal is too weak or anorectic,
or something interferes with its ability to ingest
food. However, often the increased food intake is
insufficient to compensate for the impaired ability
to use it. Thus, weight loss and poor condition
result. This paradox of increased food intake and
weight loss is classical for the malassimilation
syndrome. Some animals, however, may be able
to consume enough food to maintain normal body
weight and condition, particularly if a sufficient
quantity of good-quality food is available.

Regardless of whether or not weight loss occurs,
stool volume is increased. Often the stools are
foul-smelling, light- or gray-colored and greasy
(clay-like). However, the stools sometimes appear
normal. Thus, although weight loss and abnormal
stools typify most cases, the absence of both does
not rule out the presence of malassimilation syndrome. The main complaint in affected puppies
may be coprophagia. Affected dogs commonly eat
their feces because of their high fat content and
often because of a dietary energy deficit. To
determine the cause for excessive food intake,
weight loss, or an increased volume of generally
abnormal stools, begin by following the procedures outlined in Figure 1 (page 7-10). If the
problem is not corrected by following these procedures, the final step in this figure refers you to
Figure 5 for a more comprehensive evaluation of
the animal.

TABLE 8

CAUSES OF MALASSIMILATION AND THEIR EFFECTS

Organ Dysfunction	Assimilation Process Decreased	Nutrients Affected
Pancreas	Digestion	Fat, carbohydrate, protein
Small Intestine	Absorption	Fat, carbohydrate, protein
Liver	Micellerization	Fat
Lymphatics	Delivery	Fat

As shown in Table 8, four processes are needed
for fat assimilation and two for carbohydrate and
protein assimilation. A dysfunction in these processes results in malassimilation of the nutrient(s)
requiring that process for its assimilation. Because
all four processes are required for fat assimilation,
a dysfunction in any one of these processes results
in fat malassimilation and, therefore, steatorrhea.
Thus, all causes of malassimilation cause steatorrhea. Conversely, confirming the presence of steatorrhea or fat malassimilation confirms that one
of these dysfunctions is present. Following the
steps outlined in Figure 5 provides a simple approach for confirming the presence of the malassimilation syndrome and its cause, using the easiest,
least traumatic, and most accessible procedures first
and progressing to procedures that are progressively
more difficult, traumatic, expensive, or less available to most practitioners.

Pancreatic exocrine insufficiency is the most
common cause in dogs for the clinical signs that
occur with the malassimilation syndrome.[67] However, pancreatic exocrine insufficiency is uncommon in cats. Instead, hyperthyroidism, rather than
nutrient malassimilation, is most often responsible for these signs in cats.[194] More than 85% of
functional pancreatic tissue must be lost before
clinical signs occur.

If pancreatic exocrine insufficiency has been
ruled out as a cause of malassimilation, malabsorption caused by intestinal or hepatic dysfunctions, or lymphangiectasia should be investigated
as outlined in Figure 5. Tests useful in differentiating between pancreatic exocrine insufficiency
(maldigestion) and malabsorption are given in
Table 6 (page 7-34). See page 7-52 for diagnosis
of hepatic dysfunctions and their causes.

Lymphangiectasia is characterized by obstructed
or dilated lympatic channels in the small intestine due to a congenital insufficiency or, more
commonly, secondary to congestive heart failure,
portal hypertension, lymphosarcoma, histoplasmosis, or chronic enteropathies. Obstruction, rup-

FIGURE 5

DETERMINING PRESENCE AND CAUSE OF STEATORRHEA

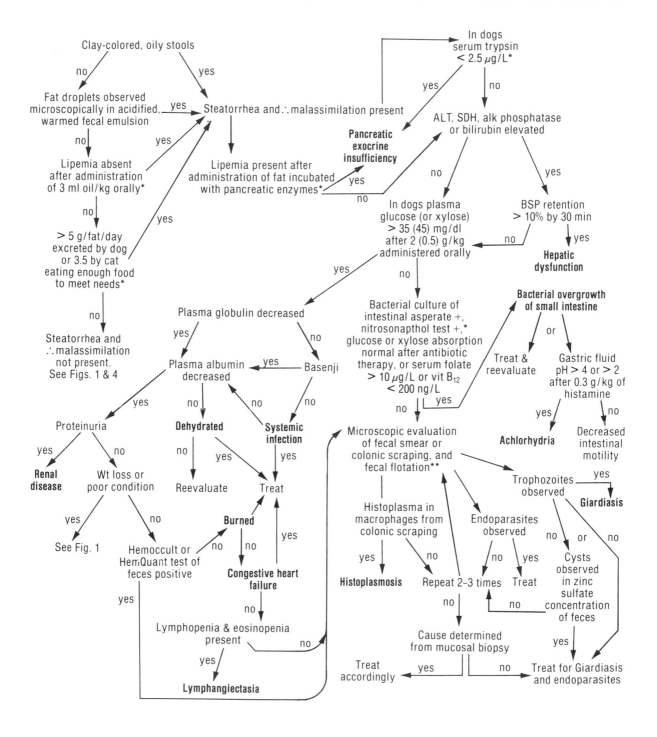

*See Table 6 page 7-34 for details on conducting and interpreting this test.
**See Table 5 page 7-30 for diagnosis of intestinal parasites.

ture or leakage of the intestinal lympatics results in the loss of lymph into the intestine lumen, abdominal cavity and/or thoracic cavity. Lymph contains substantial amounts of albumin and globulin. These losses may result in hypoproteinemia, hypocalcemia, hypocholesterolemia, lymphopenia, and eosinopenia. Diarrhea usually, but not always, occurs as do steatorrhea and effects of hypoproteinemia, including edema, ascites, and hydrothorax. Vomiting occasionally occurs. Some affected animals are anorectic and weak, whereas others may have a voracious appetite. In some, the presenting complaint may only be weight loss, and in others edema or ascites. Hypocholesterolemia may also occur because of reduced lipid absorption.

Lymphangiectasia is the most common cause of **protein-losing enteropathy.** Other causes are food allergy, chronic enteritis from any cause, chronic parasitism, histoplasmosis, diffuse intestinal lymphosarcoma, and right-sided congestive heart failure. Protein-losing enteropathy from any cause is characterized by weight loss, poor condition, and usually a chronic diarrhea. Generally both plasma albumin and globulin concentrations decrease, resulting in a generalized lessening in total plasma protein concentration and little or no change in the albumin/globulin ratio. The exception is in the Basenji, or if a systemic bacterial disease-induced increase in gamma globulin production occurs. In contrast to other breeds, Basenjis with protein-losing enteropathy usually have hypergammaglobulinemia and hypoalbuminemia, and, as a result, a decrease in the albumin/globulin ratio (see page 8-15). A decrease in both plasma albumin and globulin concentrations in other breeds with protein-losing enteropathy is similar to that occurring with blood loss and burns. It is in contrast to other causes of hypoproteinemia such as: 1) protein or calorie deficiency, or 2) hepatic disease in which albumin production is decreased, and 3) protein-losing nephropathy in which primarily albumin is lost. With these conditions, plasma albumin concentration decreases with no decrease in plasma globulin concentration. As a result, the albumin/globulin ratio is reduced. Regardless of which plasma proteins are lost, or the cause, if hypoproteinemia is sufficiently severe (albumin below 2 and often 1.3 g/dl), ascites and pitting edema may develop.

MANAGEMENT OF DIARRHEA

If water and electrolyte losses are sufficient to cause any degree of clinically apparent dehydration, correction of these deficits should always be the first objective of treatment given the diarrheic animal. Fluid and electrolyte therapy is described beginning on page 5-16.

If steatorrhea (oily, gray feces) is not evident, the following management should be instituted:[38]

1. Fast for 24-48 hours, or longer with severe intestinal disturbances such as parvovirus infection. Do not restrict water intake unless vomition occurs. Fasting allows restoration of mucosal integrity and a more rapid return of normal gastrointestinal function. In most cases, fasting reduces, or eliminates, diarrhea by removing the osmotic or irritating effects of undigested or unabsorbed nutrients.

2. Feed small amounts of food 4-6 times daily. Begin with one-third the amount needed to meet normal caloric needs. Over the next several days, gradually increase to the amount needed to maintain body weight.

3. Feed diarrheic dogs, except those in which the diarrhea is due to lymphangiectasia or colonic dysfunctions, a highly digestible, low-fiber, moderately low-fat, lactose-free diet (Prescription Diet i/d, Hill's, or Recipe 1, Appendix Table 3).

4. For dogs or cats with lymphangiectasia or colonic dysfunctions feed a high-fiber, severely restricted fat diet (Prescription Diets r/d, or instead for dogs w/d, Hill's, or Recipes 4 or 10, Appendix Table 3). If a favorable response does not occur within 1-2 weeks, or if optimal body weight and condition cannot be maintained on these diets, change to the diets recommended in number 3 above for dogs and number 5 below for cats.

5. Feed diarrheic cats, except those in which the diarrhea is due to lymphangiectasia or colonic dysfunctions, a highly-digestible, low-fiber, lactose-free diet, relatively high in a highly available fat (Prescription Diet Feline c/d, Hill's, or Recipe 8, Appendix Table 1).

6. If diarrhea has been a chronic problem, or intestinal parasites or giardiasis may be present, administer an anthelmenic and metronidazole (Table 1).

Diet is perhaps the most important factor in treating acute or chronic gastrointestinal disturbances.[37] The majority of carbohydrate in the diarrheic or post-diarrheic animal's diet should be from rice. Consumption of a diet with rice as the only carbohydrate (Prescription Diet d/d, Hill's) by healthy dogs resulted in no increase in breath hydrogen excretion, whereas it increased over eight times (800%) when corn or wheat flour were added to the diet,[227] even though the flours were cooked, which increases their digestibility. Breath

hydrogen excretion increases quantitatively with the amount of unabsorbed carbohydrate.[227] Because wheat and corn are less completely assimilated and are the main sources of calories in most commercial pet foods, dogs with small intestinal mucosal disease and carbohydrate malabsorption may become diarrheic when given these diets.[227] Differences in digestibility of carbohydrate, as well as all nutrients, is greatly magnified if there is any impairment in the ability to utilize these nutrients. For example, in one study there was nearly a six-times greater difference in digestibility (15% greater versus 89% greater) between a highly-digestible diet (Prescription Diet i/d, Hill's) and a regular commercial dog food (Purina Dog Chow, Ralston Purina) when fed to the healthy dog as compared to the dog with pancreatic exocrine insufficiency.[168] Thus, the greater digestibility of rice, than corn or wheat, would be magnified in the animal with an impairment in carbohydrate digestion or absorption. This is the reason that regular commercial diets have been reported to exacerbate diarrhea and therefore are contraindicated for the diarrheic animal.[38]

In contrast, feeding small amounts at frequent intervals of a highly-digestible diet in which rice is its only (Prescription Diet d/d, Hill's) or major (Prescription Diet i/d, Hill's) source of carbohydrate, results in a greater amount of the diet being digested and absorbed in the upper small intestine. For the animal with an impaired ability to digest or absorb nutrients, regardless of the reason, this is extremely beneficial. It not only insures that more of the food eaten is digested and absorbed, but it also decreases the amount of excess nutrients remaining in the intestinal tract, which is harmful. These excess nutrients alter gastrointestinal motility and support bacterial multiplication. This frequently results in bacterial colonization and overgrowth in the small intestine. Bacteria deconjugate bile salts, which decreases fat digestion and absorption. Bacteria also convert undigested fats and carbohydrates to fatty acids. These fatty acids and deconjugated bile salts, when present in sufficient quantities, cause diarrhea. The bacteria also produce ammonia and other nitrogenous waste products from undigested dietary protein and endogenous protein in the intestinal tract. These products may be absorbed. In excessive quantities they are toxic, particularly if the liver's ability to remove them from the circulation is impaired. Thus, the presence of excessive fat, carbohydrates, and protein in the lower intestinal tract are quite detrimental and are greatly decreased by feeding small amounts of a highly-digestible diet at frequent intervals.

For the animal with enteritis from any cause, in addition to the diet being highly digestible (with rice as its major source of carbohydrate), it should be lactose-free. Lactose may cause osmotic diarrhea in these animals (see page 7-42). For dogs and cats with lymphangiectasia a diet as low in fat as possible is preferred because absorption of the long-chain fatty acids in dietary fats increases lymph flow and therefore lymph losses. The diets recommended (item no. 4, p. 7-40) are the lowest-fat, nutritionally-adequate diets readily available.

In contrast to the long-chain fatty acids in dietary fats which are absorbed into the lymphatics, medium-chain triglycerides (MCT) are absorbed directly into the capillaries and do not increase lymphatic flow. As a result, they are occasionally recommended as a means of increasing dietary energy intake for dogs with lymphangiectasia. Although they may be helpful in some cases in many dogs, clinical response is poor (see page 7-45 for information on their use).

In addition to being highly digestible, dietary fat should also be moderately restricted for dogs with diarrhea due to causes other than lymphangiectasia. Some fat in the diet is needed for energy density, diet palatability, essential fatty acids and fat-soluble vitamin absorption. However, unabsorbed fatty acids are hydroxylated by intestinal bacteria to short-chain fatty acids. These fatty acids stimulate water secretion by the colon, which exacerbates diarrhea and fluid loss.[37] Unabsorbed fat can also form a physiochemical barrier at the mucosal surface. This barrier delays or impairs absorption of other nutrients which may induce an osmotic diarrhea.[168] Although these same factors may also apply to the cat, most diarrheic cats, except those with lymphangectasia or colitis, respond much better to a diet relatively high in highly available fat. Feeding the diarrheic cat a low-fat diet often worsens the diarrhea, whereas a diet relatively high in highly-digestible fat will generally lessen the diarrhea.

In **summary,** the animal with any impairment in the ability to digest or absorb nutrients (pancreatic exocrine, hepatic or intestinal dysfunction) should be fed small amounts, frequently, of a diet that: 1) is highly-digestible, 2) has rice as its major source of carbohydrate, 3) is lactose-free, 4) is as hypoallergenic as possible, and 5) (for the dog) is moderately restricted in highly available fat; whereas, diarrheic cats seem to do better when fed a relatively high-fat diet.

Because the majority of dogs and cats with diarrhea without steatorrhea respond to the management described on page 7-40 (steps 1-6), it has

been recommended that they be evaluated further and additional therapy be instituted only if they do not respond to this management within 2-3 weeks.[33,38] Additional therapy depends on the specific factor(s) responsible for causing the diarrhea.

Drugs, such as **anticholinergics and xylazine** (Table 1) that reduce intestinal motility,[97] are not indicated because intestinal motility is already decreased in most diarrheic animals (see page 7-24). In contrast, administration of **opiates** such as loperamide, tincture of opium or diphenoxylate (Table 1) may be beneficial. The combination of paregoric and the antiprostaglandin, bismuth subsalicylate, may be even more effective (Table 1). Although in dogs and cats, opiates paralyze intestinal motility, they increase absorption and decrease secretion. As a result, they are often beneficial.[38] Side effects, which seldom occur with dosages that produce the desired effect, are characterized by constipation or central nervous system depression. These effects may be antagonized by naloxone. In most cases, therapy should be limited to a few days due to the extreme inhibition of motility.[234] In addition, opiates are contraindicated in the presence of toxigenic infections produced by *Escherichia coli*, Salmonella spp. or Shigella spp. or an antibiotic-instigated pseudomembranous colitis.[234]

Intestinal protectants may be beneficial in some cases. They absorb bacteria, toxins, and bile acids, and provide a protective coating for inflamed or irritated mucosal surfaces. However, there is little proof of their benefit and they interfere with absorption of a number of drugs. The intestinal protectants most commonly used include kaolin-pectin, many antacids, and activated charcoal (Table 1). **Antiprostaglandin** drugs such as aspirin, bismuth subsalicylate and flunixin meglumine (Table 1) may be beneficial in reducing bacterial toxin-induced secretory diarrhea[37] (see page 7-25).

Antimicrobial drugs are often given orally to diarrheic patients. However, their value is questionable in treatment of many diarrheal diseases. Most dogs and cats appear to recover faster without them.[37] Antimicrobial drugs are best avoided except in patients in which: 1) damage to the intestinal mucosal barrier is suspected (evidenced by hemorrhagic diarrhea, fever, leukocytosis or degenerative left shift of the hemogram), 2) the protozoal diseases (such as giardiasis) are present, or 3) intestinal bacterial overgrowth is suspected. Antibiotics should be given parenterally to animals with damage to the intestinal mucosa, as this damage may allow bacteria or toxins to gain access

to the body, causing deleterious effects. Oral administration of poorly absorbed antibiotics is indicated only if there is **bacterial overgrowth** in the small intestine. The nitrosonapthol test, although not specific for bacterial overgrowth in the small intestine, indicates which dogs with chronic diarrhea may respond favorably to oral administration of antibiotics (e.g. tylosin or tetracycline[40]). This test is easily done in a few minutes using inexpensive, stable reagents and urine (Table 6, page 7-34). An increase in serum folate concentration (more than $10 \mu g/L$) and decrease in serum vitamin B-12 concentration (less than 200 ng/L) also strongly suggest that intestinal bacterial overgrowth is present.[14,15,16] These changes occur because intestinal bacteria produce folate and bind vitamin B-12. Tylosin (Table 1) is one of the more effective antimicrobial drugs for controlling inflammatory bowel disease and bacterial overgrowth in the canine small intestine.[37] Long-term treatment is sometimes required. The minimum dose required to control signs is empiric.

It has long been suggested that giving *Lactobacillus acidophilus, Bacillus* spp. or their spores, may be beneficial in treating diarrhea and other intestinal disorders; although there are no reports from well controlled studies that document this benefit. It has been speculated that benefit from *Lactobacillus acidophilus* ingestion may occur because these bacteria would partially or completely replace enteropathogenic bacteria in the small intestine. However, *Lactobacillus acidophilus* and *bulgaricus* persist in the small intestine of people for only 3-6 hours after their ingestion.[173] Therefore, it appears doubtful that less than continuous ingestion is likely to be beneficial. In a double-blind randomized study,[231] people with irritable bowel syndrome each ingested 240 ml of milk three times a day for two weeks and the same amount of *L. acidophilus* milk for two more weeks.[161] The degree of signs during the two milk-drinking periods was the same as during the control period when no milk was ingested.

Milk Intolerance—Management

Excess ingestion of milk can produce diarrhea due to lactose intolerance (see page 7-26). In one report, 3 dogs 7-9 years old were able to utilize up to 1 g of lactose/kg body weight/day,[146] an amount equivalent to 20-22 ml/kg of cow's or goat's milk. Greater amounts increased intestinal fluid lactose and lactic acid concentrations, fecal water content, and frequency of defecation. All of these parameters continued to increase with increasing lactose intake up to 1.5 g/kg/day. At that intake they plateaued. A diet providing these

same dogs 2.5 g of beta-galactosidase hydrolysed lactose/kg body weight/day was well tolerated and intestinal fluid lactic acid concentrations were insignificant. Adding beta-galactosidase to milk has also been shown to eliminate lactose malabsorption in lactase-deficient people.[191]

Milk protein or casein is well utilized, even by lactase deficient animals, because it does not contain lactose. It is an excellent dietary protein for dogs and cats and has a biological value of 78, which is similar to beef protein. When methionine, the limiting amino acid in casein, is added, the biological value of the resulting protein is 100, the same as egg protein. Dairy products such as cheese and unpasteurized yogurt, in which the lactose has either been removed or partially hydrolyzed through bacterial action, can usually be tolerated.[57] Unpasteurized yogurt has been shown to significantly decrease both mortality and reduced weight gain of Salmonella-infected rats, as compared to rats fed unfermented milk.[93] These rats presumably had decreased intestinal lactose activity because of Salmonella-induced enteritis. This suggests that in young animals with enteritis from any cause, in which it may be nutritionally benefical to give milk, it may be helpful to treat the milk with beta galactosidase (LactAid, LactAid Co, and Lactase N, GB Fermentation Inds) to hydrolyze its lactose, or instead give unpasteurized yogurt.

Neither boiling milk, which coagulates the protein, nor using skimmed milk, which decreases milk fat content, is helpful in alleviating lactose intolerance, since lactose content remains unchanged. Pasteurized yogurt, cultured milk (buttermilk), and sweet or unfermented acidophilus milk are also of no benefit.[161,183] In one study, there was no difference in tolerance to unaltered milk and to acidophilus milk by lactase-deficient people.[161]

Unfermented lactose should be eliminated from the diet of all animals with diarrhea; in sufficient quantity it will cause, and, in any quantity, worsen diarrhea.

Gluten Enteropathy—Management

An allergy to the gliadin, gluten, resulting in partial villus atrophy (also called "celiac disease" and "non-tropical sprue") and malabsorption, occasionally occurs in people and in dogs (especially Irish Setters).[14] The primary clinical sign is poor growth or weight loss, usually accompanied by intermittent chronic diarrhea. Typically onset of the condition occurs in dogs 4-7 months of age, although it may occur in adults.

Gluten is highest in wheat and, therefore, the severest signs occur when food containing wheat is fed. As a result, the condition has been referred to as "wheat-sensitive enteropathy." Gluten actually is present in all cereal grains except rice and is, therefore, present in all forms of dog food (dry, soft-moist and canned). As with any allergy, exposure to even a small amount of the allergen is detrimental. Thus, treatment is to feed a gluten-free diet (Appendix Table 1). If signs are not alleviated when one of these diets is fed, other causes are responsible for the diarrhea.

Pancreatic Exocrine Insufficiency—Management

In management of pancreatic exocrine insufficiency, both dietary management and pancreatic enzyme supplementation are needed for the best results. In some cases, enzyme replacement is not effective unless a highly-digestible diet is fed.[91] As shown in Table 9, results of controlled studies in dogs with pancreatic exocrine insufficiency have demonstrated that feeding a highly digestible dietary food is more beneficial than any other single treatment. In this study, the highly-digestible diet was only 15% more digestible than a regular dog food when fed to normal healthy dogs; but when fed to dogs with pancreatic exocrine insufficiency, this diet was almost twice as digestible, and its fat 13 times more digestible. The highly digestible

TABLE 9

EFFECT OF DIET, AND OTHER TREATMENTS IN DOGS WITH PANCREATIC EXOCRINE INSUFFICIENCY[168]

Management	Digestibility (%)		Fecal (g/kg/day)	
	Dry Matter	Fat	Dry Wt.	Fat
Dogs with Pancreatic Insufficiency:				
Regular Food[a]	36	4	12	1.6
Regular Food[a] & Treatment[b]	63	33	7	1.1
Dietary Food[c]	68	52	4	0.6
Dietary Food[c] & Treatment[b]	78	78	3	0.3
Normal Dogs:				
Regular Food[a]	78	84	4	0.3
Dietary Food[c]	90	94	1	0.1

[a]Purina Dog Chow (Ralston Purina) (8.8% fat in dry matter).

[b]Treatment was 1.3 g of Viokase-V (AH Robins), 15–20 mg/kg/body wt of cimetidine (Tagamet, Smith Kline & French) and 20–25 mg/kg/body wt of Maalox, all given three times daily.

[c]The dry form of Prescription Diet i/d (Hill's) (13.5% fat in dry matter).

dietary food fed alone, without any other treatment, was even more digestible by dogs with no pancreatic exocrine function than was the regular dog food when pancreatic enzymes, a gastric acid secretion inhibitor, and antacids were given. When pancreatic enzymes, a gastric acid secretion inhibitor, and antacids were given with the highly-digestible dietary food to dogs with pancreatic insufficiency, digestibility was the same as when the normal dogs were fed the regular dog food.

This study illustrates three major points:

1. The most effective treatment for dogs with pancreatic exocrine insufficiency is to feed a highly-digestible, low-fiber, moderate-fat diet supplemented with pancreatic enzymes, a gastric acid secretion inhibitor, and an antacid.
2. When this regimen is instituted, the digestive function of the dog with total absence of pancreatic exocrine function is returned to the same level as when a regular dog food is consumed by a normal dog.
3. Feeding dogs with pancreatic exocrine insufficiency a highly-digestible diet with no other treatment is more beneficial than continuing to feed a regular dog food and giving pancreatic enzymes, a gastric acid secretion inhibitor, and an antacid.

Another finding of this study was that in managing dogs with pancreatic exocrine insufficiency, a highly digestible diet is more important than simply a low-fat diet. The highly-digestible diet used in this study contained more than 50% more fat than the regular dog food (13.5% vs 8.8%). However, when it was fed either with or without pancreatic enzymes, to dogs with pancreatic exocrine insufficiency, its digestibility was greater than that of the lower fat regular dog food.

As demonstrated by this study and others,[148] the proper diet for the management of pancreatic exocrine insufficiency is a moderate-fat, low-fiber, highly-digestible diet. The importance of restricting fiber intake was well demonstrated in a study of 12 people with pancreatic exocrine insufficiency. In this study, decreasing dietary fiber from 4.2% to 0.7% (most commercial pet foods contain 3-5% fiber) lowered both fecal weight and fat excretion by one-third and reduced bloating and flatulence.[68] These effects were thought to occur because fiber binds bile acids and pancreatic enzymes. Adding 1.5% pectin or wheat bran to an in vitro incubation medium reduced the activity of all three of the major pancreatic enzymes (amylase, lipase, and trypsin) by 14-60%.[68]

Although the difference in digestibility between diets may be small among normal animals, this

TABLE 10

CALORIES PROVIDED BY DIFFERENT DIETS IN DOGS WITH PANCREATIC INSUFFICIENCY[168]

| Food* | Metabolizable Energy (kcal/lb) | | |
| | Normal Dogs | Pancreatic Insufficiency | |
		Untreated	Treated*
Dietary Food	1600	1135	1370
Regular Food	1390	525	1000
Difference (%)	15	116	37

*See Footnotes Table 9

TABLE 11

AMOUNT OF FOOD NEEDED AND ENERGY-SUPPLYING NUTRIENTS EXCRETED BY A 20-kg DOG WITH PANCREATIC INSUFFICIENCY[168]

| Food* | Dry Food Needed (lb/day) | Fecal Excretion (g/day) | | |
		Fat	Carbohydrate and Protein	Total
Dietary Food	1.1	22	110	132
Regular Food	2.5	87	620	707
Difference (%)	127	295	464	436

*See Footnotes Table 9

difference is greatly magnified when diseases that reduce nutrient digestion or absorption are present. In one study, a highly-digestible dietary food was only 15% more digestible than a regular dog food by normal dogs, but was 89% more digestible by dogs with pancreatic exocrine insufficiency (Table 9). As a result, as shown in Table 10, the highly-digestible diet provides more than twice as many calories (1135 vs 525). Even when dogs with pancreatic exocrine insufficiency are given pancreatic enzymes to improve the digestibility of regular dog food, the highly-digestible diet without pancreatic enzymes added still provides 13.5% more calories (1135 vs. 1000, Table 10).

Because of the differences in available calories between a highly-digestible and a regular dog food, more of the regular food must be fed to meet the animal's need. For example, as shown in Table 11, to fufill energy need a 20 kg dog with pancreatic insufficiency would need to eat 2.5 lb/day of regular dog food as compared to 1.1 lb of the dietary food, and would excrete more than 4 times more fat, carbohydrate and protein in the feces. This is why the dog with pancreatic exocrine insufficiency, fed a regular dog food, with or

without the pancreatic enzymes, eats a greater amount of food, excretes more feces and may still lose weight.

Not only are more nutrients excreted in the feces when a regular dog food is fed to dogs with pancreatic exocrine insufficiency (or other impairments in the ability to digest or absorb nutrients), but also more nutrients remain in the intestinal lumen. This is quite harmful, as described previously (page 7-41).

Summary—Management of Pancreatic Exocrine Insufficiency

Dogs with pancreatic exocrine insufficiency should be managed in the following manner. The first two treatments listed should be used first. The other treatments listed should be used only if response to the treatment preceding it is not satisfactory.

1. Feed a highly-digestible diet such as Prescription Diet i/d, Hill's, or Recipe 1, Appendix Table 3, 3-6 times daily, or free-choice. The diet dry matter should be at least 90% digestible, provide at least 1600 metabolizable kcal/lb of dry matter for the normal animal, contain 10-15% of a highly utilizable fat, and less than 1.0% fiber.

2. Add to the diet a non-enteric coated pancreatic enzyme powder (Table 1). Pancreatic enzyme activity varies greatly among different products. Giving amounts greater than recommended (Table 1) rarely improves response to treatment. Response to enzyme administration, regardless of the amount given, may not occur in some cases, unless a highly-digestible diet is fed.[91] In addition, controlled studies have shown that enzyme administration is less effective than feeding a highly-digestible diet (Table 9, page 7-43). Although 60-90% of ingested pancreatic enzyme activity is destroyed by gastric acid, enteric-coated tablets generally are of no benefit. Most of them remain coated throughout the intestinal tract and, therefore, are ineffective. It is often recommended that pancreatic enzymes be added to the food and that the food be allowed to stand at room temperature for 20 to 30 minutes for predigestion before being fed. However, in controlled studies, predigesting the food or giving antacids, bile salts, neomycin, or a larger amount of pancreatic enzymes did not improve therapeutic efficacy.[167] Giving more of the pancreatic enzymes probably did not improve the response to therapy because a highly digestible diet was not fed. For the majority of animals with pancreatic exocrine insufficiency, giving

pancreatic enzymes and feeding a highly-digestible diet is all that is needed. However, if response is not satisfactory, the following procedures may be helpful.

3. Giving cimetidene (Table 1) 5 to 30 minutes before feeding greatly reduces gastric acid secretion and has been shown to improve response to orally administered pancreatic enzymes.[167]

4. Give orally an antibiotic, such as tylosin or oxytetracycline (Table 1). In some animals with malassimilation this may be needed to treat bacterial overgrowth in the small intestine.

5. Add medium-chain triglycerides (MCT) to the dog's diet. MCT contain fatty acids that are 8-10 carbons long as compared to 16-18 for the fatty acids in most dietary fats or oils. MCT do not require micellerization and are absorbed directly into the capillaries rather than the lymphatics. Therefore, in contrast to other dietary fats, they can be digested and absorbed without hepatic bile salts or lymphatic delivery. However, only a small amount of MCT is absorbed without pancreatic lipase.[96] Thus, their utilization may be minimal in animals with pancreatic exocrine insufficiency. Even when pancreatic function is normal they may be poorly utilized because they do not stimulate cholecystokinin secretion.[96] In dogs, intestinal perfusion with fatty acids of less than 9 carbons in chain length did not stimulate secretion of pancreatic enzymes.[147] Unabsorbed MCT induce abdominal cramps and diarrhea.[96] In addition, MCT are ketogenic, so they should not be given to patients with ketosis or acidosis, or patients with severe hepatocellular damage since MCT are metabolized by the liver.[164] MCT also have a specific deleterious effect in cats resulting in a fatty liver.[137]

MCT should not be given to cats and should be given to dogs only if: 1) they can be tolerated without detrimental effects, 2) they can be utilized and 3) additional dietary energy is needed to increase weight gain or maintain condition in the animal that fails to respond to other treatments. MCT can be used to provide up to 25% of a dog's caloric need (Table 1). Because of poor palatability and frequently poor utilization, it is best to begin with small amounts and gradually increase the dose. MCT, when fully utilized, provide 8 kcal/ml, but none if they are not utilized.[164] They are an expensive source of dietary calories.

LARGE BOWEL DISORDERS

Diesases of the large-bowel are responsible for more than 50% of the cases of chronic diarrhea in dogs, (colitis being diagnosed most frequently), but are rare in cats.[34] Abnormal stools of large-bowel origin are characterized by a semiformed soft or excessively firm consistency. They may contain mucus and, less often, fresh blood. The volume of stool passed is usually reduced. Increased frequency of mucoid, bloody stools is a reliable sign of a large-bowel disorder but it does not occur in all cases. Tenesmus and a sense of urgency may be present. A description of clinical signs helpful in differentiating diarrhea induced by small intestine dysfunction from that induced by large intestine dysfunction is given in Table 3 (page 7-27).

Diseases that directly involve the colonic wall and its nerve supply induce pathologic alterations in the anatomy and physiology of the large intestine. Large-bowel diarrhea may result because fecal transit time is greatly reduced when the colon is irritated or inflamed. Because less fluid and electrolytes are absorbed, a soft or mushy malformed stool is passed, and dehydration may occur. Infiltrative diseases of the colonic wall cause large-bowel diarrhea because absorption of water and electrolytes is inhibited.

If fecal transit time is greatly prolonged, firm or hard feces may result. Excessive water is absorbed from the fecal mass and an inspissated residue results. Anatomic obstruction, pain with stool passage, or inappropriate innervation of the colon, rectum, and anus are the most common causes. Tenesmus and frequent attempts to defecate develop secondarily to constant stimulation of the defecation reflex by the inflamed rectum or anus. Because the defecation reflex is constantly stimulated, the colon seldom has time to retain normal fecal volume. Thus, small amounts of stool usually are passed in association with recurrent tenesmus. Colonic irritation produces local effects that stimulate the large goblet cells of the colonic mucosa to produce excessive mucus, which is grossly observable in the feces. Grossly detectable blood in the feces results from injury to the colonic mucosa with the release of blood that is not digested before it passes out with the feces. Because absorption or assimilation of nutrients occurs in the small bowel, large-bowel disorders seldom lead to weight loss or steatorrhea.

In consideration of large-bowel disorders, it is convenient to list the rule-outs under one of three problems. These are acute mucoid bloody diarrhea, chronic mucoid bloody diarrhea and constipation or tenesmus.

DIAGNOSIS OF LARGE-BOWEL DISORDERS

Acute Mucoid Bloody Diarrhea

The minimum data base for determining the cause of acute mucoid bloody diarrhea should include:

1. Rectal examination and, if necessary, biopsy
2. Gross stool examination
3. Microscopic stool examination and fecal flotation performed on three random stool samples (see Table 5, page 7-30, for procedures for diagnosing various intestinal parasitisms).

This diagnostic plan is based on the logic of performing simple inexpensive procedures before more detailed manipulations are employed. For the dog or cat with acute mucoid bloody diarrhea the following conditions should be considered.

1. **Trichuriasis** (whipworms) (see page 7-47)
2. **Balantidiasis**
   Pathogenic, particularly when present with trichuriasis.
3. **Foreign body** (see page 7-32)
4. **Bacterial** or **mucoid colitis** (see page 7-30)
5. **Spastic or irritable colon syndrome**
   This affects predominately larger dogs and those that are stressed or hyperexcitable. Onset of signs may be associated with a change in environment. Signs are usually intermittent and cause either acute or chronic diarrhea. Otherwise, afflicted dogs appear normal. No intestinal inflammation is present but the colon is often hyperemic. Diagnosis is made by eliminating the other causes of acute large-bowel disorders. Although the terms "spastic" or "irritable" colon implies that motility is increased, in reality it is usually decreased. It may occur in conjunction with functional or psychological diarrhea (see page 7-37). Librax administration (Table 1) and a high-fiber diet (Prescription Diets r/d, or for the dog w/d, Hill's) may be helpful.[34,203]
6. **Amebiasis**
   This is an uncommon cause of acute or chronic colitis in dogs and people. It is caused by the protozoon Entamoeba histolytica. It is characterized by punctiform ulcerations, abdominal pain, anorexia, lethargy and intermittent diarrhea, which is often bloody and mucoid. Diagnosis is made by finding trophozoites or cysts in fresh feces. Treatment is antibiotics, such as

tetracyclines, and amebacidal drugs such as diodoquin, chloroquine, and emetine.

7. **Hemorrhagic gastroenteritis** (see page 7-32)

Chronic Mucoid Bloody Diarrhea

To determine the cause of chronic mucoid bloody diarrhea the data base for acute causes (page 7-46) should be completed. If a diagnosis cannot be confirmed, on the basis of this information, more tests are indicated. These include:

1. Proctoscopic and colonoscopic examination with biopsy. This procedure has great diagnostic importance. It can establish a morphologic diagnosis, reveal the etiologic agent, and help determine prognosis.

2. Barium enemas are useful in identifying cecal inversion and lesions in the cranial colon, such as those causing strictures, which cannot be observed by proctoscopy.

3. Cytology of colonic exudates. The etiologic agent may be found.

4. Fecal culture.

5. Complete blood count and urinalysis.

The following causes of chronic bloody diarrhea should be considered:

1. **Idiopathic chronic colitis**
   This is the most common colitis in dogs.[34] There may be many causes, all resulting in a common colonic response which can be self-perpetuating long after the inciting cause is gone. Clinical signs are typical for colitis (as described on page 7-46).

2. **Trichuris** (whipworms) and **Ancylostoma** (hookworms)
   These are a common cause of diarrhea in dogs and cats. Both parasites are usually associated with the small intestine but can be in the colon, where they cause colitis. In most cases there is a nonhemorrhagic (although occasionally bloody) chronic diarrhea with minimal weight loss but often poor appearance, hypo-albuminemia, hypoglobulinemia, and anemia. Occasionally, a severely affected dog shows evidence of trichuris irritation in the cecum and colon by chewing at its flank.

3. **Ulcerative colitis** (rare)
   a. Histiocytic ulcerative colitis
      Usually occurs in Boxers of either sex, less than 2 years of age, but its occurrence in a French Bulldog and a cat has been reported.[217] It was referred to by one investigator as **granulomatous colitis**[215] and by two others as histiocytic ulcerative colitis.[34,217] Affected dogs present with a history of intractable bloody diarrhea, and, until the condition is severe, have no weight loss. Typically, they have healthy skin and coat, are afebrile, bright, alert, and eat well. Defecation occurs 8-15 times daily and is often followed by brief tenesmus and passage of frank blood. The stools are tan to light brown, blood-streaked to very bloody, and soupy to mushy in consistency. They have a granular, glistening surface and a characteristic offensive odor.[215] Hypoalbuminemia and hyperglobulinemia are usually present.

      A corrugated mucosa may be felt on rectal palpation. Diagnosis is confirmed by a mucosal biopsy, revealing thickening of the submucosa caused by plasma cells, lymphocytes, and Periodic Acid Schiff-positive histiocytes. Treatment is symptomatic and minimally successful. Corticosteroids seem to be of little benefit. Long-term tylosin therapy may be helpful (Table 1).[215]

   b. Eosinophilic ulcerative colitis
      This disease may be acute or chronic and frequently occurs with eosinophilic gastroenteritis (see page 7-36). Diagnosis is based on finding large numbers of eosinophils in the lamina propria. Oral corticosteroid therapy usually produces clinical improvement (Table 1).

4. **Histoplasma colitis** (see page 7-37)

5. **Colonic neoplasia**
   a. Benign
      1) Polyps
      2) Adenomas
      3) Leiomyomas
   b. Malignant
      1) Adenocarcinoma
      2) Lymphosarcoma
      3) Leiomyosarcoma

This is one of the more common intestinal disorders affecting older dogs. In many cases colonic neoplasms cause a loss of blood in the stool. Although this loss may be quite small, detecting its presence is helpful diagnostically. However, in 98% of clinically healthy people with asymptomatic colorectal cancer fecal hemoglobin was less than 2 mg/g of fresh stool, and from 2 to 20 mg/g are required to ensure a positive orthotoluidine (Hematest, Miles Lab) or guaiac (Hemoccult, Smith Kline Diagnostics) test.[23] A new quantitative assay (HemoQuant) for fecal blood

based on fluorescence of heme-derived porphyrin will detect levels of less than 0.1 mg/g of stools, and has been shown to be quite helpful as a screening test for colorectal cancer in people[2] and therefore may be of value in dogs and cats. However, dietary hemoglobin must be considered in interpreting the test since fecal hemoglobin is directly related to the amount of hemoglobin ingested. In one study in healthy dogs, the mg of hemoglobin/g of fresh stools varied from 0.31 ± 0.14 when a dry diet containing 0.05 mg of hemoglobin/g of diet was fed, to 4.57 ± 1.5 when a canned diet containing 1.49 mg hemoglobin/g of diet was fed.[23]

Over 80% of the heme entering the gastrointestinal tract of people is converted by bacteria and enzymes to porphyrin, which does not react with guaiac or orthotoluidine tests. It does, however, react with the HemoQuant test.[2] The ability of the HemoQuant test to measure degraded heme (porphyrin) may be useful in indicating the anatomic site of gastrointestinal bleeding, since the higher in the tract that bleeding occurs, the greater the proportion of degraded heme. However, this is of no benefit in dogs, because in this species little hemoglobin is degraded to prophyrin in the gastrointestinal tract.[23]

6. **Cecal inversion**
   Usually caused by chronic trichuriasis (see page 7-47)

7. **Spastic or irritable colon syndrome** (see page 7-46)

8. **Allergic colitis** (see page 7-32)

9. **Granulomatous colitis** or **regional enterocolitis**
   This disease may be analogous to **Crohn's disease** of people and is also called "**terminal or regional ileitis.**" It is not known to affect cats and is rare in dogs. There is no breed predilection and most affected dogs are less than 4 years of age. It affects both the small and large intestine. the cause is not known. Usual clinical signs are a severely sick malnourished dog with chronic, bloody, mucoid diarrhea, lethargy, anorexia, and often tenesmus and fever. Severe granulomatous mucosal proliferation with a narrowed lumen and failure to dilate with insufflation with air are found on colonoscopic examination. The colon mucosa appears corrugated and hyperemic. The prognosis is grave and recovery rare.

There may be some response to administration of corticosteroids and antibiotics. In one study in people, regular food was withheld and a protein-free elemental diet (Vivonex, Norwich-Eaton) was fed for 4 weeks. At that time, regular food was reintroduced. This regimen resulted in remission of signs in 9 of 11 people with Crohn's disease as compared to 8 of 10 people given corticosteroids.[152] It was speculated that the beneficial effects of the diet may be due to alteration in the bacterial flora of the gut, or because the diet contained amino acids, which are absorbed more cranial in the small intestine, away from diseased intestine, or the amino acids were less allergenic than protein. Two further studies support the latter hypothesis. When a hypoallergenic diet was fed, 7 of 10 people with Crohn's disease remained in remission for 6 months, whereas none of 10 who were fed a high-fiber diet, responded.[109] The foods most commonly implicated were wheat and dairy products. As these studies and investigators suggest, a hypoallergenic diet may be a practical strategy for long-term management of Crohn's disease. Whether a hypoallergenic diet would be of benefit to dogs with granulomatous colitis is not known; however, these studies suggest that it may be (see Appendix Table 1 for hypoallergenic diets).

10. **Lymphocytic-plasmacytic colitis** (see page 7-37)

CONSTIPATION OR TENESMUS

The minimum data base for determining the cause of constipation and/or tenesmus should include:

1. Rectal examination for pain, foreign material, or reduction in size of rectum or colon lumen, such as from pelvic fractures, perineal hernias, pregnancy, tumors, or prostatic hyperplasia. Pain associated with prostatitis, sacculitis or injury, may also cause constipation.

2. Proctoscopic examination and biopsy

3. Barium enema

4. Complete blood count and urinalysis

The following causes of constipation and tenesmus should be considered:

1. **Obstructive neoplasims** or **foreign material**
   Impactions with foreign material, such as bone and hairballs, are the most common cause of constipation in dogs and cats.[34] Rectal, colonic or pelvic tumors may also cause impaction. The frequency of impaction from both

causes increases with age. Gastrointestinal obstructions have been reported to be the major cause of constipation in cats and may also cause vomiting. One-half of these obstructions in cats are due to hairballs in the stomach, and most of the others are due to tumors—most commonly intestinal lymphosarcoma.[165]

2. **Congenital megacolon**
   Analogous to **Hirschprung's disease** in children and due to the absence of the myenteric plexi.

3. **Idiopathic megacolon**
   Occurs in cats of any age, but is especially common in older cats, where it is the most common colon lesion. It is possibly due to degeneration of the muscle or myenteric ganglion cells in the colon wall. Laxatives, a high fiber diet (Prescription Diet Feline r/d, Hill's) and weekly enemas may help in some cases, but for many this treatment is unrewarding. Total colon resection is considered the treatment of choice.[36]

4. **Pseudo** or **secondary megacolon**
   May result from any lesion or disease listed below, that prevents normal defecation over a prolonged period. It is most common in older animals.

5. **Prostatic enlargement**

6. **Pelvic abnormalities**

7. Sacral **nerve,** pudendal nerve or lumbar cord **injury**

8. **Hypothyroidism**

9. **Hyperparathyroidism**

10. **Debilitating disease**

11. **Painful defecation** from anorectal disease

12. **Perineal hernia** or **fistula** which may be obstructive

13. **Drug induced**
    Anticholinergic, antihistamine, barium sulfate, diuretic, or opiate administration

14. **Colonic perforation**
    Results in constipation in about one-half of affected dogs, depression, anorexia and emesis in most, and death within an average of less than 24 hours in all cases (see page 7-16, item 1-d).

MANAGEMENT OF LARGE-BOWEL DISORDERS

Colitis

The drug of choice in treating colitis is sulfasalazine (Table 1). Sulfasalazine contains a prostaglandin inhibitor (5-aminosalicylic acid) that appears to assist in returning colonic secretion and motility to normal.[129] It may take 2-4 weeks before a favorable response is noted.[38] An allergic response, keratoconjunctivitis, or signs of salicylate toxicity in cats is uncommon in response to sulfasalazine given at the dosages recommended.[38,129] Metronidazole (Table 1) is occasionally beneficial to patients that do not respond to sulfasalazine.[37] In addition to its antiprotozoal action, metronidazole has a protective effect against experimentally induced colitis.

Because whipworms are a common cause of colitis in many geographic areas and may be difficult to diagnose, suspected cases are often treated empirically.[203] Fenbendazole (Table 1) and fenbantel/praziaquantel (Vercom, Haver) are the safest and most effective anthelmintics and should be used to treat whipworm infections.[203] Tylosin (Table 1) is effective in many inflammatory bowel diseases. It is most useful in the treatment for bacterial overgrowth. Corticosteroids (Table 1) are the most effective therapy for eosinophilic colitis. Corticosteroid retention enemas (Table 1) are useful in achieving prompt relief in patients with tenesmus and dyschezia due to severe colitis. They are recommended in the initial treatment of these patients in conjunction with other therapy or when sulfasalazine, corticosteroid or other therapy is unsuccessful in bringing about rapid control of clinical signs.[203] Relief is often rapid when they are used. After administration, the patient's rear quarters should be elevated for 10 minutes to increase contact time of the solution with the colonic mucosa. Chlorpromazine is effective in controlling nausea and vomiting, which may occur with colitis, and may help stressed animals to rest.[203] Perianal sores, which may develop in conjunction with severe colitis and proctitis, should be treated. Balneol (Table 1) 3-4 times daily works well to soothe irritated tissue and enhance healing.[203]

Hypoallergenic diets should be fed if allergic colitis is suspected (see page 7-32). In acute cases of colitis withhold food, but not water, for 24-48 hours. Most dogs and cats with colitis respond best to frequent feedings of small amounts of a high-fiber diet (Prescription Diets r/d, Hill's). Although fiber can be added to the diet and is often recommended, it is difficult to add much fiber and at the same time maintain sufficient palatability to ensure that the animal will eat the diet. In addition, the resulting diet may not be nutritionally balanced. Fiber from some sources decreases the availability, and may result in a deficiency, of proteins, fats and certain miner-

als[5,41] unless the high-fiber diet contains sufficient amounts of these nutrients to offset their reduced availability. In contrast, cellulose is a relatively innocuous fiber source causing no deleterious effects unless it is combined with a deficient or poorly balanced diet.[41,61,149] This is not the case, however, with some other fiber sources, such as pectin[59,60] and those high in lignin.[149]

Increased dietary fiber hastens transit time in people and dogs with slow transit time, and prolongs it in those with abnormally rapid transit time.[41,180] Increased intake of fiber has been shown to decrease intraluminal pressure and clinical signs in patients with colonic disease.[180] Adding fiber to the diet in the form of 1% pectin has significantly improved healing of experimental colitis in rats and improved nitrogen balance 57%.[175] Because of these effects, increased fiber intake has alleviated both diarrhea and constipation in patients with large-bowel disorders.[76,98,99,190] Increased dietary fiber also relieves pain and bowel dysfunction in people with diverticulosis,[3] and appears to be beneficial in decreasing colonic cancer.[84] Diverticulosis, however, is not known to occur naturally in either dogs or cats.

If the animal with colitis does not respond to the consumption of a high-fiber diet within 1-2 weeks, change to a highly-digestible diet (Prescription Diets i/d for dogs or Feline c/d for cats, Hill's, or Recipes 1 or 8, Appendix Table 3). A highly digestible diet results in most of the diet being digested and absorbed in the upper small intestine. Thus, a smaller amount of undigested material reaches the diseased colon. This effect is one of the reasons this dietary management should be used for several weeks after all gastrointestinal tract surgery.

Constipation or Tenesmus

A high fiber diet is beneficial not only for most patients with colitis; it also helps prevent recurrent constipation[72] and therefore should be fed to the animal with this problem.[98,99] Constipation in older dogs is usually a problem associated with diet and lack of exercise. Because constipation usually involves the large intestine, enemas 2-3 times daily until constipation is relieved are the most beneficial therapy. Phosphate-containing enema solutions (e.g. Fleet, CB Fleet and PVL, Prof Vet Lab) should not be used in cats, or very small dogs, as they can cause a potentially fatal hyperphosphatemia, hypocalcemia, hypernatremia, hyperglycemia, hyperkalemia and metabolic acidosis.[10,110] Soapy-water enemas containing dioctyl sodium sulfosuccinate, glycerin, or both, should be used instead. Recurrence of constipation due to diet, lack of exercise, or hairballs can be prevented in many cases by feeding a high-cellulose fiber-weight reducing diet (Prescription Diets r/d, Hill's, or Recipes 4 or 10, Appendix Table 3).

High-fiber diets increase fecal output, lessen stool density and, in some cases, help maintain normal transit time through the intestine.[72] In one study in rats, stool density was reduced from 1.3 to 1.0 g/ml by adding 8% cellulose, and from 1.3 to 0.7 g by adding 21% wheat bran to a fiber-free diet, whereas adding 8% guar or 8% pectin had no significant effect on stool density.[136] In a study in dogs, increasing dietary fiber from 0.6 to 14.7% of the diet dry matter by adding cellulose to the diet, tripled fecal water excretion.[41] This study also indicated that the canine colon contracts more effectively with increasing cellulose fiber intake and, as a result, increased luminal bulk.[42] In contrast to what might be assumed, increased luminal bulk decreases colonic work.[70] These effects often alleviate constipation.[72,98,99] Vegetables high in fiber, methyl cellulose, milk of magnesia, mineral oil, petroleum jelly, psyllium hydrophilic mucilloid (Metamucil, Searle), or dioctyl sodium succinate or other fecal softeners in the diet may also be helpful. Bisacodyl (Table 1), a stimulant laxative that increases intestinal transit and inhibits electrolyte and water absorption, is useful in treating chronic intractable constipation.[37] Feeding bones is contraindicated for animals with problems of constipation. The patient should be exercised frequently to encourage defecation.

Colon Cancer

The incidence of colon cancer, which is second only to lung cancer in people, is low in dogs and cats. The incidence of this disease may be lessened with increased intake of dietary fiber.[8] The low incidence of colon cancer in dogs and cats may be due in part to their consumption of a relatively high-fiber diet in comparison to the diet of people. High-fiber diets increase total bile acid excretion and reduce the proportion of secondary bile acids in feces.[84] Many types of dietary fiber have been shown to reduce the carcinogenicity of a number of chemicals.[84] The continuous ingestion of Lactobacillus acidophilus may also reduce the incidence of colon cancer.

Continuous ingestion of Lactobacillus acidophilus has resulted in a 2 to 4-fold reduction in the activity of possible procarcinogenic bacterial enzymes in the colon.[81] Rats continually ingesting Lactobacillus acidophilus had significantly fewer

chemically induced colon cancers than those not receiving the organisms.[80]

FLATULENCE

ETIOLOGY

Flatulence is a chronic objectionable problem which occurs often in small animals, especially dogs. Although the cause of chronic flatulence in pet animals is often not established, several factors should be considered when this problem is approached diagnostically and therapeutically. Intestinal gas accumulates from four sources:

1. Swallowed air
2. Gas diffusion from the blood to the gut lumen
3. Acid-base neutralization reactions, which produce carbon dioxide
4. Bacterial fermentation of nutrients, which produce primarily hydrogen, methane, and carbon dioxide

The greatest amount of gas in the digestive tract at any time probably comes from air swallowed during eating or panting. This may be the cause of the flatulence so common in many brachycephalic breeds. A considerable amount of gas is also formed from bacterial fermentation of poorly digestible carbohydrate or fiber in the colon. Diets high in fiber may decrease nutrient digestion in the small-bowel and thus allow more fermentable substance to reach the colon. As a result, flatulence increases in animals consuming poorly-digestible or high-fiber diets[72] and can be decreased by feeding a low-fiber, highly-digestible diet. Dietary substances that contain large amounts of the non-absorbable oligosaccharides, such as raffinose, stachyose, and verbascose, are likely to produce large amounts of intestinal gas.[132] Dogs and cats lack the enzymes needed to split these sugars into absorbable monosaccharides. These sugars are fermented by clostridia and other bacteria, which produce hydrogen and carbon dioxide. Soybeans, beans, and peas contain large quantities of the non-absorbable oligosaccharides. Production of hydrogen and carbon dioxide may be greatly increased in the intestinal tract of dogs by feeding a commercial diet high in soybean meal. Wheat has also been shown to result in excessive intestinal hydrogen production in some people, but not in dogs or cats.[6]

Diseases that produce maldigestion (pancreatic exocrine insufficiency or a loss of intestinal brush border disaccharidase enzymes) or malabsorption are usually associated with excessive flatulence. Failure to digest and absorb carbohydrate, protein or fat in these disorders allows colonic bacteria to ferment these substances and produce excessive carbon dioxide, hydrogen, and volatile fatty acids.

The major components of intestinal gas are air, hydrogen, methane, and carbon dioxide, which have no odor. Odoriferous gases include ammonia, hydrogen sulfide, indole, skatole, volatile amines, and short-chain fatty acids. These gases represent less than 1% of the composition of flatus but contribute most of the objectionable odor. Many dietary substances, including onions, spices, spoiled food, and particularly high-protein foods increase the production of these gases, and thus, objectional flatus results. Oral vitamin therapy can increase intestinal microbial activity and lead to a greater quantity of bacterial by-products and odoriferous gases. Body and breath odors arise, at least partially, from odoriferous gases produced by bacterial flora in the intestine. These gases are absorbed and excreted in expired air and from the skin.[132] Some of these gases, such as those produced by garlic or onions, are detectable in the healthy animal. Others are detectable only when there is a dysfunction in the normal routes of excretion, such as failure of the liver to clear volatile bacterial metabolites (mercaptans) from the blood,[52] or failure of the kidney to excrete nitrogenous waste products, resulting in an ammonia or uremic odor.

MANAGEMENT OF FLATULENCE

1. Control aerophagia. Feed free-choice or two or more times a day to discourage gulping of air and encourage frequent consumption of smaller amounts of food. Feeding the pet in a quiet location by itself to eliminate competition for food and slow the eating process may also help.
2. Avoid diets high in fiber and those that contain soybeans or wheat. Do not feed strong-flavored sulfur-containing vegetables, milk, garbage, or high-protein diets, or give vitamin-mineral supplements.
3. Feed highly-digestible diets such as Prescription Diets i/d or k/d for dogs and Feline c/d for cats (Hill's) or diets produced from Recipes 1, 2 or 8 (Appendix Table 3).
4. If these procedures do not produce the desired response, evaluate the animal for steatorrhea (Figure 5, page 7-39) and, if present, treat accordingly.

COPROPHAGY

Although frequently encountered and disgusting to the client, coprophagy is not generally

harmful to the animal unless parasites are transmitted. The actual causes of coprophagy are not well established. It usually is due to boredom[114] or a vice.[35] An insufficiency of pancreatic enzymes occasionally may be involved. Dogs may eat their own or another animal's feces to obtain the unabsorbed nutrients contained therein. Wild canines are known to eat droppings of their herbivorous prey, which may be an important source of nutrients for them. Bitches commonly consume the feces of their pups. Thus, coprophagy is fairly natural for dogs.

The objectives in combating coprophagy are: 1) remove stools promptly from the environment to curtail opportunity, 2) create more activity for the dog, and 3) provide a highly digestible balanced diet adequate in all nutrients.

Management of coprophagy should include the following:

1. Instruct the client to spend more time with the dog and provide more opportunity for exercise.

2. Feed a good-quality diet that is nutritionally adequate for the pet's particular stage of life.

3. Sprinkling commercial meat tenderizer, such as Adolph's, on the dog's food, in the same manner as salting one's own food, may make stools less palatabile and therefore lessen or eliminate coprophagy. Unseasoned meat tenderizer should be given to dogs with known gastrointestinal disorders, as ingredients used in the seasoned type can irritate the dog's gastrointestinal tract.

4. If steatorrhea is present, determine the cause (Figure 5, page 7-39) and manage accordingly.

HEPATIC DISEASE

CLINICAL SIGNS OF HEPATIC DISEASE

The most common clinical signs in mature dogs and cats with hepatic disease are lethargy, anorexia, depression, and weight loss. Intermittent vomiting, diarrhea, polydipsia, polyuria, ascites, icterus, and, in kittens, kernicterus (conjugated bilirubin-induced encephalopathy) may occur. Central nervous system signs due to encephalopathy may also occur due to: 1) diffuse and severe hepatocellular damage from any cause, 2) enzymatic defects preventing conversion of ammonia to urea, and 3) major circulatory bypass of the liver. Circulatory hepatic bypass may be congenital or it may be acquired because of advanced hepatic fibrosis and portal hypertension, which can result in shunting.[54] Malabsorption of fat and fat-soluble

vitamins may occur due to insufficient hepatic bile salts. Blood coagulation may be impaired resulting in bleeding tendencies due to reduced synthesis of clotting factors and prothrombin, and reduced vitamin K absorption. The resulting bleeding tendencies and portal hypertension-induced rupture of varices can result in chronic blood loss, although this is uncommon in dogs or cats. With chronic liver disease, a number of conditions may occur due to decreased hepatic metabolism or excretion of several hormones. These include: 1) hypogonadism, 2) gynecomastia in males, 3) hyperadrenocorticism, and 4) hyperaldosteronism.

DIAGNOSIS OF HEPATIC DISEASE AND ITS CAUSES

In addition to clinical signs, the following factors may be helpful in diagnosing the presence of liver disease.

1. Presence of hepatic tenderness or changes in size as determined by palpation and/or ultrasonography or radiographs (plain or pneumoperitoneography, lateral view best). The normal liver is difficult to palpate in dogs and cats. It is firm and its borders are sharp; the caudal borders just reach the costochondral junction. Most cats with liver disease have hepatomegaly; decreased liver size is uncommon.

   a. Enlarged due to:

      1) Acute hepatitis—may also cause tenderness

      2) Venous congestion or edema as a result of congestive heart failure

      3) Lipidosis from obesity, caloric deficit, protein deficiency, prolonged anorexia (especially in cats and especially if they are also obese), diabetes mellitus, hypothyroidism, pancreatitis, drugs or toxins.

      4) Hepatopathy from Cushing's syndrome or glucocorticoid administration, in which hepatic changes appear similar to lipidosis, but hepatocytes do not contain excess lipids.[197]

      5) Neoplasia—may also cause tenderness

      6) Granulomatous diseases such as histoplasmosis (see page 7-37)

      7) Chronic active hepatitis—liver may be enlarged or reduced in size

      8) Bile engorgement

      9) Amyloidosis

      10) Hemochromatosis from chronic iron toxicity. The liver is large, firm, cir-

rhotic and rusty-colored or chocolate brown (see page 1-20).

11) Coombs'-positive hemolytic anemia. Treatment is corticosteroid administration.

12) Haemobartonellosis. Treatment is tetracycline administration for 2-3 weeks.

b. Small due to:

1) Cirrhosis (diffuse hepatic fibrosis)

2) Atrophy as a result of portasystemic shunts

3) Subacute necrosis

4) Chronic active hepatitis—liver may be enlarged or reduced in size

2. Alterations in plasma concentration or activity of:

a. Albumin and usually alpha globulins are decreased, and gamma globulins are often increased in dogs (but often not in cats) with chronic or advanced liver disease.

b. Total serum cholesterol is usually increased in obstructive biliary disease, and may be markedly decreased in hepatic failure (when this occurs the prognosis is grave) and protasystemic shunts.[29] Frequently it is also decreased in animals with pancreatic exocrine insufficiency and small intestinal dysfunctions because of impaired cholesterol absorption, and with lympangiectasia because of excessive loss in lymph.[29]

c. Alanine aminotransferase (ALT, formerly SGPT), aspartate aminotransferase (AST, formerly SGOT), alkaline phosphatase (AP), lactic dehydrogenase (specifically fraction 5), sorbital dehydrogenase (SDH) and gamma glutamyl transpeptidase (GGT) are increased with many liver diseases. However, animals may have profoundly reduced liver function, such as with cirrhosis or portasystemic vascular anomalies, and have normal plasma activities of all of these enzymes.[45] ALT and AP are the hepatic enzymes most commonly measured. Most hepatic disorders in dogs can be detected by measuring the plasma activity of these two enzymes.

An elevated AP activity is almost always from liver or bone, although the enzyme is also present in the uterus, intestine and kidney. An elevation from bone abnormalities is minimal in the cat, and in the dog rarely exceeds 5 times normal. In dogs, many drugs, including corticosteroids, primidone, phenobarbital, and diphenylhydantoin, cause 3 to 100-fold increases in plasma AP activity. Corticosteroids also increase plasma bile acid concentration, ALT activity, and BSP retention.[62] Plasma AP activity is elevated by any impairment in bile flow, and, in cats, only with severe cholestatic diseases.[86]

Increased plasma ALT activity indicates acute hepatocellular damage. The magnitude of this increase in plasma ALT activity is directly proportional to the number of hepatocytes affected, but not to the severity or reversibility of the damage. ALT and AP in cats do not increase as much as they do in dogs. Thus, mild increases of either in the cat are more significant than in the dog. Both may be normal in the cat with significant liver disease. In the dog, ALT is more specific for hepatic disease than is AST. ALT is often elevated (to 150) in old cats without hepatic disease. AST is present in substantial amounts in many tissues, particularly muscle. In cats, increased AST activity may be a more sensitive indicator of hepatobiliary disease than it is in the dog. An elevated GGT activity is more sensitive than ALP for detecting liver disease in cats but ALP is more specific for cholestatic disease.

An increase in SDH activity is specific for hepatocellular damage. All plasma SDH (even in hemolyzed samples) in dogs originates from the cytoplasm of the hepatocyte.[9,65] It is stable during storage when the plasma is separated from the erythrocytes.[65] Normal SDH activity in dogs is 5.8 U/L, with little variation between individuals.[65] and increases of only 20-40% above normal are easily identified.[65]

3. Bromsulphalein (BSP) (Vet-BSP solution, Vantec Labs) retention of more than 3-5% by cats, and 5-10% by dogs, 30 minutes after intravenous administration of 5 mg/kg optimum body weight is indicative of hepatic dysfunction, although it does not confirm its presence. BSP retention is always increased, regardless of hepatic function, in the icteric animal because both BSP and unconjugated bilirubin use glucuronic acid for hepatic uptake and conjugation. BSP retention also increases with conditions that lessen hepatic blood flow, such as congestive heart failure. BSP is cleared rapidly by the cat and therefore retention does not occur until liver disease is well advanced. As a result, the BSP clearance test is less valuable in cats than dogs. Ammonia clearance is a more sensitive indicator of hepatic dysfunction.

4. Ammonia clearance is reduced in animals with liver disease. Normal values must be established for each laboratory. However, for most laboratories in normal dogs and cats, fasting blood ammonia is less than 60-120 $\mu g/dl$. It increases by less than 80 $\mu g/dl$, 30 minutes after oral administration of ammonium chloride (100 mg/kg up to a maximum of 3 g/animal diluted in 20-50 ml of water to prevent vomiting). In animals with hepatic disease, blood ammonia will increase to 400-1500 $\mu g/dl$. A kit for measuring blood ammonia is available (Sigma Chemical Co). Ammonia is quite unstable in blood and therefore any delay in laboratory analysis may result in spuriously increased or decreased values.

5. Hyperbilirubinemia (jaundice), elevated serum bile acids and alterations in urine urobilinogen and bilirubin occur in animals with liver disease (Table 12). In one study, clinically detectable jaundice in cats was due to: 23% FIP, 17% toxic hepatopathy, 21% cholangitis-cholangiohepatitis, 13% idiopathic hepatic lipidosis, 8.5% diabetes mellitus induced hepatic lipidosis, 8.5% hemolytic anemia, 6% extrahepatic obstructions and 4% neoplasia.[78]

6. Prolonged prothrombin time will correct by more than 30% within 24-36 hours after parenteral administration of aqueous vitamin K-1 (Table 1) if cholestasis is present, but not if severe hepatocellular damage is present. Partial thrombosplastin time and activated clotting time are also prolonged in animals with liver disease.

7. Anemia often occurs in cats with liver disease.

8. Copper content of liver and kidney, but not plasma, may increase (from a normal of 20-70 mg/kg liver wet weight, 3-20 mg/kg kidney wet weight and 0.6-0.9 mg/L of plasma) in chronic liver disease with cholestasis in both dogs and cats and in all dogs with copper-storage disease (see page 7-58).

9. Liver biopsies are the only definitive method of accurate diagnosis and prognosis in many cases. To prevent excessive bleeding, blood coagulation should be checked and be adequate before a biopsy is taken. Blood coagulation may be corrected by giving fresh whole blood or plasma. Do not give stored blood, as its ammonia content increases with storage. For anesthesia of cats with suspected liver disease,

TABLE 12

ICTERUS[a] — DIFFERENTIATION OF CAUSES

Icterus—Causes	Hyperbilirubin-emia type[b]	Urine Urobilinogin[c]	Urine Bilirubin[d]	Serum Bile Acids ($\mu M/L$)[e] Fasting	Serum Bile Acids ($\mu M/L$)[e] 2 hr Postprandial	Stool Color
Hemolytic or Prehepatic	Both	Greatly increased	Decreased	<5	<16 dogs <10 cats	Dark or orange
Hepatocellular	Both	Increased	Increased	>10	Greatly Increased	Normal
Obstructive or Posthepatic	Conjugated	Decreased	Increased	>8	Greatly Increased	Light, if severe white to gray

[a]Icterus is present when plasma total bilirubin concentration is greater than 0.6 mg/dl in dogs and 0.2 in cats, although icterus cannot be detected clinically until plasma bilirubin is greater than 1.5-3 mg/dl. Anorexia increases plasma bilirubin, but rarely above 3 mg/dl.

[b]With prehepatic causes total plasma bilirubin rarely exceeds 3-4 mg/dl, and initially it is primarily unconjugated bilirubin, but within 1-2 days the conjugated form also increases. Unconjugated bilirubin is also called indirect reading, free, or non-protein-bound bilirubin. Conjugated is also called direct reading, bilirubin glucoronide, or protein bound. Conjugated bilirubin is both covalently and non-covalently bound to albumin. The longer plasma bilirubin concentration is elevated, the more of it that becomes covalently bound to albumin.[229]

[c]Also increased with constipation and decreased by urine dilution, antibiotic suppression of intestinal bacterial formation of urobilinogen, or reduced intestinal absorption.

[d]Normal dogs may have a 1+ urine bilirubin, whereas any bilirubin in the cat's urine is abnormal. The tablet diazo test (Ictotest, Ames Co.) is more sensitive and reliable than the reagent strip test in detecting urine bilirubin.

[e]Using direct spectrometric methods.[49] Normal in the dog and cat is less than 5 $\mu M/L$ fasting and less than 17 at 2 hours postprandial.[49] Fasting values are greater than 8 with intrahepatic and 40 with extrahepatic cholestasis.[47] Dogs with non-hepatic disease may have fasting values as high as 30-50 $\mu M/L$.[147] It was recommended that when fasting values exceed 30 in the dog and 20 in the cat, a liver biopsy is warranted.[45,47] In dogs and cats with severe impairment of hepatobiliary function (cirrhosis) or portasystemic venous anomalies, fasting values may be normal or increased, but at 2 hrs postprandial serum bile acid concentration may exceed 100 $\mu M/L$ or be greater than 10 times the fasting concentration.[45,46] Values for glyco-bile acid conjugates are not meaningful since dogs and cats conjugate bile acids mainly to taurine.[45]

10-30 mg of ketamine intravenously followed by nitrous oxide and halothane, has been recommended, and surital strongly cautioned against.[78] Inhalent induction with nitrous oxide and halothane by using a face mask has also been recommended for dogs with hepatic dysfunction.[172] If greater sedation of these dogs is necessary prior to inducing anesthesia, opioids, with diazepam (Valium, Roche Labs at 0.1-0.2 mg/kg) have been recommended.[172]

The best test for detecting liver disease in both dogs and cats has been shown to be a combination of serum bile acid and total bilirubin concentrations (Table 12), and serum activity of ALT.[45] The only exception was in animals having portasystemic vascular anomalies in whom the serum bile acid concentration and ammonia tolerance test had the best diagnostic efficacy.

MANAGEMENT OF HEPATIC DISEASE

The **initial management** of hepatic disease is to correct any fluid electrolyte, or glucose deficits or other alterations present. If ascites or edema is not present, give isotonic saline solution. If ascites or edema is present, use half-strength saline solution with 2.5% glucose (dextrose) instead of isotonic saline. From 10-30 mEq/L of potassium chloride should be added to either fluid. In addition, provide cage rest and frequently feed small amounts of a highly digestible diet, that is moderately restricted in salt, fat and high-quality protein, and that has increased amounts of B-vitamins (Table 13).

Clinical signs of **hypovitaminosis,** particularly those involving vitamins B, K, and (with cholestasis) E,[204] occur in many people with hepatic disease. This occurs because 1) water loss is increased, therefore causing greater loss of water-soluble B vitamins, if polyuria or diarrhea occur and 2) because of decreased fat and, therefore fat-soluble vitamins A, D, E, and K absorption, if excretion of bile is inadequate. It has been recommended that daily vitamin requirements be doubled for dogs and cats with liver disease.[86] This can be accomplished for the B vitamins by feeding a renal-failure type diet (e.g. Prescription Diets k/d, Hill's). These diets have greater amounts of B-vitamins to compensate for the increased B vitamin loss that occurs with polyuric renal failure. Vitamin K-1 (Table 1) should be given parenterally if blood coagulation is impaired. Oral administration of 5-10 mg of alpha-tocopherol/kg/day was needed to maintain normal plasma vitamin E concentrations in children with long-standing cholestasis and high serum bile acids.[204] Giving alpha-tocopherol may be a good safety precaution in similarly affected animals; however there are no studies indicating that it is necessary or beneficial.

Excess intake of **dietary fat** should be avoided because certain fatty acids induce encephalopathy. In addition, with hepatic disease, bile salt excretion may be reduced and as a result fat utilization impaired. However, dietary fat increases diet palatability and caloric content, and is needed to supply essential fatty acids, and for absorption of fat-soluble vitamins. Medium chain triglycerides (see page 7-45) are metabolized primarily in the

TABLE 13

NUTRITIONAL MANAGEMENT OF HEPATIC DISEASES

	Type of Diet*	Example** Dog	Example** Cat
Initially	Highly digestible, moderately salt, and protein restricted	Canine k/d or Recipe 2	Feline k/d or Recipe 9
If the following problems occur, or are not alleviated when this diet is being consumed, feed the diets indicated.			
Diarrhea or Steatorrhea	Highly digestible with moderate fat content	Canine i/d or Recipe 1	Feline c/d or Recipe 8
Ascites/Edema	Ultra-low sodium	Canine h/d or Recipe 5	Feline h/d or Recipe 8
Encephalopathy (CNS signs occur after eating)	Ultra-low protein	Canine u/d or Recipe 3	Add 1 T sucrose or 1 t salad oil per 4 oz Feline k/d

*Feed small amounts at frequent intervals (3–6 times daily).
**Prescription Diets (Hill's). For Recipes, see Appendix Table 3.

liver and therefore should not be given to patients with hepatic cirrhosis.[164]

Protein requirements may be increased with liver disease to return plasma albumin concentration to normal and for repair of hepatic tissue. But the ability of animals with liver disease to tolerate excess protein is impaired because of a decrease in the liver's ability to metabolize and excrete waste products produced from protein metabolism. Inadequate dietary protein results in hypoalbuminemia. Excessive dietary protein results in encephalopathy in animals with hepatic disease. A good quality moderate renal-failure diet usually prevents both a protein deficiency and an excess. Although lower in protein than most dog foods, a diet of this type, because of the high quality and digestibility of its protein, provides nearly twice the protein needs of normal dogs. It is, therefore, quite adequate for dogs with hepatic disease.

Ensure that the animal receives sufficient quantities of food to meet its **caloric needs.** Failure to provide adequate calories results in body protein catabolism, with the formation of ammonia and other waste products that must be metabolized and/or excreted by the liver. A caloric deficit also results in an increased release of fatty acids from storage fat. This may contribute to encephalopathy when the fatty acids are not removed by the diseased liver.[197] Prolonged anorexia also induces hepatic lipidosis, which is a major problem and cause of jaundice, particularly in cats.[78] If the animal refuses to eat enough to meet its caloric needs, force-feeding or tube-feeding should be used (see Chapter 5 for these procedures).

Secretion of bile salts and, therefore, digestion and absorption of fat, may be reduced and contribute to malnourishment in animals with liver disease. Despite this occurrence, giving hepatic bile salts is not usually beneficial and frequently causes diarrhea. Commercial preparations contain deconjugated bile salts which irritate the gastrointestinal mucosa.

Ascites or, less frequently, peripheral **edema** may develop in animals with liver disease. This occurs primarily as a result of portal hypertension, not hypoproteinemia caused by impaired hepatic protein synthesis, as was thought in the past.[237] Plasma albumin concentration correlates poorly with the appearance of ascites or edema in animals with liver disease.[237] Portal hypertension induces vascular fluid loss and activation of the renin-aldosterone system, which increases sodium and water retention.[237] A moderately restricted sodium diet may alleviate the ascites or edema. If it does not, sodium intake should be more severely restricted (Table 13). In addition, diuretics may be needed in some cases. Some have recommended against the use of furosemide because it must be metabolized by the liver and potentially may worsen hepatic damage; whereas, others recommend it.[86] Spironolactone or triamterene diuretics may be used to reduce the potassium-wasting caused by most other diuretics. The following procedures have been recommended for animals with ascites due to hepatic disease:[86]

1. Marked sodium restriction and spironolactone administration (Table 1).
2. If after 3-4 days these procedures are ineffective, add furosemide to the above regimen. If the response is ineffective within the next 4-7 days, double the furosemide dosage.

However, caution must be exercised in giving any diuretic to an animal with liver disease. Use of diuretics can result in a rapid fall in blood pressure, leading to hypovolemic shock. To prevent this the animal should be weighed daily and not more than 200-300 g of water loss/day allowed. A decrease of greater than 1-1.5% of body weight/day is due to fluid loss. With no loss of body water, without food intake, the nonobese animal's body weight will decrease at this rate and the obese animal's body weight will decrease at about one-half this rate (Figure 4, page 6-27). In addition to preventing too rapid a loss of body water, ascitic fluid should not be removed unless necessary to relieve dyspnea and patient discomfort. Then only enough should be removed to accomplish these goals. Removing a large amount of ascitic fluid can deplete albumin and cause hypovolemia. Diuretics should not be given to patients with potential encephalopathy. Diuretics can cause hypovolemia and prerenal azotemia. The elevated BUN will raise blood ammonia content. This is because urea moves into the gut, where bacteria convert it to ammonia, which is absorbed. Diuretics may also increase renal production of ammonia and induce hypokalemia and alkalosis, both of which increase intracellular trapping of ammonia.

Either one or both of two factors can cause **encephalopathy** with liver disease: 1) decreased hepatic removal of ammonia and other toxins (mercaptans, short-chained fatty acids, skatols, and indoles) from the circulation and 2) alterations in plasma amino acid concentrations resulting in false neurotransmitter production. Encephalopathy is most common in puppies with congenital vascular anomalies. It is uncommon in other hepatic dysfunctions. However, encephalopathy may occur in older dogs with cirrhosis, or it may

be due to extensive parenchymal destruction from lipidosis, neoplasia or hepatotoxicity.

The most common signs of encephalopathy are intermittent depression and, less commonly, vomiting, weight loss or retarded growth, diarrhea, polyuria, polydipsia, anorexia or polyphagia, hypersalivation, and central nervous system signs. Central nervous system signs include pacing or circling, ataxia, stupor, weakness, head pressing or drooping, transient blindness, seizures, and personality change. Head tremors, deafness, coma, bleeding, or jaundice may occur occasionally. The signs often appear intermittently—in about 25% of the cases, particularly after eating.

In animals with encephalopathy ammonia and usually BSP clearances are decreased. Generally, fasting plasma ammonia concentration, partial thromboplastin time, and alkaline phosphatase activity are increased, and the BUN, plasma protein and cholesterol concentrations are decreased. As with any condition in which blood ammonia levels are increased, large numbers of ammonium biurate crystals may be present in the urine. A definitive diagnosis can be made from positive-contrast portography.

If a **portasystemic vascular shunt** is responsible for the encephalopathy and it can be corrected surgically, it should be done. The patient should be stabilized with proper medical management before surgery and this management continued for as long as necessary after surgery. Proper medical management is to feed a moderately restricted protein diet (Table 13). Because protein requirements to regenerate hepatic tissue may be increased in animals with hepatic disease, an ultra- low-protein diet should not be used unless necessary, that is, unless signs occur when a moderately restricted protein diet is being consumed. Feeding a diet containing a high ratio of branched-chain amino acids to aromatic amino acids may be beneficial. This helps correct the alterations in plasma amino acid concentrations that may occur with hepatic encephalopathy.[200] A diet composed of equal parts of cottage cheese and boiled rice accomplished this objective. However, for long-term feeding this diet would need to be balanced with vitamins, minerals, and essential fatty acids as given in Recipe 6 (Appendix Table 3).

For patients with liver disease, the diet, in addition to being low in protein and containing a high ratio of branched-chain amino acids to aromatic amino acids—should be: 1) high in readily available carbohydrate to prevent hypoglycemia, 2) low in urate precursors (cell nuclei) and produce an alkaline urine to assist in preventing formation of

ammonium urate uroliths, and 3) low in methionine and choline. Ammonium urate uroliths are a common complication in dogs with hepatic disease. Diets properly formulated for managing renal failure (e.g. Prescription Diets k/d and u/d, Hill's, or Recipes 3 and 9, Appendix Table 3, substituting 1/4 cup of non-creamed cottage cheese per egg and per 1/4 lb of liver) meet all of these criteria.

Diuretics and lipotrophic agents such as methionine and choline should be avoided in patients at risk of encephalopathy. Methionine and choline are converted by intestinal bacteria to mercaptans, which are quite toxic. They may be absorbed, escape hepatic removal because of decreased hepatic function and induce encephalopathy and coma. Thus, diets fed to patients with severe liver disease (or to patients in which encephalopathy may occur) should be low in methionine and choline. Neither should lipotrophic agents be given to these patients. Their benefit in all cases of liver disease is questionable and they are not needed if a good diet is being fed. In one study, 5 dogs were given choline citrate orally at a dosage of 88 mg/kg twice daily for 10 days, after carbon tetrachoride-induced hepatic damage.[139] Efficacy was minimal. In contrast, silibinin given orally at a dosage of 16 mg/kg twice daily for 10 days decreased BSP retention from 11% to 4.5% and lessened the increase in serum alanine aminotransferase (ALT) and alkaline phosphatase activities.

Intestinal bacterial degradation of nutrients and production of ammonia should be reduced in animals with hepatic encephalopathy. This may be accomplished by giving poorly absorbed antibacterial agents orally (e.g. vancomycin, neomycin, or kanamycin). Enemas containing 1% neomycin and 10% vinegar may also be beneficial. Vinegar contains acetic acid which, by acidifying the intestinal contents, converts ammonia which is readily absorbed to the ammonium ion, which is not absorbed. However, antibiotics and enemas are usually necessary only in cases of massive hepatic necrosis.[197] Lactulose (Table 1) may also be given to acidify intestinal contents. Lactulose is a poorly absorbed carbohydrate that is converted by intestinal bacteria to acetic and lactic acids. The dosage used should be adjusted to produce 2-3 soft stools daily. For dogs, this is generally 5-15 ml of lactulose, three times per day.

Any gastrointestinal bleeding should be controlled as quickly as possible. This is best detected using the HemoQuant test, which is significantly more sensitive than the guaiac Hemoccult test (see page 7-47).[2,23] Digestion of blood by intestinal bacteria contributes to production of ammonia and mercaptans. It is important to control hook-

worm infestation, gastroenteritis, gastrointestinal ulcers, and bleeding disorders. The latter two are common complications of hepatic disease. If there is bleeding from the colon, cleansing enemas may be administered. Blood transfusions with stored blood should be avoided as the ammonia content of blood increases with storage.

Prednisolone, is usually considered of no benefit in the therapy of acute hepatic necrosis. It may induce hepatopathy and should not be used if suppurative cholangiohepatitis is present. Prednisolone, however, is generally considered beneficial for dogs and cats with chronic active hepatitis or fibrosis (0.5-1 mg of prednisolone/kg/day) because of its anti-inflammatory, immunosuppressive and antifibrotic effects.[44] Although this treatment is controversial, in a study in dogs it lengthened survival time from 6.5 to 18-29 months[197] and has been reported to be beneficial for affected cats.[78] Azathioprine (Table 1) also may be beneficial in treatment of chronic active hepatitis. It allows for a reduction in corticosteroid dosage because of its immuno-suppressive effects on the liver. Colchicine (Table 1) has been used experimentally in dogs with chronic active hepatitis,[197] and its use reported in one clinical case.[20] Colchicine is thought to inhibit collagen production, and increase collagenase-mediated removal of fibrous tissue from the liver.[127] It has also been reported to be beneficial to some people with cirrhosis.[113] In one dog with hepatic necrosis, fibrosis, and ascites, prednisolone worsened clinical signs and biochemical alterations. There was dramatic clinical improvement within 3 weeks after administration of colchicine. By 7 weeks, biochemical alterations improved, hepatic inflammation decreased, and hepatic fibrosis was less aggressive.[20] Four months later, after continued improvement, colchicine therapy was discontinued. Relapse and death occurred within 2 months after colchicine therapy was stopped, despite reinstitution of colchicine therapy and aggressive medical management. At necropsy, hepatic fibrosis was found to be minimal. Adverse reactions associated with either acute or chronic colchicine therapy in people were not seen in dogs.[20,197] However, colchicine is not approved for use in dogs, and should be administered with caution. There are no controlled studies of its efficacy or safety in managing canine hepatic fibrosis.[20]

Infectious conditions are one of the more common complications of liver disease. Rectal temperature should be monitored and, if elevated, systemic antibiotics should be given. Antibiotics are also indicated for animals with cholangitis or cirrhosis. Although many antibiotics are metabolized and excreted by the liver, most of them can be used at standard dosages without harmful effects. Ampicillin, cephalosporins, streptomycin, gentamicin, and kanamycin have been recommended; whereas, chloramphenicol, nitrofurans, tetracycline, novabiocin, and lincomycin may be harmful. Metronidazole (Table 1) is reported to be more effective than penicillin in treatment for suppurative cholangiohepatitis in cats.[78]

COPPER STORAGE DISEASE

A primary hepatic copper-storage disease occurs as a heredity autosomal recessive disorder in Bedlington Terriers, West Highland White Terriers, and perhaps occasionally other breeds. It resembles **Wilson's Disease** in people except that neurologic and corneal lesions (Kayser-Fleischer rings) do not develop in dogs as they do in people. As many as 50% of Bedlington Terriers may be affected, with incidence equal in both sexes.[211] The disorder involves impaired removal of copper from the liver, resulting in accumulation of abnormally large amounts of copper, which causes a chronic progressive liver disease characterized by hepatolenticular degeneration.

Abnormally high content of copper in the liver may occur secondary to any chronic liver disease that impairs bile excretion (such as primary bilary cirrhosis, bilary tract disorders, and chronic active hepatitis)[48,63] because copper is removed from the body primarily by biliary excretion. Thus, excess liver copper is the **cause** of copper-storage disease in Bedlington Terriers and Wilson's Disease in people. In people, excess liver copper is considered an **effect** of any chronic liver disease in which excretion of bile is impaired.[63] However, excess hepatic copper (more than about 2000 ppm of dry matter) causes hepatic damage.[195,205,211] Hepatic damage, if it restricts bile excretion, decreases copper excretion, further increasing hepatic copper content and resulting in a progressive reduction in hepatic function. In addition, elevated hepatic copper content at concentrations that are hepatotoxic has been found in dogs without hepatic fibrosis, cirrhosis, histologic cholestasis, an elevated plasma bilirubin, or clinical signs of liver disease. This condition affects primarily purebred dogs regardless of breed.[207,208] It has been suggested that all of this indicates that the elevated hepatic copper content does not occur as a result of, but instead is a cause of, chronic liver disease in many breeds of dogs.[207,208] However, in these dogs histologic hepatic alterations differ from those in Bedlington Terriers with primary copper-storage disease. In these dogs, the main histologic alteration is focal hepatitis, characterized by single-

cell necrosis and inflammation; whereas, primary copper-storage disease in Bedlington Terriers is characterized by hepatolenticular degeneration.[208]

High hepatic liver copper content secondary to cholestasis occurs in cats.[48] It also occurs in conjunction with chronic liver disease, particularly in middle-aged female Doberman Pinschers with chronic active hepatitis. It may, however occur in other breeds, in any aged adult, and in either sex.[56,104,207] A genetic basis for this higher incidence in female Doberman Pinschers has been suggested.[56,104] In these dogs, liver copper content is less than 2500 μg/g (ppm) of dry matter.[56,104,207,208] In dogs with primary copper storage disease, although hepatic copper content may be 2500 ppm or less, it may exceed 10,000 ppm.[211] Normal is 100-400 ppm of dry matter (20-70 ppm of wet weight).[104,207,211]

In dogs with primary copper storage disease, hepatic copper concentrations rise with age. By the time the dog is 6 months of age, the increase in hepatic copper content is evident, although clinical signs and biochemical evidence of liver disease do not generally occur until the dog is several years of age.[206] The condition manifests itself as a typical liver disease (see page 7-52).

ALT (SGPT) activity is elevated in about two-thirds of affected dogs. There is intolerance to stress with insidious deterioration. Plasma copper concentration is usually near normal (0.6-0.9 mg/L) or is only slightly elevated. Plasma ceruloplasmin concentration may be reduced (normal is 25-35 mg/dl), although if severe hepatic dysfunction is present, it may be closer to normal. The liver is swollen and hepatic cell necrosis, fibrous tissue proliferation, and brownish eosinophilic granules in the hepatocytes may be seen microscopically. Dogs with primary copper-storage disease, and those with any liver disease that may lessen bile and therefore copper excretion, should be fed a low-copper diet as described on page 13-5.

Once copper-toxicity induced hepatic damage is present, no treatment will reverse it; therefore, for breeds such as the Bedlington Terrier, in which a high percentage are affected, a low-copper diet should be fed throughout the animal's life. Zinc supplementation may also be beneficial for both prevention and treatment. Zinc reduces copper absorption and, when given 3-6 times daily at a dosage of 2-3 mg/kg/day, has caused a negative or neutral copper balance in people with primary copper storage disease (Wilson's Disease).[92] A low-copper diet should be started early in the dog's life. If this is not done and, as a result, hepatic dysfunction occurs, routine supportive therapy for decreased hepatic function should be given, in addition to feeding a low-copper diet and possibly giving zinc. D-penicillamine (Table 1) increases urinary copper excretion and therefore may be helpful for dogs with primary copper-storage disease.

D-penicillamine should be given orally at least 30 minutes before meals or at least 2 hours after eating. Food in the stomach decreases the absorption of D-penicillamine.[18] If vomiting occurs, the daily dose should be divided into smaller doses, given more often. In one trial in a single Bedlington Terrier, giving D-penicillamine at this dosage removed all excess copper from the liver in 26 months.[135] Based on results of this study, and since the drug can cause copper deficiency,[201] it may be best to decrease to a much smaller maintenance dosage after 1-2 years, or discontinue giving the drug and maintain the dog on a low-copper diet. D-penicillamine may also cause a pyridoxine deficiency;[101] therefore, when it is given, the diet should be high in this B-vitamin, or supplemental amounts should be given daily. D-penicillamine should not be given for at least 3 weeks after surgery or trauma as it decreases wound healing by interfering with topocollagen synthesis, and collagen and elastin cross-linking.[13,63,187] In addition, animals with chronic liver disease should not be given D-penicillamine as a means of decreasing or preventing excessive hepatic copper content. It seems logical, and it has been suggested[104] that D-penicillamine may be beneficial and is the treatment of choice in affected dogs,[207] but has not been demonstrated. In contrast, in two double-blind studies involving 253 people with primary biliary cirrhosis, D-penicillamine was of no benefit, and is not recommended. In 22% of people taking the drug it induced major side effects, including cytopenia, anorexia, lichen planus, dysgeusia, proteinuria, skin rash, nausea and death.[63,102,141] Instead, a low-copper diet is recommended.[102]

GLYCOGEN-STORAGE DISEASES

Glycogen-storage diseases occur due to a deficiency in one of the enzymes required for proper glycogen metabolism. Eight types have been identified in people, each type being due to the deficit of a different enzyme. All types occurring in dogs, except Type II, result in hypoglycemia, which in turn results in weakness, ataxia, a dazed appearance, muscle fasciculations, exercise intolerance, and, if sufficiently severe, hysteria, convulsions, and coma. There are three, and possibly four, types of glycogen storage diseases reported to occur in dogs. All are uncommon. These are:

1. **Generalized** glycogen-storage disease of puppies or juvenile hypoglycemia, which they outgrow. Although this is often referred to as a glycogen-storage disease, there is no supportive evidence, and it is unlikely that it is. This disease affects primarily smaller breeds and may be simply a stress-induced hypoglycemia, which is usually precipitated by cold, starvation, or excitement. Response to glucagon administration is normal.

2. **Type I** glycogen-storage disease or **von Gierke's Disease** is due to a deficiency of the enzyme (glucose-6-phosphatase) needed for converting glucose-6-phosphate, and therefore glycogen, to glucose. It occurs primarily in 6-12 week old puppies and is characterized by slow growth, hypoglycemia, hepatomegaly due to excess glycogen deposition, and decreased response to glucagon administration.[21] Elevations in plasma concentrations of lactate, uric acid, free fatty acids, triglycerides, and cholesterol may also be present.[184] Management requires frequent feedings, with dietary restriction of dextrose and fructose (such as table sugar) and galactose (milk sugar), especially early in life.[121] Ingestion of raw, but not cooked, cornstarch at 1.75-2.5 g/kg every 6 hours maintains normoglycemia in children with this disease.[51]

3. **Hunting-dog** or **functional hyopoglycemia** thought, but not confirmed, to be similar to **Cori's Disease (Type III** glycogen-storage disease or limited dextrinosis) in people. Type III glycogen-storage disease is caused by a deficiency of the debranching enzyme (amylo-t-phosphatase) required for complete glycogen utilization.[21] Hunting-dog hypoglycemia usually affects nervous, lean, eager dogs 1-2 hours after beginning a hunt. Although recovery usually occurs within a few minutes, affected dogs remain exhausted for the rest of the day. After administration of glucagon, the plasma glucose concentration increases in non-fasted but not fasted dogs. Management of the dog with functional or hunting-dog hypoglycemia and other possible causes of hypoglycemia are given on pages 3-30 and 13-12.

4. **Type II** glycogen-storage disease or **Pompe's Disease** is due to a deficiency of lysosomal acid alpha-glucosidase, which results in excessive generalized accumulation of glycogen, particularly in cardiac and skeletal muscle. All confirmed and suspected cases have been in Lapland dogs of which 4 of the 5 cases were males.[225] Clinical signs developed gradually, beginning after the dogs were 6 months of age and progressing slowly, with death or euthanasia occurring prior to 18 months of age. Clinical signs included frequent vomiting and regurgitation, megaesophagus, dysphonia, persistent panting, cardiac abnormalities, muscle weakness, and an inclination to remain recumbent although affected animals were not lethargic.

With glycogen-storage diseases, like most other causes of hypoglycemia, except **insulinomas** (insulin-secreting tumor of the pancreatic beta cells), plasma insulin concentration is reduced in the presence of hypoglycemia. Insulinomas are rare in dogs and have been reported in only two cats.[144] Hyperinsulinemia (normal is 4-50 micro Units/ml) at the time of hypoglycemia (less than 70 mg/dl) is the most accurate means of diagnosing insulinoma.[131] Simultaneous measurements of plasma glucose and insulin concentrations after an overnight fast are diagnostic in most dogs with this tumor. If fasting does not produce hypoglycemia so this test can be run, glucagon administration (0.03 mg/kg given intravenously), monitoring the plasma glucose 0, 3, 5, 15, 30, 60, 90, and 120 minutes later, and measuring plasma insulin concentration when hypoglycemia occurs, are indicated[105,131] Glucose/insulin, insulin/glucose, and amended insulin/glucose ratios provide fewer false-negative results in testing for the presence of an insulinoma, but more false-positive results, than does the presence of a lowered plasma insulin with hypoglycemia.[131]

Treatment of insulinoma is surgical removal of the tumor and enlarged regional lymph nodes. If the tumor cannot be located, if metastasis has occurred, or hypoglycemia recurs after surgery, frequent feedings may be sufficient to maintain the animal.[131] If it is not, give diazoxide (Proglycem, Schering) orally, initially at a dosage of 3 mg/kg every 8 hours and increase it gradually to a maximum of 40 mg/kg/day if necessary to control hypoglycemia.[131]

SUMMARY AND CONCLUSIONS

A highly digestible diet is indicated for conditions in which the ability to digest or absorb nutrients is impaired. These impairments greatly magnify differences in diet digestibility. For example, although a dietary food was only 15% more digestible than a regular dog food when fed to normal dogs; it was 89% more digestible when consumed by dogs with pancreatic exocrine insufficiency (Table 9, page 7-43). Magnification of differences in diet digestibility occurs with any impairment in the ability to digest or absorb

ingested nutrients, whether this impairment is caused by pancreatic, gastric, intestinal, or hepatic dysfunction. Feeding a highly digestible diet, particularly in small amounts at frequent intervals, greatly reduces the amount of undigested nutrients that remain in the intestinal tract (Table 11, page 7-44). This decrease is beneficial in lessening the osmolality of the intestinal luminal fluid, and therefore intestinal secretion, and in decreasing or preventing bacterial multiplication and overgrowth in the intestine. Intestinal bacterial overgrowth causes, maintains, or worsens diarrhea and nutrient malassimilation.

A number of treatment and management procedures may be beneficial, depending on the gastric, intestinal, pancreatic, or hepatic dysfunction present. However, with the exception of constipation, and in most dogs with colitis, regardless of which dysfunction is present or what other treatments are used, feeding a highly-digestible, low-fiber, lactose-free diet at frequent intervals is in many cases the most beneficial treatment, and should always be used in managing these cases. In contrast, a high-fiber weight reducing-type diet is beneficial for most dogs and cats with colitis, and is also beneficial in decreasing recurrence of constipation. A high-fiber diet helps normalize altered intestinal motility, helping to alleviate both diarrhea and constipation in patients with large bowel disorders.

A hypoallergenic diet should be fed in cases where food allergy or sensitivity is suspected or confirmed. In addition to food allergy, this would include eosinophalic gastroenteritis and/or colitis. A hypoallergenic diet is one consisting of ingredients the animal has not previously experienced, and contains as few ingredients as possible. A low-fat diet, such as a weight reducing diet, should be fed to animals with lymphangiectasia.

REFERENCES

1. Abbitt B, Huey RL Eugster AK, Syler J: Treatment of giardiasis in adult Greyhounds, using ipronidazole-medicated water. J Amer Vet Med Assoc 188:67-70 (1986).

2. Ahlquist DA, McGill DB, Swartz S, et al: Fecal blood in health and disease. New Engl J Med 312:1422-1488 (1985).

3. Almy TP, Howell DA: Diverticular disease of the colon. New Engl J Med 302:324-331 (1980).

4. Alroy J, Leav I, DeLellis RA, et al: Distinctive intestinal mast cell neoplasms of domestic cats. Lab Invest 33:159-167 (1975).

5. Anderson JW: Physiological and metabolic effects of dietary fiber. Feder Proc 44:2902-2906 (1985).

6. Anderson I, Levine A, Levitt MD: Use of breath hydrogen excretion to study absorption of wheat flour. Gastroent 78:1131 Abstract (1980).

7. Appel M, Meunier P, Pollock R, et al: Canine viral enteritis. Canine Pract 7:22-36 (1980).

8. Armstrong B, Poll R: Environmental factors and cancer incidence and mortality in different countries with special reference to dietary practices. Int J Cancer 15:617-631 (1975).

9. Asada M, Galambos JT: Sorbitol dehydrogenase and hepatocellular injury. Gastroent 44:578-587 (1963).

10. Atkins CE, Tyler R, Greenlee P: Clinical, biochemical, acid-base, and electrolyte abnormalities in cats after hypertonic sodium phosphate enema administration. Amer J Vet Res 46:980-988 (1985).

11. August JR: Diet hypersensitivity in the dog. Proc Amer Anim Hosp Assoc Ann Meeting pp 2-5 (1986).

12. Baker E: Food allergy in the cat. Feline Pract pp. 18-26 (May-June 1975).

13. Bardach H, Gebhart W, Niebauer G: "Jumpy-bumpy" elastic fibers in the skin and lungs of a patient with a penicillamine-induced elastosis perforans serpiginosa. J Cutan Pathol 6:243-252 (1979).

14. Batt RM: Chronic small intestinal disease in the dog. Proc Kal Kan Symp pp 93-103 (1984).

15. Batt RM, Morgan JO: Role of serum folate and vitamin B-12 concentrations in differentiation of small intestinal abnormalities in the dog. Res Vet Sci 32:17-22 (1982).

16. Batt RM, Needham JR, Carter BW: Bacterial overgrowth associated with a naturally occurring enteropathy in the German Shepherd dog. Res Vet Sci 35:42 (1983).

17. Bentinck-Smith J: A roster of normal values. In Current Vet Therapy, No. V, Editor RW Kirk, WB Saunders Co, Philadelphia, PA pp 1000 (1974).

18. Bergstrom RF: Penicillamine kinetics in normal subjects. Clin Pharmacol Therapeut 30:404-413 (1981).

19. Blum AL, Riecken EO, Dammann HG, et al: Comparison of omeprazole and ranitidine in the treatment of reflux esophagitis. New Eng J Med 314:716 (1986).

20. Boer HH, Nelwon RW, Long GG: Colchicine therapy for hepatic fibrosis in a dog. J Amer Vet Med Assoc 185:303-305 (1984).

21. Bordens JW: Glycogen storage disease in puppies. Vet Med/Small Anim Clin 61:1174-1176 (1966).

22. Boudrieau RJ, Rogers WA: Megaesophagus in the dog: A review of 50 cases. J Amer Anim Hosp Assoc 21:33-40 (1985).

23. Boulay JP, Lipowitz AJ, Klausner JS, et al: Evaluation of a fluorometric method for the quantitative assay of fecal hemoglobin in the dog. Amer J Vet Res 47:1293-1295 (1986).

24. Breitschwerdt EB: Immunoproliferaive enteropathy of Basenjis. Proc 8th Kal Kan Symp pp 111-117 (1984).

25. Breitschwerdt EB, Barta O, Waltman C, et al: Serum proteins in healthy Basenjis and Basenjis with chronic diarrhea. Amer J Vet Res 44:326-328 (1983).

26. Breitschwerdt EB, Halliwell WH, Foley CW, et al: A hereditary diarrheic syndrome in the Basenji characterized by malabsorption, protein losing enteropathy and hypergammaglobulinemia. J Amer Anim Hosp Assoc 16:551-560 (1980).

27. Brooks FP: Effect of diet on gastric acid secretion. Amer J Clin Nutr 42:1006-1019 (1985).

28. Brunner CJ, Swango LJ: Canine parvovirus infection. Comp Cont Ed 7:979-988 (1985).

29. Bunch, SE: Hypocholesterolemia in dogs. Proc Amer College Vet Int Med 2:13-7 to 13-20 (1986).

30. Burrows CF: Part II: Disease of the colon, rectum and anus in the dog and cat. In Veterinary Gastroenterology, Editor NV Anderson, Publisher Lea & Febiger, Philadelphia, PA pp 553-592 (1980).

31. Burrows CF: Chronic diarrhea in the dog. Vet Clin of N Amer 13(3):521-539 (1983).

32. Burrows CF: Concepts of gastrointestinal disease. Amer Anim Hosp Assoc Ann Proc pp 155-158 (1984).

33. Burrows CF: Diarrhea in the dog, a clinical perspective. Monograph published by Alpo Petfoods, Inc, Allentown, PA (1984).

34. Burrows CF: Diseases of the canine and feline colon and anorectum. Amer Anim Hosp Assoc Ann Proc pp 177-181 (1984).

35. Burrows CF: Approach to the gastrointestinal case and formulation of a differential diagnosis. Amer Anim Hosp Assoc Ann Proc pp 261-266 (1985).

36. Burrows CF: Gastrointestinal diseases of aging animals. Proc 10th World Small Anim Cong pp 61 (1985).

37. Burrows CF: Treatment of gastrointestinal disease in small animals. Mod Vet Pract Part 1 pp 93-97, Feb and Part 2 pp 181-185, March (1985).

38. Burrows CF: Western States Vet Med Assoc Ann Meeting. Las Vegas, NV (1986).

39. Burrows CM, Bright RM, Spencer CP: Influence of dietary composistion and canine gastric emptying and motility-potential role in acute gastric dilatation. Amer J Vet Res 46:2609 (1985).

40. Burrows CF, Jezyk PF: Nitrosonapthol test for screening of small intestinal diarrheal disease in the dog. J Amer Vet Med Assoc 183:318-322 (1983).

41. Burrows CF, Kronfeld DS, Banta CA, Merritt AM: Effects of fiber on digestibility and transit time in dogs. J Nutr 112:1726-1732 (1982).

42. Burrows CF, Merritt AM: Influence of alpha-cellulose on myoelectric activity of proximal canine colon. Amer J Physiol 245 (Gastrointest Liver Physiol 8):G301-G306 (1983).

43. Caywood D, Teague HD, Jackson DA, et al: Gastric gas analysis in canine gastric dilitation-volvulus syndrome. J Amer Anim Hosp Assoc 13:459-462 (1977).

44. Center SA: Differentil diagnosis of juandice in the cat. Amer Anim Hosp Assoc Ann Proc pp 277-287 (1986).

45. Center SA: The biochemical evaluation of liver function in the dog and cat. Proc Amer College Vet Int Med 1:1-69 to 1-83 (1986).

46. Center SA, Baldwin BH, deLahunta A, et al: Evaluation of serum bile acid concentrations for the diagnosis of portasystemic venous anomalies in the dog and cat. J Amer Vet Med Assoc 186:1090-1094 (1985).

47. Center SA, Baldwin BH, Erb HN, Tennant BC: Bile acid concentrations in the diagnosis of hepatobiliary disease in the dog. J Amer Vet Med Assoc 187:935-940 (1985).

48. Center SA, Baldwin BH, King JM, Tennant BC: Experimental extrahepatic bile duct obstruction in the cat. Proc Conf of Research Workers in Anim Dis p 46 (1982).

49. Center SA, Leveille CR, Baldwin BH, Tennant BC: Direct spectrometric determinatin of serum bile acids in the dog and cat. Amer J Vet Res 45:2043-2050 (1984).

50. Chang EB, Field M: Intestinal electrolyte transport and diarrhea disease. In: The Gastroenterology Annual I. Editors Kern F, Blum AL; Elsevier/N Amsterdam, Holland pp 148-180 (1983).

51. Chen Y-T, Cornblath M, Sidbury JB: Cornstarch therapy in type I glycogen-storage disease. New Engl J Med 310:171-174 (1984).

52. Chew S, Mahadevan V, Zieve L: Volatile fatty acids in the breath of patients with cirrhosis of the liver. J Lab Clin Med 75:622-627 (1970).

53. Clifford DH, Soifer FK, Wilson CF, et al: Congenital achalasia of the esophagus in four cats of common ancestry. J Amer Vet Med Ass 158:1554-1560 (1971).

54. Cornelius CE: Biochemical evaluation of hepatic function in dogs. J Amer Anim Hosp Assoc 15:259-269 (1979).

55. Cox VS, Wallace LJ, Anderson VE, Rushmer RA: Hereditary esophageal dysfunction in the Miniature Schnauzer dog. Amer J Vet Res 41:326-330 (1980).

56. Crawford MA, Schall WD, Jensen RK, Tasker JB: Chronic active hepatitis in 26 Doberman Pinschers. J Amer Vet Med Assoc 187:1343-1350 (1985).

57. Dairy Council Digest:Lactose intolerance. National Dairy Council, 111 N Canal St, Chicago. IL 42(No.6) (1971).

58. DeHoff WD: Medical treatment of gastroesophageal intussusceptive hiatal hernia. Tex Vet Med J 46:32 (1984).

59. Delorme CB, Gordon C: The effect of pectin on the utilization of marginal levels of dietary protein by weanling rats. J Nutr 113:2432-2441 (1983).

60. Delorme CB, Gordon C: The effect of protein levels on the response of weanling rats to dietary pectin. J Nutr 114:1797-1806 (1984).

61. Delorme CB, Wojcik J: Interaction of dietary protein with cellulose in the adaptation to caloric dilution by weanling rats. J Nutr 112:21-28 (1982).

62. DeNovo RC, Prasse KW: Comparison of serum biochemical and hepatic functional alterations in dogs treated with corticosteroids and hepatic duct ligation. Amer J Vet Res 44:1703-1709 (1983).

63. Dickson ER, Fleming TR, Wiesner RH, et al: Trial of penicillamine in advanced primary biliary cirrhosis. New Engl J Med 312:1011-1015 (1985).

64. Dietze A: Digestive tract foreign bodies of small animals. Kal Kan Forum 54-59 (Summer 1984).

65. Dooley JF: Sorbitol dehydrogenase and its use in toxicology testing in lab animals. Lab Anim J 13(4):20-21 (1984).

66. Douglas SW: Lesions involving the pyloric region of the canine stomach. Proc 1st International Conf of Vet Radiologists, Dublin, Ireland (6 Sept 1968).

67. Drazner FH: Diseases of canine and feline pancreas. Amer Anim Hosp Assoc Ann Proc pp 293-301 (1985).

68. Dutta SK, Hlasko J: Dietary fiber in pancreatic disease: Effect of high fiber diet on fat malabsorption in pancreatic insufficiency and in vitro study of the interaction of dietary fiber with pancreatic enzymes. Amer J Clin Nutr 41:517-525 (1985).

69. Eastwood GI, Castell DO, Higgs RH: Experimental esophagitis in cats impairs lower esophageal spincter pressure. Gastroent 69:146:153 (1975).

70. Eastwood MA: Fiber in the gastrointestinal tract. Amer J Clin Nutr 31:S30-S32 (1978).

71. Fleming MP: Association of Campylobacter jejuni with enteritis in dogs and cats. Vet Rec 113:372-374 (1983).

72. Fleming SE, Marthinsen D, Kuhnlein H: Colonic function and fermentation in men consuming high fiber diets. J Nutr 113:2535-2544 (1983).

73. Forbes DC, Leishman DE: Megaesophagus in a cat. Canad Vet J 26:354-356 (1985).

74. Fox JG, Krakowka S, Taylor NS: Acute-onset Campylobacter associated gastroenteritis in adult Beagles. J Amer Vet Med Assoc 1877:1268-1271 (1985).

75. Fox SM, Ellison GW, Miller GJ, Howells D: Observations on the mechanical failure of three gastropexy techniques. J Amer Anim Hosp Assoc 21:729-734 (1985).

76. Frank HA, Green LS: Successful use of a bulk laxative to control the diarrhea of tube feeding. Scand J Plast Reconstr Surg 13:193-194 (1979).

77. Gabbert NH, Nachreiner RF, et al: Serum immunoreactive gastrin concentrations in the dog: Basal and postprandial values measured by radioimmunoassay. J Vet Res 145:2351-2353 (1984).

78. Garvey MS: The jaundiced cat. Amer Anim Hosp Ann Proc pp 214-224 (1985).

79. Glickman LT, Domanski LM, Patronek GJ, Visintainer F: Breed-related risk factors for canine parvovirus enteritis. J Amer Vet Med Assoc 187:589-594 (1985).

80. Goldin BR, Gorbach S: Effect of Lactobacillus acidophilus dietary supplements on 1,2-dimethylhydrazine dihydrochloride-induced intestinal cancer in rats. Natl Cancer Inst 64:263-265 (1980).

81. Goldin BR, Gorbach SH: The effect of milk and lactobacillus feeding on human intestinal enzyme activity. Amer J Clin Nutr 39:756-761 (1984).

82. Goldstein F: Bacterial populations of the gut in health and disease: Clinical aspects. In Gastroenterology, 3rd edition, Editor Brockus HL, Publisher WB Saunders Co, Philadelphia, PA 2:152-169 (1974).

83. Goodall RJR, Temple JG: Effect of cimetidine on lower oesophageal sphincter in oesophagitis. Brit Med J 280:611-612 (1980).

84. Gyory CP, Chang GW: Effects of bran and deoxycholic acid on the permeability of the rat cecum and colon. J Nutr 113:2300-2307 (1983).

85. Hardy RM: Esophageal disorders. Proc Amer Hosp Assoc Midwest Regional Meeting (9 Dec 1978).

86. Hardy RM: The diagnosis and therapy of hepatic disease. Amer Anim Hosp Assoc Ann Proc pp 384-397 (1986).

87. Harvey CE, O'Brien JA, Durle VR, et al: Megaesophagus in the dog: A clinical survey of 79 cases. J Amer Vet Med Asooc 165:443-446 (1974).

88. Hawkins EC, Meric SM, Washabau RJ, et al: Digestion of bentiromide and absorption of xylose in healthy cats and absorption of xylose in cats with infiltrative intestinal disease. Amer J Vet Res 47:567-569 (1986).

89. Hayden DW, Van Kruinigen HJ: Control values for evaluation of gastrointestinal function in the dog. J Amer Anim Hosp Assoc 12:31-36 (1976).

90. Henderson RD, Mugashe F, Jeejeebhoy KN, et al: the role of bile and acid in the production of esophagitis and the motor defect of esophagitis. Ann Thorac Surg 14:465-473 (1972).

91. Hill FWG: Malabsorption syndrome in the dog: a study of thirty-eight cases. J Sm Anim Pract 13:575-594 (1972).

92. Hill GM, Brewer GJ, Prasad AS, et al: Oral zinc therapy for Wilson's disease patients. Clin Res 31:466A (1983).

93. Hitchins AD, Wells P, McDonough FE, Wong NP: Amelioration of the adverse effect of a gastrointestinal challange with Salmonella enteritidis on weanling rats by a yogurt diet. Amer J Clin Nutr 41:92-100 (1985).

94. Hoenig M: Intestinal malabsorption attributed to bacterial overgrowth in a dog. J Amer Vet Med Assoc 176:533-535 (1980).

95. Hoffer RE, MacCoy DM, Quick CB et al: Management of acquired achalasia in dogs. J Amer Vet Med Assoc 175:814-818 (1979).

96. Hopman WPM, Jansen BMJ, Rosenbusch G, Lamers CBHW: Effect of equimolar amounts of long-chain triglycerides and medium-chain triglycerides on plasma cholecystokinin and gall bladder contraction. Amer J Clin Nutr 39:356-359 (1984).

97. Hsu WH, McNeel SV: Effect of yohimbine on xylazine-induced prolongation of gastrointestinal transit in dogs. J Amer Vet Med Assoc 183:297-300 (1983).

98. Hull C, Greco RS, Brooke DL: Alleviation of constipation in the elderly by dietary fiber supplementation. J Amer Geriatr Soc 28:410-414 (1980).

99. Iseminger M, Hardy P: Bran works! Geriatr Nurs pp 402-404 (Nov/Dec 1982).

100. Jaffe BM, Kopen DF, DeSchryver-Keck-kemeti K, et al: Indomethacin-responsive pancreatic cholera. N Engl J Med 297:818-821 (1977).

101. Jaffe I, Altman K, Merryman P: The antipyridoxine effect of penicillamine in man. J Clin Invest 43:1869-1873 (1964).

102. James SP: Primary biliary cirrhosis. New Engl J Med 312:1055-1057 (1985).

103. Jarroll EA, Hoff JC, Meyer EA: Resistance of cysts to disinfection agents. In Giardia and Giardiasis, Editors SL Erlandsen, EA Meyer, Plenum Press, New York, NY pp 311-328 (1984).

104. Johnson GF, Zawie DA, Gilbertson SR, Sternlieb I: Chronic active hepatitis in Doberman Pinschers. J Amer Vet Med Assoc 180:1438-1442 (1982).

105. Johnson RK, Atkins CE: Hypoglycemia in the dog. In Current Vet Therapy VI, Editor RW Kirk, publisher WB Saunders Co, Philadelphia, PA pp 1010-1016 (1977).

106. Johnson SE: Clinical pharmacology of antiemetics and antidiarrheals. Proc 8th Kal Kan Symp, 7-15 (1984).

107. Jones BD: The medical problem of vomiting. Amer Animal Hosp Assoc Ann Proc, pp 270-281 (1985).

108. Jones BD: The malassimilation syndromes. J Amer Anim Hosp Assoc Ann Proc, pp 335-353 (1986).

109. Jones VA: Diet therapy for Chrohn's disease. Lancet II (8448): 177-180 (July 27, 1985).

110. Jorgenson LS, Center SA, Randolph JF, Brum D: Electrolyte abnormalities induced by hypertonic phosphate enemas in two cats. J Amer Vet Med Assoc 187:1367-1368 (1985).

111. Kagan KG, Schaer M: Gastric dilatation and volvulus in a dog—A case justifying electrolyte and acid-base assessment. J Amer Vet Med Assoc 182:703-706 (1983).

112. Kasprzah W, Mazur T, Matylla W: Resistance of Giardia cysts to physical and chemical agents. Biul Inst Med Morsh 31:239-249 (1980).

113. Kershenobich D, Uribe M, Suares GI, et al: Treatment of cirrhosis with colchicine: A double-blind randomized trial. Gastroent 77:532-536 (1979).

114. Kirk RW: Pediatrics. In Canine Medicine, First Catcott Edition, Amer Vet Publications Inc, Santa Barbara, CA (1968).

115. Kirk RW, Bistner SI: In Vet Procedures & Emergency Treatment, publisher WB Saunders Co, Philadelphia, PA pp 119 (1985).

116. Kirkpatrick CE: Giardiasis in a cattery, J Amer Vet Med Assoc 187:161-162 (1985).

117. Kirkpatrick CE, Farrell JP: Giardiasis. Comp Cont Ed 4:367-378 (1982).

118. Kirkpatrick CE, Farrell JP: Feline giardiasis: Observations on natural and induced infections. Amer J Vet Res 45:2182-2188 (1984).

119. Kitchell BE, Strombeck DR, Cullen J, Harold D: Clinical and pathologic changes in experimentally induced acute pancreatitis in cats. Amer J Vet Res 47:1170-1173 (1986).

120. Knowles JO: Provocative exposure for the diagnosis and treatment of certain canine allergies. J Amer Vet Med Assoc 149:1303-1306 (1966).

121. Kogut MD: Hypoglycemia: Pathogenesis, diagnosis and treatment. Curr Probl Pediatr 4:1-59 (1974).

122. Kretchmer N: Lactose and Lactase. Scientific Amer 227:70-78 (1972).

123. Kwitko AO, Pieterse AS, Hecker R, et al: Chronic radiation injury to the intestine: A clinico-pathological study. Aust NZ J Med 12:272-277 (1982).

124. Lauritsen K, Rune JS, Bytzer P, et al: Effect of omeprazole and cimetidine on duodenal ulcer. New Engl J Med 312:958-961 (1985).

125. Lee T: Food allergies. The Med Forum pp 3-4 (Dec 1983).

126. Leib MS, Blass CE: Gastroesophageal intussusception in the dog: A review of the literature and a case report. J Amer Anim Hosp Assoc 20:783-790 (1984).

127. Leib MS, Hall RL: Megaesophagus in the dog Part II. Clinical aspects. Comp Cont Ed 6:11-17 (1984).

128. Leib MS, Konde LJ, Wingfield WE, Twedt DC: Circumcostal gastropexy for preventing recurrence of gastric dilatation—volvulus in the dog: An evaluation of 30 cases. J Amer Vet Med Assoc 187:245-248 (1985).

129. Leib MS, Sponenberg DP, Wilcke JR, et al: Suppurative colitis in a cat. J Amer Vet Med Assoc 188:739-741 (1986).

130. Leib MS, Wingfield WE, Twedt DC, Bottoms GD: Plasma gastrin immunoreactivity in dogs with acute gastric dilatation—volvulus. J Amer Vet Med Assoc 185:205-208 (1984).

131. Leifer CE, Peterson ME, Matus RE: Insulin-secreting tumor: diagnosis and medical and surgical management in 55 dogs. J Amer Vet Med Assoc 188:60-64 (1986).

132. Levitt MD: Intestinal gas production-recent advances in flatology. New Engl J Med 302:1474-1475 (1980).

133. Lewis LD Boulay JP, Chow FHC: Fat excretion and assimilation by the cat. Feline Pract 9:46-49 (1979).

134. Lewis LD, Phillips RW: Pathophysiologic changes due to coronavirus-induced diarrhea in the calf. J Amer Vet Med Assoc 173:636-642 (1978).

135. Ludwig J: The liver in the inherited copper disease of Bedlington Terriers. Lab Invest 43(1):82-87 (1980).

136. Lupton JR. Ferrell RG: Using density rather than mass to express the concentration of gastrointestinal tract constituents. J Nutr 116:164-168 (1986).

137. MacDonald ML, Anderson BC, Rogers QR, et al: Essential fatty acid requirements of cats: Pathology of essential fatty acid deficiency. Amer J Vet Res 45:1310-1317 (1984).

138. Martin DT: Crystalloid versus colloid resuscitation in pancreatitis. Surg Gyn & Obstet 159:445-449 (1984).

139. Martin R, Wittwer F, Thibaut J, et al: Hepatic regenerative drugs in dogs: effect of choline and silibinin in dogs with liver damage. Vet Med pp 504-510 (April 1984).

140. Masoero G, Andriulli A, Bianco A, et al: Diagnostic accuracy of serum cationic trypsinogen estimation for pancreatic disease. Dig Dis Sci 27:1089-1094 (1984).

141. Matloff DS, Alpert E, Resnick RH, Kaplan MM: A prospective trial of D-penicillamine in primary biliary cirrhosis. New Engl J Med 306:319-326 (1982).

142. Mattheeuws D, Rottiers R, Kaneko JJ, Vermeulen A: Diabetes mellitus in dogs: relationship of obesity to glucose tolerance and insulin response. Amer J Vet Res 45:98-103 (1984).

143. Matthiesen DT, Walter MC: Surgical treatment of chronic hypertrophic pyloric gastropathy in 45 dogs. J Amer Anim Hosp Assoc 22:241-247 (1986).

144. McMillan FD, Barr B, Feldman EC: Functional pancreatic islet cell tumor in a cat. J Amer Anim Hosp Assoc 21:741-746 (1985).

145. Merritt AM, Duelly P: Phloroglucinol microassay for plasma xylose in dogs and horses. Amer J Vet Res 44:2184-2185 (1983).

146. Meyer H, Kienzle E, Hannes M, Mundt H-C: Nutrition in dogs with hydrolyzed milk. Kleintierpraxis 29:301-308 (1984).

147. Meyer H, Jones RS: Canine pancreatic responses to intestinally perfused fat and products of fat. Amer J Physiol 226:1178-1187 (1974).

148. Meyer H: Feeding dogs with pancreatic insufficiency. Wien tierarztl Mschr 72:91-95 (1985).

149. Mitaru BN, Blair R, Reichert RD, Roe WE: Dark and yellow rapeseed hulls, soybean hulls and a purified fiber source: Their effects on dry matter, energy, protein and amino acid digestibilities in cannulated pigs. J Anim Sci 59:1510-1518 (1984).

150. Moore RW, Carpenter J: Intestinal sclerosis with pseudo-obstruction in three dogs. J Amer Vet Med Assoc 184:830-833 (1984).

151. Moore RW, Withrow SJ: Gastrointestinal hemorrhage and pancreatitis associated with intervertebral disk disease in the dog. J Amer Vet Med Assoc 180:1443-1447 (1982).

152. Morain CO, Segal AW, Levi AJ: Elemental diet for Crohn's disease. Brit Med J 288:1859-1862 (1984).

153. Muir WW: Gastric dilatation—volvulus in the dog, with emphasis on cardiac arrythmias. J Amer Vet Med Assoc 180:739-742 (1982).

154. Muller GH, Kirk RW, Scott DW: Small Animal Dermatology, 3rd ed, publisher WB Saunders Co, Philadelphia, PA pp 420-425 (1983).

155. Mulvany MH, Feinberg CK, Tilson DL: Clinical characterization of acute necrotizing pancreatitis. Comp Cont Ed 4:394-407 (1982).

156. Murtaugh RJ, Jacobs RM: Serum amylase and isoamylases and their origins in healthy dogs and dogs with experimentally induced acute pancreatitis. Amer J Vet Res 46:742-747 (1985).

157. Murtaugh RJ, Lawrence AE: Feline Campylobacter jejuni-associated enteritis. Feline Practice 14:37-42 (1984).

158. Nelson RW, Dimperio ME, Long GG: Lymphocytic-plamacytic colitis in the cat. J Amer Vet Med Assoc 184:1133-1135 (1984).

159. Nesbitt GH, Kedan GS: Differential diagnosis of feline pruritus. Comp on Cont Ed 7:163-172 (1985).

160. Netter FH: Aerophaia and eructation. In the Ciba Collection of Medical Illustrations—Digestive System—Upper Digestive tract. Ciba pharmaceutical Co, Summit, NJ p 94 (1959).

161. Newcomer AD, Park HS, O'Brien PC, McGill DG: Response of patients with irritable bowel syndrome and lactase deficiency using unfermented acidophilus milk. Amer J Clin Nutr 38:257-263 (1983).

162. Newman A, Blendis LM, Katsaris J, et al: Small intestinal injury in women who have had pelvic radiotherapy. Lancet 2:1471-1473 (1973).

163. Nimni ME, Deshmukh K, Gerth N: Collagen defect induced by penicillamine. Nature (New Biol) 240:220-221 (1972).

164. Nutrition and the M.D.: Medium-chain triglycerides. Van Nuys, CA 9(9):3-4 (Sept 1983).

165. Osbaldiston GW, Greve T, Mosier JE: Disorders of the digestive system in cats. Feline Pract, pp 8-16 (Sept-Oct 1972).

166. Perman JA, Waters LA, Harrison MR, et al: Breath hydrogen reflects canine intestinal ischemia. Pediatr Res 15:1229-1233 (1981).

167. Pidgeon G: Malassimilation syndrome: Maldigestion/malabsorption. In Current Veterinary Therapy VII, Editor RW Kirk, Publisher WB Saunders Co, Philadelphia, PA p 930 (1980).

168. Pidgeon G: Effect of diet on exocrine pancreatic insufficiency in dogs. J Amer Vet Med Assoc 181:232-235 (1982).

169. Pitts RP, Twedt DC, Mallie KA: Comparison of duodenal aspiration with fecal flotation for diagnosis of giardiasis in dogs. J Amer Vet Med Assoc 182:1210-1211 (1983).

170. Pollock RVH: Viral enteritis update. Proc Amer Anim Hosp Assoc Ann Meeting pp 241-242 (1984).

171. Pollock RVH, Zimmer JF: Canine viral enteritis. Proc 8th Kal Kan Symp pp 105-110 (1984).

172. Raffe MR, Hardy R: Anesthetic management of the hepatic patient. Comp Cont Ed 4:841-850 (1982).

173. Robins-Browne RM, Ch B, Path FF, Levine MM: The fate of ingested lactobacilli in the proximal small intestine. Amer J Clin Nutr 34:514-519 (1981).

174. Rojkind M, Kershenobich D: Hepatic fibrosis. In Progress in Liver Diseases. Editors Grune and Stratton, New York, NY 5:294-310 (1976).

175. Rolandelli RH, Settle G, Sand S, et al: A comparison of parenteral nutrition and enteral feeding with pectin in experimental colitis. Amer J Clin Nutr 41:849 (1985).

176. Rollin RE, Mero KN, Kozisek PB, Phillips RW: Diarrhea and malabsorption in calves associated with therapeutic doses of antibiotics: Absorptive and clinical changes. Amer J Vet Res 47:987-991 (1986).

177. Rollin RE, Mero KN, Levine K, et al: Antibiotic-induced malabsorption syndromes. Fed Proc 43:Abst 2360 (1984).

178. Rosin E: Quantitation of the pharyngoesphageal sphincter in the dog. Amer J Vet Res 47:660-662 (1986).

179. Roudebush P, Delivorias MH: Duodenal aspiration via flexible endoscope fr diagnosis of giardiasis in a dog. J Amer Vet Med Assoc 187:162-163 (1985).

180. Royal College of Physicians of London: Report on medical aspects of dietary fiber. Pitman Medical Ltd, Kent, England (1980).

181. Ruben P, Casarett R: Alimentary tract. In Clinical Radiation Pathology. Editors Rubin P, Casarett R, WB Saunders Co, Philadelphia, PA pp 193-240 (1970).

182. Rutgers C, Herring DS, Orton CE: Pancreatic pseudocyst associated with acute pancreatitis in a dog: Ultrasonographic diagnosis. J Amer Anim Hosp Assoc 21:411-416 (1985).

183. Savaiano DA, AbouElAnouar A, Smith DE, Levitt MD: Lactose malabsorption from yogurt, pasteurized yogurt, sweet acidophilus milk, and cultured milk in lactase-deficient individuals. Amer J Clin Nutr 40:1219-1223 (1984).

184. Schwenk WF, Haymond MW: Optimal rate of enteral glucose administration in children with glycogen storage disease type I. New Engl J Med 314:682-685 (1986).

185. Scott FW: Gastroenteritis outbreaks: Cornell Feline Health Center News. 6:1 (1982).

186. Sherding RG: A clinical approach to diagnosis of intestinal disease. Proc 8th Kal Kan Symp, pp 73-79 (1984).

187. Siegal RC: Collagen cross-linking: effect of D-penicillamine on cross-linking in vitro. J Biol Chem 252:254-259 (1977).

188. Sikes RI, Birchard S, Patnaik A, Bradley R: Chronic hypertrophic pyloric gastropathy: A review of 16 cases J Amer Anim Hosp Assoc 22:99-104 (1986).

189. Sherding RG: Acute medical diseases of the small intestine. Proc Amer Anim Hosp Assoc Ann Meeting, pp 163-167 (1984).

190. Smalley JR, Klish WH, Campbell MA, Brown MR: Use of psyllium in the management of chronic non-specific diarrhea of childhood. J Pediatr Gastroenterol Nutr 1:361-363 (1982).

191. Solomons NW, Guerrero AM, Torun B: Effective in vivo hydrolysis of milk lactose by beta-galactosidases in the presence of solid foods. Amer J Clin Nutr 41:222-227 (1985).

192. Sorjonen DC, Dillon AR, Powers RD, Spano JS: Effects of dexamethasone and surgical hypotension on the stomach of dogs: Clinical endoscopic and pathologic evaluations. Amer J Vet Res 44:1233-1237 (1983).

193. Stann SE, DiGiacomo RF, Giddens WE, Evermann JF: Clinical and pathologic features of parvoviral diarrhea in pound-source dogs. J Amer Vet Med Assoc 185:651-655 (1984).

194. Stein B: The cat versus its GI tract. Ohio Vet Med Assoc Ann Meeting (24 Feb 1984).

195. Sternlieb I: Copper and the liver. Gastroenterol 78:1615-1628 (1980).

196. Stogdale L, Bomzon L, Bland van den Berg P: Food allergy in cats. J Amer Anim Hosp Assoc 18:188-194 (1982).

197. Strombeck DR: Gastrointestinal diseases: rational diagnosis and therapy. Proc DC Academy June 6 (1985).

198. Strombeck DR, Harrold D: Effects of atropine, acepromazine, meperidine, and xylazine on gastroesophageal sphincter pressure in the dog. Amer J. Vet Res 46:963-965 (1985).

199. Strombeck DR, Harrold D: Effect of gastrin, histamine, serotonin, and andrenergic amines on gastroesophaged sphincter pressure in the dog. Amer J Vet Res 46:1684-1690 (1985).

200. Strombeck DR, Rogers Q: Plasma amino acid concentrations in dogs with hepatic disease. J Amer Vet Med Assoc 173:93-96 (1978).

201. Takeda T: D-penicillamine toxicity in mice 1. Pathological findings. Toxicol Appl Pharmacol 55(2):324-333 (1980).

202. Tams TR: Reglan—Clinical applications in GI disorders. Proc Amer Anim Hosp Assoc Ann Meeting p 207 (1984).

203. Tams TR: Medical diseases of the canine and feline colon. Amer Anim Hosp Assoc Ann Proc pp 357-363 (1986).

204. Tazawa Y, Nakagawa M, Yamada M, et al: Serum vitamin E levels in children with corrected biliary atresia. Amer J Clin Nutr 40:246-250 (1984).

205. Thornburg LP, Postnecrotic canine cirrhosis—6: Suspected causes. Vet Med/Small Anim Clin 78:886-891 (1983).

206. Thornburg LP, Ebinger WL, McAllister D, Hoekema DJ: Copper toxicosis in dogs. Part 1: Copper-associated liver disease in Bedlington Terriers. Canine Practice 12:41-46 (1985).

207. Thornburg LP, Rottinghaus G: What is the significance of hepatic copper values in dogs with cirrhosis? Vet Med pp 50-54 (May 1985).

208. Thornburg LP, Rottinghaus G, Koch J, Hause WR: High liver copper levels in two Doberman Pinschers with subacute hepatitis. J Amer Anim Hosp Assoc 20:1003-1005 (1984).

209. Toombs JP, Collins LG, Graves GM, et al: Colonic perforation in corticosteroid-treated dogs. J Amer Vet Med Assoc 188:145-150 (1986).

210. Trier JS, Browning TH: Morphologic response of the mucosa of human small intestine to X-ray exposure. J Clin Invest 45:194-204 (1966).

211. Twedt DC, Sternlieb I, Gilbertson SR: Clinical, morphologic, and chemical studies on copper toxicosis of Bedlington Terriers. J Amer Vet Med Assoc 175:269-275 (1979).

212. Twedt DC: Chronic gastritis. Proc Kal Kan Symposium 41-48 (1984).

213. Twedt DC: Disorders of gastric retention. Proc Kal Kan Symp 87-92 (1984).

214. Twedt DC, Wingfield WE: Medical diseases of the stomach. In Canine and Feline Gastroenterology. Editors BD Jones and WD Liska, publisher WB Saunders Co, Philadelphia, PA pp 126 (1986).

215. Van derGaag I, Toorenburg JV, Voorhout G, et al: Histocyte ulcerative colitis in a French Bulldog. J Small Anim Pract 19:283-290 (1978).

216. Van derGagg I, Happe RP: Zollinger-Ellison syndrome. Comp Path Bulletin, Armed Forces Institute, Washington DC XVI (2) pg 2 (May 1984).

217. Van Kruiningen HJ: Granulomatous colitis of dogs. Proc Gains Vet Symp pp 19-26 (1966).

218. Van Kruiningen HJ: Multifocal eosinophilic gastroenteritis. In Gastroenteric Pathology Course Syllabus. Tufts Univ, Boston, MA pp 132-135 (1985).

219. Venker-van Haagen AJ, Hartman W, Wolvekamp WTC: Contributions of the glossopharyngeal nerve and the pharyngeal branch of the vagus nerve to the swallowing process in dogs. Amer J Vet Res 47:1300-1307 (1986).

220. Wald A, Tunuguntla AK: Anorectal sensorimotor dysfunction in fecal incontinence and diabetes mellitus. New Engl J Med 310:1282-1287 (1984).

221. Walsh JH, Grossman MI: Gastrin. New Engl J Med 292:1324-1384 (1975).

222. Walter MC, Matthiesen DT, Stone EA: Pylorectomy and gastroduodenostomy in the dog: Technique and clinical results in 28 cases. J Amer Vet Med Assoc 187:909-914 (1985).

223. Walton GS: Skin responses in the dog and cat to ingested allergins. Observations on 100 confirmed cases. Vet Rec 81:709-713 (1967).

224. Walton GS: Allergic responses to ingested allergens. In Current Vet Therapy VI, Editor RW Kirk, Publisher WB Saunders Co, Philadelphia, PA pp 576-579 (1977).

225. Walvoort HC, van Nes JJ, Stokhof AA, Wolvekamp WTC: Canine glycogen storage disease type II: A clinical study of four affected lapland dogs. J Amer Anim Hosp Assoc 20:279-286 (1984).

226. Washabau RJ, Strombeck DR, Buffington CA, Harrold D: Use of pulmonary hydrogen gas excretion to detect carbohydrate malabsorption in dogs with chronic diarrhea. Univ of Calif, Davis CA, research report (1985).

227. Washabau RJ, Strombeck DR, Buffington CA, Harrold D: Evaluation of intestinal carbohydrate malabsorption in the dog by pulmonary hydrogen gas excretion. Amer J Vet Res 47:1402-1405 (1986).

228. Watters JW: Esophagraphy in the dog and cat. Calif Vet 34:10 (1980).

229. Weiss JS, Gantam A, Lauff JJ, et al: The clinical importance of a protein-bound fraction of serum bilirubin in patients with hyperbilirubinemia. New Engl J Med 309:147-150 (1983).

230. White SD: Food hypersensitivity in 30 dogs. J Amer Vet Med Assoc 188:695-698 (1986).

231. Willard MD: Some newer approaches to the treatment of vomiting. J Amer Vet Med Assoc 184:590-592 (1984).

232. Williams DA: Exocrine pancreatic insufficiency—What's new? Western States VMA Annual Meeting. Las Vegas, NV (1986).

233. Williams DA, Batt RM: Reduced serum trypsin-like immunoreactivity detected severe exocrine insufficiency in a dog with a normal BT-PABA test. Abstract Amer College Vet Int Med Ann Proc pp 50 (1984).

234. Wilson RC: Antimotility drugs used in treatment of diarrhea. J Amer Vet Med Assoc 180:776-777 (1982).

235. Wingfield WE: Vomiting in small animal patients. Proc Amer Anim Hosp Assoc, pp 179-181 (1983).

236. Wingfield WE, Twedt DC, Moore RW, et al: Acid-base and electrolyte values in dogs with acute gastric dilatation—volvulus. J Amer Vet Med Assoc 180:1070-1072 (1982).

237. Witte CL, Witte MH: Splanchnic circulatory and tissue fluid dynamics in portal hypertension. Feder Proc 42:1685-1689 (1983).

238. Zeldis JB, Friedman LS, Isselbacher KJ: Ranitidine: A new H2-receptor antagonist. New Engl J Med 22:1368-1373 (1983).

239. Zimmer JF: Canine esophageal foreign bodies: Endoscopic, surgical and medical management. J Amer Anim Hosp Assoc 20:669-677 (1984).

240. Zimmer JF, Burrington DB: Comparison of four techniques of fecal examination for detecting canine giardiasis. J Amer Anim Hosp Assoc 22:161-167 (1986).

241. Zimmer JF, Burrington DB: Comparison of four protocols for the treatment of canine giardiasis. J Amer Anim Hosp Assoc 22:168-172 (1986).

242. Zimmer JF, Todd SE: Further evaluation of bentiromide in the diagnosis of canine exocrine pancreatic insufficiency. Cornell Vet 75:426-440 (1985).

243. Youngberg CA, Wlodyga J, Schmaltz S, Dressman JB: Radiotelemetric determination of gastrointestinal pH in four healthy Beagles. Amer J Vet Res 46:1516-1522 (1985).

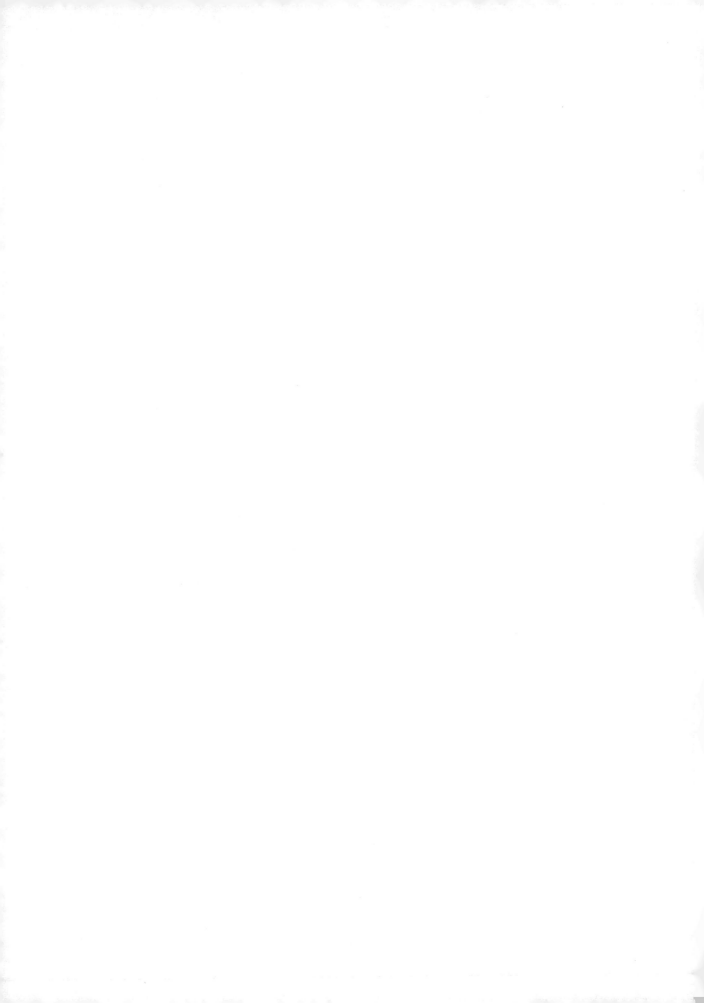

CHAPTER 8

Renal Failure

CONTENTS

CHRONIC RENAL FAILURE SUMMARY OF MANAGEMENT RECOMMENDATIONS

ALL CASES

1. Drugs and nutrients useful in management of renal failure, including their source, dosage, mode of action, reasons for administration, contraindications and complications are given in Table 1 (page 8-4).

2. Collect urine and blood for analysis.

3. If dehydration is evident, give fluids as described in step 3 page 8-6.

4. Avoid all stress possible (such as hospitalization and surgery) and use of corticosteroids, antibiotics and other drugs which can cause adverse reactions in patients with renal disease (Table 9, page 8-29). When an antibiotic is needed, ampicillin may be the drug of choice if organisms are sensitive to it. Avoid urinary catheterization as it may cause urinary tract infection in the immuno-suppressed animal. Use cystocentesis to obtain urine samples.

5. Ensure free access to clean fresh water. There is an inability to concentrate the urine, resulting in polyuria, which will cause dehydration and death if water is not available.

6. Ensure adequate caloric intake to prevent body protein catabolism and maintain optimal body weight. Most dogs eat better at home; therefore, use minimal hospitalization. If the animal is anorectic, any or all of the following may help:
   a. Giving potassium chloride, vitamin B, and zinc (Table 1)
   b. Correcting an energy deficit by force, tube, or intravenous feeding (Chapter 5)
   c. Correcting uremia by diuresis or peritoneal dialysis (page 8-45)
   d. Treating vomiting and stomatitis, as described below

7. At **first sign** of renal dysfunction, feed a restricted protein, phosphorus and sodium diet (Prescription Diets Canine k/d or Recipe 2 for the dog, and Feline k/d or Recipe 9 for the cat-Tables 13 and 14, page 8-44). If the canine diet does not maintain the BUN at less than 60 mg/dl after 10 to 14 days feeding, change to a lower protein diet (Prescription Diet Canine u/d or Recipe 3). The objective is to maintain the BUN consistently below 60 mg/dl since clinical signs occur above this level. Do not supplement with any source of sodium, such as sodium chloride (table salt) or sodium bicarbonate (baking soda), unless sodium bicarbonate is needed to treat metabolic acidosis.

8. Feed several times daily. Small meals fed more frequently enhance food consumption and may reduce body protein catabolism.

9. Periodically assess the animal's condition. The following parameters should be determined and used in instituting and monitoring response to therapy and progression of the disease:
   a. Owner's impression of therapeutic response
   b. Hydration
   c. Body weight
   d. Plasma concentrations of urea, creatinine, albumin, potassium, calcium, phosphate, glucose, and bicarbonate or total carbon dioxide
   e. Hematocrit
   f. Blood pressure
   Check these parameters at 1-4 week intervals until the animal is stabilized; then check two or three times a year to monitor progression of the disease. Calcium, vitamin D, potassium and bicarbonate should **not** be given routinely or without close monitoring of the animal. Both the plasma urea and creatinine concentrations should be measured. A fall in urea with a stable creatinine is favorable; whereas, a rise in creatinine, regardless of urea, suggests progression of the disease.

CONSIDERATIONS

1. If vomiting or diarrhea occur, administer cimetidine orally, or intravenously if the patient is severely uremic or if necessary because of vomition (Table 1). If vomiting is not controlled, administer centrally-acting antiemetics (Table 1, page 7-4). Withhold food for 1-2 days. If vomiting, diarrhea or severe uremia persist, institute osmotic diuresis or peritoneal dialysis (page 8-45), and feed intravenously (page 5-35) until vomiting stops.

2. If gingivitis, stomatitis, glossitis or oral ulcers are present, administer cimetidine orally and a topical anesthetic (Table 1).

3. If the plasma bicarbonate or total carbon dioxide concentration is less than 18 mEq/L, add sodium bicarbonate to the food (Table 1). Do not give bicarbonate when the plasma concentration is above 18 mEq/L; stop giving it if the fasting urine pH becomes alkaline.

4. If the plasma phosphorus concentration exceeds 5.0 mg/dl in the mature animal eating a re-

TABLE 1

DRUGS AND NUTRIENTS USEFUL IN MANAGEMENT OF RENAL FAILURE

Chemical Name	Product Name	Source	Dosage	Mode of Action
Aluminun Carbonate or Hydroxide	Amphojel, Basaljel, or Dialume	Wyeth Wyeth Armour	2 ml or 0.1 g/kg orally 3 ×/day	decreases phosphorus absorption
Calcium Carbonate	Limestone, TUMS, ground egg shells	grocery and feed stores	100 mg/kg (¼ t /10 kg) day *mixed in food*	compensate for reduced calcium absorption
Cimetidine	Tagamet	Smith Kline & French	5–10 mg/kg IV, or 5 mg/kg orally twice daily	decreases uremia reduces gastric acid secretion decreases $[PTH]_p$
Dihydrotachy-sterol	Dihydrotachy-sterol Hytakeral	Phillips Roxan, Winthrop	0.03 for 2 days, 0.02 next 2, then 0.01 mg/kg/day (Table 10, pg 8-38)	compensate for reduced activation of vitamin D
Dopamine	Dopamine Intropin	Elkins-Sinn Amer. Critical Care	2–5 μg/kg/min continuous IV drip	inotropic vassopressor
Furosemide	Lasix	Hoechst-Roussel	2–4 mg/kg 1–4 ×/day	diuretic
Lidocaine HCl	Xylocaine Viscous	Astra Phar-maceutical	2–10 ml orally before meals	topical anesthetic
Nandrolone Decanoate	Deca-Durabolin	Organon	3–5 mg/kg to max. 200 mg/dog once/wk IM	anabolic steroid, increase erythropoiesis
Potassium Chloride	Salt Substitute	most grocery stores	2–5 g (½–1 t)/day *mixed in food*	replaces body losses
Sodium Bicarbonate	Baking Soda	most grocery stores	100 mg/kg (¼ t/10 kg) 2 ×/day *mixed in food*	treats acidosis
Sodium Poly-styrene Sulfonate	Kayexalate	Breon Labs	1 g/kg 2–3 ×/day orally or high enemas	ion exchange resin
Sucralfate	Carafate	Marion Labs	Dissolve in water and rinse oral cavity	protective barrier
Thiazide	many	many	as indicated on product	diuretic
Vitamin B-complex	many	many	as indicated on product	} replaces body losses
Vitamin C	many	many	50–100 mg/ animal/day	
Vitamin D (1,25-dihydroxy)	Rocaltrol	Roche	0.02 μg/kg/day orally (Table 10)	compensates for reduced activation of vitamin D
Zinc	many	many	1 mg/kg/day orally	corrects deficiency

TABLE 1—Continued

DRUGS AND NUTRIENTS USEFUL IN MANAGEMENT OF RENAL FAILURE

Reasons for Administration*	Contraindications	Complications
$[P]_p > 5$ mg/dl	none	ineffective without dietary P restriction, unpalatable, reduced calcium absorption, dementia, constipation
$[Ca]_p < 10$ mg/dl and $[Ca]_p \times [P]_p < 55$	$[Ca]_p > 10$ mg/dl or $[Ca]_p \times [P]_p > 55$	soft tissue calcification**
severe uremic crisis vomiting, diarrhea, stomatitis $[P]_p > 5$ mg/dl	none	none
same as calcium	same as calcium	soft tissue calcification,** generally hypercalcemia
initiate urine excretion in oliguria		nausea, tachycardia, dyspnea, hypotension
edema, ascites, pleural effusions, hyperkalemia	dehydration	increases potassium and Ca excretion
oral ulcers, stomatitis, glossitis	none	none
hematocrit < 30%		virilization and reversible liver damage
lethargy, weakness, anorexia, $[K]_p < 3.5$ or < 5 mEq/l if diuretics are being given	anuria and hyperkalemia	cardiotoxicity if hyperkalemia occurs**
$[HCO_3]_p$ or $TCO_2 < 18$ mEq/L	$[HCO_3]_p > 20$ mEq/L or urine pH > 8	alkalosis,** cerebral hypoxia,** gastric gas production
unresponsive hyperkalemia	hypokalemia	lethargy, weakness, anorexia**
oral ulcers, stomatitis, glossitis	none	none
instead of furosemide if $[Ca]_p < 10$ mg/dl	dehydration	potassium excretion and deficit
anorexia, or if additional amounts are not already present in the diet	none	none
	none	none
same as calcium	same as calcium	soft tissue calcification,** generally hypercalcemia
anorexia	none	none

*Not recommended unless the situations given are present.

**Does not occur unless the product is given when contraindicated or above recommended dosage.

stricted phosphorus diet, give cimetidine (Table 1). After two weeks, if plasma phosphorus concentration still exceeds 5.0 mg/dl, give one of the phosphate binders, aluminum carbonate or hydroxide, in the food or before feeding (Table 1). Phosphate binders are not effective unless the patient is fed a restricted phosphorus diet.

5. Do not supplement prepared dietary foods with calcium or vitamin D unless the plasma calcium concentration is less than 10 mg/dl and, **in addition,** the plasma calcium times phosphorus concentration (both in mg/dl) is less than 55. If this is not the case, treat as described in step 4 above until the plasma phosphorus concentration is no longer elevated. Then, if the plasma calcium concentration remains less than 10 mg/dl, add calcium carbonate to the diet and give the active form of vitamin D (Table 1). If the plasma calcium concentration does not increase by at least 0.5 mg/dl within four weeks, double the amount of vitamin D given until the plasma calcium reaches 10 mg/dl. If therapy includes diuretics and the plasma calcium concentration is decreased, give thiazide rather than furosemide or ethracrynic acid. Furosemide and ethracrynic acid diuretics increase urinary excretion of calcium; whereas, thiazide diuretics reduce it by enhancing distal renal tubular reabsorption of calcium.

6. When the hematocrit is less than 30% and the animal is fully hydrated, give nandrolone decanoate (Table 1).

7. If the plasma potassium concentration is less than 3.5 mEq/L or if nonpotassium-sparing diuretics are being given for more than a few days and it is less than 5.0 mEq/L, add potassium chloride to the diet (Table 1).

8. If a diet specifically formulated for chronic renal failure is not being fed, give vitamins B and C daily to compensate for the excessive losses of these vitamins due to polyuria (Table 1). Avoid supplements containing vitamin A.

9. If edema, ascites or pleural effusions are present, follow the treatment regimen described in Figure 3 (page 8-31).

ACUTE RENAL FAILURE SUMMARY OF MANAGEMENT RECOMMENDATIONS

1. Find out how much the client really wants to save the affected animal and proceed only if interest is sufficient to support the extensive cost and effort that may be necessary.

2. Collect urine and blood for analysis.

3. Rehydrate the animal by giving fluids intravenously. Correct the initial fluid deficit (% dehydration x kg body wt) with equal parts isotonic saline and isotonic glucose (dextrose) solutions, or isotonic saline solution (0.9%) containing 2.5% glucose (50 ml of 50% dextrose/L) (page 8-25). Add 20 mg/dl of calcium (10 ml of 23% calcium gluconate/L) to either fluid. Rehydration should be completed within the first several hours to enhance renal perfusion and prevent further renal damage. If additional fluid is needed, give Ringer's lactate.

4. If rehydration does not initiate urine excretion, give furosemide intravenously (2 mg/kg; if there is no response, double dose and repeat it in 1-2 hours). If necessary, institute osmotic diuresis (page 8-46) and give dopamine by continuous intravenous infusion at the rate of 2-5 μg/kg/min. If these procedures are not successful, metabolic wastes should be removed by peritoneal dialysis (page 8-46).

5. If the animal is severely uremic, give cimetidine intravenously (Table 1) and nothing by mouth for 1-2 days.

6. Treat or remove any specific cause of renal damage if one is present. This includes insuring patency of the urinary tract. Oliguria is usually, though not always, present with acute renal failure.

7. Following the previous procedures which will correct a uremic crisis, if present, insure adequate intake of a low protein and phosphorus diet (Prescription Diet Canine u/d or Recipe 3 for the dog, and Feline k/d or Recipe 9 for the cat-Tables 13 and 14, page 8-44) to meet caloric needs. Feed at least three times daily. If the animal refuses to eat enough food voluntarily, force feed. If this is unsuccessful, tube feed (see Chapter 5). If vomiting occurs, administer cimetidine orally or intravenously (Table 1). If caloric requirements cannot be met orally, feed intravenously (page 5-35).

8. Monitor body weight, plasma concentrations of urea, creatinine, potassium, bicarbonate (or total carbon dioxide), calcium, phosphorus, albumin, and glucose, and adjust therapy as indicated. No food, but adequate fluid intake, results in a 0.5-1%/day decrease in body weight. A greater decrease indicates dehydration and therefore inadequate fluid administration or consumption.

9. Recovery from acute renal failure usually takes two to three weeks, but the time varies. Follow-

ing recovery many animals will have permanently impaired renal function and therefore require the management described for chronic renal failure.

INTRODUCTION

Renal failure is an inability of the kidney to perform its many functions sufficiently to prevent clinical signs. After renal injury there is hypertrophy of remaining nephrons but no formation of new nephrons to replace those damaged. Thus, the amount of water and solute excreted by the remaining renal mass must increase directly in proportion to the amount of renal damage; if 1/2, 1/4 or 1/10 of renal function remains, the amount of water and solute excreted by the remaining renal mass must increase two, four, and ten times respectively to maintain homeostasis. When the increase in needed solute excretion exceeds the functional capacity of the remaining renal mass, solute retention occurs, unless solute intake or production is reduced to lessen the amount which must be excreted. The amount of solute the remaining renal mass is able to excrete differs for different solutes.

These same factors apply to solutes that the kidney must retain or produce. Thus, renal dysfunction results in excesses or deficits of fluids, electrolytes, hormones and metabolic waste products, whose excretion, retention, production or degrada-

tion are altered (Table 2). With a decrease in renal function of:

50% there is a decreased ability to excrete parathyroid hormone, causing hyperparathormonemia.[182]

67% there is a reduced ability for the dog to concentrate urine, resulting in isosthenuria, polyuria and polydipsia. In contrast to dogs, many cats become uremic before they lose the ability to concentrate urine.[170]

75% there is a reduced ability to excrete urea, creatinine, phosphorus, and sodium resulting in uremia, hyperphosphotemia and hypertension.

80% there is reduced ability to degrade or excrete gastrin and decreased production of erythropoietin, resulting in gastroenteritis and anemia.

90% there is a reduced ability to excrete potassium and hydrogen ions resulting in hyperkalemia and acidosis.

INCIDENCE

The major causes of non-accidental death in the dog, in order of occurrence, are the many different types of cancer, renal failure, and heart disease. Renal failure is more common in male than female dogs and is also a major cause of death in cats.

TABLE 2

DYSFUNCTIONS, EFFECTS AND SIGNS OF RENAL FAILURE

Renal Dysfunction	Effect	Clinical Signs and Manifestations
1. Leakage of filtered blood constituents 〉	excess loss of body constituents and decreased ability to concentrate or dilute the urine 〉	polyuria, pollakiuria, nocturia, polydipsia
2. ↓ tubular absorption		
3. ↓ synthesis of erythropoietin	↓ erythropoiesis	anemia
4. ↓ tubular secretion and renal excretion	retention of body wastes (e.g. nitrogen compounds), ⟶ uremia 〉 hormones (e.g. gastrin), ⟶ ↑ gastric acid and excesses (e.g. P) 〉	gastroenteritis, vomiting, diarrhea, stomatitis, hypophagia, weight loss
5. ↓ activation of vitamin D	↓ calcium absorption	bone de-mineral-ization 〉 ↑ $([Ca]_p \times [P]_p)$
6. ↓ degradation of parathyroid hormone	hyperparathormonemia	nephrocalcinosis
7. ↓ total glomerular filtration rate (GFR)	compensatory ↑ in GFR of remaining nephrons 〉	renal damage

Except for congenital causes, renal failure is not limited to animals of any particular age or breed but is more prevalent among older animals. In one study, interstitial nephritis was present in 10% of dogs less than 1 year old, in 60% of those 1-5 years old and in over 85% of all dogs more than 5 years of age.[126] In another study 59% of dogs over 4 years old had interstitial nephritis present.[180] Glomerular lesions were also present in 43-78% of these dogs.

CAUSES

There are many causes of renal damage. As shown in Table 3 these include diseases that directly damage the kidney or cause either pre-renal or post-renal alterations that result in renal damage. Diseases that directly damage the kidney include many infectious diseases, toxins, and congenital, neoplastic, and immunologic disorders.

INFECTIOUS CAUSES

Infectious diseases that can result in renal failure may be localized in the kidney, causing pyelonephritis—or they may be systemic. Organisms causing pyelonephritis may come from the circulation; however most of them are from ascending lower urinary tract infection.[4] Leptospirosis, a common cause of renal damage in dogs in the past, is no longer common in most areas because of wide-

TABLE 3

CAUSES OF RENAL DAMAGE

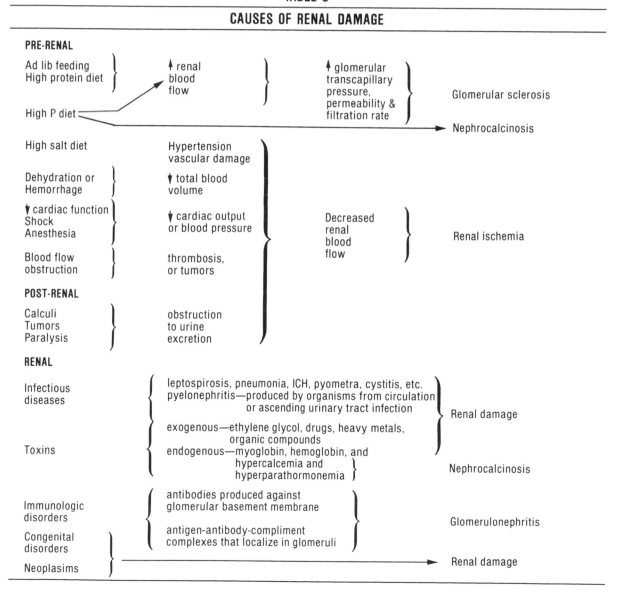

PRE-RENAL

| Ad lib feeding, High protein diet | → ↑ renal blood flow | } ↑ glomerular transcapillary pressure, permeability & filtration rate | Glomerular sclerosis |

High P diet → Nephrocalcinosis

High salt diet	Hypertension vascular damage		
Dehydration or Hemorrhage	↓ total blood volume		
↓ cardiac function, Shock, Anesthesia	↓ cardiac output or blood pressure	Decreased renal blood flow	Renal ischemia
Blood flow obstruction	thrombosis, or tumors		

POST-RENAL

| Calculi, Tumors, Paralysis | obstruction to urine excretion | | |

RENAL

Infectious diseases	leptospirosis, pneumonia, ICH, pyometra, cystitis, etc. pyelonephritis—produced by organisms from circulation or ascending urinary tract infection	Renal damage
Toxins	exogenous—ethylene glycol, drugs, heavy metals, organic compounds / endogenous—myoglobin, hemoglobin, and hypercalcemia and hyperparathormonemia	Nephrocalcinosis
Immunologic disorders	antibodies produced against glomerular basement membrane	Glomerulonephritis
Congenital disorders	antigen-antibody-compliment complexes that localize in glomeruli	
Neoplasims		Renal damage

spread vaccination. Bacterial pneumonia, pyometra, cystitis, infectious canine hepatitis (adenovirus), and herpes viruses may also cause renal damage.

TOXIC CAUSES

Toxins that may cause renal damage include ethylene glycol (antifreeze), other organic compounds, many heavy metals (arsenic, lead, thallium, bismuth, mercury and uranium) and many drugs. These include three- to ten-fold overdoses of tetracyclines,[186] adriamycin in cats,[36] amphotericin B, cephaloridine, polymyxin B, colistimethate, and aminoglycoside antibiotics (such as neomycin and gentamicin) whose nephrotoxicity is potentiated by furosemide, cephalosporin, other aminoglycosides, cytotoxic drugs, and dehydration.[25,79,162] After anesthesia renal failure may occur because of renal ischemia or direct nephrotoxicity of the anesthetic agent (particularly chloroform and methoxyflurane). Endogenous substances or effects that may cause renal damage include myoglobin, hemoglobin, hypercalcemia, and hyperparathormonemia.

NEOPLASTIC CAUSES

Of the many neoplastic diseases that may affect the kidney, lymphosarcoma is the most common.[137] It may be primary[202] or metastatic, in which case it is most commonly from the alimentary tract.[136] Renal neoplasms are characterized by marked bilateral renal enlargement and are usually diagnosed from a renal biopsy.[202]

CONGENITAL CAUSES

Dogs of all of the following breeds have been reported to have hereditary or congenital tendencies to develop chronic irreversible renal disease: Norwegian Elkhound, Alaskan Malamute, Cocker Spaniel, Samoyed, Lhasa Apso, Beagle, Keeshond, Golden Retriever, Doberman Pinscher, Standard Poodle, Wheaton Terrier, Blue Merle Collie and, perhaps most commonly, Shih Tzu.[37,52,87,131,138] It has been reported that the majority of Shih Tzu are affected to some extent.[17] The congenital disorders in these breeds result in the typical signs of renal failure. The kidneys are reduced in size and have irregular capsular surfaces. The disease is usually manifest in animals less than 1 year of age, although some cases may not become apparent until the victim is several years old. It usually leads to death within one year. Affected dogs should not be used for breeding.

A renal disease resembling **Fanconi syndrome or primary renal glucosuria** in people occurs in approximately 30% of adult Basenjis in North America. It has also been reported to occur in Norwegian Elkhounds, Shelties and Whippets and,

at least in Basenjis, appears to be a hereditary disease.[19,23,115,205] With this disease there is a reduction in active reabsorption of glucose, amino acids, sodium, potassium, phosphorus, and bicarbonate by the proximal tubules, resulting in increased urinary excretion of these solutes. The clinical presentation usually begins with young adults, 2-4 years of age, showing signs of polyuria, polydipsia and glucosuria. The plasma urea and creatinine concentrations initially are normal but increase as renal failure progresses. Progression to death may occur within a few months to several years.[17] The principal difference of diagnostic benefit in differentiating between this disease and other causes of glucosuria is the presence of a normal blood glucose concentration. Affected dogs may also have hypercortisolism, nephrogenic diabetes insipidus and gastroenteropathy.[23] Signs do not appear until adulthood and the course of the disease may run months or years.

The occurrence of an apparent hereditary membranoproliferative glomerulonephritis in 13 Doberman Pinscher dogs has been reported. All of the dogs were from the same sire.[204] In these and 22 others severe interstitial lesions, fibrosis, and focal mineralization were also present.[31] There was no predilection by sex. All were diagnosed before they were 2 years of age; usually they were less than 1 year of age. The most common manifestations noted by owners were anorexia, weight loss or poor growth, vomiting and lethargy. Diarrhea, polyuria and polydipsia also occurred. Azotemia, hyperphosphatemia, hypercholesterolemia, and proteinuria were almost always features, although hypoalbuminemia (less than 2.1 g/dl) was not usually present.

IMMUNOLOGIC CAUSES

Two distinct immunologic mechanisms may cause renal disease; both cause glomerular damage: 1) antibodies produced against the glomerular basement membrane, for which the cause is not known; and 2) circulating non-renal antigen-antibody-complement complexes that become localized in the glomeruli. These may be produced secondary to such diseases as systemic lupus erythematosus, endocarditis, pyometra, dirofilariasis, adenoviral infections, feline leukemia, feline infectious peritonitis, neoplasia, and chronic exposure to mercury and treatment with drugs such as D-penicillamine (Cuprimine, Merck) and captopril (Capoten, ER Squibb).[5]

AMYLOIDOSIS

Glomerular damage may also be caused by deposition of amyloid in the glomerular basement

membrane, where it narrows and finally obliterates the capillaries. Amyloid is insoluble protein fibrils found as abnormal localized or systemic deposits in various organs. Systemic amyloidosis may be primary, secondary (reactive) or hereditary. Primary amyloidosis is associated with immunoglobulin; whereas, secondary amyloidosis may occur as a late development in chronic suppurative, granulomatous, neoplastic, or inflammatory diseases.[11] However, amyloidosis may occur without any discernible pre-existing illness. In some cases, it may be hereditary, as has been reported in Abyssinian cats, in which it appears to be an autosomal recessive trait.[30]

Amyloidosis is uncommon in cats with the exception of the Abyssinian breed. In affected Abyssinian cats, renal amyloidosis manifests with clinical signs typical of chronic renal failure. These signs include polyuria, weight loss, lethargy and anorexia; generally manifest at 1 to 5 years of age. Both sexes are affected.[30] Small irregular kidneys, hyperphosphatemia, hyperglobulinemia with the alpha-2 globulins elevated, metabolic acidosis, and nonregenerative anemia are generally present. Proteinuria varies in cats with amyloidosis.

In contrast to dogs, amyloid in cats (Abyssnian as well as other breeds) is deposited primarily in the renal medulla. The result is medullary fibrosis, papillary necrosis and renal tubular damage leading to polyuric renal failure.[30,101] The glomeruli are often spared in cats. Therefore, proteinuria does not occur in cats with renal amyloidosis except in cases of advanced renal failure where amyloid-induced tubular damage has progressed to the point of causing glomerular damage. In dogs, renal amyloidosis is primarily a glomerular disease that allows proteins to pass through the damaged glomerular membrane and be lost in the urine. This results in the hypoalbuminemia, hypocholesterolemia, and frequently hyperglobulinemia.[51]

PRE- AND POST-RENAL CAUSES

Pre- and post-renal causes of renal damage include anything that either decreases or increases renal blood flow or pressure (Table 3, page 8-8). A sufficient reduction in renal blood flow causes renal ischemia and damage. A prolonged sustained increase in renal blood flow or pressure also results in renal damage by causing glomerular sclerosis. This has been demonstrated in several different animal species and in people,[22,90] and is in contrast to the belief that increased renal blood flow and glomerular filtration rate are beneficial. These increases cause glomerular hypertrophy and ultrastructural alterations, including vacuolation and deposition of osmophilic droplets in glomerular epithelial cells and fusion of foot processes. These are followed by expansion of mesangial matrix and denudation of cells from areas of glomerular basement membrane. These ultrastructural alterations herald progressive hyalinization and ultimately sclerosis of the glomeruli. Nephrosclerosis is the primary renal lesion in aged azotemic dogs.[41] Circulating plasma proteins are deposited in the damaged glomerular capillaries and may be excreted in the urine. Two major factors have been shown to cause an increase in renal blood flow and pressure and, as a result, renal damage; they are diets high in protein, salt and/or phosphorus, and *ad libitum* feeding. These effects are illustrated in Figure 1.

Dietary Protein Excess

More than 50 years ago increased protein intake by the dog was found to increase glomerular filtration rate.[98] Recently it was found that this effect may be mediated by glucagon whose secretion is stimulated by amino acids from ingested protein.[144] Some investigators have assumed that the increase in renal blood flow and glomerular filtration rate induced by increased protein intake is beneficial. In contrast, evidence in all species of animals studied indicates that these changes cause renal damage and therefore are detrimental. Although these studies in dogs and people are quite recent, more than 60 years ago feeding high protein diets to rabbits over a long period were shown to result in renal disease.[129] Nearly 50 years ago this was also demonstrated in rats.[57]

An increase in both proteinuria and glomerulosclerosis with increased protein intake has been demonstrated in dogs with reduced renal function. In one study, although the degree of renal dysfunction and proteinuria were the same at the beginning of the study, after 40 weeks urinary protein excretion was 10 times higher in dogs consuming a 44% protein diet than in those consuming a 17% protein diet.[155] In another study in dogs in which 75% of the renal mass had been removed surgically, glomerulosclerosis, mesangial proliferation, and thickening of the glomerular basement membranes, as determined by light, but not by electron, microscopy was significantly higher in those fed a 56% protein diet for 48 months than those fed a 27% or 19% protein diet.[15,20]

Dietary Phosphorus Excess

Diets high in phosphorus cause renal damage by two different mechanisms: 1) by increasing glomerular filtration rate[90] and 2) by promoting calcium and phosphorus deposition in the kidney.[199] High phosphorus diets increase and low phosphorus diets decrease glomerular filtration rate.[90] A sus-

tained increase in glomerular filtration rate may cause renal damage as described previously.

As shown in Table 2 (page 8-7), when renal damage is present there is a decrease in the kidney's ability to excrete phosphorus, to produce the active form of vitamin D (1,25 dihydroxycholecalciferol), and to degrade parathyroid hormone (PTH). These effects result in the condition referred to as renal secondary hyperparathyroidism (Figure 4, page 8-35). Hyperparathyroidism causes bone demineralization or osteodystrophy which, in conjunction with reduced renal phosphorus excretion and high dietary phosphorus intake, may increase the plasma phosphorus concentration. If plasma calcium and phosphorus concentrations exceed their solubility product, calcium phosphate deposition occurs. This deposition may occur in damaged tissues even at normal plasma calcium and phosphorus concentrations. Thus, with renal insufficiency, calcium and phosphorus are deposited in the damaged renal tissue even when plasma calcium and phosphorus concentrations are normal, and to a much greater extent if either is increased. This causes a progressive reduction in renal function, which can be prevented or substantially reduced by lessening phosphorus intake.

Dietary Sodium Excess

High sodium intake causes hypertension in animals and people.[35,121,128,195] Hypertension increases with age in animals on a high sodium diet but not on a low sodium diet. The severity of hypertension becomes greater with increased sodium intake and increased duration of excessive sodium consumption. Hypertension causes vascular damage and has been shown to be a major risk factor in the development of many diseases, including renal disease, heart disease, and peripheral vascular disease.[44,169] In addition, a high sodium diet has been shown to cause renal damage even without an increase in blood pressure.[196] As this and other data (page 8-32) emphasize, supplementation with dietary salt, as was widely advocated in the past for managing renal failure, is contraindicated.[40]

FIGURE 1

MECHANISM FOR RENAL DAMAGE CAUSED BY HIGH PROTEIN, SODIUM AND PHOSPHORUS DIETS, AND AD LIBITUM FOOD INTAKE[22,90]

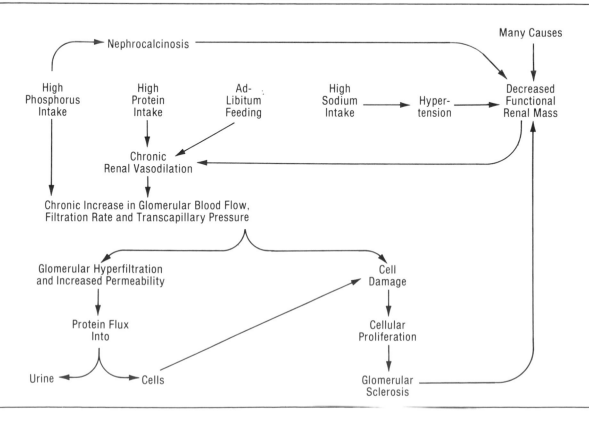

Ad Libitum Feeding

When food is available *ad libitum*, there is a sustained elevation of renal blood flow and glomerular filtration rate resulting in perfusion of superficial nephrons, which occurs in the meal-fed animal only after the meal.[22] Thus, as shown in Fig. 1, *ad libitum* feeding, and an increased dietary intake of protein or phosphorus increases glomerular blood flow, filtration rate, and transcapillary pressure.[22] When these are chronically increased, renal damage results.[90]

PREVENTION

Once renal damage from any cause occurs, renal function deteriorates steadily at rates peculiar to the individual patient but not related to the initial insult.[124,173] In some cases the disease or initial insult may remain active throughout the progression of renal failure, but in most instances renal failure progresses even when a well-defined initiating process is no longer evident. This occurs because, with a loss of renal function, a compensatory increase in glomerular filtration occurs in the remaining functional nephrons, which is referred to as increased "single-nephron glomerular filtration rate" (SNGFR). This increase in SNGFR eventually causes sclerosis of that nephron's glomeruli, leading to a further increase in SNGFR of other nephrons and their subsequent destruction. This process results in a progressive deterioration of renal function.

Consumption of diets low in protein, phosphorus, and sodium, as described on page 8-10, lessens the increase in SNGFR. Growing evidence in many species, including dogs, indicates that this slows or prevents the progression of renal failure.[153,168] It seems probable that meal feeding clinically normal animals and feeding diets containing adequate, but not excessive, amounts of protein, phosphorus, and sodium would also greatly assist in slowing the decline in renal function that occurs with age. This would help prevent renal failure.

It has been shown in people and rats that, from a peak at early maturity, renal weight, volume, and glomerular numbers decrease 20-30% with aging.[76,110] Older people have a reduced renal reserve and are more sensitive to subtle or overt renal insults. Usually, functional renal loss in elderly persons is more likely to be permanent than in younger people.[107] Similar information is not available on dogs or cats, but azotemia and morphologic changes have been reported to occur in the kidneys of geriatric dogs in response to extra-renal diseases.[41]

As stated recently, "The well recognized decline in glomerular filtration rate with age could be the consequence of a lifetime of eating too much protein"[22] and, as stated by others, "This hypothesis provides a powerful argument for a preventive role of dietary management for kidney disease."[94] This has not been demonstrated in controlled studies in dogs and cats, but it has in other species. In one study in rats a 40% reduction in protein, but not calories, phosphorus or salt intake, throughout life markedly slowed the progression of age-induced chronic nephropathy and cardiomyopathy, although life span was increased only 3%.[206] Restricting total food, and therefore protein, phosphorus, salt, and calorie intake throughout adult life, but not during growth, had an even more profound effect on retarding these diseases, as well as neoplastic diseases, and increased life span 38%.[206] Because:

1. Of studies of this type
2. Of the well-demonstrated benefits of protein, phosphorus, and sodium restriction in managing of renal failure
3. Of the well-demonstrated decrease in renal function with increased age[41,76,107,110]
4. Reports that from 59% to more than 85% of dogs past 5 years of age have interstitial nephritis[126,180]
5. Once sufficient renal damage occurs, renal function deteriorates steadily.[124,173]
6. Regeneration of damaged renal nephrons does not occur.
7. Renal failure is one of the major causes of nonaccidental death of dogs.
8. No studies have suggested any harm from the following procedures.

It is recommended that **to assist in preventing renal failure excess protein, phosphorus and salt intake should be prevented throughout life** by feeding as described in Chapters 3 and 4.

CLINICAL SIGNS

Despite the uniform changes that develop with renal failure, clinical signs vary and may be vague and nonspecific. Overt manifestations of uremia may appear suddenly or develop gradually over many months. The presenting manifestations may be obscured by concurrent disease such as congestive heart failure, diabetes mellitus, hypo- or hypercorticosteroidism, hypothyroidism, and others.

Because of renal adaptive responses, the more rapidly renal damage occurs the more profound the clinical signs and biochemical alterations as compared to the same degree of renal damage developing at a slower rate. Thus, clinical signs and increases in

TABLE 4

PARAMETERS USEFUL IN DIFFERENTIATING ACUTE AND CHRONIC RENAL FAILURE

Parameter	Renal Failure*	
	Acute	Chronic
Urine volume**	Generally ↓ but can be N & rarely ↑	↑ until terminal
Urine concentration	Generally ↑ but can be N & rarely ↓	↓
Anemia	Rare	When severe
Glucosuria	Often	Rare
Cr$_p$ (mg/dl)	> 1.5	> 1.5
BUN (mg/dl)	> 35 regardless of diet, > 10 if < 18% protein in diet dry matter	
Unthrifty appearance from renal disease	No	Often
Renal pain on palpation	Frequently in dog rarely in cat	Rare
Plasma albumin	N	N to ↓ with tubular, ↓ with glomerular
Hyperphosphatemia	Generally	When severe
Hyperkalemia	Generally	When severe
Leukocytosis	Occasionally	Uncommon
Lymphopenia	Often	Often
Eosinopenia	Often	Often
Neutrophilia	Often	Often

* ↑ indicates increased, ↓ decreased, N normal, > greater than and < less than. Plasma concentrations should be evaluated in samples obtained from non-dehydrated patients as dehydration increases plasma concentrations.

**Anuria is generally indicative of urinary tract obstruction. When urine volume is increased (> 50 ml/kg/day), polydipsia (> 100 ml/kg/day of water consumed in food and drink), pollakiuria and nocturia occur. Upon recovery from acute renal failure polyuria generally occurs and oliguria generally occurs when chronic renal failure is terminal.

plasma concentrations of phosphorus and potassium, and acidosis are more severe at lower plasma creatinine and urea concentrations with acute renal failure than with chronic renal failure. With chronic renal failure plasma urea and creatinine concentrations may increase greatly with minimal changes in other plasma concentrations; whereas, with acute renal failure plasma urea and creatinine concentrations may increase only moderately with substantial changes in other plasma concentrations. Clinical signs and laboratory tests useful in differentiating between acute and chronic renal failure are given in Table 4.

If renal damage is rapid and severe, the animal usually, but not always, will be oliguric or anuric. This is referred to as anuric, oliguric, or acute renal failure. Nonoliguric acute renal failure occurs occasionally. If the renal failure develops over a more prolonged time span, polyuria routinely occurs. In addition, weight loss and a coarse lusterless hair coat may also be present, giving the overall appearance of an unthrifty, poorly nourished animal. This is referred to as polyuric or chronic renal failure. The animal with polyuric renal failure may become oliguric terminally, and the animal with oliguric renal failure will usually become polyuric upon recovery. Polyuria results in greater water consumption. Thus, both water intake and excretion exceed the normal of 45-65 ml of water/kg/day consumed (in food and drink) and 20-45 ml of urine/kg/day excreted when the healthy dog or cat is in a thermoneutral environment with good-quality water always easily accessible. Although polyuria and the resulting polydipsia are routinely present in animals with chronic renal failure, they may be unnoticed by the owner. Frequent urination (pollakiuria) and nocturia, which usually result from polyuria, are more commonly observed. Polyuria and, as a result, polydipsia, pollakiuria and nocturia are important clinical signs of renal failure, but they

TABLE 5

POLYURIA — DIFFERENTIAL DIAGNOSIS OF CAUSES

Disease	Cause of Polyuria	Differential
Renal Failure	Loss of functional nephrons	Can't concentrate urine, ↑ BUN and plasma creatinine
Diabetes Mellitus	↓ insulin secretion or effect resulting in hyperglycemia exceeding renal threshold	Can concentrate urine, glucosuria and hyperglycemia after eating
Diabetes Insipidus (DI)	↓ ADH (pituitary DI) or response to ADH (nephrogenic DI)	Can't concentrate urine until ADH is given, unless its nephrogenic then still cannot
Inappropriate ADH Secretion[24,46]	↓ urine excretion initially resulting in hyponatremia which may cause renal medullary washout	Cannot dilute urine to maximum, hyponatremia, normal to ↓ plasma K and Cl
Hyperadrenalism (Cushing's Disease or Syndrome)	↑ corticosteroids which inhibit ADH release, ↑ GFR and ↓ tubular permeability to water	Can concentrate urine, mild neutrophilia, lymphopenia, eosinopenia, ↑ blood corticosteroids, pendulous abdomen, thin skin and hair coat
Chronic Hypoadrenalism	↓ aldosterone which ↑ sodium excretion causing renal medullary washout	Clearance of Na ↑ and K ↓ which ↓ plasma Na/K concentration ratio to < 27, ↓ response to ACTH
Hyperthyroidism	Unknown	Palpate enlarged thyroid, ↑ T_3 and T_4, weight loss, polyphagia
Pyometra or Endometritis	Unknown, ovarian cysts, persistent corpus luteum, or endotoxin decreasing response to ADH	± vaginal discharge, pyometra, leukocytosis, depression, anorexia, often occurs in estrous or 1–12 wks after
Chronic Hepatic Disease	Unknown, ↓ urea production which ↓'s urine concentrating ability or ↓ metabolism of corticosteroids or aldosterone?	↑ bilirubin, ↓ BSP clearance, ↑ liver enzymes, ↓ albumin, ↑ prothrombin time
Primary renal glucosuria or Fanconi synd.[19,23,115,205]	Decreased renal tubular reabsorption of glucose, amino acids, PO_4, Na, K, uric acid, and occasionally bicarbonate resulting in renal tubular acidosis	Glucosuria, hyposthenuria, amino aciduria, normal glucose tolerance test and blood glucose concentration, most common in Basenjis
Renal tubular acidosis[50,154]	↓ renal tubular secretion of hydrogen ions	Hyperchloremia, hypokalemia, metabolic acidosis nonazotemic, can concentrate urine somewhat, fasting alkaline urine not due to urinary tract infection
Hypercalcemia	Calcium interferes with renal response to ADH	Weakness, depression, anorexia, vomiting, BUN and creatinine normal
Hypokalemic Nephropathy	↓ renal tubular function or ADH secretion	Hypokalemia
Excess Sodium Intake (salt supplementation)	↑ sodium and water intake which ↑'s their excretion	Can concentrate urine, history, urine sodium > 4 mEq/kg/day or $(Na_u/Na_p) \times (Cr_p/Cr_u)$ > 0.01[50]
Psychogenic Water Consumption	Normal response to excess water intake	Elimination of other causes, can concentrate urine
Low protein diet	↓ renal medullary urea concentration	↓ BUN, ↓ plasma albumin, ↓ A/G ratio, ↑ plasma alkaline phosphatase

also occur as a result of several other diseases as given in Table 5. Use of the procedures in the sequence diagramed in Figure 2 may help in determining the cause of polyuria.

With either acute or chronic renal failure, the dog or cat is usually depressed, listless, often dehydrated and anorectic. Vomiting, unrelated to food intake,

may occur with increasing frequency with worsening uremia in some animals (30 of 35 cats in one study[135]) and not at all in others. The same is true of diarrhea, which may or may not be hemorrhagic and occurs more often in uremic dogs than cats. If the animal is severely uremic, its breath may smell like ammonia; or halitosis, gingivitis, oral ulcers, glos-

sitis, stomatitis, or loose teeth may be noted. Occasionally, neurologic disturbances, including lethargy, drowsiness, behavioral changes, neuro-muscular twitches, coma and convulsions may occur. If prolonged extensive proteinuria is present, edema, ascites, and pleural effusion may occur. The pleural effusion may cause dyspnea and coughing, which initially occur without exercise. These signs rarely develop unless the plasma albumin concentration falls below 1.5 g/dl or a significant degree of hypertension is present.

Typically, with end-stage chronic renal failure the kidneys are small, firm, and their surface is irregular. However, in one report bilateral renal enlargements were detected in 9, and a reduction in 14, of 31 cats with renal failure.[135] With acute renal failure or active renal disease, frequently in dogs, but rarely in cats,[135] there is evidence of pain on palpation over the kidney. An enlarged irregular kidney may indicate neoplasia, cystic disease, hydronephrosis, intracapsular hemorrhage, or acute inflammation. As can be compared radiographically or sonographically the normal kidney in dogs and cats is 2.5 to 3.5 times the length of the second lumbar vertebra.[58]

DIAGNOSIS

The diagnosis of renal failure is derived from the history, clinical signs, physical examination, hemograms, and urinalysis. Renal function tests, radiographs and renal biopsies may be needed in some cases. The factors given in Table 4 (page 8-13) are useful in differentiating between acute and chronic renal failure. The factors in Table 5 are useful in differentiating renal failure from the many other diseases that cause polyuria, polydipsia, polla-kiuria or nocturia. Before treatment is started, blood and urine samples should be taken for diagnostic purposes and to establish a base line for therapy. The following blood parameters are needed for either diagnosis or therapy, or both: white blood cell count and differential, hematocrit and the plasma concentration of total protein, albumin, potassium, calcium, phosphate, bicarbonate or total carbon dioxide, glucose, urea nitrogen, and creatinine.

LEUKOCYTES

Leukocytosis in an animal with renal failure suggests an acute disease such as leptospirosis or pyelonephritis but is atypical of chronic renal failure. Lymphopenia often occurs with either acute or chronic renal failure and appears to be due to a specific uremic effect on lymphoid tissue.[38] An eosinopenia and neutrophilia are also common features.[135]

PLASMA PROTEINS

A lessening in the plasma protein or albumin concentration may suggest their loss in the urine due to glomerular damage. Large quantities of protein may be lost in the urine in the absence of azotemia.[38] However, the plasma protein and albumin concentrations will decrease only when their loss exceeds the liver's ability to synthesize them. Thus, their concentration decreases only if: 1) proteinuria or other body losses are fairly severe, 2) hepatic function is reduced, or 3) dietary protein or caloric intake is inadequate. In addition, a reduced plasma concentration is masked by dehydration, which is often present in animals with renal failure. Full rehydration of the animal may be necessary before a decrease in plasma concentration can be recognized.

The plasma concentrations of both total protein and albumin should be determined. Albumin, because of its smaller size, is the main protein lost as a result of glomerular damage. Its loss decreases the plasma oncotic pressure, which results in the loss of fluids from the vascular compartment. This fluid loss increases the concentration of all plasma solutes so that little change in the plasma concentration of either total protein or albumin may occur. Total plasma protein concentration may be further increased by greater globulin production in response to an infectious disease process. Assessing the plasma concentration of total protein, albumin, and particularly the albumin/globulin ratio (A/G)* alleviates many of these problems in interpretation.

In the fully hydrated dog or cat a plasma concentration of less than 5.5 g protein/dl, 2.3 g albumin/dl or an A/G ratio of less than 1 are abnormal.[10] Even though these parameters will not fall below these levels unless proteinuria exceeds hepatic protein synthesis and their decrease may be caused by many other factors, they are useful in diagnosing renal disease, in prognosis, and particularly in instituting therapy and monitoring the animal's response.

PLASMA CREATININE AND UREA

Reduced renal function impairs the ability to excrete metabolic waste products, which causes their accumulation in the body. This is called uremia (meaning urine in the blood) or, because most of these metabolic waste products are nitro-

---

*If globulin concentration is not measured, the albumin/(total protein minus albumin) ratio may be used instead. Albumin and globulin generally make up greater than 90% and fibrinogen less than 10% of the plasma protein.

FIGURE 2

POLYURIA — DETERMINING CAUSE

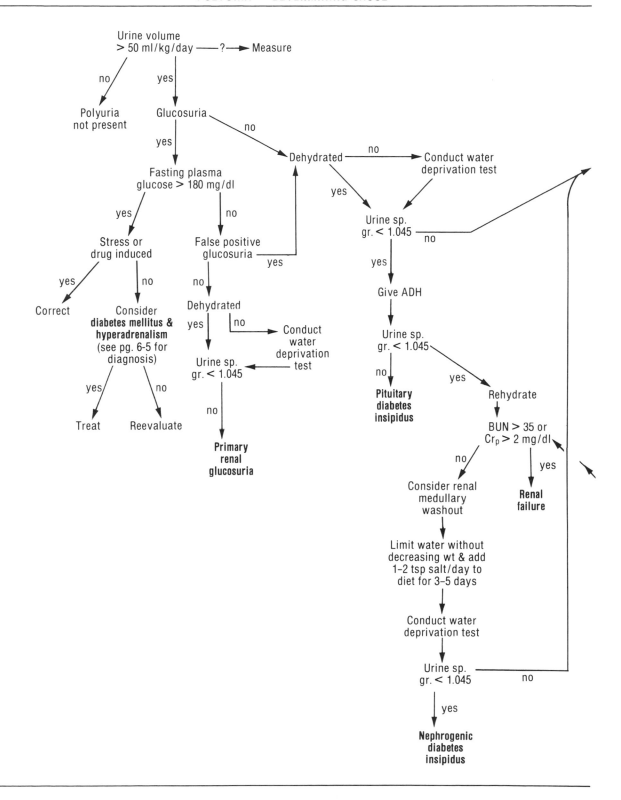

FIGURE 2 — Continued

POLYURIA — DETERMINING CAUSE

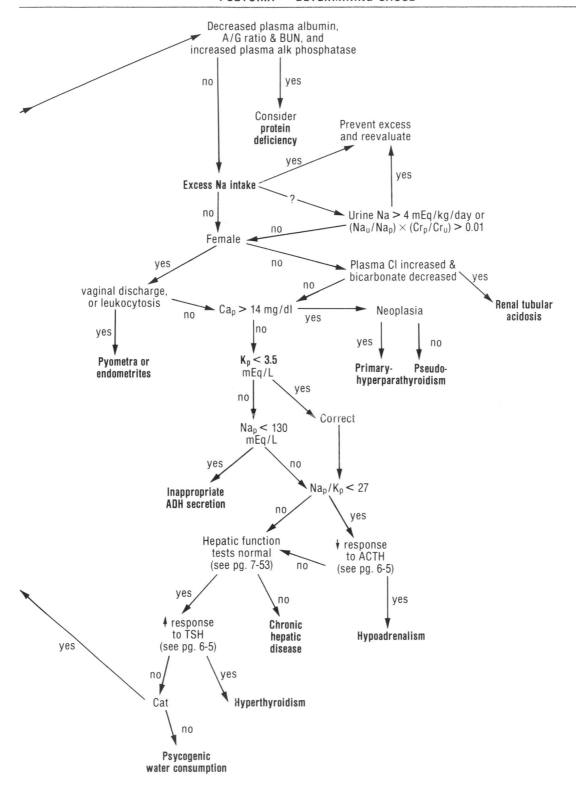

genous compounds, azotemia. Measurement of the plasma concentration of these metabolic waste products is therefore useful in determining the presence of reduced renal function and measuring response to therapy. The two most useful are creatinine and urea.

Neither compound is more sensitive than the other for detecting renal dysfunction.[63] An elevation of plasma creatinine above 3.5 mg/dl is a more sensitive indicator of the degree of renal dysfunction and is not affected by dietary protein intake. However, plasma concentration of urea correlates more directly than creatinine with clinical signs of uremia.[170] Patients with a high blood urea nitrogen (BUN) value have more uremic signs than those with a low BUN, even though the plasma creatinine may be similar. The urea concentration is the same in blood and plasma. Although plasma, rather than blood, urea concentration is usually measured by historical habit it is frequently referred to as the BUN.

The plasma concentrations of both creatinine and urea are altered for as long as 12 to 24 hours after a meal;[56,208] therefore, it is best to measure them after an overnight fast. The plasma creatinine concentration (Cr_p) in the dog can increase as much as 50% from 1-4 hours after the ingestion of cooked meat, which increases creatinine intake because cooking enhances the conversion of creatine to creatinine. In contrast the Cr_p is decreased by 10 to 20% for 4-16 hours after ingestion of raw meat or commercial soft-moist or canned dog foods.[208] These foods do not contain creatinine. The decrease in Cr_p after they have been consumed is due to the increase in glomerular filtration rate and, therefore, creatinine excretion that occurs after eating food not containing creatinine. The BUN may increase 100% by 4-8 hours, 40-100% by 16 hours, and return to pre-meal levels by 20 hours after eating canned or soft-moist dog food in an amount sufficient to provide daily caloric needs.[56,208]

Plasma Creatinine Concentration (Cr_p)

Creatinine is produced at a constant and uniform rate by muscle conversion of creatine to creatinine and is excreted only by the kidney. The greater the muscle mass the more creatinine produced. In the cat, creatinine is excreted only by glomerular filtration.[66] It is not reabsorbed or secreted by renal tubules; and the ureter and bladder, even under moderate distention, are relatively impermeable to creatinine. Thus, excretion of creatinine is a direct indication of total glomerular filtration rate (GFR). In the dog, and to a greater extent in males, there is

some tubular secretion of creatinine which becomes greater as the Cr_p increases; and, therefore, the measurement of creatinine excretion in the dog overestimates the GFR. However, tubular creatinine secretion is quite small and rarely alters clinical interpretation or the evaluation of canine patients.[38]

A decrease in GFR occurs with any decrease in renal function regardless of the cause. However, the Cr_p and the BUN do not increase until the GFR is reduced by more than 75%. When this occurs, the Cr_p increases as the GFR decreases. However, this relationship is not linear until the Cr_p is equal to or greater than 3.5 mg/dl.[38] Small changes in the Cr_p between 1-2 mg/dl indicate much greater losses of renal function than similar Cr_p changes at modest or severely elevated concentrations. Therefore, careful interpretation of Cr_p in the range of 1.0 to 2.0 mg/dl is necessary. Although a Cr_p of less than 2.0 mg/dl is often considered normal, many animals have significant renal damage at or below this concentration. In addition, older animals may have markedly reduced renal function without a significant increase in plasma creatinine concentration. This has been reported to occur in elderly people.[164] It occurs because the rate of muscle conversion of creatine to creatinine becomes less with age.

A Cr_p of greater than 1.2 mg/dl should be viewed suspiciously, and these patients should be more closely evaluated. Although other factors must be considered, a Cr_p of greater than 2.0 and an inability to concentrate the urine (specific gravity less than 1.035 in the dehydrated animal) indicates renal failure is present. A Cr_p of more than 5 indicates a poor prognosis; more than 10 a grave prognosis. Caution should be used in evaluating the Cr_p in the ketotic animal. If the measurement is made using the alkaline picrate (Jaffe) method, acetoacetate will increase the value obtained.[75]

Blood Urea Nitrogen Concentration (BUN)

Since urea is rarely present in the dog's or cat's diet and urea is not degraded in the body, the BUN therefore depends on the rate at which it is produced and excreted. Urea is produced in the liver from the metabolism of either body or dietary protein and is excreted primarily by the kidney. Although substantial amounts of urea passively diffuse into the intestinal lumen and are degraded by bacteria to ammonia, almost all of the ammonia is absorbed and resynthesized to urea. Thus, a futile cycle occurs and enteric loss of urea is minimal.[122] The BUN decreases with a severe reduction in liver function or decreased protein intake. Conversely,

TABLE 6

BLOOD UREA NITROGEN (BUN) CONCENTRATION INTERPRETATION

BUN (mg/dl)	Dietary Protein (% in dry matter)	Urea Excretion
100 or above	any	Renal or post-renal dysfunction present
50-100	any	Pre-renal, renal, or post-renal dysfunction present
35-50	any	} Pre-renal, renal, or post-renal dysfunction probably present
15 or more	18% or less	
10-35	25% or more	Normal
10 or less	18% or less	Normal

the BUN increases with reduced renal excretion or increased protein metabolism. The amount of protein metabolized increases with increasing protein intake and with inadequate caloric intake. Inadequate caloric intake causes body proteins to be broken down and used for energy.

In healthy dogs, when caloric intake is adequate to meet the dog's requirement, the BUN may vary from 1 to 35 mg/dl with dietary protein levels of 5 to 55% (in the diet dry matter), respectively. Protein intake must be considered when the BUN is used to evaluate renal function. BUN values of 10-25 mg/dl, are normal in a dog consuming commercial dog foods with protein contents of 25-40% in their dry matter. But these BUN concentrations

TABLE 7

DIFFERENTIATION BETWEEN PRE-RENAL AND RENAL INDUCED AZOTEMIA

Parameter	Pre-Renal	Renal
[Sodium]$_u$mEq/L	< 10	> 25
Max. Urine Sp. Gr.	> 1.030	< 1.030
[Na]$_u$/[Na]$_p$ × ([Cr]$_p$/[Cr]$_u$)*	< 0.01	> 0.03
Response to fluid therapy (decrease in azotemia)	Large & rapid	Minimal
Kidney size & pain	Normal	May be abnormal
[Urea]$_u$/[Urea]$_p$**	> 20/1	< 10/1
[Cr]$_u$/[Cr]$_p$**	> 20/1	< 5/1

Abbreviations used: [ ] = concentration, u = urine, p = plasma, < = less than, > = greater than.

*Valid only in oliguric dogs.[177]

**In contrast to humans these may be unreliable in dogs.[68]

are abnormally high if the dog is eating one of the restricted-protein dietary foods that contain 10-18% protein and are commonly used to manage renal failure. Normal BUN values for dogs eating restricted-protein dietary foods are less than 10 mg/dl. In addition, because the BUN may increase by more than 100% after a meal,[56,208] it should be measured after an 18 to 24-hour fast. As shown in Table 6, a BUN greater than 50 mg/dl is almost always due to a decrease in urea excretion; a BUN greater than 80-100 mg/dl is due to renal or post-renal causes. Rarely does the BUN rise above this amount as a result of pre-renal causes.[38]

In contrast to the BUN, the Cr_p is not affected by the amount of protein metabolized. Thus, decreasing protein metabolism by decreasing dietary protein intake, and ensuring adequate food intake to prevent the use of body protein for energy needs, will reduce the BUN but will not affect the Cr_p. In contrast to creatinine, up to 40% of the filtered urea may be reabsorbed.[10] As the speed glomerular filtrate moves through the tubules slows, more urea is absorbed. Thus, with diuresis, less urea is reabsorbed and the BUN is lower with respect to the Cr_p; whereas, with a decrease in urine excretion, such as with pre-renal diseases, more urea is reabsorbed and the BUN is higher with respect to the Cr_p. Because of these factors, the BUN/Cr_p ratio is often used in human medicine to distinguish between pre-renal and renal azotemia. However, it is not useful for this purpose in the dog.[68] The major factors useful in differentiating between pre-renal and renal azotemia in the dog are given in Table 7.

PLASMA AMYLASE AND LIPASE

Plasma amylase or lipase activities are increased and azotemia is present, in most dogs and cats with either chronic renal failure or acute pancreatitis. This may make differentiation difficult. Although both enzymes are excreted by the kidney, the amount of increase in their plasma activities is not related to the degree of renal dysfunction present, or to the diet.[159] The plasma activity of both enzymes has been reported to be increased in 81% of dogs with acute pancreatitis and in 37% with chronic renal failure.[159] Plasma amylase has also been reported to be increased in 73%, and alkaline phosphatase in 53% of cats with renal failure.[135] In renal failure without pancreatitis, the amount of increase is usually less than in the case of acute pancreatitis with or without renal failure.

The following factors suggest the presence of primary renal failure rather than acute pancreatitis with secondary pre-renal azotemia:

1. Both amylase and lipase plasma activities are not increased.

2. Plasma amylase activity is less than 4000 diamyl units and lipase activity is less than 1-2 Sigma-Tietz Units.
3. Urine specific gravity in the dehydrated animal is less than 1.030.
4. The BUN is more than 80 mg/dl.
5. There is no abdominal pain or distention.

URINALYSIS

For urinalysis a first morning sample is best. It is usually more concentrated and free from influences of feeding and exercise. A voided sample is acceptable unless cultures are required. In cases where cultures are needed, the samples should be obtained by cystocentesis. Avoid catching the first part of a urine stream; it will contain cellular debris, leukocytes, and exudate flushed from the urethra, prepuce, and genital tract. Catheterization of the uremic animal to obtain a urine sample should be avoided because it may result in urinary tract infection, particularly in animals that are immunosuppressed as a result of uremia.

The urine should be examined for casts, erythrocytes, leukocytes, and other cells. The presence of occult blood and glucose should be determined; and urine protein/creatinine ratio and specific gravity or osmolality should be measured. The presence of hematuria with few leukocytes suggests neoplasia, trauma, or uroliths. More than a few erythrocytes or leukocytes in the urine indicates an active urinary tract disease. Pyuria, bacteriuria, proteinuria, hematuria and particularly many leukocytes or white blood cell casts suggest pyelonephritis. With chronic pyelonephritis, however, the urine may be sterile.[4] With acute pyelonephritis, pain on renal palpation, fever, and leukocytosis may be present. The presence of most types of casts in the urine suggests renal tubular damage, although a few hyaline casts in the urine may be normal.[10] Renal tubular casts in the urine however, occur infrequently in cats with renal failure.[135] Red blood cell casts usually indicate acute glomerular inflammation.[181]

Proteinuria

Proteinuria without hematuria or inflammatory urine sediment is suggestive of glomerular disease. It may occur, however, as a result of passive renal congestion, such as caused by cardiac insufficiency. A transient, mild proteinuria may occur after strenuous exercise, seizures, fever, and extreme stress. Proteinuria without glomerular injury is usually limited to excretion of inflammatory proteins, or Bence Jones proteins produced by neoplasms; whereas, with glomerular damage albumin is the main protein lost. The presence of many neutrophils in the urine suggests urinary tract inflammation as the cause of proteinuria.

The hemoglobin detection pads on reagent test strips (e.g. Bili-Labstix, Ames and Chemstrip 9, Boehringer Mannheim) indicate the presence of hemoglobin at a concentration of 0.1 mg/dl or more, whereas the protein detection pads on these strips do not give a positive reaction from hemoglobin until its concentration exceeds 5 mg/dl.[95] Because of this difference in sensitivity, if these test strips indicate less than the highest value possible for a strip for hemoglobin, a positive reaction for protein is due to protein exceeding that from blood. A protein reaction of greater than 100 mg/dl is also due to protein exceeding that from blood, if blood cannot be detected visibly.[95] Blood cannot be detected visibly in clear, light-colored urine until its hemoglobin concentration exceeds 30-50 mg/dl.[95] If the urine is visibly reddened, another sample visibly free of blood must be obtained, or electrophoresis must be conducted to identify the type of protein present and to determine if proteinuria is due to hematuria or is primarily albumin and, therefore, due to glomerular damage. The sulfosalicylic acid turbidity test is much less sensitive than reagent test strips; it detects hemoglobin only at concentrations of 40 mg/dl or more.[95]

Huge amounts of albumin may be lost without azotemia, or a reduction in the ability to concentrate or dilute the urine. However, as glomerular injury progresses, renal tubular damage often occurs, resulting in azotemia and isosthenuria (urine with the same concentration as plasma). The reverse also occurs. That is, tubular damage leads to glomerular damage. Renal tubular damage resulting in loss of functional nephrons causes an increase in the glomerular transcapillary pressure, permeability and filtration rate of other less-affected nephrons, causing glomerular damage, proteinuria, and a progressive decrease in renal function.[22,90] Thus, glomerular disease results first in proteinuria and later in polyuria and azotemia; whereas, renal tubular disease results in polyuria and azotemia first and proteinuria later. The degree of proteinuria often correlates poorly with the degree of renal damage.[38]

In one study, 76% of azotemic cats without glomerulonephropathies were proteinuric, with 20% due to blood, 40% due to inflammation, and 40% thought to be due to glomerulosclerosis secondary to renal tubular disease caused by hyperfiltration of remaining functional nephrons.[135] This hyperfiltration causes a progressive impairment in renal function.

The major causes of a persistent proteinuria are glomerulonephritis, amyloidosis, or renal tubular disease that has become severe and causes glomerular sclerosis. The treatment and prognosis of these diseases may be quite different; however, they often cannot be differentiated on the basis of clinical or laboratory findings and a renal biopsy is needed (see page 8-23).

A dipstick colorimetric test is usually used as a screening test for detecting proteinuria. However, false-positives may be caused by a highly alkaline urine or leaving the dipstick in the urine too long.[77] False-negatives may occur if the urine is quite dilute or acidic.[77] The dipstick test must therefore be interpreted with respect to urine dilution and pH. A quantitative measurement of urine protein concentration must also be evaluated with respect to urine dilution, i.e. urine specific gravity or osmolality.

A more accurate means of detecting and quantitating proteinuria is the measurement of the amount of protein excreted daily, or the urine protein/creatinine ratio. This ratio may be measured in a single randomly obtained voided urine sample.[78] It is much faster and easier to obtain, and is also more sensitive in detecting mild glomerular disease than is the amount of urinary protein excreted daily.[28] In three studies in dogs, the urine protein/creatinine ratio (both expressed in mg/dl) was found to be less than 0.2 in 40 of 43 healthy dogs, less than 0.4 in 42 of 43 healthy dogs, and greater than 0.6 in 60 of 62 dogs with renal disease.[28,78,203] A protein/creatinine ratio of 1 was equal to 20-30 mg of protein/kg/24 hours. The mg of urinary protein/kg/24 hours in these dogs was less than 10 in 42 of 43 healthy dogs and greater than 12 in those with renal disease. In the dogs with renal disease these values were lowest in those with primary tubular dysfunction, ranging from a urine protein/creatinine ratio of 1-11 and urine protein excretion of 12-150 mg/kg/day.[28,53] All dogs with amyloidosis had values greater than these. In those with glomerulonephritis, both values were extremely variable. Although they tended to be lower than in dogs with amyloidosis, and higher than those in dogs with primarily renal tubular dysfunction, neither value was beneficial in determining which dogs had glomerulonephritis and which had either amyloidosis or primarily renal tubular dysfunction. A renal biopsy is therefore necessary for this differentiation.

In 12 healthy cats urinary protein excretion ranged from 4 to 43 mg/kg/day and varied as much as 25 mg/kg/day in the same cat on consecutive days.[177]

Urine Specific Gravity and Osmolality

As renal tubular function decreases, the animal's ability to either dilute or concentrate the urine is decreased; thus, regardless of body needs, the urine specific gravity and osmolality will move closer to that of the plasma, which is 1.008-1.012, or 280-310 mOsm/kg. A urine concentration within these ranges is called isosthenuric. Values obtained from nondehydrated animals either outside or within the isosthenuric ranges gives no indication of renal function. There may be a decrease in the kidney's ability to concentrate maximally or dilute the urine; complete loss of this ability does not usually occur. As a result, the urine specific gravity and osmolality may be outside of the isosthenuric values, even though a decrease in renal function is present. Conversely, if the animal is not dehydrated, a urine specific gravity or osmolality within the isosthenuric range does not necessarily indicate that any degree of renal dysfunction is present, since these values are within the range that occurs in animals with normal kidney function. Thus, the urine specific gravity and osmolality are meaningless unless the animal's state of hydration is assessed which, if dehydration is not present, requires a water-deprivation test. Dehydration, a BUN above 35 mg/dl and a urine specific gravity of less than 1.030 in dogs and 1.035 in cats confirms that renal failure is present, i.e. greater than 75% of renal function has been lost.[133]

RENAL FUNCTION TESTS

The history, clinical signs, physical examination, BUN, plasma creatinine concentration (Cr_p), and urinalysis may be all that is needed to determine if renal failure is present and the type. However, the Cr_p and BUN may be normal or only equivocally elevated, and renal dysfunction may still be present. Conversely, a significant azotemia may be present in the animal with normal renal function due to pre-renal or post-renal causes (Tables 5 and 6, pages 8-14 and 19). In addition, renal function may be normal in a dog or cat with urine in the isosthenuric range. There are two reasons for this: 1) because the animal is adequately hydrated and does not need to concentrate its urine, or 2) in the dehydrated animal, because of a lack of antidiuretic hormone (ADH) or renal medullary washout from any cause. Thus, neither the presence nor absence of azotemia or an isosthenuric urine in either the fully hydrated or dehydrated animal confirms or rules out the presence of renal disease. In some cases, to confirm the presence of renal disease, renal function tests are needed. The most useful and meaningful tests

are water deprivation and creatinine clearance. Phenosulfonphthalein (PSP) and sodium sulfanilate clearance are occasionally used but they provide less specific information than does creatinine clearance.[38] In addition, in many dogs there is a reduced ability to concentrate the urine, or proteinuria occurs before sodium sulfanilate clearance is significantly reduced.[112]

Water Deprivation Test

The water-deprivation test is conducted to determine if when sufficiently dehydrated the animal can concentrate the urine. If clinically apparent dehydration is already present, water deprivation is unnecessary; if it is not, the water-deprivation test is helpful in determining if renal dysfunction is present—particularly in dogs—and in differentiating between the various causes of polyuria, polydipsia, and pollakiuria, as given in Table 5 (page 8-14). This test is less useful in cats because many azotemic cats with primary renal failure retain considerable urine concentrating ability.[170] In one report, only 42% of 109 azotemic cats with renal failure were polyuric, and therefore presumably had a reduced ability to concentrate the urine, although this was not tested.[135]

Before the water-deprivation test is conducted, renal medullary washout, if present, should be corrected. Renal medullary washout is a decrease in the high concentration of primarily sodium and urea normally present in the renal medulla. It is necessary for water reabsorption from the glomerular filtrate. Renal medullary washout results in an impaired ability of the kidney to concentrate the urine even if renal function is normal. Polyuria from any cause, if present for more than a few days, can cause renal medullary washout. Therefore, if polyuria has existed for more than a few days, ensure that renal medullary washout is corrected before conducting a water-deprivation test. This is accomplished by limiting water intake without causing dehydration, as would be indicated by a decrease in body weight, and adding 1 to 2 teaspoonfuls of salt to the diet daily for several days.

The water-deprivation test is conducted in the following manner:

1. Ensure that the animal is fully hydrated and weigh it. If the animal is dehydrated, the test is unnecessary.
2. Withhold water until the animal's body weight decreases by 5%. If the animal is unable to concentrate the urine, this may take only a few hours; whereas, in the normal animal it may take from 1-3 days.
3. Empty residual urine from the bladder, then

obtain a urine sample and measure its specific gravity or osmolality. The maximum urine concentrating ability of human beings, dogs, and cats is to a specific gravity of 1.040, 1.065, and 1.080, respectively.[63,140] If the urine can be concentrated to at least 1.030 by the dog, renal function is sufficient to prevent azotemia.[140] However, if the urine specific gravity is below this level and the BUN exceeds 35 mg/dl, renal failure is present. In contrast to dogs, many cats become severely azotemic before their urine concentration is significantly reduced.[170]

a. If the urine concentration exceeds 1.045 or 1600 mOsm/kg in either dogs[85] or cats[170] renal urine concentrating ability is normal (1.025-1.030 is often used but is applicable to people, not dogs or cats).

b. If the urine concentration is less than these levels, give 2-5 units of antidiuretic hormone (Pitressin, Parke-Davis) subcutaneously or intramuscularly and remeasure the urine specific gravity or osmolality 2-4 hours later. If urine concentration is still below these levels and renal medullary washout is not present, renal function is decreased, or ability to respond to ADH is decreased, i.e. nephrogenic diabetes insipidus is present.[127] If the urine concentration increases within 2-4 hours after ADH is given, the animal has diabetes insipidus due to inadequate ADH secretion by the pituitary.

Creatinine Clearance

Creatinine clearance is determined by measuring the amount of creatinine excreted in the urine over time (mg/min) divided by its plasma concentration (mg/ml). The creatinine clearance in dogs with normal renal function is 50-70 ml/min/(kg body wt)$^{0.75}$ or 2.8-3.7 ml/min/kg.[63] A value less than 40 suggests renal dysfunction, and a value less than 25 is diagnostic of the disease. Values of less than 10 dictate a grave prognosis.[18,63] Creatinine clearance in the cat with normal renal function is 1.3-3.1 ml/min/kg and may vary as much as 30% in the same cat on different days.[172]

For this test, Cr_p should be measured using Lloyd's reagent rather than the alkaline picrate (Jaffe) method. Lloyd's reagent separates creatinine from other chromogens, whereas alkaline picrate does not and therefore gives an erroneously high Cr_p.[38] If the alkaline picrate method is used, the creatinine clearance measured underestimates the GFR by about 30%, although this is quite variable.[67] Nearly all Cr_p measurements from commercial laboratories are by the alkaline picrate method because the procedure utilizing Lloyd's reagent does

not adapt to automated equipment.[63] Instead of using Lloyd's reagent to measure the Cr_p, exogenous creatinine may be given to elevate the Cr_p so that interfering chromogens constitute an insignificant fraction of what is measured.[67]

Although measuring the creatinine clearance is the best indication of the GFR and, therefore, renal function, it requires an accurately timed measurement of urine volume. The longer the period over which urine volume is measured the less accurate the measurement needs to be. However, carefully conducted 20-minute measurements of urine volume from dogs and cats have given creatinine clearance values similar to those obtained when 24-hour urine volume was measured.[18,62,172]

Several factors are important in conducting the creatinine clearance test:

1. The bladder must be emptied immediately before and at the end of the urine collection period.
2. The urine must not be contaminated with feces or food.
3. The animal must be eating and drinking normally.
4. The animal must be in a steady state, i.e. not gaining or losing weight.

Dehydration, volume expansion, or oliguria will cause widely varying and spurious clearance values. Because of these factors and because an accurate assessment of the degree of renal dysfunction is usually not needed for managing the animal with renal failure, creatinine clearance is not usually measured clinically.

RADIOGRAPHY AND ULTRASONOGRAPHY

Survey radiographs and ultrasonographic evaluations of the ureters, urinary bladder and size, shape, location and surface contours of the kidneys may be quite helpful in determining the site of, and diagnosing various disorders of the kidneys and urinary tract, including hydronephrosis, uroliths, neoplasms, polycystic disease, renal agenesis, etc. An excretory urogram is helpful in evaluating portions of the urinary tract that cannot be adequately seen by survey ultrasonography or radiography.[27,58,59] It is particularly useful for detecting upper urinary tract obstruction. The urinary system proximal to the site of obstruction is characteristically dilated. Dilation of a portion of the urinary tract, however, does not invariably indicate obstruction. Other findings characteristic of urinary tract obstruction include:[152]

1. Delayed appearance of the nephrogram

2. Prolonged nephrogram which becomes progressively more dense with time
3. Faint pyelogram especially when the renal pelvis is markedly dilated
4. Renomegaly with acute obstruction
5. A rim sign representing the thin remnant of functional renal mass remaining in chronic hydronephrosis

RENAL BIOPSY

Renal biopsies are associated with risk of complications, particularly when performed by persons inexperienced with the technique. Few renal lesions for which proven specific therapy exists require renal biopsy for diagnosis.[150] Therefore, renal biopsy rarely leads to alteration of therapy and is not justified in most cases.[150] It is best to institute intensive symptomatic and supportive therapy and monitor patient response. When response to treatment is unsatisfactory a biopsy may be indicated to determine reversibility before instituting more aggressive therapy, such as dialysis,[150] and to differentiate between the six major causes of nephrogenic proteinuria. These six causes are terminal chronic renal tubular disease and the five different **types of primary glomerular disease,** which are:

1. Membranous nephropathy characterized by severe proteinuria. It is distinguished from other glomerulopathies by thickening of the capillary wall without primary proliferative changes or inflammation, and the absence of mesangial involvement.[5] It has an insidiously progressive course leading to renal tubular damage and, as a result, polyuria and uremia. With the exception of Abyssinian cats, which may be affected with a familial renal amyloidosis, membranous nephropathy is the most common glomerular disease in cats and also is common in dogs. Glomerulopathies, however, are uncommon in cats.[42] When they do occur, it is primarily in adults and may be associated with feline leukemia or hematopoetic neoplasia.[42] It affects dogs of all ages and breeds, and appears to occur with equal incidence in both sexes.[5] Presenting manifestations vary, with anorexia, weight loss, lethargy, depression, azotemia and hypertension being most common.

2. Proliferative glomerulonephritis, which often has a rapidly progressive course and a tendency to be fulminating

3. Membranoproliferative or mesangiocapillary glomerulonephritis which is the most common glomerular disease in dogs and people

4. Glomerulosclerosis, which occurs secondary to renal tubular disease

5. Amyloidosis

These five different types of glomerular diseases can be differentiated only with a renal biopsy. Treatment and prognosis as described on pages 8-31 and 32 are quite different for the different types, making their differentiation important.

A renal biopsy may be obtained percutaneously using Franklin-Silverman, Metcoff or true-cut needles.[96,141] Blood coagulation should be adequate before a biopsy is taken (see page 8-30). Diagnosis from biopsy is quite accurate. In one study, the antemortem diagnosis from a needle biopsy correlated with the necropsy diagnosis in 80 of 82 dogs and 17 of 19 cats with a variety of renal dysfunctions.[96] However, in cats, in contrast to dogs, amyloid deposits usually localize in the inner medulla, making them difficult to detect.[51]

PATHOPHYSIOLOGIC BASIS FOR DISEASE EFFECTS AND THEIR TREATMENT

Treatment for renal failure must be tailored to the individual patient and be comprehensive enough to correct all recognized or anticipated disorders. The principles of therapy are the same regardless of the underlying cause of the renal damage. Such therapy is primarily designed to relieve clinical signs and prevent or slow progression of the disease. Rarely will it reverse established renal dysfunction. When a definite cause can be established, specific therapy can be combined with supportive measures to halt the progression or renal injury. A summary of the major dysfunctions occurring in the animal with renal failure, their causes, and management are given in Table 8.

OLIGURIA

If renal damage is rapid and severe, or in cases of terminal renal failure, oliguria may occur. Oliguria, however, is uncommon in the azotemic cat.[135] Oliguria results in severe uremia and often hyperkalemia. Both of these conditions cause lethargy and depression, often to the point of coma. There is usually a complete absence of food and water intake, resulting in dehydration.

Treatment of the oliguric patient is rehydration, stimulation of urine excretion if possible, removal of metabolic wastes and provision of nutritional support. If rehydration doesn't initiate urine excretion, institute the following in the order given: 1) give furosemide intravenously (2 mg/kg, double dose and repeat in 1-2 hours if no response), 2) induce osmotic diuresis using either a hypertonic glucose solution or mannitol (page 8-46), and 3)

administer dopamine (Dopamine HCl, Elkins-Sinn and Intropin, American Critical Care) by continuous intravenous infusion at a rate of 2-5 $\mu g/kg/$minute.[29,150] Stimulating urine excretion removes metabolic waste products which are responsible for the clinical signs and effects of the disease. Nutritional support, with sufficient calories, protein, water, electrolytes, and vitamins to meet the animal's needs are necessary to support life, provide the nutrients required for recovery, and prevent body protein catabolism, which worsens the uremia and all of its effects. In one study in dogs, when both kidneys were removed and no treatment was given, death occurred in 4 days. Maintaining nutrition prolonged life for 9 days. With both nutritional support and the removal of metabolic wastes by peritoneal dialysis, the dogs were still doing well after 120 days, when the study was terminated.[111]

Metabolic wastes may be removed by inducing diuresis as described. If diuresis cannot be accomplished, peritoneal dialysis is necessary (page 8-46). Nutritional support, as described on page 8-42, usually requires intravenous, tube, or force feeding, since oliguric animals rarely eat voluntarily. Because uremia induces gastroenteritis and vomiting, intravenous feeding (page 5-35) may be required in the initial management until food can be tolerated orally.

DEHYDRATION, ACIDOSIS OR HYPERKALEMIA

Dehydration, acidosis, and hyperkalemia are uncommon in dogs with polyuric renal failure, but are common in polyuric cats[135] and are often present in both species if oliguria develops. In one study in polyuric azotemic cats, when the cats were first examined, 94% were dehydrated. Their average blood pH was 7.24 ± 0.14 and (in mEq/L, mean $\pm$ standard deviation) plasma bicarbonate was 16.1 ± 6.1, potassium was 4.6 ± 1.1, chloride was 120 ± 10.5 and sodium was 159 ± 6.6 with more than one-third being hypernatremic due to dehydration.[135]

Dehydration causes poor renal perfusion and may cause further renal damage, thus **rehydration** with intravenously administered fluids should be accomplished within a few hours (3-6). However, fluid should not be given any faster than 20 ml/kg body wt/hr unless the central venous pressure is monitored. Caution must be used to prevent overhydration of the oliguric patient. Clinical signs of overhydration include serous nasal discharge, mild coughing, dyspnea, restlessness, abdominal distention, diarrhea, and hypothermia. Insertion of an indwelling catheter to monitor urine output often helps in determining when rehydration has been

TABLE 8

RENAL FAILURE INDUCED DYSFUNCTIONS, THEIR CAUSES AND MANAGEMENT

Dysfunction	Cause	Management Recommended
Uremia	↓ excretion	Insure intake of sufficient food low in high quality protein to meet caloric needs (p. 8-39).
Dehydration	↑ water loss &/or ↓ water intake	Correct initial fluid deficit with parenteral administration of equal parts isotonic saline & glucose, or isotonic saline with 2½% glucose if not hypernatremic. If additional fluid is needed, give Ringer's lactate.
Acidosis	↓ acid excretion	Add sodium bicarbonate to food if eating (Table 1, p. 8-4); if not, to rehydration fluids to increase plasma bicarbonate or total CO_2 to 18–22 mEq/L (p. 8–26).
Hyperkalemia	Acidosis and ↓ K^+ excretion	Treat dehydration and acidosis, and add 10 ml 23% calcium gluconate/L of rehydration fluid. If necessary, give furosemide, osmotic diuresis, dialysis, decrease potassiun intake or give Kayexalate (Table 1, p. 8-4).
Vomiting or Diarrhea	Excess gastric acid due to hypergastrinemia	Administer cimetidine (Table 1, p. 8-4). If vomiting continues, give phenothiazine or trimethobenzamid (Table 1, p. 7-4).
Oral inflammation or lesions	same as vomiting	Administer cimetidene, a topical anesthetic and sucralfate (Table 1, p. 8-4).
Anorexia, weight loss, lethargy	All of above dysfunctions	Correct all of above dysfunctions. Give potassium, zinc and B-vitamins (Table 1, p. 8-4).
Polyuria, polydipsia, pollakiuria, nocturia	↑ in GFR in remaining nephrons	Free access to good quality water and increased vitamin B complex intake (Table 1, p. 8-4).
Oliguria	Dehydration or severe renal damage	Treat dehydration, provide nutritional support (p. 8-42) and, if necessary, remove wastes by diuresis or dialysis (p. 8-45).
Hyperhpospha-temia	PTH induced bone demineralization & ↓ renal P excretion	Feed low phosphorus diet. If 2 weeks later plasma P exceeds 5 mg/dl, give cimetidine & if 2 weeks later it still does give aluminum salt P binders (Table 1, p. 8-4).
Hypertension	See page 8-32	Feed low sodium diet. If ineffective, treat as described on page 8-33.
Edema, ascites or hypoproteinemia	↑ urine albumin loss & hypertension	As given in Figure 3 (page 8-31).
↑ Blood coagulation & thrombosis	Glomerulopathy allowing loss of coagulation inhibi-tors & albumin	Specific therapy given in Figure 3 (page 8-31).
↓ Blood coagulation	↓ platelet aggregation & ↓ thromboplastin	Treat uremia.
Anemia	↑ RBC loss & ↓ RBC life & synthesis	Administer nandrolone decanoate (Table 1, p. 8-4).
Hypocalcemia	↓ abs. ↑ excretion & ↑ plasma P	If Ca < 10 mg/dl **and** Ca × P < 55 give calcium carbonate and vitamin D (Table 1, p. 8-4).
Hyperglycemia	Insulin resistance	Treat uremia.
Hyperlididemia	↑ glucagon &/or ↑ hepatic synthesis	Treat uremia.
↓ Immunity	Uremic toxins	Treat uremia. Monitor for infectious disease, e.g. rectal temperature. Use caution in administration of antimicrobials (Table 9, p. 8-29).

achieved. Failure to induce a urine flow of 0.5-2 ml/kg/hr indicates either inadequate hydration or renal damage so severe that urine cannot be produced. When normal hydration is obtained, body weight should be monitored twice daily and this weight maintained by giving more fluids if necessary. If the body weight decreases by more than 0.5-1%/day, dehydration is occurring. Body weight will decrease this amount without dehydration occurring in the absence of intake of energy supplying nutrients (Figure 4, page 6-27).

A solution of one-half isotonic saline and one-half isotonic glucose is preferred if hypernatremia is present; if it is not, isotonic saline with 50 ml of 50% glucose (dextrose) added to each liter is recommended. These are preferred to extracellular replacement fluids, such as Ringer's lactate, because extracellular replacement fluids contain potassium and hyperkalemia is often present in oliguric animals. Administration of glucose results in movement of potassium into the cell, helping correct hyperkalemia. If the plasma potassium concentration exceeds 6-7 mEq/L or hyperkalemic EKG changes are noted (bradycardia, decreased amplitude of the P wave, prolonged Q-T interval and increased amplitude and peaking of the T wave), add 10 ml/liter of 23% calcium gluconate to the fluid given. This will produce a fluid with a calcium concentration of 20 mg/dl. This is almost twice the normal plasma calcium concentration but less than that which may cause any detrimental effects, even if hypocalcemia is not present. Administration of calcium is beneficial because hypocalcemia is often present and because calcium antagonizes the cardiac depressive effects of hyperkalemia.

Osmotic diuresis or peritoneal dialysis (page 8-46) will correct **hyperkalemia.** If these procedures do not correct hyperkalemia, or if they are not needed to correct a severe uremia, but hyperkalemia persists after rehydration, prolonged control can be achieved by restricting potassium intake and giving furosemide to increase potassium excretion (Table 1). If necessary, the ion-exchange resin, sodium polystyrene sulfonate may be given (Table 1). However, after rehydration, and particularly when renal function and urine excretion return, the animal will often become hypokalemic. If this occurs, potassium chloride should be given (Table 1, p. 8-4).

Metabolic acidosis may develop with oliguria or severe polyuric renal failure. It is caused by a reduced renal excretion of sulfate, phosphate, organic acids, hydrogen, and ammonium ions. Retention of these ions decreases the plasma bicarbonate concentration, resulting in metabolic acidosis. Metabolic acidosis may also occur as a result of the uncommon disease, renal tubular acidosis. With renal tubular acidosis there may be either a decrease in distal tubular secretion of hydrogen ions or a decrease in proximal tubular reabsorption of bicarbonate, which frequently occurs in conjunction with primary glucosuria (Fanconi syndrome) (Table 5, page 8-14).[154] In either case, sufficient alkalinizing agents must be given to maintain a normal plasma bicarbonate or total carbon dioxide concentration. Sodium or potassium bicarbonate may be added to the food. Large quantities (0.1-1 g/kg/day, 4 g/tsp) may be necessary. Urinary bicarbonate wasting results in potassium wasting; therefore, potassium bicarbonate may be helpful.

Metabolic acidosis enhances osteodystrophy and protein catabolism.[200] In addition acidosis results in movement of hydrogen ions into the cell, which causes potassium ion movement out of the cell. When combined with reduced renal excretion of potassium, as may occur in advanced renal failure, hyperkalemia results. Correcting acidosis decreases uremia and increases potassium movement back into the cell. This helps to correct hyperkalemia, if present. In one study, giving sodium bicarbonate (84 mg/kg/day) to 6 uremic people increased their plasma bicarbonate concentration from 15.8 ± 0.7 to 23.4 ± 1.2 mEq/L and lowered their BUN from 86 to 53 mg/dl.[146] The decrease in BUN was not due to increased excretion of urea in the urine, but instead was thought to be due to increased synthesis of body protein.

If **acidosis** is sufficiently severe that the plasma bicarbonate concentration is less than 18 mEq/L, enough sodium bicarbonate should be given to increase it to 18-22 mEq/L. The approximate amount needed, as shown below, is the bicarbonate concentration deficit times the bicarbonate's volume of distribution. The bicarbonate volume of distribution is approximately twice the extracellular fluid volume of 25-30% of body weight.[108]

mEq bicarbonate needed = (18 minus the patient's plasma bicarbonate or total carbon dioxide concentration) × 0.3 × 2 × kg body weight

This amount of bicarbonate should be given in the quantity of fluid needed to correct the patient's fluid deficit, which in liters is the percent dehydration/100 times kilograms body weight. Bicarbonate should not be given as a bolus. Care should be taken not to raise the plasma bicarbonate concentration above 22-24 mEq/L. Increasing body fluid pH impairs release of oxygen from erythrocytes, respiratory drive, vasodilation, and ionized calcium concentration.

If the animal is eating, and the plasma bicarbonate or total carbon dioxide concentration is less than 18

mEq/L, add sodium bicarbonate to the diet (Table 1, p. 8-4) and monitor the urine pH. If the urine pH exceeds 7 before the animal consumes any food, stop giving bicarbonate. If hypertension, congestive heart failure or edema is present and hyperkalemia is not present, use potassium bicarbonate instead of sodium bicarbonate. If both hyperkalemia and acidosis are present, give calcium lactate or calcium carbonate (limestone) orally instead of sodium or potassium bicarbonate.

POLYURIA, POLLAKIURIA, NOCTURIA AND POLYDIPSIA

Although oliguria is common in animals with acute renal failure and it occurs terminally in animals with chronic renal failure, polyuria occurs before there is this degree of decrease in renal function. Polyuria induces pollakiuria, nocturia, and polydipsia. Diseases that cause these clinical signs, and factors useful in their differential diagnosis are given in Table 5 (page 8-14). The procedures given in the flow diagram in Figure 2 (page 8-16) may help in determining their cause.

Polyuria occurs in animals with renal failure because, as the number of functional nephrons decreases, a compensatory increase occurs in the glomerular filtration rate per remaining nephron. Thus, an increase occurs in the quantity of fluid presented to the distal tubule of the remaining functional nephrons. In addition, the renal medullary concentration gradient is reduced because there are fewer functional nephrons and, hence, fewer functioning sodium pumps in the loop of Henle. Polyuria results from the increased fluid presented to the remaining functional tubules and the decreased renal medullary solute concentration gradient required for its reabsorption.

Treatment for polyuria is unnecessary. However, it is extremely important that the animal have free access to water. Since the animal cannot concentrate the urine even when dehydrated, death ensues rapidly if water is not available. When polyuria is present, a larger amount of water-soluble B complex vitamins are lost,[88] and are needed, especially if food intake is reduced. The dietary foods specifically formulated for animals with renal failure, given in Tables 13 and 14 (page 8-44), contain adequate amounts of these vitamins, so that additional supplements are not needed. If these diets are **not** used, give daily a B complex vitamin supplement. Because of its protein content brewer's yeast should not be given to supply B vitamins.

VOMITION OR DIARRHEA

Vomition occurs with increasing frequency as renal failure worsens. It is not associated with food intake. Rather, it develops as a result of excessive gastric acid secretion stimulated by gastrin. Impaired renal function decreases excretion of gastrin, resulting in an increase in its plasma concentration.[99] Increased gastrin stimulates secretion of gastric acid. Excessive gastric acid secretion may cause gastroenteritis, vomiting, and diarrhea. The diarrhea may be hemorrhagic. Although vomiting commonly occurs in uremic cats (51% in one study) diarrhea rarely occurs.[135] In contrast to dogs, cats may have constipation.[135]

Treatment is the reduction of gastric acid secretion by giving cimetidine (Table 1, p. 8-4). In one report uremia-induced vomiting in the dog stopped 3-6 hours after administration of cimetidine.[193] Cimetidine is also beneficial in reducing hyperparathormonemia-induced progression of renal damage and osteodystrophy. It has been shown in uremic dogs to lessen plasma parathormone and phosphorus concentrations and bone reabsorption; and to increase plasma calcium and 1,25-dihydroxy vitamin D concentrations, and calcium balance.[93] Vomiting may also be due to uremic toxin stimulation of the chemoreceptor trigger zone, in which case giving phenothiazine or trimethobenzamide (Table 1, page 7-4) may be beneficial.[45]

GINGIVITIS, STOMATITIS, GLOSSITIS OR ORAL ULCERS

Oral lesions may develop as a result of gastritis and the effect of uremic toxins on mucosal membranes. Gingivitis and halitosis were present in 20% of 109 uremic cats in one study, whereas only 3% had oral ulcers. The recommended treatment for the oral lesions is cimetidine (Table 1). Also, decrease uremia, give a topical anesthetic (Table 1) to relieve oral discomfort and increase food intake, and rinse the mouth with a sucralfate solution (Table 1, p. 8-4). Sucralfate coats and protects the oral cavity.

ANOREXIA, WEIGHT LOSS OR LETHARGY

These are often the most prevalent signs in both dogs and cats with renal failure. In one study of uremic cats, 100% were anorectic, 70% had weight loss, 67% were depressed and 53% were weak.[135] All of these signs are worsened by vomiting, gingivitis, stomatitis, glossitis, oral ulcers and diarrhea. Vomition and diarrhea cause excessive loss of water and electrolytes, including potassium. Potassium losses are further increased if diuretics are given and if acidosis is present. A potassium deficit results in lethargy, anorexia, and weakness and may be pres-

ent even if the plasma potassium concentration is increased, normal, or decreased.

A zinc deficiency also may develop in animals with renal failure and causes anorexia. This deficiency is more likely to occur if aluminum salts are given. They are commonly given to reduce phosphorus absorption. However, they also decrease zinc absorption and result in depressed food intake and other signs of zinc deficiency.[143] Impaired taste acuity and gonadal dysfunction, which result from zinc deficiency, and a low concentration of zinc in plasma, hair, and leukocytes have been seen in animals with polyuric renal failure.[113] Zinc supplementation (0.7 mg/kg of elemental zinc daily) to people with polyuric renal failure has been shown to correct these alterations; whereas, these factors remained unchanged in persons given placebos.[113] This amount of zinc is added to the prepared dietary foods recommended for managing renal failure (Tables 13 and 14, page 8-44). Thus, zinc supplementation is unnecessary if one is being fed.

The effect of accumulated uremic toxins on the nervous system also may be at least partially responsible for causing lethargy, weakness and anorexia. Drowsiness, behavioral changes, neuromuscular twitches, coma, and convulsions may also occur.

Treatment of these signs is designed to:

1. Ensure that the animal is fully hydrated and that the plasma bicarbonate concentration is 18 mEq/L or greater.
2. Actively manage vomition, diarrhea, stomatitis and glossitis if present.
3. Ensure intake of an adequate amount of a restricted protein diet to meet caloric needs.
4. Add potassium chloride to the diet daily (Table 1, p. 8-4) if diuretics are being given for a prolonged period or if hypokalemia is present.
5. Add B vitamins and zinc to the ration daily if the diet does not already contain additional quantities.

IMPAIRED REPRODUCTIVE ABILITY

Uremic animals lose libido, and show signs of impotence, sterility, decreased testicle size, spermatogenic damage, decreased plasma testosterone, and reduced ovarian function.[86,89,187] Treatment is to correct the uremia.

HYPERGLYCEMIA

In uremic animals, hyperglycemia usually occurs in the presence of normal or slightly elevated insulin secretion and blood concentration. The response to exogenous insulin is decreased[47] due to the insensitivity of peripheral tissue to insulin.[48] Unlike diabetes, there is an elevated insulin/glucagon ratio. The insulin intolerance is thought to result from elevated levels of insulin antagonists such as growth hormone, glucagon, catecholamines, parathyroid hormone, cortisol, urea, creatinine, potassium, or acidosis.[88] Occasionally, uremia inhibits beta cell sensitivity to glucose, resulting in decreased insulin secretion.[48] Hyperglycemia is also promoted by an increase in alanine conversion to glucose, which may occur in animals with chronic azotemia[114] although total hepatic glucose production remains unchanged.[48] Ketosis is not usually present.

Treatment of uremia-induced hyperglycemia is to reduce uremia. When this is accomplished, administration of insulin is not usually needed. It may be used initially in severe cases if glucosuria is present.

HYPERLIPIDEMIA

Protracted renal failure is often accompanied by hyperlipidemia characterized by elevated free fatty acids, triglycerides, and cholesterol. Two mechanisms have been proposed as being responsible. One is that elevated glucagon values (which occur because of reduced renal glucagon excretion) cause lipolysis and depress lipoprotein lipase which clears triglycerides from very low-density lipoproteins. The second proposed mechanism is that a reduction in plasma albumin concentration or oncotic pressure (which occurs because of protein loss in the urine and/or malnutrition) stimulates an increase in hepatic synthesis of cholesterol and low-density lipoprotein cholesterol.[7] Detrimental effects of renal-failure induced hyperlipidemia have not been demonstrated in dogs or cats with renal failure. **Treatment** is to decrease uremia.

IMPAIRED IMMUNITY

Impaired immune response to infectious agents occurs in uremic animals. The inflammatory response is altered. Lymphopenia occurs, and a defect in cellular immunity has been demonstrated. As a result, uremic animals are more susceptible to infectious diseases. **Treatment** is to correct uremia.

Caution should be used in giving antimicrobial drugs to animals with renal failure as many are cleared by the kidney. After initial administration at the normal dose the dosage of many drugs should be reduced or the interval between administration lengthened as described in Table 9. Ampicillin has been recommended as a good antibiotic to use in animals with renal failure because it is not nephrotoxic, is concentrated in the urine, and decreases azotemia.[176] If severe life-threatening sepsis is pres-

ent, microbiologic efficacy should take precedence over fear of nephrotoxicosis because, in this situation, the sequelae of the infectious disease are often more serious than is an episode of nephrotoxicosis.[167] However, the guidelines given in Table 9 should be followed. Drug-induced nephrotoxicosis is often difficult to detect and may not be manifest during drug administration. In one report, nephrotoxicosis was not detected in 8 of 10 dogs without known prior renal dysfunction until 1-7 days after cessation of 3-11 days of gentamicin administration at a dosage of 2.2-12 mg/kg every 6-12 hours.[25] Despite extensive therapy, 8 of these 10 dogs died or failed to respond and were euthanized. Even serial urinalysis, BUN, and creatinine clearance monitoring during administration of gentamicin does not detect polyuric acute renal failure until damage sufficient to cause death has occurred.[25,79]

ANEMIA

A progressive normocytic, normochromic, non-regenerative anemia is a common problem in uremic dogs, but it occurs less frequently in uremic cats. In the early stages of the diseases, it may be a minor factor. In the dog, but not the cat, it becomes more important as renal failure becomes more severe. Typical laboratory findings reveal reduced hemoglobin, hematocrit, and red blood cell count. Dehydration can mask these changes and cause erythrocyte indices to be within normal limits. There may be bizarre-shaped erythrocytes. Serum iron concentration is usually normal, but iron utilization is decreased;[38] and there is usually no reticulocyte response.

The anemia is due to three defects: 1) shortened lifespan of erythrocytes in uremic plasma, 2) decreased production of erythrocytes, and 3) blood loss. The erythrocytes in uremic plasma have a fragile cell membrane and are quickly removed from the circulation. The toxic factor responsible for this is assumed to be increased creatinine or guanidine in the plasma. It has been suggested that these substances interfere with the normal sodium-potassium pump in the erythrocyte membrane because the stability of the membrane quickly returns to normal after dialysis and removal of these two substances.

The second and probably primary factor in the pathogenesis of uremic anemia is the decreased production of erythrocytes. Uremic toxins may have a direct effect on inhibiting erythrocyte production. In addition, in the dog, only the kidney produces erythropoietin—a hormone that stimulates production of erythrocytes by the bone marrow. As renal failure progresses, production of erythropoietin, and as a result bone marrow stimu-

TABLE 9

ANTIMICROBIAL DRUG DOSAGE ADJUSTMENTS IN ANIMALS WITH RENAL DISEASE[167]

PRECISE MODIFICATION REQUIRED

Amikacin	Sisomicin
Colistimethate*	Tobramycin
Gentamicin	Vancomycin
Kanamycin	

HALF DOSE OR DOUBLE INTERVAL

Ampicillin	Lincomycin‡
Amoxicillin	Methicillin
Carbenicillin	Penicillin G
Cefamandole*	Penicillin V
Cephalothin+	Ticarcillin

CREATININE CLEARANCE (ML/MIN/KG) BETWEEN: 1.0 TO 0.5 USE 2 × INTERVAL; 0.5 TO 0.3 USE 3 × INTERVAL; < 0.3 USE 4 × INTERVAL**

Cephalexin	Streptomycin
Cephaloridine	Sulfisoxazole
Cephalothin	
Trimethoprim/sulfamethoxazole§	

NO DOSAGE CHANGE REQUIRED

Cefaclor	Doxycycline
Chloramphenicol§	Erythromycin
Clindamycin	Nafcillin
Cloxacillin	Oxacillin
Dicloxacillin	Tylosin

CONTRAINDICATED

Mandelamine	Nitrofurantoin
Nalidixic acid	Polymyxin B
Neomycin	Tetracyclines (except doxycycline)

*Reduce dose

+Increase interval

‡3 × interval

§Avoid in animals with severe renal failure

**If creatinine clearance is unknown, it may be estimated as (1/plasma creatinine concentration) although this results in an overestimate as plasma creatinine concentration increases above 4 mg/dl.

lation of erythrocyte production, decrease. However, in cats erythropoietin is produced by both the kidney and the carotid bodies.[197] This quite likely is why anemia is less common in uremic cats than dogs, and that in contrast to dogs, in cats there is no correlation between the degree of renal failure and the degree of anemia.[135]

The third factor responsible for anemia in the uremic animal is blood loss, most commonly from the gastrointestinal tract. Bleeding results from increased blood pressure, decreased platelet aggregation, and decreased thromboplastin generation by platelets.

Treatment for uremic anemia is anabolic steroids. They increase production of erythropoietin, potentiate erythropoietin's effect, directly stimulate erythropoiesis, and increase erythrocyte, 2,3-diphosphoglycerate concentration (which decreases hemoglobin's affinity for oxygen so that greater amounts of oxygen are released to the tissue).[111,139] Response to therapy may not be detected for 2-3 months. This response may be an increase, maintenance, or slowing in the decline of the hematocrit. In the fully hydrated animal, the hematocrit should be maintained above 30% and the hemoglobin concentration above 10%.

In addition to helping correct anemia, anabolic steroids have been purported (but not demonstrated in uremic dogs or cats) to enhance calcium deposition in bones and increase nitrogen utilization if energy intake is adequate; thus, urea production and uremia are decreased.[111,139] However, in one study in dogs with experimentally induced renal failure, a testosterone derivative (Boldenone undecylenate, ER Squibb & Sons) had no effect on food intake, body weight, plasma creatinine or albumin concentrations, nitrogen balance, lean body mass, or limb circumference.[65] Side effects of long-term use of anabolic steroids in people include virilization, cholestatic liver damage manifested by icterus, and increased bromsulphalein (BSP) retention. The liver damage is reversible with discontinued use of the anabolic steroid. In young animals, anabolic steroids may also cause premature metaphyseal closure, thus decreasing mature size.

Anabolic steroids considered most effective in promoting erythropoiesis in animals with renal failure are:

1. Nandrolone decanoate (Deca-Durabolin, Organon) is considered to be the most effective (Table 1, p. 8-4).[111,134]
2. Testosterone enanthate (Delatestryl, Squibb), 50-150 mg/dog intramuscularly repeated every 1-4 weeks.
3. Testosterone proprionate (Oreton, Schering), 10-15 mg/dog day given orally.

BLOOD COAGULATION DISORDERS

In the absence of proteinuria, in uremic animals blood coagulation is decreased which, in conjunction with hypertension, may result in hemorrhage. The decrease in blood coagulation is due to a reduction in platelet aggregation and a decrease in thromboplastin production by platelets caused by uremic toxins. Bleeding time is the most useful platelet function test with uremia.[116] A synthetic derivative of antidiuretic hormone, diamino-8-D-arginine vasopressin, shortens bleeding time when given to people with uremic-induced prolonged bleeding time.[116] It may, therefore, be useful in temporarily restoring hemostatic competency in patients with spontaneous hemorrhage or undergoing biopsies or surgery. The dosage used is 0.3 g/kg in 50 ml of isotonic saline solution given intravenously over 30 minutes. It shortens bleeding time for up to 4 hours with a peak effect at 1-2 hours. There are no reports of its use in animals.

In uremic animals with prolonged proteinuria, increased coagulation and thrombosis, particularly pulmonary, may occur.[80] In one study, thrombosis was found at necropsy in 14 of 44 dogs with renal amyloidosis.[183] It occurs most often in the early stages of glomerulonephropathies.[53] The thrombosis is due to selective retention of high molecular weight hemostatic factors such as fibrinogen and clotting factor VIII, and a loss of low molecular weight coagulation inhibitors such as antithrombin III by the damaged glomeruli.[80] Hypoalbuminemia induced by loss of albumin also contributes to thrombosis because it increases platlet sensitivity for aggregation.[81] Hyperfibrinogenemia is consistently present and plasma antithrombin III concentration is usually decreased in dogs with hypoalbuminemia due to persistent proteinuria.

Treatment: Heparin and warfarin have been used in an attempt to prevent excessive blood coagulation and fibrin deposition. However, controlled studies have shown no benefit from their use.[13] Continual administration of the platlet inhibitors, aspirin and dipyridamole, for as long as 8.4 months have decreased urinary protein loss, rate of decline in renal function, and development of end-stage renal failure in people.[54] Similar studies in dogs and cats have not been reported.

EDEMA, ASCITES OR HYPOPROTEINEMIA

Edema, ascites, and pleural effusion may develop as a result of either hypoalbuminemia or hypertension or both. The plasma albumin concentration must fall below 1.5% before these effects occur. However, they may occur at a higher plasma albumin concentration if hypertension is present, as it is in most dogs with renal failure.[38] Hypoalbuminemia may be due to persistent proteinuria occurring as a result of glomerular damage (page 8-15 and 8-20). Hypoalbuminemia reduces the plasma oncotic pressure, and hypertension increases hydrostatic pressure. Either factor, if of sufficient magnitude, causes loss of fluid from the vascular compartment. The resulting decrease in blood volume reduces renal arterial blood pressure which, via the renin-

angiotensin system, stimulates increased aldosterone secretion. Aldosterone increases sodium and water retention. Sodium retention may be further increased by a reduction in the glomerular filtration rate and enhanced distal nephron reabsorption due to undefined factors.[38] Because of the decreased oncotic and frequently increased hydrostatic blood pressures, sodium and water cannot be retained in the vascular compartment; therefore, their retention worsens edema. Sodium and fluid retention are consistent features of glomerulonephropathies.[38]

Edema may be pulmonary, resulting in dyspnea and coughing. Initially, this occurs only after exercise; but as it worsens, it may occur at any time.

There may be abdominal distention due to ascites and diarrhea due to intestinal edema. Subcutaneous edema may develop and is most notable in the dependent portions of the limbs, ventral thorax, and scrotum. These signs must be differentiated from other causes of edema, including trauma, cardiovascular disease, obstructive hepatic diseases, and other causes of hypoproteinemia, which include nutrient malassimilation, protein deficiency, protein-losing enteropathy and certain hepatopathies. With nephrotic hypoproteinemia, the plasma lipids and cholesterol concentrations may be elevated. The combination of these alterations, hypoalbuminemia, hyperlipidemia, hypercholesterole-

FIGURE 3

EDEMA, ASCITES, PLEURAL EFFISIONS OR PROTEINURIA TREATMENT

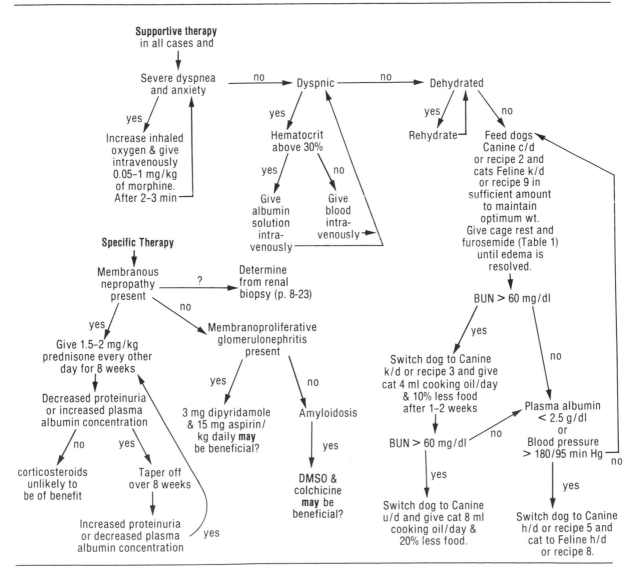

mia, proteinuria, and edema are referred to as the **nephrotic syndrome.** A plasma albumin concentration of 1.5% or less and a urine protein/creatinine ratio of 1 or greater is highly indicative of the nephrotic syndrome.[28] It may occur with or without azotemia. Azotemia occurs only if there is renal tubular involvement which, until the advanced stage, results in polyuria with minimal proteinuria. Nephrotic syndrome simply indicates a sufficiently severe proteinuria to cause these effects. It is nearly always due to glomerular disease. Even with advanced renal tubular disease urinary protein losses are less than 150 mg/kg/24 hr.[28,53] With primary glomerular disease, losses may be many times greater than this.

Supportive therapy, as described in Figure 3, is indicated for all patients with edema, ascites, or proteinuria. It is aimed at enabling affected animals to live in equilibrium with their damaged glomeruli. The major goal is to prevent sodium and water retention by restricting sodium intake, reducing hypertension, increasing the plasma albumin concentration, and maintaining a BUN of less than 60 mg/dl to prevent uremia-induced effects.

For all cases, restrict sodium intake and ensure that water is available. Sodium restriction is the most beneficial aspect of therapy.[38] Initially dietary sodium should be reduced to 0.2-0.3% in the diet dry matter.[38,134] This is the amount present in Prescription Diets w/d, k/d, u/d and Recipes 2, 3 and 9, and is 25-50% that in commercial pet foods (Tables 13 and 14, page 8-44).

Ensure that food intake is sufficient to maintain the animal at optimal body weight. If the animal weighs less than optimum, as is often the case when proteinuria is present, enough food should be fed to correct the weight deficiency. If food intake is not adequate, body proteins, including albumin, are broken down and used to meet energy needs. In addition, sufficient nutrients are not available for albumin synthesis to correct the hypoalbuminemia. The diet must contain sufficient protein to meet these needs and to replace the proteins being lost in the urine. However, if azotemia is present, excessive protein intake must be prevented.

If membranous nephropathy is present, high alternate-day doses of corticosteroids, as described in Figure 3, are beneficial.[34,97] Chlorambucil (Leukeran, Burroughs Wellcome) may also be of benefit. A six-month course of methylpredisolone alternated with chlorambucil every other month resulted in complete or partial remission of membranous nephropathy in 23 of 32 people, as compared to 9 of 30 untreated control patients.[161] Cytotoxic or immunosuppresive drugs are of no benefit in treatment of membranous nephropathy.

Neither they nor corticosteroids are effective in treating membranoproliferative or proliferative glomerulonephritis.[38] These causes of proteinuria are usually progressive and unresponsive to treatment. Recent studies, however, suggest that continual daily administration of 3 mg/kg of dipyridamole (Dipyridamole, Danbury, Geneva or Schein) and 15 mg/kg of aspirin slow the deterioration of renal function and the development of end-stage renal failure in people with membranoproliferative glomerulonephritis.[54]

Corticosteroids are contraindicated for animals with amyloidosis as they may enhance amyloid formation and deposition, thus worsening the disease.[96] Dimethyl sulfoxide (DMSO) (Dermassay, Pittman-Moore or Domoso, Syntex) and colchicine (Lilly or Danbury) have both been used with varying degrees of benefit in treatment for amyloidosis.[51] DMSO may mobilize amyloid deposits and reduce their deposition. However, in 3 of 4 dogs with renal failure due to amyloidosis, DMSO was of no benefit.[83] Colchicine may be useful in delaying amyloid deposition but is less useful in patients with established renal disease.

It has been suggested that anabolic steroids may be beneficial in treating proteinuric animals. However, no effect on food intake, body weight, plasma albumin concentration, nitrogen balance or lean body mass were demonstrated in dogs with experimentally induced renal failure.[65] Captopril (Capoten, ER Squibb) has promptly decreased proteinuria without a fall in systemic blood pressure in people with diabetic nephropathy.[189] Whether it would be effective in other forms of glomerulopathy or in animals is unknown.

HYPERTENSION

Hypertension is present in 58-93% of dogs with renal failure.[38,209] The major causes include:[38,169]

1. Inability to excrete enough sodium to maintain sodium balance. This results in fluid retention and circulatory congestion which activates the renin-angiotensin-aldosterone axis, leading to greater vascular resistance and a further increase in salt retention.

2. Stiffening of venous capacitance

3. Alterations in adrenergic activity

4. Stimulation of renopressor systems

5. Suppression of renodepressors or prostaglandins

6. Increased total peripheral resistance secondary to anemia

7. Hyperparathormonemia due to an unknown mechanism

Hypertension causes renal necrosis, fibrinoid lesions, hyalinization, and capillary occlusion.[38] These changes cause atrophy and sclerosis of the renal cortex, renal ischemia, and progressive parenchymal loss.[169] A direct and consistent correlation exists between renal insufficiency, hypertension, and development of renal vascular pathology.[38] Hypertension also causes left ventricular hypertrophy, which is a constant feature of renal insufficiency in dogs.[38] The hypertrophy reduces cardiac reserve, predisposes to myocardial ischemia, and may progress to cardiac failure.

Treatment: To prevent the sodium and water retention and the hypertension present in most dogs—and probably cats—with renal failure, sodium intake must be reduced.[3] A 20-kg dog being fed most commercial rations, which contain 0.5-0.8% sodium in their dry matter (Table 8, page 11-30), will consume more than 2 g of sodium daily. To excrete 2 g of sodium, the kidney must filter 300 g.[38] If renal function is decreased 90%, the remaining functional nephrons must filter and excrete 10 times more sodium per nephron. Failure to do this results in accumulation of sodium. If the ability of the remaining renal mass to filter and excrete sodium was able to increase only five-fold, 1 of the 2 g of sodium ingested daily would be retained. Retention of 1 g of sodium/day, as shown below, would increase the extracellular fluid (ECF) volume by 310 ml/day. To prevent retention, sodium intake must be reduced, in this example to 1 g or less daily, which would require a diet containing 0.3% sodium or less.

$$\left(\frac{1\ g\ Na}{day\ retained} \right) \times \left(\frac{1000\ mg}{g} \right) \times \left(\frac{1\ mEq\ Na}{23\ mg\ Na} \right) \times$$

$$\left(\frac{1\ liter\ ECF}{145\ mEq\ Na} \right) \times \left(\frac{1000\ ml}{liter} \right) = \quad \begin{array}{l} 310\ ml\ of\ ECF/ \\ day\ retained \end{array}$$

In dogs with chronic renal failure, reduced sodium intake resulted in less sodium excretion without dehydration or other adverse effects.[175] However, animals with renal insufficiency have an impaired ability to adjust sodium excretion rapidly in response to sudden changes in sodium intake.[200] Thus, a sudden decrease in sodium intake may result in salt-wasting and dehydration. The resulting decrease in glomerular filtration rate and renal blood flow may worsen renal damage. To prevent this reducing salt intake gradually is often recommended. This is a good recommendation; however there appears to be no harm in abruptly reducing

sodium intake from the amount in most commercial pet foods (0.5-0.8% in dry matter) to that recommended for dogs and cats with renal disease(0.1-0.3% in dry matter).

In one study in dogs in which 40% of the renal mass had been removed surgically, there was no net loss of sodium (sodium dumping) when first measured one week after an additional 40% of renal mass was removed (which decreased glomerular filtration rate from 83 to 54 ml/min), and dietary sodium intake was decreased abruptly from 120 to 77 mEq/day (equivalent to 0.95 and 0.62% sodium in diet dry matter).[175] Sodium dumping did not occur when again measured 1 week after one-half of the remaining renal mass was removed surgically (which decreased glomerular filtration rate from 54 to 11 ml/min) and sodium intake was abruptly decreased from 77 to 16 mEq/day (equivalent to 0.62 and 0.13% sodium in diet dry matter). Thus, in dogs with only 12% of renal mass remaining, abruptly reducing dietary sodium from 0.62 to 0.13% of diet dry matter did not result in sodium dumping when the measurement was first taken one week later. These dogs maintained sodium balance on their low sodium intake and showed neither evidence of volume depletion nor any other adverse effects.

Changing the diet of dogs with renal disease from regular commercial foods to Prescription Diet k/d (Hill's), which contains 0.23% sodium in its dry matter, has been shown to reduce mean blood pressure from a hypertensive 132 mmHg to a normotensive 108 mmHg.[38] The benefit gained from restricting sodium intake in preventing hypertension induced by renal failure was well demonstrated in a study of rats in which seven weeks after removing 75% of renal mass, systolic blood pressure was 172, 138 and 131 mmHg when the diet contained 3.2, 0.35 or 0.05% sodium, respectively; as compared to 129 mmHg in healthy rats fed the same diets.[32] Dogs consuming a low-sodium diet have a reduced sensitivity of the renal vasculature to the potent vasoconstrictor angiotensin II and bradykinin without an alteration in the percent conversion of angiotensin I to angiotensin II.[61] In contrast, in the superior mesenteric vasculature the percent conversion is reduced and the sensitivity to angiotensin II and bradykinin remain unaltered.

Reducing sodium intake is the most effective treatment for hypertension and is the only treatment needed in most hypertensive dogs and cats with renal disease. If sodium restriction does not control hypertension, prognosis for long-term survival is poor. If hypertension is severe or if after reducing sodium intake the systolic/diastolic blood pressure exceeds 180/95 mmHg, additional ther-

apy should be instituted in the order given. Continue the previous therapy and only if hypertension is severe or if after several weeks the blood pressure remains elevated institute the next treatment.[3,39]

1. Restrict sodium intake to 0.1-0.3% in diet dry matter.

2. Give thiazide diuretics if plasma creatinine is less than 4; if it is 4 or more give furosemide (Table 1, p. 8-4). Diuretics should be used only after the animal is fully hydrated, then with caution in animals with renal insufficiency in order to prevent hypotension, hypovolemia, and decreased renal perfusion.

3. Give 2 or 3 times daily 5-20 mg of the beta-adrenergic blocking agent propranolol (Inderal, Ayerst). It generally takes several days of therapy before a reduction in blood pressure occurs.

4. Give the vasodilator captopril (Capoten, ER Squibb) at a dosage of 1-2 mg/kg every 8-12 hours. Captopril may be preferable to other vasodilators for the patient with renal failure because it inhibits the formation of angiotensin II thus reducing aldosterone levels and therefore sodium retention. Its effects are increased by sodium restriction.[3] See page 11-28 for a discussion of vasodilator therapy.

Monitor arterial pressure at two-week intervals and adjust the therapy as needed.

Sodium supplementation is contraindicated for dogs and cats with renal failure. In the past sodium supplementation has been recommended based on the assumptions that: 1) the resulting increase in diuresis from supplementation increases urinary excretion of nitrogenous wastes, thus helping to correct uremia, and 2) sodium-wasting nephropathy was present. The first assumption has been disproven in dogs[21] and the second assumption has never been verified in either dogs or cats with chronic renal failure.[139] In contrast, salt supplementation may induce a number of harmful effects. These include increased hypertension, which may result in edema and, in conjunction with a uremia-induced decrease in blood coagulation, may result in hemorrhage from body openings and into the retina. High salt intake also worsens the signs and progression of renal failure and congestive heart failure, and exacerbates hypernatremia, metabolic acidosis, and osteodystrophy as bone buffer reserves are excreted to maintain acid base balance.[40]

OSTEODYSTROPHY

Osteodystrophy occurring with renal failure may be referred to as "renal secondary hyperparathyroidism," which indicates one of the major causes of the bone demineralization that occurs; or it may be called "renal rickets" or "rubber jaw," because the mandible is the skeletal structure most noticeably affected clinically. Although there is generalized bone demineralization, alveolar bone and the lamina dura dentes are often affected first and are most noticeable. The cancellous bone of the maxilla and mandible are especially affected, resulting in loose teeth. In severe cases, the bone may become flexible. The long bones of the abaxial skeleton are less affected. Although bone demineralization shows up radiographically as decreased bone density, this cannot be detected until quite late in the disease process. From 30-60% of the mineral content of the bone must be lost before demineralization can be detected radiographically.[106]

Renal osteodystrophy is caused by a decrease in the kidney's ability to:

1. Degrade parathyroid hormone (PTH)

2. Excrete phosphorus

3. Convert vitamin D to the active form

As shown in Figure 4, this not only results in osteodystrophy; but is also one of the major factors responsible for a progression or worsening of renal dysfunction. With a progressive decrease in renal function, there is an increase in PTH followed by an increase in phosphorus, and later by either an increase or decrease in plasma calcium concentration.[158] Plasma PTH concentration is increased with only a 50% loss in glomerular filtration rate; it increases progressively as renal function decreases.[182] In one study, plasma PTH concentration was elevated from a normal of 2 to 11 μEq/ml in dogs in which 75% of the renal mass was removed surgically. This elevation occurred even though the plasma creatinine concentration was less than 2 mg/dl.[16] When the plasma creatinine was greater than 4 mg/dl, plasma PTH concentration was 24 μEq/ml. A similar increase in plasma PTH concentration in clinical cases has also been reported.[210] The plasma phosphorus concentration usually remains normal until the plasma creatinine concentration exceeds 4-5 mg/dl.[38] The plasma calcium concentration usually remains normal until the plasma creatinine concentration is greater than 5 and often greater than 8 mg/dl.

The kidney is the main site of PTH degradation. Therefore, as renal function decreases, PTH plasma concentration increases (Figure 4). It is further increased if the plasma phosphorus concentration is increased or the plasma ionized calcium concentration is decreased, since these changes stimulate an increase in PTH secretion. The increase in the plasma PTH concentration causes bone demineralization or osteodystrophy.

Because the urine is the main route for excretion

FIGURE 4

VICIOUS CYCLES THAT RESULT IN OSTEODYSTROPHY AND THE PROGRESSION OF RENAL FAILURE

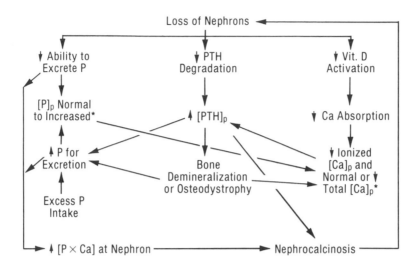

*Although plasma P and Ca concentrations are normal initially, as renal function decreases the ability to excrete P decreases and as a result the $[P]_p$ increases. An increase in $[P]_p$ and decrease in intestinal Ca absorption may decrease the ionized $[Ca]_p$ which stimulates increased PTH secretion, thus further increasing $[PTH]_p$, bone demineralization and nephrocalcinosis.

of phosphorus and alkaline phosphatase, continued reduction in renal function leads to increased plasma phosphorus concentration and alkaline phosphatase activity (Figure 4). In assessing both plasma phosphorus concentration and alkaline phosphatase activity in the young, it is important to realize that these values are normally much higher during growth. Normal plasma phosphorus concentration is 8 ± 2 mg/dl during peak growth (from birth to 6-12 months of age, depending on breed) and 4.0 ± 1 mg/dl in adults.[38] It also is slightly higher after a meal.

The plasma calcium concentration is generally normal until the advanced stages of renal failure; at which time it may be increased, decreased or remain normal.[158] Plasma calcium concentration is decreased due to decreased intestinal calcium absorption, increased plasma phosphorus concentration and increased calcium excretion. A decrease in calcium absorption occurred in 3 of 6 dogs with chronic renal failure in one study.[198] It occurs due to a lack of the active form of vitamin D (1,25 dihydroxycholecaliciferol), which is necessary for intestinal calcium absorption. The active form of vitamin D is produced in the kidney. Its production is decreased in renal insufficiency. Intestinal vitamin D absorption is also decreased, at least in azotemic rats.[198] An increase in the plasma phos-

phorus concentration decreases the plasma ionized calcium concentration by combining with it to form calcium phosphate. Although this has no effect on the total plasma calcium concentration, which is the amount routinely measured in the laboratory, it does decrease ionized calcium concentration, which is the biologically active form. Increased calcium excretion may occur due to impaired renal tubular reabsorption of calcium. All of these factors tend to decrease the plasma ionized calcium concentration.

In advanced renal insufficiency, the plasma calcium concentration may be increased. This increase is thought to be due to an excessive plasma PTH concentration due to decreased renal degradation and parathyroid gland hypertrophy. As a result of the hypertrophy, PTH secretion by the parathyroid gland is no longer inhibited by an elevated plasma calcium concentration.[190]

In one study in cats that had an average plasma creatinine concentration of 7.4 ± 3.6 mg/dl, their mean plasma phosphorus and calcium concentrations were both 9.5 mg/dl.[135] There was a direct correlation between plasma creatinine and phosphorus concentrations. Alkaline phosphatase was increased in over one-half of these cats and there was increased calcium and phosphorus deposition in their kidneys.

As plasma calcium and phosphorus concentrations exceed their solubility product, mineral deposition occurs—even in healthy tissue (Figure 4). Mineral deposition also occurs in damaged tissues at normal plasma calcium and phosphorus concentrations. With renal insufficiency, calcium and phosphorus are deposited in the damaged renal tissue, causing nephrocalcinosis and a further reduction in renal function. It is important to realize that this occurs **before** there is a change in the plasma calcium or phosphorus concentration.

Nephrocalcinosis is an early morphologic abnormality in dogs and cats with renal insufficiency. It often exists in the absence of clinical or biochemical evidence of renal insufficiency. It occurs to an even greater extent if either the plasma calcium or phosphorus concentration is increased, and may then result in calcification of previously healthy soft tissues. Calcification of soft tissue occurs, particularly in periarticular and vascular tissues. Visceral and vascular calcification are early consistent lesions in the uremic animal.[38,135] In severe cases with an elevated plasma calcium times phosphorus concentration, large tumorous calcified masses may develop around tendon sheaths and in foot pads. As these masses develop, they cause pain, dysfunction, and disfigurement.[38] Areas of predilection include the gastric mucosa, lungs, bronchial walls, myocardium, endocardium, intercostal muscles, posterior capsule of the eye, and the renal tubules, and glomeruli.

Treatment: To prevent a progressive decrease in renal function and osteodystrophy, dietary phosphorus should be restricted. Restricting dietary phosphorus is beneficial in reducing osteodystrophy and nephrocalcinosis, even in mild renal insufficiency with no increase in the plasma phosphorus concentration.[118] It is important that the plasma concentrations of calcium times phosphorus be maintained at less than their solubility product. Their solubility product for damaged tissue appears to be approximately 55 (when both are expressed in mg/dl).[119] Although it may be approximately 70 for healthy tissue, it is recommended that to prevent nephrocalcinosis it be maintained below 55 in mature animals with renal damage. Everything possible should be done to maintain the plasma phosphorus concentration in adult animals at 5.0 mg/dl or less, the plasma calcium concentration at 10 mg/dl or more, and the product of the two at 55 or less. However, regardless of what the plasma calcium concentration is, no attempt should be made to increase it unless the plasma concentration of calcium times phosphorus is less than 55. Generally these goals can be accomplished by

reducing phosphorus intake. **Calcium supplementation is rarely necessary.**

If renal insufficiency is mild, these goals may be accomplished by feeding the dog a mildly restricted phosphorus diet such as Prescription Diets Canine c/d or g/d (Hill's) that provides about 1 mg of phosphorus per kilocalorie. If renal insufficiency is more severe, treatment may require feeding diets such as Prescription Diets k/d and u/d that provide 0.5 mg or less of phosphorus per kilocalorie (Table 13, page 8-44). Although phosphate binders are ineffective when phosphorus intake is not restricted,[9,64] if a severely restricted phosphorus diet is fed and the plasma phosphorus concentration in the adult still exceeds 5.0 mg/dl, phosphate binders may be given. The most effective phosphate binders available are the antacids aluminum carbonate and aluminum hydroxide (Table 1, p. 8-4).

The aluminum in these antacids binds phosphorus decreasing its absorption, at least initially. However, people adapt to these phosphate binders and phosphorus absorption returns to normal within 12 days after beginning their administration.[82] In addition, even without adaptation, doses about 10 times greater than are usually given are needed for the binders to be effective if a low-phosphorus diet is not being consumed. Maximal phosphate-binding capacity of these aluminum salts is 130 mg of phosphorus/g of dry product.[184] Thus, 1.3 g of phosphate binder/kg body wt/day would be needed to reduce phosphorus absorption as much as does the dietary restriction described above (i.e. when dietary phosphorus is reduced from the amount in commercial pet foods, 1.3%, to that in the restricted-phosphorus diets, 0.3%). In actual practice the effect of aluminum salts on phosphorus absorption is probably considerably less than this, since only a portion of dietary phosphorus exists as, or is absorbed as, inorganic phosphate. The absorption of phosphorus in phosphopeptides, nucleic acids, phospholipids, and other organic phosphates may not be susceptible to inhibition by phosphate binders.[200] As stated by Walser, "the use of phosphate binders with no attempt to restrict dietary phosphorus is analogous to the use of diuretics with no attempt to reduce dietary salt. Both practices are indefensible."[200]

It has been demonstrated in both clinical studies in cats and controlled research studies in dogs that phosphate binders given at the dosage commonly used are ineffective when unrestricted phosphorus diets are fed.[9,64] In hyperphosphatemic dogs with renal failure (plasma creatinine of 3.1 mg/dl) fed regular commercial dog foods and a phosphate binder (1.5-2.5 g/day/dog of Basaljel, Wyeth), the

plasma phosphorus concentration did not change or it increased, and the plasma creatinine concentration increased 13-19% during the 90-day study.[64] In contrast, during the same period the plasma phosphorus concentration fell from 6.0 to 4.1 and creatinine from 3.5-3.4 mg/dl in dogs fed a phosphorus-restricted diet (Prescription Diet k/d, Hill's) without any phosphate binder.

Not only are the aluminum-salt phosphate binders ineffective without dietary phosphorus restriction; they are unpalatable, they reduce intestinal calcium[185] and zinc[143] absorption, and a small amount of aluminum is absorbed.[6] Administration of aluminum salts reduced food intake and caused other signs of a zinc deficiency in uremic rats, whereas these effects did not occur in rats fed the same diet without aluminum salts.[143] Aluminum absorption is enhanced by the elevated PTH associated with renal failure and renal excretion of aluminum is reduced.[120] The retained aluminum causes anemia,[132] impairs bone formation or mineralization causing osteomalacia,[142] and a severe progressive fatal encephalopathy.[2] As one of these investigators stated, "Alternative methods of phosphate control should be sought."[6] Antacids containing magnesium are less effective than aluminum salts as phosphate binders, and magnesium is more readily absorbed. Administration of magnesium-containing antacids to patients with renal failure may induce dangerous hypermagnesemia because of defective renal magnesium excretion.[163]

Results of studies in dogs,[174] cats,[171] rats,[91] and people[60] with renal insufficiency have shown that reduction of dietary phosphorus delays or prevents hyperphosphatemia, hyperparathyroidism, osteodystrophy, renal mineralization, and the progression of renal failure. In 4 dogs in which glomerular filtration rate (GFR) was reduced from 66 to 18 ml/min by nephrectomy and in which phosphorus intake was restricted, PTH was only slightly greater after 2 years and no bone abnormalities were present. In contrast, in 4 dogs with a similar decrease in GFR and in which phosphorus intake was not restricted, plasma PTH concentration progressively increased more than 15 times and extensive bone lesions were present after 2 years.[174]

Surgically removing most of the renal mass in one group of rats fed a normal phosphorus diet resulted in an increase in the plasma phosphorus concentration.[91] These rats progressed to death. At necropsy, the remaining renal mass showed degeneration and contained 20 times more calcium than similar rats fed a low-phosphorus diet. On the low-phosphorus diet, the plasma phosphorus concentration remained normal. In addition, there was no decrease

in renal function, and the remaining renal mass was normal at necropsy.

When a normal phosphorus diet was fed to cats in which two-thirds of their renal mass was surgically removed, their plasma phosphorus concentration progressively increased and GFR decreased.[171] After 12 months, the remaining renal mass showed degeneration and mineralization. In contrast, in similar cats fed a restricted phosphorus diet, the remaining renal mass was normal, and neither GFR nor plasma phosphorus concentration changed. When protein and phosphorus intake were restricted and calcium supplementation given, there was no progression of renal disease in 2 years in 27 people with polyuric renal failure. Without this dietary alteration, 70% of a similar number with initially the same degree of renal dysfunction had died within one year, and 90% had died within 2 years, with death resulting from the progression of the renal disease.[199] In another study, osteomalacia was more severe and plasma PTH concentration was 2.5 times greater in people that did not receive a diet low in protein and phosphorus as compared to those that did.[199]

In addition to restricting dietary phosphorus, cimetidine (Table 1, p. 8-4) appears to be quite beneficial. Although the chief reason for using cimetidine is to decrease the secretion of gastric acid, it also dramatically reduces the concentration of plasma PTH, both in uremic people[92] and dogs.[93] In uremic dogs, it decreased PTH secretion, bone demineralization, and plasma phosphorus concentration, increased plasma concentrations of calcium and the active form of vitamin D, and increased total body calcium balance.[93]

If the plasma calcium concentration is less than 10 mg/dl **and** the calcium times phosphorus concentration is less than 55, vitamin D and calcium administration is indicated. However, neither should be given unless this is the case. If this supplementation is required, add calcium carbonate to the ration and give vitamin D (Table 1, p. 8-4).

Vitamin D administration to patients with renal disease is associated with marked beneficial effects including relief of bone pain, increased muscle strength, amelioration and healing of bone lesions of renal osteodystrophy, and increased plasma calcium concentration.[119] Unfortunately vitamin D also promotes intestinal absorption of phosphate, so that the net effect is often to increase plasma phosphorus concentration.[200] Vitamin D administration is potentially very dangerous when employed in the presence of hyperphosphatemia or in near-end stage renal failure patients. Under these conditions vitamin D administration may accelerate

TABLE 10

VITAMIN D PREPARATIONS[147]

Product	Dosage Form*	Commercial Name	Dosage** (kg body wt/day)	Time for Response After	
				giving	discontinuing
Vitamin D$_2$	Capsules (50,000 units)	Calciferol (K-U) Drisdol (Winthrop) Deltalin (Lilly)	Until response 4,000–6,000 units then 1,000–2,000	2 weeks	1 week
	Oral solution (8,000 units/ml)	Drisdol (Winthrop)			
	IM injectable (50,000 units/ml)	Calciferol (K-U) Vitadee (Gotham)			
Dihydro-tachy-sterol	Tablets (0.12–0.4 mg)	Dihydrotachy-sterol (P-R)	0.03 mg for 2 days, 0.02 mg next 2 days, then 0.01 mg	1 week	several days
	Capsules or Oral solution (0.125 mg/ml & /capsule	Hytakeral (Winthrop)			
1,25 dihydroxy Vitamin D$_3$	Capsules (0.25 & 0.5 mg)	Rocaltrol (Roche)	0.002 micrograms	1–4 days	1 day

*40,000 units has an activity of 1.0 mg.

**Dosage must be adjusted to each individual patient to maintain a plasma calcium concentration of 9 to 11 mg/dl. If it does not increase by at least 0.5 mg/dl within 4 weeks, double the dosage. Don't give vitamin D at all if the plasma calcium concentration exceeds 10 mg/dl or the plasma calcium times phosphorus concentration exceeds 55.

the progression of renal failure. This effect is usually associated with hypercalcemia but occasionally occurs even when hypercalcemia does not occur.[200]

The forms and dosages of available vitamin D preparations are given in Table 10. The active form of Vitamin D (1,25 dihydroxy vitamin D$_3$), which does not require renal metabolism, offers the advantage of a rapid onset of action and a short half life. If hypercalcemia results from overdosage, it can be rapidly corrected by discontinuing the drug for 24 to 48 hours. However, dihydrotachysterol and 1-alpha-hydroxy Vitamin D, which also do not require renal conversion to the active form, have been reported to be just as effective.[200] 24,25 Dihydroxy vitamin D may have beneficial effects on bone mineralization without the propensity to induce renal damage.[33] It decreases PTH concentration in uremic dogs and people, and has little tendency to cause hypercalcemia.[26,33,84] The requirement for and tolerance to vitamin D may decrease progressively during treatment of animals with renal failure. Therefore, after a period of therapy, the dose may need to be decreased.

FEEDING

The goal in feeding the animal with renal failure is to meet all nutritional needs while preventing the intake of nutrients in excess of the animal's ability to utilize or excrete them, therefore preventing their accumulation in the body. The major factors needed to accomplish this goal are:

1. Have water available at all times.
2. Ensure sufficient food intake to maintain optimum body weight and thus prevent body protein catabolism.
3. Feed a diet sufficiently restricted in high-quality protein to prevent uremia.
4. Feed a restricted-phosphorus diet.
5. Feed a restricted-sodium diet.

In some cases supplementation with, bicarbonate, potassium, calcium, and vitamins B, C, or D may be beneficial.

Ingestion of phosphorus in excess of the animal's ability to excrete it causes osteodystrophy and progression of the disease (Figures 1 and 4, pages 8-11 and 35). Sodium ingestion in excess of the animal's ability to excrete it causes hypertension, which contributes to the development of ascites or edema in those with protein-losing nephropathy. Ingestion of protein in excess of the animal's ability to excrete nitrogenous waste products results in uremia. Uremia in turn is responsible for most of the signs and effects of the disease. In addition,

excess intake of protein and phosphorus increases glomerular blood flow, filtration rate, and trans-capillary pressure, which leads to glomerular sclerosis and progression of the disease[22,90] (Figure 1, page 8-11).

Glomerular blood flow, filtration rate, and trans-capillary pressure also increase in nephrons that remain functional when there is damage from any cause to other nephrons[22,90] (Figure 1). For example, if renal function is decreased by 50%, the glomerular blood flow and filtration rate in the remaining nephrons must double in order to excrete the same amount of solutes. These increases result in damage to these nephrons leading to their ultimate destruction and renal failure. However, if when total renal function is decreased by 50% the amount of solutes the kidney must excrete is also decreased by 50% by reducing their intake, the amount of solutes each remaining functional nephron must excrete remains the same and there is no progressive decrease in renal function. Thus, as illustrated in this example, as the decrease in renal function worsens; an increase in the restriction of protein, sodium and phosphorus is necessary to prevent disease progression and to alleviate their accumulation and the resulting signs and effects.

The beneficial effects of sodium and phosphorus restriction were described in the treatment for hypertension (page 8-33) and osteodystrophy (page 8-36). Protein requirements and restriction in renal failure are described below.

PROTEIN

There is general agreement that to control clinical signs of uremia, reduced protein diets should be given to azotemic, hyperphosphatemic animals with moderate to severe renal failure. The value of initiating diet therapy for animals that do not require dietary protein restriction for amelioration of clinical signs of uremia has been controversial. One school of thought suggests that diet therapy should be withheld until clinical signs of uremia are apparent, because 1) protein restriction limits renal function, and 2) a therapeutic role for low-protein diets in early chronic renal failure has not yet been proven.[105] It is true that higher protein diets enhance glomerular filtration rate and renal blood flow,[21,179] but there is no evidence to suggest that this is beneficial. In contrast, as previously described (page 8-10) current information indicates that it is harmful. For this reason, and those described on page 8-12, dietary protein restriction is recommended for all patients with reduced renal function regardless of the severity of the dysfunction. The potential benefits of restricting dietary protein intake include:[151]

1. The quantity of proteinaceous waste products in the body are reduced

2. The progression of renal failure may be slowed or stopped

3. Hyperparathyroidism and osteodystrophy may be minimized as a result of reduced dietary phosphate. Dietary phosphorus increases with increasing protein in the diet.

A potential risk in reducing protein intake is induction of a protein deficiency. This risk is prevented by not restricting protein intake too severely and monitoring the patient. Protein deficiency is indicated by a decrease in the plasma albumin concentration and albumin/globulin ratio, and an increase in alkaline phosphatase activity.

The minimum amount of a dietary protein needed to meet the animal's requirement depends on the digestibility and quality of the protein. Proteins are many different amino acids bound together (Figure 1, page 1-3). The body needs all of the different amino acids. However, many amino acids can be produced in the body and, therefore, are not essential in the diet. These are called "non-essential" or "dispensable" amino acids. The other amino acids, however, cannot be produced in the body and, therefore, are essential in the diet. These are called "essential" or "indispensable" amino acids (EAA).

Proteins are needed in the diet to provide EAA. The amount of the most limiting EAA in a protein, with respect to the animal's EAA requirements, determines the amount of that protein needed. The lower the amount of the most limiting EAA in a protein, the more of that protein that must be ingested. For example, if a diet containing 10% protein when ingested in the amount required to meet the animal's caloric needs provides 0.5 to 1.5 times the amount of all of the EAA needed, 20% of that protein would be needed in that diet to provide the amount of the most limiting EAA required. When the diet contained 20% of that protein and enough was ingested to meet the animal's caloric needs, it would provide from 1 to 3 times the amount of all the EAA needed. Thus, it would just meet the animal's requirements for the most limiting EAA, but in doing so it would provide three times more of its most abundant EAA than the animal needs.

Amino acids (both essential and non-essential) in excess of body needs are deaminated and used for energy. This occurs with any protein regardless of its quality, or any amino acid ingested in excess of the body needs. This increases the quantity of metabolic waste products that must be excreted. If the kidney is unable to excrete this increased

amount of metabolic waste products, uremia and all its accompanying signs and effects result.

It has been shown that people[201] and dogs[133] with renal failure need more protein than do normal subjects. Healthy dogs need 1.25 g/kg body wt/day of a protein that is highly digestible (85% or greater) and contains EAA in the same quantity as in egg.[139] Egg protein is one of the highest quality dietary proteins available. In one study, however, dogs with the degree of renal dysfunction being studied were found to need 2.0 g/kg/day of a protein of this type.[133] If both the digestibility and quality of the protein fed were 75% of the protein used in this study, these dogs would need 3.5 g of that protein/kg/day (2.0 divided by both 75% digestibility and 75% protein quality).

The increased protein need by animals with renal failure may be due to increased urinary amino acid losses, increased body protein breakdown or altered metabolism of individual amino acids.[90] The amount of dietary protein needed varies with the degree of renal dysfunction and its effect on these factors, as well as the digestibility and quality of the protein ingested. Thus, the best procedure is to feed a diet known to contain more high-quality protein than needed but low enough to maintain the BUN at 60 mg/dl or less. The clinical signs and effects that occur as a result of uremia become clinically evident at a BUN exceeding 60-90 mg/dl.

Protein restriction sufficient to prevent uremia has been shown in many studies in rats,[91,103,166,188] people[12,70,72,74,104,173] and dogs,[55,148,149,155,160,165] to result in marked clinical improvement, increased survival, and preserved renal function. A dramatic illustration of this is a study in dogs in which renal mass was removed surgically, resulting in a plasma creatinine concentration of 2-4 mg/dl.[155,156] During the 40-week study, 6 of 6 dogs died that were fed a canned dog food containing 44.4% protein in its dry matter (Ken L Ration, Quaker Oats); as compared to no death losses in 6 dogs fed a diet containing 17% protein in its dry matter (Prescription Diet Canine k/d, Hill's) and 1 of 6 deaths in those fed a diet containing 8.2% protein in its dry matter (Prescription Diet u/d, Hill's, as formulated at that time). These results cannot be attributed entirely to the lower protein content of the diets since the lower protein diets also contained only 9-25% as much calcium, 6-18% as much phosphorus, and 20% as much sodium as the regular dog food.

The benefit of a low-protein diet was well demonstrated in 149 people with various renal diseases. In these people the progression of renal failure was 3 to 5 times slower than in 139 people consuming a conventional diet.[168] In another study, the rate at which renal function was lost was 20 times faster in people when their protein intake was not restricted.[117] In another study, the average time until dialysis or transplantation was required was prolonged from 16 months to 7.6 years by restricting protein and phosphorus intake.[1] As stated "these results are impressive, especially since no adverse effects of the dietary regimen were noted."[123] The same appears to be true for dogs.[157]

The amount of dietary protein animals with decreased renal function can tolerate without increasing the BUN depends on the amount of renal dysfunction present. The best clinical indication of the amount of renal dysfunction is the plasma creatinine concentration (Cr_p). As renal function or GFR decreases, the Cr_p rises regardless of protein intake. If protein intake remains constant, the BUN also rises with decreasing renal function. However, the increase in the BUN can be prevented or corrected by reducing protein intake. The greater the impairment in renal function, the higher the Cr_p, and the lower the protein intake required to prevent a rise in the BUN. The relationship between the Cr_p and the protein needed in the diet to maintain a constant BUN is linear at a Cr_p above 3.5 mg/dl. The percent protein in the diet that will result in a BUN of 60 mg/dl when the Cr_p is 3.5 mg/dl or more can be determined as shown in equation 1 (adapted from reference 38).

Equation 1:
$$\% \text{ protein in diet dry matter} = 3 (BUN/Cr_p) - 26$$

The amount of dietary protein a dog with various degrees of renal dysfunction can consume while maintaining a BUN of 60 mg/dl, as determined from equation 1, is shown in Table 11. At the Cr_p shown in Table 11, a dietary protein above the amounts given will result in a BUN greater than 60 mg/dl, and below the amounts given, a BUN less than 60 mg/dl. Dietary protein intake should not exceed these amounts and preferably should be less. Since the elevation in the Cr_p associated with decreasing renal function is not linear at a Cr_p of less than 3.5 mg/dl, the amount of dietary protein that can be tolerated at a Cr_p less than 3.5 mg/dl cannot be determined. However, since excess protein intake causes a progressive decrease in renal function (Figure 1, page 8-11), it is recommended that a diet containing a high-quality, highly digestible protein content of 14-17% in its dry matter be fed to dogs with a Cr_p of greater than 1.5-2 mg/dl.

Feeding a diet containing 17% protein maintained body weight, plasma albumin concentration, and hematocrit in 6 dogs with Cr_p of 2-3 mg/dl. In contrast, these parameters became smaller by 10 to 30% in 40 weeks in 12 dogs with a similar Cr_p fed

TABLE 11

AMOUNT OF DIETARY PROTEIN THAT WILL RESULT IN A BUN OF 60 mg/dl IN THE DOG WITH RENAL FAILURE

Plasma Creatinine (mg/dl)	Protein* (% in dry matter)
3.5	25
4.0	19
4.5	14
5.0	10
5.5	7

*To prevent clinical signs dietary protein should be equal to or less than the amount given. For example, if the dog's plasma creatinine is 4.5 consumption of a diet containing more than 14% protein will result in a BUN above 60 mg/dl.

diets containing either 44 or 8% protein.[160] Dogs should be maintained on a diet providing 14-17% high-quality, highly digestible protein in its dry matter as long as the BUN remains less than 60 mg/dl. If the BUN increases above 60 mg/dl when this is the only diet being consumed, a diet lower in protein should be fed. If the Cr_p exceeds 5 to 5.5 mg/dl, it may be impossible to maintain a BUN of less than 60 mg/dl and still meet the dog's protein needs. To meet its needs, a dog with severe renal dysfunction needs 9-12% of a high-quality, highly digestible protein in the diet dry matter. A diet containing less of this type of protein appears to be adequate to meet the normal dog's protein requirements but not those of a dog with renal failure.[160]

By rearranging equation 1, it can be shown that:

$$BUN = [(\% \text{ protein in diet dry matter} + 26) \div 3] \times Cr_p$$

From this relationship it can be determined that for each increase of 1 mg/dl above 3.5 in the Cr_p, provided that protein intake remains constant, the BUN will increase by 10-20 mg/dl (approximately 10 on a diet containing 5% protein and 20 on one containing 34% protein). This calculation correlates well to clinical results. For example, in one study it was found that on a diet containing 5% protein, dogs with a Cr_p of 8-10 had a BUN of 80-100 mg/dl.[38] From this equation a BUN of 83-103 would be predicted.

USE OF ESSENTIAL AMINO ACIDS AND KETO ACIDS

Essential amino acids (EAA) and essential keto acids (EKA) have been used in nutritional management of renal failure in people. Severely uremic human patients appear to have an increased requirement for some EAA.[71] As a result, nitrogen balance can be achieved only by supplementing the diet to provide a higher proportion of EAA to total nitrogen than found in natural proteins. A diet containing only EAA has been studied in cats with experimentally induced renal failure.[49] In these azotemic cats the BUN and urine nitrogen excretion were less and nitrogen retention more when an EAA diet was fed than when an isonitrogenous protein diet containing both essential and nonessential amino acids was fed. These effects were thought to occur because of endogenous nitrogen use for non-EAA synthesis when the EAA diet was fed. However, a pure EAA diet is unnecessary and impractical for most clinical situations.

The rationale for using EKA is that these compounds reduce production of urea by diverting nitrogen toward protein syntheses, as shown below. The net result is that they permit the use of either body or dietary non-EAA for energy without production of urea.

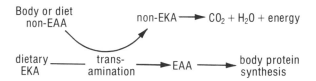

The major keto analogues of EAA used are valine, leucine, isoleucine, phenylalanine, and the hydroxy analogue of methionine. However, current data do not demonstrate any benefit of EKA that cannot be achieved with EAA.[73] In contrast, weight gain and nitrogen balance favor the use of EAA rather than EKA.[73] Thus, EKA appear to be of little benefit in managing renal failure in people. The use of these products in the nutritional management of renal failure in animals has not been reported; therefore, recommendations on their use cannot be given.

DIETARY ENERGY

An important requirement in managing animals with renal failure, in addition to restricting protein, phosphorus and sodium intakes, is to ensure adequate caloric intake. The amount of food required to meet an animal's caloric needs are shown in Table 12. These amounts are guidelines for short-term feeding only. The amount fed should be adjusted to obtain and maintain optimal body weight. Recovery cannot occur or will be greatly slowed without sufficient dietary energy.

If the dietary energy consumed is inadequate, body proteins are used for energy. This may worsen the uremia. Malnutrition and wasting commonly develop in renal disease and may contribute to many aspects of the uremic syndrome, including increased

TABLE 12

CALORIES AND FOOD NEEDED FOR CANINE AND FELINE MAINTENANCE*

Body Wt (lbs)	kcal ME /lb	Amount of Food	
		Cans**	Cups**
5	50	0.5	1
30	30	1.5	3
75	25	3	6

*Minimum amount. If animal is thin feed up to 50% more.
**15–16 oz cans providing 600 kcal and 8 oz volume cup providing 300 kcal.

susceptibility to infection, impaired wound healing, and reduced strength and vigor. If the animal is anorectic, as many uremic animals are, force- or tube-feeding may be needed until uremia is decreased to the extent that the animal will voluntarily eat an adequate quantity of food. Regardless of the method used, feed several times daily—ideally three or more. Small amounts of food at frequent intervals increase total food intake and decrease between-meal protein catabolism. For the severely uremic dog, Prescription Diet u/d and for the cat Feline k/d (Hill's) are recommended. If persistent vomiting unresponsive to treatment (described on page 8-27) occurs, intravenous feeding, and induction of diuresis or peritoneal dialysis are necessary (page 8-46). Procedures for intravenous, force- and tube-feeding are described in detail in Chapter 5. If intravenous feeding is necessary, electrolytes may be added to the feeding fluid as needed, depending on plasma values. Five mg of vitamin K and the vitamin B complex requirements should be given daily.

When glucose is given intravenously to the uremic patient, glucose intolerance may occur. It has been recommended that small doses (1 IU/2-3 kg) of crystalline insulin be included in intravenous feeding fluids for uremic patients. The blood glucose should be closely monitored daily and insulin given (0.5 IU/kg) if the blood glucose exceeds 350 mg/dl. Hyperglycemia can be monitored by measuring urine glucose values. If the test shows a 0 to +2 glucose level, no insulin is needed. If a +3 or greater reaction is shown, give insulin or slow down the rate of fluid administration. Fructose may be better used by uremic animals since fructose does not depend on insulin for entering the cell. In addition, hypertonic fructose solutions are reported to be less irritating to the vein than glucose and, as a result, cause less thrombophlebitis. It is best if fluids used for intravenous feeding of uremic animals, in addition to containing glucose or fructose, also contain essential amino acids rather than protein

hydrolysates. Early and vigorous intravenous feeding is tremendously beneficial and is often required for successful treatment of patients with acute renal failure. It should be used only until the animal can tolerate food orally.

MINERALS AND ELECTROLYTES

Sodium intake should be restricted in animals with renal failure, hypertension, ascites or edema. As much as 93% of all dogs with renal failure are hypertensive.[38] Ascites or edema may occur if glomerular damage is present. Thus, sodium intake should be restricted in dogs with renal failure by feeding a low-sodium diet and not supplementing with any source of sodium, such as sodium chloride (table salt) or sodium bicarbonate (baking soda). A sodium concentration of 0.2-0.3% in the ration dry matter is recommended.[38,134]

Bicarbonate supplementation, however, is needed if acidosis is present, but it should not be given unless the plasma bicarbonate concentration is less than 18 mEq/L. This may occur in some animals with advanced, severe renal failure. If it does occur, add sodium bicarbonate to the food (Table 1, p. 8-4) until the plasma bicarbonate concentration or urine pH increases. Although hypochloremia is often present in the acidotic renal failure dog, correcting the acidosis corrects the hypochloremia. **Chloride** administration is neither needed nor beneficial.

A total body **potassium** deficit, which often is not reflected by the plasma potassium concentration, may occur after long-term diuretic administration, or rehydration of the anuric animal. Potassium deficit causes weakness, depression and anorexia. It is worsened by acidosis which increases potassium movement out of the cells (see page 8-26). This is reversed and total body potassium balance improved by correcting the acidosis.[146] In addition to correcting acidosis, if hyperkalemia is not present, add 2-5g of potassium chloride to the ration daily:

1. If diuretics (other than triamterene or spironolactone, which are potassium-sparing) are given for more than a few days
2. For 5-10 days after recovery from anuria
3. If the plasma potassium concentration is less than 3.5 mEq/L.

A **zinc** deficiency also causes anorexia and may be present in animals with polyuric renal failure.[113] It is more likely to occur if aluminum salts are given to decrease phosphate absorption, as they also decrease zinc absorption.[143] Adding 1 mg/kg body weight of zinc to the diet may be helpful in correcting anorexia but is not recommended if the animal is not anorectic.

Both **magnesium** and **phosphorus** intake by the animal with renal failure should be restricted to the lowest level possible with natural foods. Hypermagnesemia and hyperphosphatemia may occur in animals with renal failure because of decreased renal excretion.[158] Retention of either magnesium or phosphorus enhances osteodystrophy and soft-tissue mineralization, including the kidneys, thus causing a progression of the disease. In addition, marked hypermagnesemia (6 to 10 mg/dl) may cause a loss of deep tendon reflexes, muscle weakness, and abnormal cardiac conduction. Phosphorus retention by the animal with renal failure is one of the major factors responsible for osteodystrophy and a progressive decrease in renal function (Figure 4, page 8-35). A low phosphorus diet should be fed to all animals at, and preferably before, the first sign of decreased renal function occurs.

Diets containing less than 1.5 mg phosphorus/kcal (Table 13, page 8-44) are recommended for:

1. Larger dogs more than 5 years of age
2. Smaller dogs more than 7 years of age
3. All dogs, regardless of age, with a decreased ability to concentrate the urine.[38,41]

If the signs of decreased renal function are clinically evident, diets containing not more than 0.5 mg of phosphorus/kcal are recommended. If the plasma phosphorus concentration in the adult remains above 5.0 mg/dl when these diets are fed, cimetidine and phosphate binders should be given (Table 1, p. 8-4), but are not recommended otherwise.

Neither **calcium** nor **vitamin D** supplementation are routinely necessary or beneficial and may be harmful to the animal with renal failure. If the plasma calcium concentration is greater than 10 mg/dl or if plasma calcium concentration times the plasma phosphorus concentration exceeds 55, supplementation with either calcium or vitamin D may cause soft-tissue calcification. However, if—but only if—**both** of these values are less than these levels, calcium and vitamin D supplementation is indicated (Table 1, p. 8-4).

VITAMINS

In addition to vitamin D, additional quantities of vitamins B and C may be beneficial and vitamin A harmful for the animal with renal failure. Any condition, such as polyuric renal failure, which results in increased water loss from the body, also results in increased loss of the water-soluble vitamins B and C. These losses may be a contributing cause of anorexia, and the replacement of these losses may be beneficial in correcting or preventing anorexia. The rations specifically formulated for dogs and cats with renal failure, given in Tables 13 and 14, contain additional amounts of these vitamins. Vitamin supplementation is not required if these diets are fed. If these diets are not used, a B-complex vitamin supplement and 50 to 100 mg of vitamin C daily may be beneficial.

Supplements containing vitamin A should be avoided.[200] With renal dysfunctions, renal excretion is decreased, and as a result there is an increase in retinal-binding protein, which increases plasma vitamin A concentration.[201] However, there is no increase in free or unbound vitamin A; therefore, it appears unlikely that elevated plasma vitamin A contributes to osteodystrophy in renal failure.[43]

RATIONS

Prescription Diets c/d, h/d, k/d, u/d and Feline h/d, c/d and k/d (Hill's) are the diets most useful in managing dogs and cats with renal disease. As shown in Tables 13 and 14, these diets contain, in the order given above, decreasing amounts of protein and phosphorus. Because an animal should eat or be given enough food to meet its caloric needs, the critical value to use in comparing rations of differing caloric densities is the mg/kcal they contain. It is this value that determines the amount of all nutrients in the diet that will be ingested.

Canine k/d is indicated for the older dog, and Feline k/d the older cat. The majority of dogs more than 5 years of age have interstitial nephritis[126,180] and, as a result, a decreased ability to tolerate excess dietary protein, sodium, and phosphorus. Hyperparathyroidism is present with a 50% reduction in renal function,[182] whereas clinical signs of renal failure do not appear until loss of 70-75% of renal function is present. Hyperparathyroidism causes progressive osteodystrophy and deterioration in renal function (see page 8-34).

More than 15% of older dogs have a BUN which is significantly increased,[41] and many have reduced cardiac function and hypertension. Sodium restriction is indicated for animals with any of these conditions.

H/d is severely restricted in sodium and is higher in protein than the protein- and phosphorus-restricted diets k/d and u/d. H/d is indicated in management of the non-azotemic animal with proteinuria (see Figure 3, page 8-31 for further management recommendations). The protein-restricted diets also contain a reduced sodium content, as is indicated in management of renal dysfunction.

Canine k/d is recommended for any dog, and Feline k/d for any cat, showing clinical or biochemical signs of impaired renal function. If the dog's BUN increases above 60 mg/dl when Canine

TABLE 13

DOG FOODS — PROTEIN, PHOSPHORUS AND SODIUM CONTENTS

Ration	Protein		Phosphorus		Sodium	
	dry wt (%)	mg dig./kcal*	dry wt (%)	mg/kcal*	dry wt (%)	mg/kcal*
Commercial:						
Canned Meat**	57	109	1.4	2.7	0.88	1.7
Dry**	27	74	1.3	3.6	0.55	1.5
Dietary:						
Canine c/d	22	43	0.48	1.0	0.27	0.6
Canine g/d	19	40	0.47	1.1	0.28	0.6
Canine h/d	17	34	0.49	1.1	0.07	0.2
Canine k/d	15	29	0.28	0.6	0.23	0.5
Canine u/d	10	18	0.13	0.3	0.26	0.5
Homemade: (see Appendix Table 3)						
Recipe 2	20	41	0.29	0.6	0.26	0.5
Recipe 3	10	20	0.22	0.5	0.32	0.6

*The most important value to consider since the amount of the diet needed depends on its caloric content. The amount of nutrients ingested therefore depends on the amount/kcal of metabolizable energy in the diet.

**Average of the three top selling brands.[125]

TABLE 14

CAT FOODS — PROTEIN, PHOSPHORUS AND SODIUM CONTENTS

Ration	Protein		Phosphorus		Sodium	
	dry wt (%)	mg dig./kcal*	dry wt (%)	mg/kcal*	dry wt (%)	mg/kcal*
Commercial:						
Canned	45	100	1.4	3.1	0.7	1.6
Dry	34	89	1.1	2.9	0.6	1.6
Dietary:						
Feline h/d	43	79	0.8	1.7	0.2	0.5
Feline c/d (dry)	35	61	0.7	1.4	0.5	0.9
Feline k/d	29	50	0.5	0.9	0.3	0.5
Homemade: (see Appendix Table 3)						
Recipe 9	24	52	0.5	1.0	0.2	0.4

*The most important value to consider since the amount of the diet needed depends on its caloric content. The amount of nutrients ingested therefore depends on the amount/kcal of metabolizable energy in the diet.

k/d is being fed, u/d should be fed.

A recent study demonstrated the benefit of Canine k/d and u/d in enhancing gain in body weight and survival in dogs with naturally occurring chronic renal failure.[8] However, hyperchloremic metabolic acidosis developed in the dogs with renal failure fed both of these diets as they were formulated at that time. Since this does not occur in dogs without renal failure fed these diets, it indicates that the diets were unable to buffer the metabolic acidosis that commonly occurs with renal failure (see page 8-26). This is because both of the diets used in the study were low in buffers. In addition, u/d at that time was high in chloride and, as a result, hypercholoremic acidosis was worse when it was fed. The diets used in this study were as formulated

in 1979, at which time u/d was high in sodium chloride (1.2% sodium and 1.8% chloride in its dry matter). The high dietary salt content was in concurrence with what was widely advocated at that time.[14,111] In 1981 the consensus of the Society of Veterinary Urologists was that based on current information moderate sodium restriction was indicated.[134] As a result, the sodium chloride content of u/d was reduced to its present level of 0.24% sodium and 0.37% chloride. This action along with an increase in the buffering capacity of k/d and u/d, will help prevent hyperchloremic metabolic acidosis induced by renal failure.

Another study published in 1984 indicated that the protein content of u/d, which at that time was 8.2% in its dry matter, was too low for the dog with

renal failure.[160] Studies we have conducted demonstrate that this amount of protein of the quality and digestibility in this diet is adequate for long-term maintenance of healthy adult dogs. However, after dogs with renal failure had been consuming this diet for 40 weeks, their plasma albumin concentrations were decreased from 3.0 to 2.0%, hematocrits decreased from 42 to 30%, and body weights and hind-limb circumferences both decreased 16%. All of these changes indicate a protein deficiency and demonstrate an increased protein requirement with renal failure, as also occurs in people.[201] Thus, animals with renal failure have an increased protein requirement but a decreased ability to tolerate excess protein because of a decreased ability to excrete metabolic wastes resulting from protein metabolism. As a result of this study, the protein content of u/d was increased by 27% (i.e. from 8.2 to 10.4%). A further increase may be untenable for preventing uremia in dogs with severe renal dysfunction.

It has been suggested that the protein-restricted diets are deficient in arginine, and that it is the most limiting amino acid in these diets. This suggestion, however, is based on a comparison with the arginine in two ordinary commercial diets, not with the animal's requirements. Canine k/d contains 228% and u/d 131% of the arginine needed by mature, healthy dogs. Much of the arginine needed by the animal is synthesized in the kidney. For this reason, it has been speculated that with a decrease in renal function, less arginine is produced and, therefore, more is needed in the diet. Studies in uremic rats demonstrate that this speculation is incorrect[207] There was no difference in growth rate, food intake, brain or muscle arginine concentrations, or health when an 18% protein diet, with and without arginine, was fed to uremic rats with 85-90% of their renal mass removed surgically.[207] In addition, plasma arginine concentration did not differ between uremic and normal rats fed either the arginine-supplemented or arginine-free diet. Renal arginine concentration was higher in uremic rats than normal rats with or without arginine in the diet. In addition, a diet deficient in arginine results in increased concentrations of plasma ammonia and urine orotic acid. These changes have not been demonstrated in dogs fed either of the protein-restricted diets designed for dietary management of renal failure.

Most people prefer to feed prepared diets. However, some pet owners want to make the pet's diet at home. Recipes for this purpose are given in Appendix Table 3. All of the ingredients are available in most grocery stores. Do not use a vitamin or mineral supplement that contains phosphorus, magnesium,

or vitamin A for animals with renal failure. The nutrient contents of these homemade and prepared diets are given in Tables 13 and 14.

REMOVING METABOLIC WASTES

If the animal is severely uremic (BUN greater than 150 mg/dl), for initial stabilization—in addition to ensuring intake of sufficient quantities of a severely restricted protein diet (Prescription Diet u/d for the dog and Feline k/d for the cat, Hill's or Recipes 3 or 9, Appendix Table 3) fed to decrease production of metabolic wastes—administration of luminal fluid acidifiers orally and rectally to increase intestinal excretion of urea may be helpful. Although there are no studies to demonstrate the benefit derived from this procedure, it is known that a substantial amount of urea diffuses passively into the intestinal lumen. The higher the BUN, the more this occurs. Bacteria degrade urea in the intestinal lumen to ammonia, which is reabsorbed and synthesized by the liver to urea. Oral and rectal administration of luminal-fluid acidifiers (as described on page 7-57) converts ammonia to the ammonium ion ($NH_3 + H^+ \rightarrow NH_4^+$) preventing its absorption. This effect may help lessen uremia. Although oral and rectal administration of antimicrobial drugs to retard bacterial degradaton of urea may help lower the BUN, administration of antibacterial agents may increase plasma creatinine concentration. Metabolism of creatinine by intestinal bacteria appears to be a major method for removing creatinine from the body. Decreasing this with antimicrobials may result in increased reabsorption of the creatinine excreted into the intestinal lumen. From 16-66% of creatinine in azotemic people is excreted via non-renal routes.[100]

If the animal is anuric, other procedures for removing metabolic wastes are needed to prevent progressive worsening of uremia and death. In veterinary medicine there are two clinically practical ways to do this: diuresis and peritoneal dialysis. Diuresis is usually preferred if renal function is sufficient for it to be used. However, before either of these procedures is carried out in animals with acute renal failure, the following steps should be taken in the order given:

1. Find out if the client wants **that** specific dog or cat, or just any dog or cat. This can greatly alter the therapy used.

2. If possible, determine if lesions will heal spontaneously. Therapy will not eliminate lesions but may allow them to heal sufficiently to prevent clinical signs. However, whether or not the lesions will heal spontaneously often cannot

be determined until the animal has been stabilized. This may require somewhat extensive procedures such as intravenous feeding and peritoneal dialysis.

3. Take blood and urine samples before treatment in order to assist in diagnosis and to establish a base for determining response to therapy.

4. Detect and eliminate the cause, if possible, to halt progression of the disease. Make sure the urinary tract is patent, and stop administration of any potentially nephrotoxic drugs.

5. Detect and correct extra-renal components that are discernible and reversible.

6. Support life by correcting deficits and excesses. Kidney function may return to normal if the animal is kept alive with proper care. This often requires tube feeding or intravenous feeding, and osmotic diuresis or peritoneal dialysis. In animals with anuric renal failure, 1-3 weeks or more may be necessary before renal function returns sufficiently so that diuresis or peritoneal dialysis is no longer necessary.

DIURESIS

If renal function can be established, metabolic wastes can be removed by osmotic diuresis or giving diuretics, or both. However, this should be done only after rehydration is completed (page 8-26). Osmotic diuresis may be instituted in the following manner:

1. Fully hydrate the animal, then weigh it.

2. Catheterize the bladder and check for glucose.

3. Give 5-20 ml of a 10-20% glucose solution/kg body wt intravenously over a period of 10-15 minutes. This will increase the plasma glucose concentration above the renal threshold.

4. Check the urine for glucose:

   a. If no glucose is present after 10-15 minutes, the kidney cannot excrete the glucose and therefore renal damage is extensive. Administer 4-6 mg/kg of furosemide (Lasix, Hoechst-Roussel) intravenously. Wait 15 minutes, and recheck the urine for glucose. If none is present, stop attempts to induce osmotic diuresis.

   b. If glucosuria occurs, give the fluid used for intravenous feeding or a 10-20% glucose solution by steady drip to attain a urine flow of 2 ml/min or more. The fluid usually must be given at a rate of 1-5 ml/min.

5. Give a maximum of 20-60 ml of the fluid/kg over 20-25 minutes, then stop.

6. Wait several hours and repeat if needed. During this period, it may be necessary to give an extracellular replacement fluid to prevent dehydration and excessive depletion of electrolytes.

7. Monitor the BUN, urine output, and body weight, and check for glucosuria. If weight increases, stop osmotic diuresis. If it decreases, give more extracellular replacement fluid.

Mannitol can be used as an alternative osmotic agent. Give an initial dose of 0.25-0.50 g/kg body wt (1.3 ml/kg of a 20-25% solution) intravenously over 3-5 minutes to initiate diuresis. Diuresis should occur within 20-30 minutes. The same parameters described above should be monitored, except that there is no practical way to measure the appearance of mannitol in the urine. To maintain diuresis, 2-5 ml/min of a 5-10% mannitol solution can be given. Mannitol may be diluted with a solution containing equal parts of isotonic saline solution (0.9%) and isotonic glucose solution (5%), or an extracellular replacement fluid such as Ringer's lactate or acetate. The total dose of mannitol should not exceed 2 g/kg/day. Mannitol may be superior to glucose in initiating diuresis in cases of renal failure where cellular swelling may be an important factor in maintaining oliguria. Glucose equilibrates with the intracellular and extracellular fluids; whereas, mannitol stays within the extracellular compartment and consequently may have a more dramatic effect on reversing cellular swelling.

Furosemide and ethacrynic acid (Edecrin, Merck Sharpe & Dohme) are natruretic diuretics that may promote diuresis when glucose and mannitol have failed to do so. These drugs may also be used initially in place of glucose or mannitol. Furosemide generally is used at a dose of 2-4 mg/kg intravenously. Diuresis is expected within 5-15 minutes and may last as long as two hours. Administration of furosemide may be repeated every eight hours to maintain diuresis. If diuresis does not occur within 30 minutes of the initial injection, double the dose of furosemide and give it intravenously. If necessary, the dose may be tripled. To prevent fluid and electrolyte deficits, administration of an extracellular replacement fluid is usually required during diuresis.

PERITONEAL DIALYSIS

Peritoneal dialysis is achieved by infusing a fluid into the peritoneal cavity, allowing it to equilibrate with the extracellular fluid, and then removing it; thus, the metabolic wastes that have diffused into the fluid are removed. If glucose- and diuretic-induced diuresis cannot be used or are not effective—as indicated by the absence of glucosuria, adequate urine volume (1-3 ml/min), or an increase in body weight—peritoneal dialysis should be in-

stituted. However, it should not be used after abdominal surgery, or if peritonitis or a ruptured diaphragm are present, or renal damage has progressed to a terminal stage.

Metabolic wastes should be removed by continuous peritoneal dialysis over the first 2-3 days of treatment and, subsequently, by intermittent dialysis as needed to maintain a BUN of less than 60-90 mg/dl. This may require dialysis once daily or two or three times a week. Procedures for peritoneal dialysis are described elsewhere.[102,145,191,192,194] Pleural dialysis has been suggested as an alternative to peritoneal dialysis, the advantage being that the catheter does not become obstructed by omentum, abdominal fat or intestines.[178]

CONCLUSIONS

Many infectious, toxic, immunologic, congenital, neoplastic and nutritional factors may cause renal damage, either directly or indirectly (Table 3, page 8-8). Regardless of the cause of the initial damage, without proper nutritional management this damage gradually progresses. Once renal function is less than needed to maintain homeostasis, clinical signs of renal failure appear (Table 8, page 8-24). With proper nutritional management, a progressive decrease in renal function can be prevented or slowed, thus, the affected animal's life is prolonged. In addition, the effects and, therefore, the clinical signs of the disease can be alleviated, and thus the patient's quality of life made more enjoyable during the added years. The proper nutritional management necessary to accomplish this differs in each case. However, in all cases the following four items are necessary:

1. **Calories** sufficient to maintain near optimal body weight

2. **Protein** intake restricted to meet requirements but maintain a BUN of less than 60 mg/dl
3. **Sodium** intake restricted and no sodium supplements given unless sodium bicarbonate is needed to correct a significant metabolic acidosis
4. **Phosphorus** intake severely restricted.

Thus a diet low in protein, sodium, and phosphorus should be fed. The greater the impairment of renal function, the more severe the dietary restriction necessary.

When the patient is unresponsive to dietary and medical management, and to osmotic diuresis or dialysis, a renal transplant may be a possible. Although done commonly in people, renal transplantation is not used clinically in veterinary medicine for two reasons: 1) a lack of studies demonstrating its feasibility and success, and 2) the expenses of surgical procedures, postoperative treatment (immunosuppresive drugs), and monitoring the patient. A recent experimental study of healthy dogs indicated that it may be a feasible procedure. In this study, 4 of 6 dogs were healthy one year after both of their kidneys had been replaced with one kidney from a sibling.[69] One dog died from septicemia and one from renal vein thrombosis. Neither had graft rejection. To prevent rejection of the graft, the donor and recipients were:

1. Siblings
2. Matched by mixed lymphocyte-culture reactions and erythrocyte antigen
3. Given pretransplantation blood transfusions from the donor
4. Given azathioprine and prednisone postoperatively

REFERENCES

1. Ahlmen J: Incidence of chronic renal insufficiency. A study of the incidence and pattern of renal insufficiency in adults during 1966-1971 in Gothenburg. Acta Med Scand (Suppl) 582 (1975).

2. Alfrey AC, LeGendre GR, Kaehny WD: The dialysis encephalopathy syndrome: Possible aluminum intoxication. New Engl J Med 294:184-188 (1976).

3. Allen TA: The treatment of hypertension. Proc Amer College Vet Int Med 1:3-105 to 2-107 (1986).

4. Allen TA, Jaenke RS: Pylonephritis in the dog. Comp Cont Educ 7:421-431 (1985).

5. Allen TA, Jaenke RS: Clincopathologic correlations in membranous nephropathy. Proc Amer College Vet Int Med 2:13-49 to 13-52 (1986).

6. Andreoli SP, Bergstein JM, Sherrard DJ: Aluminum intoxication from aluminum-containing phosphate binders in children with azotemia not undergoing dialysis. New Engl J Med 310:1079-1084 (1984).

7. Appel GB, Blum CB, Chien S, et al: The hyperlipidemia of the nephrotic syndrome: Relation to plasma albumin concentration, oncotic pressure, and viscosity. New Engl J Med 312:1544-1548 (1985).

8. Barsanti JA, Finco DR: Dietary management of chronic renal failure in dogs. J Amer Anim Hosp Assoc 21:371-376 (1985).

9. Barsanti JA, Gitter ML, Crowell WA: Long-term management of chronic renal failure in the cat. Feline Pract, 11:10-20 (1981).

10. Benjamin MM: Outline of Veterinary Clinical Pathology, 3rd Ed. publisher Iowa State Univ Press, Ames, IA (1978).

11. Benson MD: Pathogenesis of amyloidosis. Proc Kal Kan Symp 47-52 (1983).

12. Berlyne GM, Shaw AB, Nilwarangkur S: Dietary treatment of chronic renal failure: Experience with a modified Giovanetti diet. Nephron 2:129 (1965).

13. Border WA, Wilson CB, Dixon FJ: Failure of heparin to affect two types of experimental glomerulonephritis in rabbits. Kidney Int 8:140-148 (1975).

14. Bovee, KC: Medical management of polyuric primary renal failure. In Current Veterinary Therapy VI, Editor RW Kirk, Publisher WB Saunders, Philadelphia, PA, pp 1137-1141 (1977).

15. Bovee KC: The role of dietary protein in the pathogenesis and management of chronic renal failure in the dog. In Proc 7th Annual Kal Kan Symp for Treatment of Small Animal Diseases. Editor E van Marthens Publisher Kal Kan Foods Inc, Vernon CA 27-34 (1984).

16. Bovee KC: In Canine Nephrology. Editor Bovee KC, Harwal Publishing, Media, PA: pp 589 (1984).

17. Bovee KC: Renal dysplasia and renal Fanconi syndrome in the dog. Proc Amer College Vet Int Med 2:13-41 to 13-43 (1986).

18. Bovee KC, Joyce T: Clinical evaluation of glomerular function: 24-hour creatinine clearance in dogs. J Amer Vet Med Assoc 174:488-491 (1979).

19. Bovee KC, Joyce T, Blazer-Yost B, et al: Characterization of renal defects in dogs with a syndrome similar to Fanconi Syndrome in man. J Amer Vet Med Assoc 174:1094-1099 (1979).

20. Bovee KC, Kronfeld DS, Ramberg C, et al: Long-term measurement of renal function in partially nephrectomized dogs fed 56, 27 or 19% protein. Invest Urol 16:378-384 (1979).

21. Bovee KC, Kronfeld DS: Reduction of renal hemodynamics in uremic dogs fed reduced protein diets. J Amer Anim Hosp Assoc 17:277-285 (1981).

22. Brenner BM, Meyer TW, Hostetter TH: Dietary protein intake and the progressive nature of kidney disease: The role of hemodynamically mediated glomerular injury in the pathogenesis of progressive glomerular sclerosis in aging, renal ablation, and intrinsic renal disease. New Engl J Med 307:652-659 (1982).

23. Breitschwerdt EB, Ochoa R, Waltman C: Multiple endocrine abnormalities in Basenji dogs with renal tubular dysfunction. J Amer Vet Med Assoc 182:1343-1353 (1983).

24. Breitschwerdt EB, Root CR: Inappropriate secretion of antidiuretic hormone in a dog. J Amer Vet Med Assoc 175:181-186 (1979).

25. Brown SA, Barsanti JA, Crowell WA: Gentamicin-induced acute renal failure in the dog. J Amer Vet Med Assoc 186:686-690 (1985).

26. Canterbury JM, Gavellas G, Bourgoignie JJ, Reiss E.: Metabolic consequences of oral administration of 24,25-dihydroxycholecalciferol to uremic dogs. J Clin Invest 65:571-576 (1980).

27. Cartee RE, Selcer BA, Patton CS: Ultrasonographic diagnosis of renal disease in small animals. J Amer Vet Med Assoc 176:426-430 (1980).

28. Center SA, Wilkinson E, Smith CA, et al: 24-hour urine protein/creatinine ratio in dogs with protein-losing nephropathies. J Amer Vet Med Assoc 187:820-824 (1985).

29. Chew DJ: Acute renal failure. Proc Kal Kan Symp 9-17 (1983).

30. Chew DJ, DiBartola SP, Boyce JT, Gasper PW: Renal amyloidosis in related Abyssinian cats. J Amer Vet Med Assoc 181:139-142 (1982).

31. Chew DJ, DiBartola SP, Boyce JT, et al: Juvenile renal disease in Doberman Pinscher dogs. J Amer Vet Med Assoc 182:481-485 (1983).

32. Chi MS: Effects of sodium intake on blood pressure and urinary excretion of prostaglandins in reduced renal mass rats. Fed Proc 44:abstr 4430 (1985).

33. Christiansen C, Rodbro P, Naestoft J, Christiansen MS: A possible direct effect of 24,25-dihydroxycholecalciferol on the parathyroid gland in patients with chronic renal failure. Clin Endocrinol 15:237-242 (1981).

34. Coggins CH, Pinn V, Glassock RR, et al: A controlled study of short-term prednisone treatment in adults with membranous nephropathy. New Engl J Med 301:1301-1306 (1979).

35. Corbett WT, Kuller LH, Blaine EH, Damico FJ: Utilization of swine to study the risk factor of an elevated salt diet on blood pressure. Amer J Clin Nutr 32:2068-2075 (1979).

36. Cotter SM, Kanki PJ, Simon M: Renal disease in five tumor-bearing cats treated with adriamycin. J Amer Anim Hosp Assoc 21:405-409 (1985).

37. Cottrell BM, Franklin JR: Congenital nephrocalcinosis in a Lhasa Apso. VM/SAC, pp 1221-1223 (Aug 1983).

38. Cowgill LD: Renal insufficiency and diseases of the glomerulus. Proc Calif Vet Med Assoc 94th Annual Scientific Seminar. Oct 14-17 (1982).

39. Cowgill LD, Kallet AJ: Recognition and management of hypertension in the dog. In Current Veterinary Therapy VIII, Editor RW Kirk, Publisher WB Saunders Co, Philadelphia, PA, pp 1025-1028 (1983).

40. Cowgill LD, Low DG: Medical management of polyuric renal failure: Salt and sodium bicarbonate. In Current Veterinary Therapy VII, Editor RW Kirk, Publisher WB Saunders Co, Philadelphia, PA 1094-1096 (1980).

41. Cowgill LD, Spangler WL: Renal insufficiency in geriatric dogs. Vet Clin N Amer 11:727-747 (1981).

42. Crowell WA, Barsanti JA: Membranous glomerulopathy in two feline siblings. J Amer Vet Med Assoc 182:1244-1245 (1983).

43. Cundy T, Earnshaw M, Heynen G, Kanis JA: Vitamin A and hyperparathyroid bone disease in uremia. Amer J Clin Nutr 38:914-920 (1983).

44. Dairy Council Digest: Dietary factors and blood pressure. 52(No.5) National Dairy Council, 6300 N River Rd, Rosemont, IL (Sept-Oct 1981).

45. Davis LE: Pharmacologic control of vomiting. J Amer Vet Med Assoc 173:241-242 (1980).

46. Decaux G, Waterlot Y, Genitle F, Mockel J: Treatment of the syndrome of inappropriate secretion of antidiuretic hormone with furosemide. New Engl J Med 304:329-330 (1981).

47. DeFronzo RA, Andres R, Edgar P, Walker GW: Carbohydrate metabolism in uremia: A review. Medicine 52:469 (1973).

48. DeFronzo RA, Alvestrand A: Glucose intolerance to uremia: Site and mechanism. Amer J Clin Nutr 332:1438-1445 (1980).

49. Deguchi E, Morizono M: Clinical pathophysiology in cats with azotemia and effect of a diet containing only essential amino acids. Proc of World Small Anim Cong, Tokyo. pp 137 (1985).

50. DiBartola SP: Renal tubular acidosis in a dog. J Amer Vet Med Assoc 180:70-73 (1982).

51. DiBartola SP: The diagnosis and management of renal amyloidosis in the dog and cat. Proc Kal Kan Symp 87-93 (1983).

52. DiBartola SP, Chew DJ, Boyce JT: Juvenile renal disease in related Standard Poodles. J Amer Vet Med Assoc 183:693-696 (1983).

53. DiBartola SP, Spaulding GL, Chew DJ, Lewis RM: Urinary protein excretion and immunopathologic findings in dogs with glomerular disease. J Amer Vet Med Assoc 177:73-77 (1980).

54. Donadio JV, Anderson CF, Mitchell JC, et al: Membranoproliferative glomerulonephrites: A prospective clinical trial of platelet-inhibitor therapy. New Engl J Med 310:1421-1426 (1984).

55. Edney ATB: Observations on the effects of feeding a low protein diet to dogs with nephritis. J Small Anim Pract 11:281 (1970).

56. Epstein ME. Barsanti JA, Finio DR, Cowgill LM: Postprandial changes in plasma urea nitrogen and plasma creatinine concentrations in dogs fed commercial diets. J Amer Anim Hosp Assoc 20:779-782 (1984).

57. Far LE, Smadel JE: The effect of dietary protein on the course of nephrotoxic nephritis in rats. J Exp Med 70:615-627 (1939).

58. Feeney DA, Barber DL, Johnston GR, Osborne CA: The excretory urogram: Part I techniques, normal radiographic appearance, and misinterpretation. Comp Cont Ed 4:233-240 (1982).

59. Feeney DA, Thrall DE, Barber DL, et al: Normal canine excretory urogram: Effects of dose, time and individual dog variation. Amer J Vet Res 40:1596-1604 (1979).

60. Fiaschi E, Maschio G, et al: Low protein diets and bone disease in chronic renal failure. Kidney International 13:79-82 (1978).

61. Fiksen-Olsen MJ, Opgenorth TJ, Keiser J, Romero JC: Changes in responses to angiotensin I (AI), angiotensin II (AII) bradykinin and AI-AII conversion induced by sodium restriction. Fed Proc 43:Abstr 728, pg 409 (1984).

62. Finco DR: Simultaneous detremination of phenolsulfonphthalein excretion and endogenous creatine clearance in the normal dog. J Amer Vet Med Assoc 159:336-340 (1971).

63. Finco DR: Clinical evaluation of renal function. Proc Kal Kan Symp:95-99 (1983).

64. Finco DR: The role of phosphorus restriction in the management of chronic renal failure in the dog and cat. As reported at Kal Kan Symposium for Treatment of Small Animal Diseases, Columbus, Ohio (Sept.25, 1983).

65. Finco DR, Barsanti JA, Adams DD: Effect of an anabolic steroid on acute uremia in the dog. Amer J Vet Res 45:2285-2288 (1984).

66. Finco DR, Barsanti JA: Mechanism of urinary excretion of creatinine by the cat. Amer J Vet Res 43:2207-2209 (1982).

67. Finco DR, Coulter DB, Barsanti JA: Simple accurate method for clinical estimation of the glomerular filtration rate in the dog. Amer J Vet Res 42:1874-1877 (1981).

68. Finco DR, Duncan JR: Evaluation of blood urea nitrogen and serum creatinine concentrations as indicators of renal dysfunction: A study of 111 cases and a review of related literature. J Amer Vet Med Assoc 168:593-601 (1976).

69. Finco DR, Rawlings CA, Barsanti JA, Crowell WA: Kidney graft survival in transfused and nontransfused sibling Beagle Dogs. Amer J Vet Res 46:2327-2331 (1985).

70. Franklin SS, Gordon A, Kluman CR, et al: Use of a balanced low-protein diet in chronic renal failure. J Amer Med Assoc 202:141 (1967).

71. Furst P, Ahlberg M, Alvestrand A, Bergstrom J: Principles of essential amino acid therapy in uremia. Amer J Clin Nutr 13:1744-1755 (1978).

72. Giordano C: Use of exogenous and endogenous urea for protein synthesis in normal and uremic subjects. J Lab Clin Med 62:231 (1963).

73. Giordano C: Ketoacids advantages and pitfalls. Amer J Clin Nutr 33:1649-1653 (1980).

74. Giovannetti S, Maggiore Q: A low-nitrogen diet with proteins of high biological value for severe chronic uremia. Lancet 1: 1000 (1964).

75. Glick MR, Moorehead WR, Oii TO, Moore GR: Acetoacetate an "ketone" interference in kinetic and continuous-flow methods for creatinine. Clin Chem 26:7626 (1980).

76. Goldman R: Aging of the excretory system: kidney and bladder. In Handbook of the Biology of Aging, Editors EE Finch, L Hayflick, Publisher Van Nostrand, New York, NY, p 409 (1977).

77. Grauer GF: Clinicopathologic evaluation of early renal disease in dogs. Comp Cont Ed 7:32-39 (1985).

78. Grauer GF, Thomas CB, Eicker SW: Estimation of quantitative proteinuria in the dog, using the urine proetin-to-creatinine ratio from a random, voided sample. Amer J Vet Res 46:2116-2119 (1985).

79. Greco DS, Turnwall GH, Adams R, et al: Urinary gama-glutamyl transpeptidase activity in dogs with gentamicin-induced nephrotoxicity. Amer J Vet Res 46:2332-2335 (1985).

80. Green RA, Kabel AL: Hypercoagulable state in three dogs with nephrotic syndrome: Role of acquired antithrombin III deficiency. J Amer Vet Med Assoc 181:914-917 (1982).

81. Green RA, Russo EA, Greene RT, Kabel AL: Hypoalbuminemia-related platelet hypersensitivity in two dogs with nephrotic syndrome. J Amer Vet Med Assoc 186:485-488 (1985).

82. Greger JL, Baier MJ: Effect of dietary aluminum on mineral metabolism of adult males. Amer J Clin Nutr 38:411-419 (1983).

83. Gruys E, Syens RJ, Biewenga WJ: Dubious effects of dimethylsul-foxide (DMSO) therapy on amyloid deposits and amyloidosis. Vet Res Comm 5:21-32 (1981).

84. Gueris JL, Bordier PJ, Rassmussen H, et al: Control of secondary hyperparathyroidism by 1,25 DHCC and 24,25 DHCC in adult nutritional osteomalacia. 6th Parathyroid Conf, Vancouver, Abstr 127 (1977).

85. Hardy RM, Osborne CA: Water deprivation test in the dog: Maximal normal values. J Amer Vet Med Assoc 174:479-483 (1979).

86. Hartitzsch B, Kerr DNS, Morley G, et al: Androgens in the anemia of chronic renal failure. Nephron 18:13 (1977).

87. Hawe, RS, Loeb WF: Caudal vaginal agenesis and progressive renal disease in Shih Tzu. J Amer Anim Hosp Assoc 20:123-130 (1984).

88. Hayes KC: Nutrition in kidney function. In Nutritional Aids. Published by Quaker Oats Co, Fall (1980).

89. Holsworth S, Atkins RC, deKretser DM: The pituitary-testicular axis in men with chronic renal failure. N Engl J Med 296:1245 (1977).

90. Hostetter TH, Rennke HG, Brenner BM: Compensatory renal hemodynamic injury: A final common pathway of residual nephron destruction. Amer J Kidney Dis I:310-314 (1982).

91. Ibels LS, Alfrey AC, Haut L, et al: Preservation of function in experimental renal disease by dietary restriction of phosphate. New Engl J Med 298:122 (1978).

92. Jacob AL, Lanier D, Canterbury J, et al: Reduction by cimetidine of serum parathyroid hormone levels in uremic patients. New Engl J Med 302:671 (1980).

93. Jacob AL, Lambert PW, Canterbury JM, et al: Further studies with cimetidine in uremic dogs. Kidney Int 19:111 (1981).

94. Jamison RL: Dietary protein, glomerular hyperemia, and progressive renal disease. Ann Int Med 99:849-850 (1983).

95. Jansen BS, Lumsden JH: Sensitivity of routine tests for urine potein to hemoglobin. Can Vet J 26:221-223 (1985).

96. Jeraj KP, Osborne CA, Stevens JB: Evaluation of renal biopsies in 197 dogs and cats. J Amer Vet Med Assoc 18:367-369 (1982).

97. Jeraj KP, Vernier RL, Polzin DJ, et al: Idiopathic immune complex glomerulonephritis in dogs with multisystem involvement. Amer J Vet Res 45:1699-1705 (1984).

98. Jolliffe N, Smith HW: The excretion of urine in the dog II. The urea and creatinine clearance on craker-meal diet. Amer J Physiol 99: 101-107 (1931).

99. Jonas LD, Twedt DC: Serum gastrin concentrations in dogs with acute and chronic renal failure. Amer Coll Vet Int Med Scientific Proceedings. Salt Lake City, Utah July (1982).

100. Jones JD, Burnett PC, Creatinine metabolism in humans with decreased renal function: Creatinine deficit. Clin Chem 20:1204-1212 (1974).

101. Jubb KVF, Kennedy PC: Pathology of domestic animals. NY, Academic Press 2:296 (1970).

102. Kaufman GM: Peritoneal dialysis. Proc Amer College Vet Int Med 1:4-123 to 4-130 (1986).

103. Kleinknect C, Salusky I, Broyer M, et al: Effects of various protein diets on growth, renal function and survival of uremic rats. Kidney Int 15:534 (1979).

104. Kopple JD, Sorensen MK, Coburn JW, et al: Controlled comparison of 20-g and 40-g protein diets in the treatment of chronic uremia. Amer J Clin Nutr 21:553 (1968).

105. Kronfeld DS: Geriatric diets for dogs. Comp Cont Ed 51:136-142 (1983).

106. Krook L, Lowe JE: Nutritional secondary hyperparathyroidism in the horse. Pathol Vet 1:44-87 (1964).

107. Levinsky NG, Alexander EA, Venkatachalam MA: Acute renal failure. In The Kidney, 2nd ed, vol 1, Editor BM Brenner, FC Rector. Publisher WB Saunders, Philadelphia p 1181 (1981).

108. Lewis LD, Phillips RW: Diarrheic induced changes in intracellular and extracellular ion concentrations in neonatal calves. Ann Rech Veter 4:99-111 (1973).

109. Lim VS, Henniquez C, Sievertsen G, et al: Ovarian function in chronic renal failure: evidence suggesting hypothalamic anovulation. Ann Intern Med 93:21 (1980).

110. Lowenstein LM: The rat as a model for aging in the kidney. In Development of the Rodent as a Model System of Aging. Editors DC Gibson, RC Adelman, C Finch. Publisher US Dept of Health, Education and Welfare, Washington DC, p 233 (1978).

111. Low DG: Medical management of polyuric renal failure: Anabolic agents. In Current Veterinary Therapy VII, Editor R W Kirk, Publisher WB Saunders Co. Philadelphia, PA 1102 (1980).

112. Maddison JE, Pascoe PJ, Jansen BS: Clinical evaluation of sodium sulfanilate clearance for the diagnosis of renal disease in dogs. J Amer Vet Med Assoc 185:961-965 (1984).

113. Mahajan SK, Prasad AS, Lambujon J, et al: Zinc deficiency a reversible complication of uremia. Amer J Clin Nutr 36:1177-1183 (1982).

114. Maillet C, Garber AJ: Skeletal muscle amino acid metabolism in chronic uremia. Amer J Clin Nutr 33:1343-1353 (1980).

115. Mainka SA: Fanconi syndrome in a Basenji. Can Vet J 26:303-305 (1985).

116. Mannucci P, Remuzzi G, Pusineri F, et al: D-Amino-8-D-Arginine Vasopressin shortens the bleeding time in uremia. New Engl J Med 308: 8-12 (1983).

117. Maschio G, Oldrizzi L, Tessitore N, et al: Effects of dietary protein and phosphorus restriction on the progression of early renal failure. Kidney Int 22:371-376 (1982).

118. Maschio G, Tessitore N, D'Angelo A, et al: Early dietary phosphorus restriction and calcium supplementation in the prevention of renal osteodystrophy. Amer J Clin Nutr 33:1546 (1980).

119. Massry SG: Requirements of vitamin D metabolites in patients with renal disease. Amer J Clin Nutr 33:1530-1535 (1980).

120. Mayor GH, Burnatowska-Hledin MA: Impaired renal function and aluminum metabolism. Feder Proc 42:2979-2983 (1983).

121. Meneely GR, Ball COT: Experimental epidemiology of chronic sodium chloride toxicity and the protective effect of potassium chloride. Amer J Med 25:713 (1953).

122. Mitch WE, Lietman PS, Walser M: Abstr 65, Proc 85th Ann Meet Amer Soc Nephrol, Washington DC (1975).

123. Mitch WE, Steinman TI: Can the course of chronic renal failure be altered by diet? The Kidney 16:31-35 (1983).

124. Mitch WE, Walser M, Buffington GA, Lemann J Jr: A simple method for estimating progression of chronic renal failure. Lancet 2:1326-1328 (1976).

125. Morris ML Jr, Doering GG: Dietary management of chronic renal failure in dogs. Canine Practice 5(1): 46-52 (1978).

126. Muller-Peddinghaus R, Trautwein G: Spontaneous glomerulonephritis in dogs. II Correlation of glomerulonephritis with age, chronic interstitial nephritis and extrarenal lesions. Vet Pathol 14:121 (1977).

127. Mulnix JA, Rijnberk A, Hendriks HJ: Evaluation of a modified water-deprivation test for diagnosis of polyuric disorders in dogs. J Amer Vet Med Assoc 169:1327-1330 (1976).

128. Murray RH, Luft FC, Block R, Weyman AE: Blood pressure responses to extremes of sodium intake in normal man. Proc Soc Exptl Biol Med 159:432 (1973).

129. Newburgh LH: The production of Brights disease by feeding high protein diets. Arch Intern Med 24:359-377 (1919).

130. Norrdin RW, Miller CW, LoPresti CA, et al: Observations on calcium metabolism, ^{47}Ca absorption and duodenal calcium-binding activity in chronic renal failure: studies in Beagles with radiation-induced nephropathy. Amer J Vet Res 41:510-515 (1980).

131. O'Brien TD, Osborne CA, Yano BL, Barnes DM: Clinicopathologic manifestations of progressive renal disease in Lhasa Apso and Shih Tzu dogs. J Amer Vet Med Assoc 180:658-664 (1982).

132. O'Hare JA, Murnaghan DJ: Reversal of aluminum-induced hemodialysis anemia by a low-aluminum dialysate. N Engl J Med 306:654-656 (1982).

133. Osborne CA: Symp on Polyuric Renal Disease in the Dog presented at Annual Amer Vet Med Assoc Meeting Washington, DC July 22 (1980).

134. Osborne CA (Chairman): Recommendations for management of primary polyuric renal failure, based on Soc of Vet Urology Meeting St. Louis, Mo July 22 (1981).

135. Osborne CA, Abdullahi S, Polzin DJ, O'Brien TD: Manifestations of feline renal failure. Proc of and as reported at World Small Animal Cong, Tokyo, pp 55 (1985).

136. Osborne CA, Finco DR, Low DG: Renal Failure: Diagnosis, treatment and prognosis. In: Textbook of Veterinary Internal Medicine, WB Saunders Co, Philadelphia, PA pp 1493-1495 (1975).

137. Osborne CA, Johnson KH, Kurtz HJ, Hanlon GF: Ranal lymphomas in the dog and cat. J Amer Vet Med Assoc 158:2058-2070 (1971).

138. Osborne CA, Low DG, Finco DR: Canine and Feline Urology. Publisher WB Saunders Co. Philadelphia, PA (1972).

139. Osborne CA, Polzin DJ: Strategy in the diagnosis, prognosis, and management of renal disease, renal failure and uremia. Amer Anim Hosp Assoc Proc (1979).

140. Osborne CA, Polzin DJ: Azotemia: A review of what's old and what's new Part I. Definition of terms and concepts. Comp Cont Ed 5:497-508 (1983).

141. Osborne CA, Stevens JB, Perman V: Kidney biopsy. Vet Clin N Amer 4:351-365 (1974).

142. Ott SM, Maloney NA, Coburn JW, et al: The prevalence of bone aluminum deposition in renal osteodystrophy and its relation to the response to calcitrol therapy. N Engl J Med 307:709-713 (1982).

143. Owsiany CS, Reber EF, Ross DH: Symptoms of zinc deficiency associated with excess aluminum intake. Fed Proc 44:Abstr 64-2 (1985).

144. Palmore WP: Glucagon and alanine-induced increases of the canine renal glomerular filtration rate. J Exp Phys 319-327 (1983).

145. Parker HR: Current status of peritoneal dialysis. In Current Veterinary Therapy VII Small Animal Practice, Editor RW Kirk, Publisher WB Saunders Co Philadelphia, PA 1106-1111 (1980).

146. Papadoyannakis NJ, Stefanidis CJ, McGeown M: The effect of the correction of metabolic acidosis on nitrogen and potassium balance of patients with chronic renal failure. Amer J Clin Nutr 40:623-627 (1984).

147. Peterson ME: Treatment of canine and feline hypoparathyroidism. J Amer Vet Med Assoc 181:1434-1436 (1982).

148. Polzin DJ, Osborne CA: Management of chronic primary polyuric renal failure with modified protein diets: Concepts, questions and controversies. In Proc of the 19th Gaines Symp, White Plains, NY, Gaines Dog Research Center (1979).

149. Polzin DJ, Osborne CA: Conservative management of polyuric primary renal failure: Diet therapy. In Current Veterinary Therapy VII, Editor RW Kirk, Publisher WB Saunders Co Philadelphia, PA 1097-1101 (1980).

150. Polzin DJ, Osborne CA,: Improving survival of the patient with an acute uremic crisis. Proc Amer College Vet Int Med 1:4 51 to 4-53 (1986).

151. Polzin DJ, Osborne CA,: Conservative medical management of canine chronic renal failure concepts and controversies. Proc Amer College Vet Int Med 1:4-55 to 4-58 (1986).

152. Polzin DJ, Osborne CA,: Urinary tract obstruction. Proc Amer College Vet Int Med 1:4-59 to 4-62 (1986).

153. Polzin DJ, Leininger JR, Osborne CA,: Can self-perpetuation of renal dysfunction be delayed? Proc Amer College Vet Int Med 1:4-63 to 4-65 (1986).

154. Polzin DJ, Osborne CA,: Detection and management of canine renal tubular acidosis. Proc Amer College Vet Int Med 1:4-67 to 4-69 (1986).

155. Polzin DJ, Osborne CA, Hayden DW, Stevens JB: Influence of modified protein diets on morbidity, mortality, and renal function in dogs with experimental chronic renal failure. J Amer Vet Med Assoc 183:980-986 (1983).

156. Polzin DJ, Osborne CA, Hayden DW, Stevens JB: Influence of reduced protein diets on morbidity, mortality and renal function in dogs with induced chronic renal failure. Amer J Vet Res 45:506-517 (1983).

157. Polzin DJ, Osborne CA, Leininger JR: The influence of diet on progression of canine renal failure. Comp Cont Ed (scheduled for Dec 1986).

158. Polzin DJ, Osborne CA, Stevens JB, Hayden DW: Influence of modified protein diets on electrolyte, acid-base, and divalent ion balance in dogs with experimentally induced chronic renal failure. Amer J Vet Res 43:1978-1986 (1982).

159. Polzin DJ, Osborne CA, Stevens JB, Hayden DW: Serum amylase and lipase activities in dogs with chronic primary renal failure. Amer J Vet Res 44:404-410 (1983).

160. Polzin DJ, Osborne CA, Stevens JB, Hayden DW: Influence of modified protein diets on the nutritional status of dogs with induced chronic renal failure. Amer J Vet Res 44:1694-1702 (1983).

161. Ponticelli C, Zucchelli P, Imbasciati E, et al: Controlled trial of methylprednisolone and chlorambucil in idiopathic membranous nephropathy. N Engl J Med 310:946-950 (1984).

162. Raisbeck MF, Hewitt WR, McIntyre WB: Fatal nephrotoxicosis associated with furosemide and gentamicin therapy in a dog. J Amer Vet Med Assoc 183:892-893 (1983).

163. Randall RE, Cohen MD, Spray C, Rossmeissl EC: Hypermagnesemia in renal failure. Etiology and toxic manifestations. Ann Int Med 61:73-99 (1964).

164. Reidenberg MM: Kidney function and drug action. N Engl J Med 313:816-818 (1985).

165. Richards MA, Hoe CM: A long-term study of renal disease in the dog. Vet Rec 80:640 (1967).

166. Ritz E, Mehls O, Gilli G, et al: Protein restriction in the management of uremia. Amer J Clin Nutr 31:1703 (1978).

167. Riviere JE: Calculation of dosage regimens of antimicrobial drugs in animals with renal and hepatic dysfunction. J Amer Vet Med Assoc 185:1094-1097 (1984).

168. Rosman JB, Meyer S, Sluiter WJ, et al: Prospective randomised trial of early dietary protein restriction in chronic renal failure. Lancet, pp 1291-1296 (8 Dec 1984).

169. Ross LA: Hypertension. Proc Amer College Vet Int Med 1:3-99 to 3-103 (1986).

170. Ross LA, Finco DR: Relationship of selected clinical renal function tests to glomerular filtration rate and renal blood flow in cats. Amer J Vet Res 42:1704-1710 (1981).

171. Ross LA, Finco DR, Crowell WA: Effect of dietary phosphorus restriction on the kidneys of cats with reduced renal mass. Amer J Vet Res 43:1023-1026 (1982).

172. Russo EA, Lees GE, Hightower D: Evaluation of renal function in cats, using quantitative urinalysis. Amer J Vet Res 47:1308-1312 (1986).

173. Rutherford WE, Blondin J, Miller JP, et al: Chronic progressive renal disease: Rate of change of serum creatinine. Kidney Int 11:62-70 (1977).

174. Rutherford WE, Bordier P, Marie P, et al: Phosphate control and 25-hydroxycholecalciferol administration in preventing experimental renal osteodystrophy in the dog. J Clin Invest 60:332-341 (1977).

175. Schmidt RW, Bourgoignie JJ, Bricker NS: On the adaptation in sodium excretion in chronic uremia. J Clin Invest 53:1736-1741 (1974).

176. Senior DF: Drug therapy in renal failure. Vet Clin N Amer 9: 805-817 (1979).

177. Senior DF: Acute renal failure in the dog: A case report and literature review. J Amer Anim Hosp Assoc 19:837-845 (1983).

178. Shahar R, Holmberg DL: Pleural dialysis in the management of acute renal failure in two dogs. J Amer Vet Med Assoc 187:952-954 (1985).

179. Shannon JA, Jolliffe N, Smith HW: The excretion of urine in the dog, IV. The effect of maintenance diet, feeding, etc., upon the quantity of glomerular filtrate. Amer J Physiol 101:625-638 (1932).

180. Shirota K, Takahashi R, Fiyiuara K, et al: Canine interstital nephritis with special reference to glomerular lesions and filariasis. Jpn J Vet Sci 41:119 (1979).

181. Sigala JF, Biava CG, Hulter HN: Red blood cell casts in acute interstitial nephritis. Arch Intern Med 138:1419-1421 (1978).

182. Slatopolsky E, Caglar S, Pennell JP, et al: On the pathogenesis of hyperparathyroidism in chronic experimental renal insufficiency in the dog. J Clin Invest 50:492 (1971).

183. Slauson DO, Gribble DH: Thrombosis complicating renal amyloidosis in dogs. Vet Pathol 8:352-363 (1971).

184. Sparks RE, Mason NS, Rutherford WE, Slatopolsky E: Maximizing phosphate capacity of aluminum-based gels. Kidney Int 13 (Suppl 8):S160-S162 (1978).

185. Spencer H, Kramer L, Norris C, Osis D: Effect of small doses of aluminum-containing antacids on calcium and phosphorus metabolism. Amer J Clin Nutr 36:32-40 (1982).

186. Stevenson S: Oxytetracyline nephrotoxicosis in two dogs. J Amer Vet Med Assoc 176:530-531 (1980).

187. Steward-Bentley M, Gans D, Horton R: Regulation of gonadal function in uremia. Metabolism 23:1065 (1974).

188. Swendseid ME, Wang M, Vyhmeister I: Amino acid metabolism in chronically uremic rats. Clin Nephrol 3:240 (1975).

189. Taguma Y, Kitamoto Y, Futaki G, et al: Effect of captopril on heavy proteinuria in azotemic patients. N Engl J Med 313:1617-1620 (1985).

190. Thier SO: Renal insufficiency and hypercalcemia. Kidney Int 14:194-200 (1978).

191. Thornhill JA: Peritoneal dialysis in the dog and cat. An update. Comp of Cont Ed, 3:20-33 (1981).

192. Thornhill JA: Peritonitis associated with peritoneal dialysis: diagnosis and treatment. J Amer Vet Med Assoc 182:721-724 (1983).

193. Thornhill JA, Bottoms GD: Hypergastrinemia as a proposed mechanism for uremic gastritis in the dog with clinical improvement following cimetidine therapy. Amer Coll Vet Int Med Scientific Proc, Salt Lake City, UT July (1982).

194. Thornhill JA, Hartman J, Boon GD, et al: Support of an anephric dog for 54 days with ambulatory peritoneal dialysis and a newly designed peritoneal catheter. Amer J Vet Res 45:1156-1161 (1984).

195. Tobian L: Dietary salt (sodium) and hypertension. Amer J Clin Nutr 32:2659-2662 (1979).

196. Tobian L. Hanlon S, Wilke T, et al: Salt fading induces renal lesions and reduced GFR & RBF in borderline pre-hypertensive rats. Fed Proc 44 (no.3):Abstr 124 (1985).

197. Tramezzani JH, Morita E, Chiocchio SR: The carotid body as a neuroendocrine organ involved in control of erythropoiesis. Proc Nat Acad Sci 68:52 (1971).

198. Vaziri ND, Hollander D, Hung EK, et al: Impaired intestinal absorption of vitamin D3 in azotemic rats. Amer J Clin Nutr 37:403-406 (1983).

199. Walser M: Does dietary therapy have a role in the predialysis patient. Amer J Clin Nutr 33:1629-1637 (1980).

200. Walser M: Nutrition in renal failure. Ann Rev Nutr 3:125-154 (1983).

201. Walser M, Mitch W: Dietary management of renal failure. The Kidney 10:13 (1977).

202. Weller RE, Stann SE: Renal lymphosarcoma in the cat. J Amer Anim Hosp Assoc 19:363-367 (1983).

203. White JV, Olivier B, Reimann K, Johnson C: Use of protein-to creatinine ratio in a single urine specimen for quantitative estimation of canine proteinuria. J Amer Vet Med Assoc 185:882-885 (1984).

204. Wilcock BP, Patterson JM: Familial glomerulonephritis in Doberman Pinscher dogs. Can Vet J 20:244-249 (1979).

205. Wright RP, Wright HJ: Paradoxic glucosuria (canine Fanconi syndrome) in two Basenji dogs. Vet Med, pg 199-202 (Feb 1984).

206. Yu BP, Maida H, Murata I, Masoro EJ: Nutritional modulation of longevity and age-related disease. Fed Proc 43:858 (1984).

207. Wang M, Kopple JD, Swendseid ME: Effects of arginine-devoid diets in chronically uremic rats. J Nutr 107:495-501 (1977).

208. Watson ADJ, Church DB, Fairburn AJ: Postprandial changes in plasma urea and creatinine concentrations in dogs. Amer J Vet Res 42:1878-1880 (1981).

209. Weiser WG, Spangler WL, Gribble DH: Blood pressure measurement in the dog. J Amer Vet Med Assoc 171:364-368 (1971).

210. Weller RE, Cliver S: Renal secondary hyperparathyroidism. Mod Vet Pract pp 117-120 Feb (1981).

CHAPTER 9

Feline Urologic Syndrome (FUS)

CONTENTS

SUMMARY OF MANAGEMENT RECOMMENDATIONS

OBSTRUCTED CATS

1. **Stabilize the cat's condition.** If the bladder is severely distended, relieve it by cystocentesis. If the cat is visibly dehydrated, lethargic, or comatose, warm fluids to 37-40° C and give intravenously over three to six hours a mixture of equal parts isotonic saline and isotonic dextrose (0.45% saline and 2.5% dextrose) in the amount necessary to replace the estimated initial fluid deficit (% dehydration x kg body wt). Based on the severity of clinical signs, add to this fluid 2.5-10 mEq of bicarbonate/kg body wt (Table 10, page 9-20). After initial rehydration give either intravenously or subcutaneously 60-80 ml/kg/day of an extracellular replacement fluid, such as Ringer's lactate, with 10-20 mEq/L of potassium chloride added if the plasma potassium concentration is less than 3.5 mEq/L. Palatable water and food should always be available. Continue giving fluids until the cat is drinking and eating well.

2. Following, if necessary, relief of severe bladder distention by cystocentesis and stabilization of the cat's condition, **relieve obstruction** by flushing the urolith or plug out of the urethra (page 9-22). Be gentle and use the minimum anesthesia necessary. If a urethral catheter is passed, do it aseptically, lubricate the catheter well and use one that is as soft and short as possible (15 cm or less). Do not leave it in place unless necessary (page 9-23).

3. **Hospitalize** the cat for at least five to seven days as the obstruction often recurs during this period. When the cat is sent home, instruct the client to palpate the cat's bladder several times daily and observe for normal urination for the first several weeks after obstruction. Newspaper in the litter pan under the litter may permit better monitoring of urination.

ALL CASES

1. To all cats showing any clinical signs of FUS (Table 9, page 9-19) **feed the calculolytic diet** (Prescription Diet Feline s/d, Hill's) exclusively for two to three months. Urinary acidifiers are contraindicated when the calculolytic diet is being fed.

2. **If clinical signs persist** beyond 10-14 days, something besides the calculolytic diet is being consumed, or the signs are not due to struvite crystals or calculi—in which case a complete urinalysis, including culture and antimicrobial sensitivity, and radiographic evaluation of the urinary tract should be considered. Struvite crystals in the urine strongly suggest that something other than the calculolytic diet is being consumed. For success nothing should be consumed besides the calculolytic diet, water and, if a urinary tract infection is present, an antimicrobial drug. Continue feeding the calculolytic diet and treat any abnormalities noted. Identifiable calculi that enlarge or do not dissolve within three months should be removed surgically as 3-10% of uroliths occurring in cats are not struvite (Table 2, page 9-7).

3. **To prevent recurrence** feed **exclusively** a diet that contains 20 mg magnesium/100 kcal or less and that maintains a urine pH of 6.4 or less (Table 5 and 13, pages 9-10 and 27). Failure to follow this recommendation, such as giving vitamin-mineral supplements or cat foods that do not meet these criteria, is a common cause of recurrence. In the vast majority of cases, when this recommendation is followed, urethrostomy is unnecessary, as are feeding supplemental salt to increase urine volume and the administration of a urinary acidifier.

4. **If obstruction recurs** when these recommendations are followed, manage as described except to continue feeding the calculolytic diet on a permanent basis. Take a urine sample by cystocentesis and obtain a culture and antimicrobial sensitivity. If the culture is positive, give the appropriate antimicrobial agent for two to three weeks or, if calculi are present, until two to three weeks after the calculi are gone. Wait for five to seven days after the drug was last given and obtain another urine culture and sensitivity. If it is positive, reinstitute appropriate therapy.

5. **To prevent occurrence** in cats that have never shown any signs of FUS, a low-magnesium urine-acidifying diet may be fed, although it is unnecessary for most cats. From 90-99% of the cats fed other diets are not affected. However, a low-magnesium urine-acidifying diet is an inexpensive preventive measure (Table 13, page 9-27) that helps ensure that the disease does not occur.

6. **For prevention** or to prevent recurrence **in all cats,** encourage frequent urination by making palatable water and a clean litter box easily accessible. A litter box for each cat is beneficial and in some instances is a necessity. Encourage the cat to exercise and control food intake to prevent obesity.

INTRODUCTION

Feline urologic syndrome (FUS) is the clinical condition that occurs as a result of cystitis and/or urethritis. It is characterized by either or both the frequent voiding of often-times bloody urine or partial or complete obstruction of the urinary tract. The cystitis and urethritis are caused by mucosal irritation. This irritation may be caused by bacteria, viruses, calculi, or crystals in the urinary tract. Bacteria and viruses, however, are rarely involved as causative factors. Calculi or mucoid plugs may cause urethral obstruction. Mucoid urethral plugs may result from excessive mucus secretion induced by irritation of the mucosal lining of the urinary tract by crystals or calculi.

Different names and definitions have been applied to the clinical syndrome characterized by these clinical signs. Different causative factors have been hypothesized and it is popular to refer to the condition as a multifactorial disease syndrome. However, the vast majority of clinical cases respond to relief of obstruction, if present, and dietary management that dissolves and prevents formation of stuvite microcalculi or crystals in the urinary tract. Some of the names applied to this clinical syndrome are cystitis, urethritis, feline urologic syndrome, FUS, urolithiasis, urinary calculi, bladder stones and kidney stones. Currently the name most in vogue is "lower urinary tract disease of the cat" with the idea that this name is more explanatory or better implies a multitude of possible—no matter how uncommon—causes.

INCIDENCE

Cats are particularly susceptible to urinary calculi formation because they normally have prolonged intervals between urinations and a highly concentrated urine.[30,68,77] Although the ability to concentrate its urine is helpful for the cat to conserve water, it greatly increases the risk for the development of uroliths, microcalculi and crystals, and as a result, FUS. A summary of the incidence of FUS and factors affecting its occurrence and recurrence are given in Table 1.

FUS is one of the more troublesome problems affecting cats. Reports of incidence range from less than 1% to 13.5% of all cats.[47,83,104,110] In a recent survey the **yearly** occurrence of never previously affected cats in the U.S.A. was found to be 0.85%.[55] Unfortunately this was reported as the incidence. In contrast, the incidence in a population is the yearly occurrence of never previously affected individuals times the average life span in years of the individuals comprising that population. In this case, if the average life span of cats kept as pets is 10 years

TABLE 1

INCIDENCE OF FUS

Population:

< 1 to 13.5% of all cats[47,83,104,110]
0.85% of population affected for the first time **yearly**[55]
4-10% of cats admitted to veterinary hospitals[23,111,114]
Feline disease of major concern to cat owners[67]
Incidence may be increasing[2,47,100,114]

Sex:

Equal incidence in both sexes
  Obstruction most common in males
  Pollakiuria and hematuria without obstruction most
    common in females

Neutering, Obesity, Confinement & Cold Weather:

May increase incidence due to decreased physical activity

Age:

Most common at 1-6 years but may occur at any
  age[5,23,45,47,111]

Recurrence Without Proper Dietary Management or Surgery:

50-70% of all cases[6,29,83]
Higher, the younger the cat when first affected[6]
Not affected by severity, initial nonsurgical treatment, or
  water content of diet[6]

and the yearly occurrence of never previously affected cats is 0.85%, then 8.5% of cats kept as pets would be affected at least once during their life. FUS has been reported responsible for 4-10% of all cats admitted to veterinary hospitals.[23,111,113,114]

Regardless of the true incidence of FUS **it is the feline disease of greatest concern to cat owners.** Nearly twice as many cat owners indicated they felt that FUS was the main health problem affecting the cat as compared to the next highest health concern.[67] Another concern is that the incidence of FUS may be rising. Some observers refute this, but in a study of several thousand cases admitted to veterinary school clinics in the United States and Canada, it was found that the risk of a cat becoming affected during the period from 1964 to 1974 nearly doubled.[114] Results of many other studies have also shown an increasing incidence of FUS.[2,47,100] Better diagnosis and reporting of affected cats, increased confinement[83] and increased feeding of dry diets[30,47,56,59,83,112] (for reasons described on page 9-12) have all been suggested or incriminated as causes, it is likely that all of them contribute in varying degrees.

SEXUAL STATUS EFFECT

Although it is often stated that the incidence of FUS is higher in males than females,[111] and higher in neutered than intact cats of both sexes,[114] there are a number of reports to the contrary. The ratio of

intact to castrated cats in the entire population of normal cats has been shown to be the same as the ratio of intact to castrated cats with FUS.[29] In another study, when cats with cystic calculi were compared to the total number of cats presented to a veterinary clinic, the incidence was higher in females than in males; there was no difference in the incidence between intact and neutered cats.[5]

Because the male's urethra is longer and narrower it is more likely to become obstructed than is the female's urethra. Obstruction is uncommon in females. The most common manifestations of FUS in females are cystitis and urethritis without obsruction. Obstruction creates the most dramatic clinical signs, perhaps giving the false impression that FUS occurs primarily in the male. Thus, **FUS appears to occur with equal frequency in both sexes, but the clinical manifestations differ.**

A hypothosis is that **castration** before puberty increases the incidence of FUS by causing the persistence of a juvenile penis with a smaller urethral diameter. This theory has been disproved in cats.[41,45] In addition, no difference was found in the percent of castrated versus intact males that developed FUS, or between affected and nonaffected cats with respect to the age of castration.[83] Laboratory studies have also failed to demonstrate any direct effect of either castration or obesity on FUS.[21] However, several surveys of clinical cases have revealed an increased risk of FUS with increased weight,[30,114] and with castration.[111] This may be as a result of decreased physical activity, as both neutering (of either the male or female) and obesity decrease physical activity.

PHYSICAL ACTIVITY AFFECT

A lessening of physical activity may reduce the frequency of urination allowing more time for formation of crystals and uroliths. Decreased physical activity resulting from confinement has been shown to increase the incidence of FUS.[83] The disease occurs primarily in cats housed indoors, and is uncommon in those that are outdoors most of the time.[83] This difference could be due either to differences in physical activity or diet. Studies have shown that the incidence is highest during late winter and early spring after several months of reduced physical activity because of cold weather; lowest incidence occurred in late summer after several months of warm weather more conducive to physical activity.[111,114] Increased physical activity and warmer weather both increase water consumption and as a result urine volume. An increase in urine volume decreases the concentration of calculi forming constituents in the urine and increases the

frequency of urination, both of which would assist in preventing FUS.

AGE EFFECT

FUS is most common in young adults, although it may occur in very young (less than 2 months) or old cats (more than 13 years).[5,45] In most cases the first episode occurs in cats 1 to 3 years of age; more than 80% occurs in cats 1 to 6 years of age.[5,23,47,111] It is probable that the low incidence of FUS in cats less than 1 year of age is because during bone growth as calcium, and dibasic and monobasic hydrogen phosphate precipitate as calcium apatite, hydrogen ions are produced and excreted which lowers urine pH.[14] Lowering urine pH retards struvite crystallization and, as a result, FUS (as described on page 9-26).

BREED EFFECT

There appears to be a greater incidence of FUS in Persians and a lower incidence in Siamese, compared to all other breeds.[5,111,114] This difference most likely reflects a difference in the degree of confinement and physical activity of these two breeds rather than genetic factors.

RECURRENCE INCIDENCE

Without surgery or proper dietary management FUS recurs in 50-70% of the cases.[6,29,83] It recurs more than twice as often in cats first affected at less than 4 years of age, than cats that are older when first affected.[6] The interval between recurrences does not vary between additional episodes; it ranges from 2 to 52 months with a mean of 21 months.[5] However, recurrences can be prevented or greatly reduced in number with proper dietary management (as described on page 9-25). According to one report[6] the probability of recurrence **cannot** be predicted based on:

1. The severity of signs
2. The initial nonsurgical treatment
3. The form of food fed—dry or canned

In one study 75% of the cases that recurred were being fed a canned food exclusively,[83] whereas in another study the incidence of recurrence was three times greater in cats fed a dry food exclusively.[112]

CAUSES

The array of clinical signs referred to as FUS are caused by cystitis, urethritis and/or intraluminal or extraluminal urethral obstruction. Many factors, as given in Figure 1, may induce these effects and therefore cause FUS. These include infectious

FIGURE 1

CAUSES OF FUS

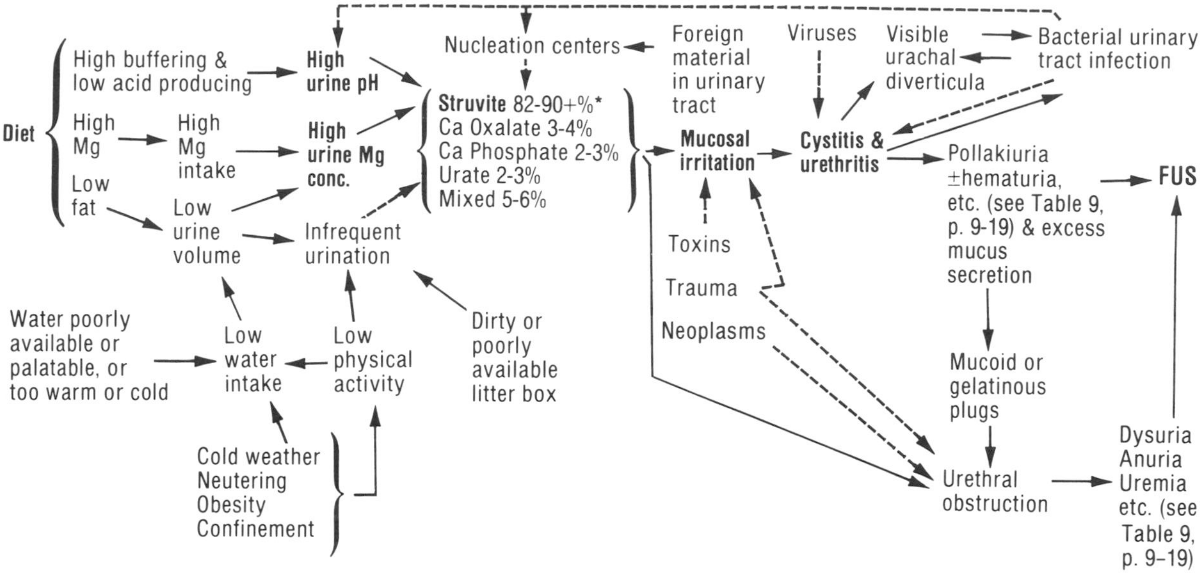

FIGURE 1: Items in bold print are responsible for causing the vast majority of cases of FUS. Solid arrows indicate factors that are necessary for that effect and/or are common causes of it. Dashed arrows indicate factors that contribute to that effect if they are present but are an unnecessary or uncommon cause of that effect.

*The percent of feline uroliths analyzed that are composed primarily or exclusively of that substance (see Table 2, page 9-7).

organisms, urachal anomalies, neoplasms, trauma, toxins, and mucosal irritation from urinary crystals or calculi. Neoplasia, trauma, and toxin induced causes are rare.

Bacteria, viruses, and other infectious organisms are not factors in most clinical cases. When a urinary tract infection does occur, it generally results from cystitis and urethritis and is not a cause.[5,56,57] A vesicourachal diverticulum has been thought to be a cause of FUS and, in some cases, to be a congenital disorder amenable only to surgical excision. This has recently been disproved.

The **vesicourachal diverticulum** is an embryonic remnant of the urachus histologically evident (but not radiographically or grossly visible) in 40-80% of all cats.[117] Theoretically it may become inflamed and enlarged, resulting in cystitis and FUS. In a recent study, radiographically visible vesicourachal diverticula were detected in 33 of 149 cats with FUS.[74] Females and males were affected, both those with and those without urethral obstruction. There was no correlation between the size or occurrence of the diverticulum and the presence or absence of urethral obstruction. Only one cat had a urinary tract infection; 42% of the diverticula extended beyond the serosal surface. The diver-

ticula resolved in 7 of 7 of these cats within 19 days after they were fed a calculolytic diet (Prescription Diet Feline s/d, Hill's). In 6 of these 7 cats the diverticulum had extended beyond the serosal surface. These results suggest that, **like urinary tract infection, enlargement of the vesicourachal diverticula occurs as a result, and not as a cause, of FUS.**

The one factor present in the great majority of cats with FUS are calculi, microcalculi, or crystals in the urinary tract. Treatment that allows these calculi to dissolve alleviates clinical signs of the disease. The calculi or crystals may obstruct the flow of urine or irritate the lining of the urinary tract. This irritation causes cystitis, urethritis, and/or excessive mucus secretion. The mucus may form a plug that obstructs the urethra. Thus, the formation of these plugs appears to be somewhat analogous to the formation of renal tubular casts,[70] i.e. they are produced in response to an irritation.

Formation of urinary calculi or crystals requires:

1. A sufficiently high concentration of calculi-forming constituents in the urine
2. A favorable pH for crystallization

3. Adequate time in the urinary tract

What these constituents are and what pH is favorable for them to form crystals and calculi depends on the type of calculi. However, regardless of what other factors may be involved, urinary calculi cannot form; therefore, the vast majority of cases of FUS would not occur without the presence of these three factors. Although not required, formation of crystals or calculi is enhanced by the presence of a nucleation center or nidus on which to form. Anything that enhances any of these factors predisposes to urolith or crystal formation and therefore FUS. Conversely, anything that suppresses these factors assists in preventing FUS. In addition, a decrease in crystallization inhibitors in the urine would also predispose to or cause FUS. However, currently there is no evidence that urine contains any struvite crystallization inhibitors,[89] which is the main type of calculi affecting cats.

NUCLEATION CENTER

Substances that may serve as a nucleation center or nidus, and thus enhance urolith formation, include sloughed epithelial cells, casts, bacteria, viruses, and cellular debris resulting from any inflammation or irritation of the urinary tract. Foreign items, such as nonabsorbable suture material and even grass seeds,[93] may also serve as a nucleation center. Stainless steel buttons and zinc beads inserted into the bladder have led to urolith formation and chronic cystitis, which resolve when the foreign material is removed.[66,107] However, a nucleation center alone is not sufficient to cause urolith formation and cystitis, as demonstrated in a cat with a lead pellet in the bladder,[1] and in 11 cats with sterile zinc implants inserted surgically.[44] Cystitis did not occur and no uroliths were present in any of these 12 cats after almost two years.

Viruses and Bacteria

Viruses have long been implicated in the etiology of FUS. Urinary obstruction has been induced in cats inoculated with a calicivirus or picornavirus.[86] A myxovirus was isolated from the urinary tract of the cats that became obstructed. It was theorized that the picornavirus might be a triggering agent that activates a latent myxovirus in the urinary tract. The activated myxovirus then produces cellular damage leading to calculi formation. A herpes virus that may play the same role as the myxovirus also was isolated. However, neither the initial investigators nor others have been able to reproduce these results, or induce urinary calculi formation with any virus, or combination of viruses.

Although a viral cystitis can be induced experimentally, the following factors suggest that **viruses are rarely a cause of naturally occurring FUS.**

1. Viruses are rarely found in clinical cases.
2. Viruses have never been isolated from experimentally induced cases of FUS although extensive efforts have been made to do so.
3. When a calculi inducing diet was fed, the incidence of obstruction in specific-pathogen-free (SPF) cats, free of all bacteria and all viruses associated with FUS, was similar to that occurring in non-SPF cats.[53]
4. There is no difference in the incidence of FUS between cats kept in single or multiple cat households, or those with or without previous respiratory disease.[83]
5. More than 90% of cases occur in cats kept primarily or exclusively indoors.[83]
6. FUS is uncommon in cats that are always outdoors where contact with infectious organisms is greater.[83]

All of these factors suggest that neither a viral nor bacterial urinary tract infection is needed for FUS to occur. However, bacteria or viruses, either by themselves or by causing urinary tract damage or inflammation and the resulting tissue debris, may predispose to FUS by increasing the material available to serve as a nucleation center for forming calculi. Urease-producing bacteria also predispose to formation of magnesium-ammonium-phosphate (struvite) calculi by increasing the urine pH and the amount of ammonium ion available for calculi formation (as described on page 10-7).

A urinary tract infection (UTI) is present in a large percentage of dogs with struvite uroliths, and is an important factor in their formation,[54] but this does not apply to most cats. A UTI is present in only 29-33% of cats with FUS.[5,56] However, **even when a UTI is present, it is generally secondary and not a factor in causing FUS.**[5,57] A UTI is rarely present at the onset of the first episode of FUS.[57] When a UTI is present, its causes as a percent of the total are:[5]

50% *Staphylococcus spp.*
18% *Escherichia coli*
11% *Streptococci spp.*
 7% *Proteus spp.*
 7% *Pseudomonas*
 7% other bacteria

These same bacteria are the major causes of UTI in dogs with urolithiasis.

Vitamin A Deficiency

Vitamin A is needed to maintain the integrity of epithelial and mucosal surfaces. A vitamin A deficiency increases squamous metaplasia and the sloughing of epithelial cells lining the urinary tract. This would increase cellular debris available to serve as a nucleation center for urolith formation. Although a vitamin A deficiency has been associated with struvite uroliths in rats,[42] it is extremely uncommon in cats and dogs; it is not considered a causative or predisposing factor for the clinical disease in either of these two species. In addition, vitamin A has never been shown to be beneficial in treating or preventing urolithiasis in cats or dogs.

URINE VOLUME AND FREQUENCY OF URINATION

The greater the urine concentration and the less frequently urination occurs, the greater the opportunity for urinary calculi formation. Increased urine concentration results in infrequent urination and allows more time for calculi to develop. Infrequent urination may occur because of a dirty, or not easily accessible litter box, or a low level of physical activity. Some cats will not share a litter box. In this situation separate litter boxes are needed to encourage urination. Confinement, castration, obesity, cold weather and most illnesses and locomotion problems reduce physical activity, and thus the

frequency of urination. Decreased frequency of urination and increased urine concentration also may result from a decrease in water intake. A decrease in water intake may occur because water is not readily available, is too cold or warm, or is of poor quality or palatability (see page 10-8 for effect of water mineral content). All these factors may predispose a cat to FUS.

DIET AS A CAUSATIVE FACTOR

Magnesium, Phosphorus and Calcium

Increased intake of urolith-forming constituents increases their excretion and concentration in the urine, thus enhancing the formation of uroliths.[58] The vast majority of uroliths, microcalculi, and crystals in cats are struvite, which is composed of magnesium, ammonium and phosphate (Table 2). At a constant pH and concentration of other solutes, formation of struvite crystals depends only on urine concentration of magnesium times ammonium times phosphate.

Because the cat requires high dietary protein and relatively high dietary phosphorus compared to its magnesium requirement, cat urine usually contains enough ammonium and phosphate for magnesium-ammonium-phosphate formation. Whether the urine contains sufficient magnesium, however, depends on the amount of magnesium consumed.

TABLE 2

CALCULI COMPOSITION IN CATS WITH FUS[72]*

% of All Calculi Analyzed**	Types of Calculi
81.9**	Struvite (magnesium-ammonium-phosphate-hexahydrate)
3.7	Calcium oxalate
2.6	Calcium phosphate (apatite)
2.6	Ammonium urate or uric acid
4.1	Mixed—did not contain at least 70% of any single type
1.5	Had a nucleus and one or more surrounding layers of different types
0.1	Cystine—only 1 case reported in cats
0.0	Calcium carbonate—have been reported in cats[45]
0.0	Silicate—not reported in cats
3.5	Gelatinous plugs of which
	5% are almost entirely organic matrix
	95% contain varying amounts of mineral of which
	76–85% are 100% struvite[70,72]
	13–14% are 70–90% struvite[70,72]
	1– 4% are primarily one of the other 4 most common calculi types

*Based on the analysis of 657 feline uroliths

**Following the introduction and widespread use of diets that dissolve struvite uroliths (first available 6/84) and prevent their formation, the percent of feline uroliths analyzed that are composed of struvite has decreased from 90–97% reported in 1971–1982[5,45,69] to 81.9% in 1986.[72] Thus, the percent of different types of calculi that actually occur in cats is quite likely more for struvite and less for non-struvite calculi than that obtained from cats for analysis as given here.

FIGURE 2

EFFECT OF MAGNESIUM CONSUMPTION ON URINE MAGNESIUM CONCENTRATION
(adapted from[27])

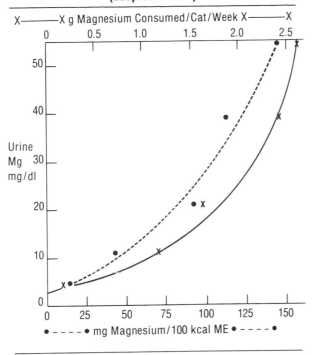

Results of several studies have shown that concentrations and excretion of urinary magnesium and phosphorus relate directly to the cat's magnesium and phosphorus intakes.[58,92,108] As shown in Figure 2, as the amount of magnesium/kcal in the diet increases, and therefore the amount of magnesium

TABLE 3

EFFECT OF DIETARY MAGNESIUM ON FUS[17,21,37,58,85,102]

Mg (% in Diet Dry Matter)	Number of Cats	Time	Affected (%)
0.75	72	8–12 mo	76*
0.37	43	11 mo	70*
0.12–0.29**	total population	lifetime	1–10
0.08	43	8–12 mo	0*

*The urine pH was greater than 6.7 in the majority of all cats in the experimental studies regardless of the amount of magnesium in the diet.

**Amount present in regular commercial cat foods (see Table 5, page 9-10).

consumed increases, there is an even greater increase in urine magnesium concentration.

Since the urine already contains sufficient ammonium and phosphate for struvite formation, if urine pH is also sufficiently high (more than about 6.6), an increase in urine magnesium concentration enhances struvite crystallization. As shown in Table 3, which summarizes many studies conducted by one group of investigators, the percentage of cats that develop struvite calculi and obstruct becomes greater as dietary magnesium content increases. In addition to magnesium, the calcium and phosphorus content of these diets was varied. Variations in calcium and phosphorus had only slight effects on struvite calculi formation.

At least three other groups of investigators have also shown that the risk of incurring struvite urolithiasis is related directly to dietary intake of magnesium.[27,46,47,48,53] Results of one of these studies are shown in Table 4. In another study 7 of 14 cats consuming a diet containing 0.75% magnesium obstructed within six weeks.[53] Another group demonstrated that feeding cats ox heart, which contained 0.20% magnesium and 0.15% calcium, resulted in urolith formation within one month.[47] They also reported that urethral obstruction developed within 23 days in 3 of 5 cats fed a dry diet containing 0.31% magnesium and 0.77% calcium.[48]

In contrast to what has been stated previously,[26] and later found to be incorrect,[27] the experimental uroliths produced in these studies were composed of struvite with a small amount of calcium phosphate. These are identical in chemical composition, crystal structure, and appearance to those occurring in clinical cases in cats eating regular commercial cat foods.[53,102]

In **summary,** several studies have shown that high dietary levels of magnesium, and to a much lesser extent phosphorus, will cause formation of struvite uroliths in cats and clinical signs of FUS. Additional support of the concept that the risk of developing FUS increases with increasing magnesium intake is derived from the numerous studies and reports in both cats and rats of the reduced incidence of struvite urolithiasis when magnesium intake is restricted (see page 9-25).

Commercial cat foods contain in their dry matter an average of 0.16% magnesium. Some contain as much as 0.29% (Table 5). When the dietary magnesium content was only slightly more (0.37%) than that in some commercial cat foods, and urine pH was similar, 70% of 43 cats developed struvite uroliths and obstructed within 11 months (Table 3). The amount of magnesium in commercial cat foods (Table 5) ranges from 4 to 18 times the

TABLE 4

EFFECT OF MAGNESIUM CONSUMPTION ON FELINE URETHRAL OBSTRUCTION[27]

Diet*	Magnesium			Cats with Calculi Present by 40 wk (%)
	% in Diet Dry Matter	mg/100 kcal ME	mg Consumed /cat/day	
c/d	0.05	14	30	0
PCC	0.17	43	157	25
c/d + MgO + H$_2$PO$_4$	0.46	94	233	75
PCC + MgO + H$_2$PO$_4$	0.45	121	334	88
c/d + MgO + H$_2$PO$_4$	0.72	147	366	75

*Canned Prescription Diet Feline c/d (Hill's) or dry Purina Cat Chow (PCC) (Ralston Purina). The pH of the magnesium oxide (MgO), phosphoric acid (H$_2$PO$_4$) mixture was adjusted to 7.2–7.3 with hydrochloric acid. In addition to magnesium, urine pH is also important in struvite calculi formation. Although it was measured in this study the values obtained are not meaningful since they were obtained after fasting the cats, at which time urine pH is acidic regardless of diet.

amount needed to fulfill the cat's dietary magnesium requirement (0.016% in diet dry matter) even during growth, a period of increased need.[95,96]

The reason that commercial cat foods contain these high amounts of magnesium is that many of the ingredients commonly used to supply protein in cat foods have a high magnesium content. For example, soybean meal contains 0.3% magnesium. Meat meal, meat and bone meal, fish meal and poultry by-products all contain a substantial amount of bone and therefore high levels of calcium, phosphorus and magnesium. Their magnesium contents range from 0.2-1.2% unless the bone is removed before it is used, which is not economically feasible in most cases. Palatable, nutritious, low-magnesium ingredients are both expensive and difficult to obtain.

In contrast to popular belief, there is little difference in the average magnesium and phosphorus contents between the different flavors of cat food (Table 6). There is little difference because many flavors of cat food are made from the same basic formula, with only the flavoring agent or "digest" being varied. Therefore, no specific flavor, without regard to brand, is any more or less likely than any other to cause or to prevent FUS.

Recently it has been stated that what is important is not the amount of magnesium in the diet, but instead the form of magnesium, i.e. magnesium oxide, magnesium carbonate or magnesium chloride.[11] The form of magnesium is important only with respect to the effect that these different magnesium salts have on urine pH. Adding magnesium oxide or carbonate to a food increases, and adding magnesium chloride decreases, the urine pH that will occur when that food is consumed.[11,66] A higher urine pH enhances struvite crystallization (see page 9-14). This effect on urine pH is important

only when magnesium is added to the diet, such as in experimental studies on the effect of magnesium on FUS. However, **the form of magnesium in the diet is meaningless when clinical cases are considered,** since magnesium is not added in any form to most commercial cat foods. Instead, magnesium in these products is an integral part of the ingredients used to provide protein and other nutrients. Thus, manufacturers have no control over the form of magnesium in their cat foods. All they can do is use ingredients that minimize their food's magnesium content and the cat's urine pH when the food is consumed.

Magnesium chloride is a poor urine acidifier. In one study a diet containing 3.4% magnesium chloride resulted in a urine pH of 6.87 and increased the diet's magnesium content from 0.19 to 0.58%.[24] Considering the detrimental effects of increased dietary magnesium, it does not appear to be a good dietary ingredient.

Although a high magnesium intake enhances formation of struvite uroliths in cats, it has been shown to help prevent formation of calcium oxalate uroliths in people,[32,52] and in rats fed ethylene glycol.[31,94] Magnesium suppresses intestinal absorption of both calcium and oxalate. Thus, low-magnesium diets increase calcium and oxalate absorption. As a result, low-magnesium diets, in conjunction with high calcium and phosphorus intake, have been shown to enhance formation of experimentally induced calcium phosphate (apatite) nephroliths in cats[58] and rats.[31,94] Thus, low-magnesium diets enhance the formation of apatite nephroliths, and high-magnesium diets help prevent the formation of calcium oxalate nephroliths. However, apatite nephroliths do not occur naturally in cats and calcium oxalate uroliths are uncommon in cats. In addition, a high magnesium intake has not

TABLE 5

MINERAL CONTENT OF CAT FOODS[a]

Food	Form	Magnesium mg/100 kcal ME[b]	Magnesium (% in Food Dry Matter)	Calcium	Phosphorus	Ash
Recommended for Struvite Urolith Dissolution:						
Prescription Diet Feline s/d (Hill's)	dry & can	11	0.06	0.7	0.6	5.8
Recommended for FUS Prevention[c]:						
Homemade (Recipe 8—pg. A3-3)	wet	7	0.04	0.8	0.4	3.9
Fancy Feast Beef & Liver (Carnation)	can	14	0.07	1.3	1.3	8.0
Prescription Diet c/d (Hill's)	dry & can	15	0.07	0.8	0.7	4.7
Science Diet Feline Maintenance (Hill's)	dry & can	16	0.08	0.9	0.6	5.2
Friskies Buffet Beef & Liver Dinner (Carnation)........	can	17	0.08	3.0	1.8	12.0
Average in Foods Available in Grocery Stores:						
Mean (n=26)	can	38	0.16	2.1	1.5	9.4
Range...	can	14-84	.07-.29	0.2-4.3	0.7-2.4	4.5-17
Mean (n=6)	S-M	34	0.14	2.9	1.9	11.8
Range...	S-M	26-51	.12-.19	1.4-4.1	1.8-3.2	9-18
Mean (n=16)	dry	45	0.16	1.6	1.1	8.0
Range...	dry	40-59	.14-.20	1.2-1.9	0.9-1.3	6.9-10
Foods With An Inverse Calcium:Phosphorus Ratio (listed in order of severity)[d]:						
Old Mother Hubbard—avg. of 4 flavors (Hubbard Milling)	can	14	0.08	0.2	0.6	4.6
9 Lives Tuna (Star-Kist Distributors)	can	33	0.15	0.5	0.9	6.1
Figaro Tuna (Bumble Bee Seafoods)	can	37	0.14	0.6	1.0	7.0
Theradiet Feline (Rogar/STB)	can	58	0.29	0.5	0.7	5.4
Moist & Tender (Benco)	S-M	26	0.12	1.4	1.8	9.1
Triumph Low Ash (Triumph Ind.)	can	24	0.13	0.6	0.8	5.4
Tami Ami (Ross Wells)	dry	32	0.14	0.6	0.7	5.6
Optimum Feline Diet (Nature's Recipe)	can	12	0.07	0.6	0.7	4.4
Tender Vittles (Ralston Purina)	S-M	28	0.12	1.8	2.0	10.0
Happy Cat (Ralston Purina)	S-M	29	0.12	2.1	2.2	10.4
Other Canned Foods (listed in decreasing order of mg Mg/100 kcal ME):						
Puss N Boots Tuna (Quaker Oats)		84	0.25	2.2	1.6	10.6
Puss N Boots Fish (Quaker Oats)		79	0.29	1.8	1.7	10.6
Kozy Kitten (Mavar Distributors).....................		71	0.27	4.3	2.4	15.6
Strongheart Fish Flavor (Strongheart Products)		64	0.22	1.8	1.3	10.0
Pet's Choice (IGA Distributors)......................		53	0.22	1.2	0.9	7.2
Friskies Fish Flavor (Carnation)		51	0.20	2.0	1.6	8.5
Safeway Chicken Flavor (Safeway Distributor)		49	0.20	1.0	0.8	6.9
Purina 100 Tuna (Ralston Purina)		45	0.17	1.7	1.5	16.9
Bright Eyes Seafood Dinner (Carnation)		39	0.17	2.6	1.8	12.0
Bolo (Simmons Industries, Distributors)		33	0.16	1.5	1.1	9.0
Fancy Feast Seafood Feast (Carnation)................		32	0.14	3.5	2.3	15.2
Safeway Tuna (Safeway Distributors)		31	0.14	1.5	1.3	7.2
Friskies Buffet Seafood Supper (Carnation)		29	0.14	1.8	1.6	10.2
9 Lives Liver (Star-Kist Distributors)		27	0.13	1.2	0.9	6.9
Cornucopia Super Stars Poultry (Vet Nutrition Assoc.)		27	0.13	2.7	1.5	9.4
Cornucopia Super Stars Plain (Vet Nutrition Assoc.)		26	0.13	0.8	0.8	5.1
9 Lives Super Supper (Star-Kist Dist.)		25	0.12	2.5	1.8	12.1
Cadillac F (Cadillac Pet Foods)		24	0.11	1.8	1.3	8.1
Friskies Buffet Turkey & Giblets (Carnation).....................		24	0.12	3.4	2.2	13.1
Kal Kan Mealtime (Kal Kan)		23	0.12	2.5	1.8	10.4
Science Diet Feline Growth		21	0.11	1.1	0.8	7.3
Other Soft-Moist Foods (listed in order of mg Mg/100 kcal ME):						
Generic (Rockford Farms)		51	0.19	4.1	3.2	17.6
Generic (Generic Products, Ft. Worth)		36	0.14	3.0	2.2	13.1
9 Lives (Star-Kist Distributors)		35	0.14	2.1	1.9	10.5
Other Dry Foods (listed in order of mg Mg/100 kcal ME):						
Generic (Rockford Farms)		59	0.20	1.9	1.3	10.0
9 Lives Tuna & Egg (Star-Kist Dist.)		53	0.18	1.7	1.3	8.3
Bonnie (Wells Pet Food Corp.)		50	0.17	1.6	1.2	7.5
Pet's Choice (IGA Distributors)......................		50	0.17	1.4	1.0	8.0

(Continued on next page)

TABLE 5—Continued

MINERAL CONTENT OF CAT FOODS[a]

Food	Magnesium mg/100 kcal ME[b]	Calcium	Phosphorus	Ash
		(% in Food Dry Matter)		
Crave (Kal Kan Foods)	48	0.17	1.4	1.2	7.7
Fish Ahoy (Carnation)	46	0.16	1.7	1.2	8.5
Kitten Chow (Ralston Purina)	44	0.16	1.6	1.3	8.9
Meow Mix (Ralston Purina)	43	0.15	1.8	1.2	6.9
Friskies Ocean Fish (Carnation)	43	0.15	1.8	1.3	8.9
Cat Chow Original Blend (Ralston Purina)	43	0.16	1.3	1.0	7.2
Chef's Blend 4 Flavors (Carnation)	43	0.15	1.5	1.1	7.5
Thrive (Ralston Purina)	43	0.17	1.6	0.9	7.9
Kozy Kitten Fish & Shrimp (Mavar Dist.)	41	0.15	1.2	1.2	7.3
Cat Chow Ocean Blend (Ralston Purina)	41	0.15	1.2	0.9	7.0
Cornucopia Super Stars (Vet Nutrition Assoc.)	41	0.15	1.8	1.4	7.5
Special Dinner Tuna & Herring (Ralston Purina)	40	0.15	1.5	1.1	8.0
Generic (K-9 Ration)	40	0.14	1.4	0.9	7.6
Iams (Iams Food Co.)	24	0.10	1.4	1.0	6.4
Science Diet Feline Growth	20	0.10	1.4	0.9	6.7

[a]Based on the average of two analyses. Energy digestibility estimated at 80% for dry and 90% for canned and soft-moist foods unless known.

[b]The most important value to consider since it determines the amount of magnesium consumed when that diet is fed.

[c]Foods consistently found to contain 20 mg, or less, magnesium/100 kcal ME, constantly maintain the urine pH below 6.4 and have a positive Ca:P ratio.

[d]An inverse Ca:P ratio may cause bone demineralization. 3 of 6 soft-moist, 9 of 35 canned and 1 of 22 dry foods analyzed had an inverse Ca:P ratio.

TABLE 6

MAGNESIUM AND PHOSPHORUS CONTENTS OF DIFFERENT FLAVORS OF CANNED CAT FOODS (% in Dry Matter)

Flavor	n	Magnesium mean	Magnesium range	Phosphorus mean	Phosphorus range
Fish	8	0.17	0.11–.24	1.5	1.0–2.3
Tuna	7	0.14	0.11–.17	1.0	0.7–1.5
Chicken	5	0.15	0.09–.20	1.4	1.2–1.7
Kidney	2	0.18	0.16–.20	1.1	1.0–1.2
Liver	7	0.15	0.08–.20	1.1	0.5–1.5
Meat	3	0.15	0.14–.17	1.2	1.1–1.6
Mixed	14	0.16	0.05–.25	1.2	0.5–2.1
All	46	0.15	0.05–.25	1.2	0.5–2.3

been shown to be beneficial in preventing calcium oxalate uroliths in cats or dogs. As these studies demonstrate, in assessing the effect of diet on urolithiasis, it is important to know:

1. The type of urolith
2. The species of animal
3. The specific minerals involved

Lack of familiarity with these factors has led to much confusion and erroneous information on urolithiasis. One of the best examples is the widespread advertising and confusion concerning the ash content of cat foods.

Ash as a Causative Factor

Ash consists of all non-combustible materials, one of which is magnesium. The facts that the incidence of FUS is enhanced by increased magnesium intake and that FUS is the major health concern of cat owners[67] are the reasons for advertising and concern regarding the ash content of cat foods. However, the ash content of a cat food may or may not correlate to its magnesium content, and therefore its likelihood of predisposing to or preventing FUS.

Ash may consist primarily of salt or any number of other minerals. A diet high in ash because of a high salt content may be beneficial in preventing struvite crystallization as is well known in ruminants,[16,105] and as is suggested by a decrease in hematuria in cats.[43] A diet high in ash because of a high calcium content, but low in magnesium, actually may be helpful in preventing feline urolithiasis.[58] In contrast, a diet low in ash because of a low calcium content is likely to enhance urolith formation and FUS if its magnesium content is high. If the dietary calcium content is low enough, and particu-

larly if the diet contains substantially more phosphorus than calcium, i.e. has a sufficiently severe inverse calcium:phosphorus ratio (Ca:P), it will cause nutritional secondary hyperparathyroidism and bone demineralization.

As shown in Table 5, 3 of 6 soft-moist, 9 of 35 canned and 1 of 22 dry cat foods analyzed had an inverse Ca:P ratio. This nutritional imbalance was most common in cat foods advertised as having a low ash content. The amount of ash in some of these foods was low because of its low calcium content, not a low magnesium content. This would be expected to enhance, not reduce, struvite crystallization. Within grocery store marketed cat foods, the presence of an inverse Ca:P ratio, and magnesium content, varied widely within brand categories, i.e. nationally distributed, regional, generic (no brand name given on the product) or private label (those in which the distributor, but not the manufacturer, is identified) (see page 2-15 for a discussion of types of pet foods). This suggests that **the common practice of recommending "any good national brand," does not increase the likelihood of obtaining a better quality cat food,** at least with respect to the food's mineral content.

The confusion surrounding the effect of dietary ash content on FUS is well demonstrated in one study in which diets containing 8, 22, or 30% ash were fed to 8-week-old kittens for 10 to 14 weeks, without causing FUS.[20] This study is widely cited as demonstrating that the ash content of the diet plays no role in FUS, which it does not, if the ash is low in magnesium. The diets used in this study were all extremely low in magnesium (0.03% or less) and high in calcium (1.6, 5.6 and 8.1%), exactly the type of diet shown in controlled studies to prevent FUS.[58] Even if the diets had been high in magnesium, it is doubtful that feeding them to kittens for such a short time would cause FUS, since FUS rarely occurs in cats less than 1 year old.[5,45] Thus, it is the magnesium, not the ash content of the diet that is important. However, the magnesium content of many cat foods is not known, but the ash content is. The question then is: How does the ash content of cat foods relate to their magnesium content?

As shown in Figure 3, the magnesium content of dry and soft-moist, but not canned, cat foods relate directly to their ash content. Thus, the greater the amount of ash in a dry or soft-moist cat food, the greater its magnesium content; therefore, everything else being constant (such as urine pH) the more likely FUS will occur when the food is consumed. In contrast, the ash content of a canned food is not correlated to its magnesium content and, therefore, its FUS-inducing potential.

The correlation between ash and magnesium

contents in dry and soft-moist cat foods, and lack of this correlation in canned foods, is due to the difference in ingredients used in these different forms of cat food. The ingredients commonly used to provide the protein in dry and soft-moist foods are soybean meal and poultry, meat and bone, or fish meal that contain varying amounts of bone. All of these meat meals provide large amounts of both ash and magnesium. In contrast, a wider variety of animal tissues, many of which do not contain bone, are used in making canned cat foods.

Thus, some canned cat foods are extremely high in magnesium, while others are quite low. The magnesium content varies less among different dry and soft-moist, than between different canned cat foods (Table 5, page 9-10). This is due to the similarity of ingredients used in the different brands of these foods. Thus, some canned cat foods may predispose to FUS, while others may be beneficial in preventing it. However, the average mg magnesium/kcal in dry cat foods marketed in grocery stores is nearly 20% more than in canned foods (Table 5).

Dry Cat Foods as a Causative Factor

Most cats kept as pets are fed commercial cat foods. In 1985 on a caloric basis, dry foods accounted for 63% of all commercial cat food sold in the United States.[90] Thus, dry commercial cat foods supply the greatest part of the food intake for the majority of cats kept as pets in United States. These foods became popular only within the past 10 to 15 years, with their popularity increasing yearly. From 1969 to 1982, on a caloric basis, sales of dry cat foods in North America rose 270% while sales of canned foods increased only 32%.[22,90] Several studies conducted during this period suggest that the incidence of FUS has increased (page 9-3).

Although there are many factors such as better diagnosis and reporting of affected cats, and increased confinement,[83] that could play a role in causing a growing incidence of FUS, many investigators have suggested that the increasing incidence results primarily from increased feeding of dry cat foods.[30,47,56,59] Two studies support the hypothesis that the risk of FUS occurring is greater when a regular commercial dry food is fed. Workers in Denmark found that the risk of developing FUS was seven times greater when a regular dry cat food made up most of the diet, as compared to when it was never fed.[112] In the United States the risk of developing FUS was found to be 1.7 times greater when a regular commercial dry food made up 50-75% of the diet, 3.1 times greater when it made up 75-99% of the diet, and 6.7 times greater when only a dry food of this type was fed.[83]

FIGURE 3

RELATIONSHIP BETWEEN ASH AND MAGNESIUM CONTENTS IN CAT FOODS

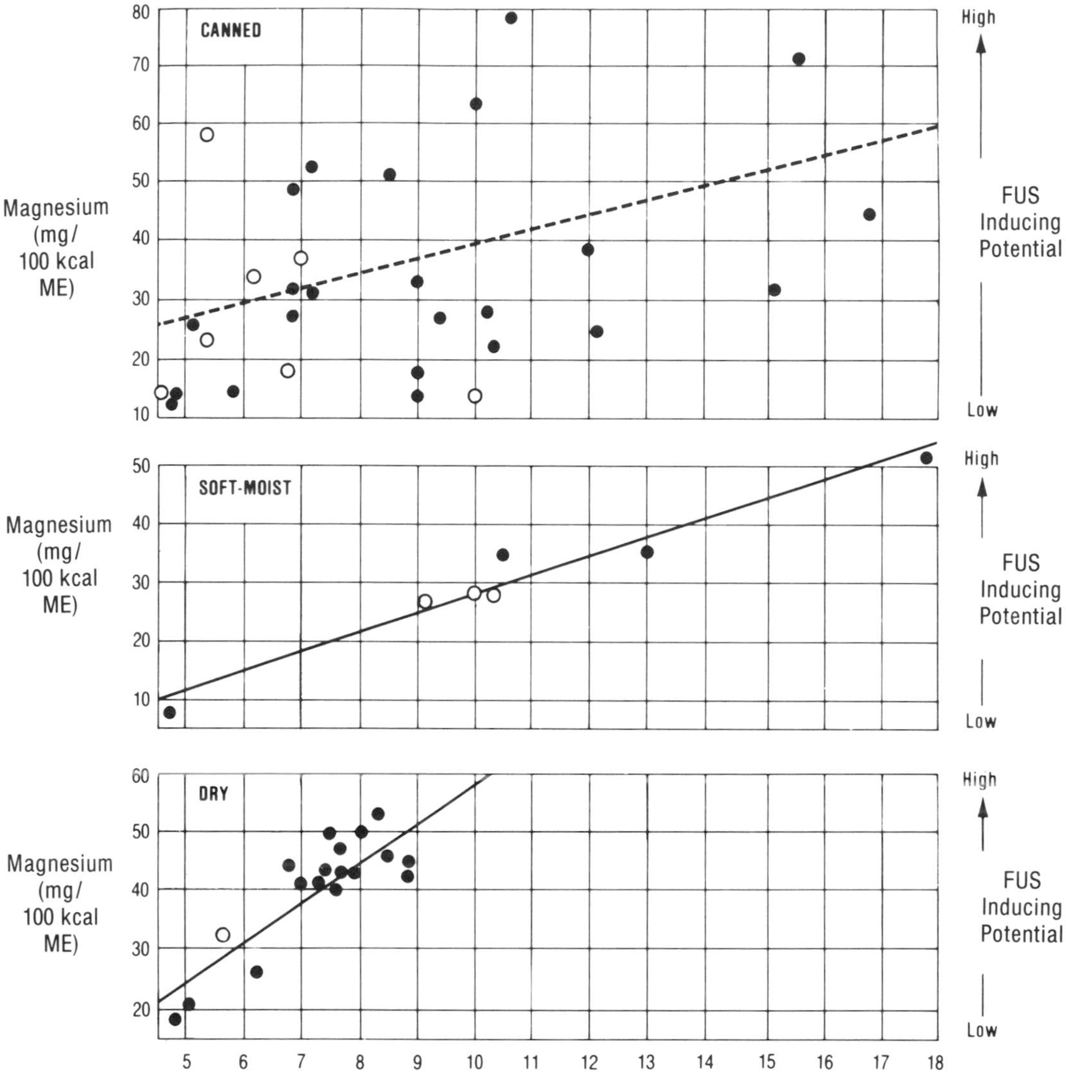

FIGURE 3: o indicates foods with an inverse Ca:P ratio. As shown, the ash content of dry and soft-moist, but not canned, foods are directly correlated to their magnesium content. The lower the ash content of dry and soft-moist cat foods, the more likely they are to assist in preventing FUS, and conversely, the higher their ash contents, the more they predispose to FUS (see Tables 3 and 4, 9-8 and 9). In contrast, the ash content of a canned food gives little indication of its potential to predispose to or prevent FUS. The correlation coefficients (R) and equations for the lines shown are: canned foods R = 0.42 and the mg Mg/100 kcal = (2.52 × % ash in dry matter) + 14.22; soft-moist foods R = 0.98 and the mg Mg/100 kcal = (3.28 × % ash in dry matter) − 4.97; dry foods R = 0.89 and the mg Mg/100 kcal = (6.73 × % ash in dry matter) − 8.81.

A number of reasons have been proposed for dry foods predisposing to FUS. One is that dry foods contain larger amounts of magnesium. As shown in Table 5 (page 9-10), when the magnesium content of the different forms of cat food are compared on a dry matter basis (all water removed), there is no significant difference, but when expressed on a caloric basis, there is a difference. Thus, regular commercial dry cat foods contain no more magnesium than do other forms of cat foods; instead, their

caloric density is less. The lower the caloric density of a food, the more the cat must eat to meet its energy need. Thus, although the magnesium contents of regular commercial dry and canned foods are the same on a dry matter basis, the cat consumes nearly 20% more food dry matter and, therefore, magnesium when eating the dry form.

A second reason proposed for dry cat foods predisposing to FUS is a lower total water intake and body water turnover per gram of dry matter consumed.[97] Because of the difference in the water content of dry and canned foods, when the cat is fed a dry food it drinks more water and ingests less water in the food. However, total water intake, but not necessarily urine volume, is the same.[49,92,103] In two studies no correlation was found between urine volume and the form of the diet;[92,103] whereas in another study urine volume was less when a dry diet was fed because a greater percentage of the water ingested was excreted in the feces.[49] The conflicts in these data appear to be because urine volume is not affected by differences in water content of the diet, but instead by other nutrient differences in the diets.

The less the fat and greater the fiber content the lower the diet's digestibility. The lower the food's digestibility, the more the cat must eat to meet its caloric needs, and the greater the quantity of feces produced. The greater the quantity of feces, the larger the percentage of ingested water retained in the intestinal tract and excreted in the feces and, as a result, the less the percentage of ingested water excreted in the urine.[91,92]

Most commercial dry cat foods have less fat and more fiber, and as a result are less digestible and have less caloric density than do most canned cat foods. Thus, even though they do not differ in dry matter magnesium content, more food, and therefore magnesium, is ingested and urine volume is less than when canned foods are consumed. Both of these factors increase urinary magnesium concentration and thus predispose to FUS. In one study the urinary magnesium concentration was three times higher when cats consumed a dry food than when they ate a canned diet, even though the magnesium content in the dry matter of the diets was the same.[47]

In **summary,** when most commercial dry cat foods are eaten, there is greater urinary magnesium concentration and therefore predisposition to FUS than when canned foods are eaten. This difference is due to the fat, fiber, digestibility and caloric density of the two forms of food, and is not due to differences in their water or dry-matter magnesium contents. A few dry cat foods are as high, or higher, in fat and caloric density, and as low, or lower, in

magnesium as any canned food. They therefore contain a low concentration of magnesium/100 kcal ME (Table 5, page 9-10). These dry diets do not predispose to FUS and are more likely to prevent FUS than are those canned diets that are low in fat, caloric density, and digestibility and high in magnesium, therefore containing a high concentration of magnesium/100 kcal ME. Another reason FUS may be more likely to occur when some dry foods are fed is that they may produce a higher urine pH than do some canned foods.

Urine pH As A Causative Factor

In addition to a sufficiently high concentration of urolith-forming constituents in the urine, a favorable pH for crystallization is necessary. Cystine and urate calculi form best in an acid urine (see pages 10-28 and 31).[64] However, they constitute less than 3% of all uroliths occurring in cats (Table 2, page 9-7). Oxalate and calcium phosphate are not affected significantly by urine pH.[75] In contrast, struvite, which constitute between 82-97% of feline uroliths, form best at a pH of 7.0 or greater.[64,88] The solubility of struvite increases as urine pH decreases below 6.6. The amount of struvite crystals in the urine of healthy cats is directly related to urine pH.[13,87] When a low magnesium diet is not being consumed, struvite crystals are almost always present in the cat's urine at a pH above 6.8 and are rarely present at a pH of 6.4 or less.[13]

Urine pH is affected by both the method of feeding and the diet. When fed free-choice, most cats eat every few hours, 24 hours a day.[40] In our colony, when 20 cats were fed individually, either a dry or a canned food free-choice, the amount consumed by each cat each five to eight hour period throughout the day and night was the same, except during the afternoon when it was decreased by approximately 50%.

As shown in Figure 4, after a cat has fasted for 18 hours or longer, its urine pH is near 6.0. Ingestion of food stimulates secretion of gastric acid. Unless sufficient acidifying ions are absorbed to offset this acid secretion, the kidney will excrete alkaline ions to prevent body fluids from becoming alkaline, which increases urine pH. This occurs in all animals and is called the "postprandial alkaline tide." The greater the amount of food consumed, the more gastric acid secreted[7] and the greater the elevation in urine pH. Thus, when the cat eats all of its food in a single daily meal, the increase in urine pH is greater than if the same food is fed free-choice, but the increase remains for only a few hours (Figure 4). Which is more important in inducing formation of struvite calculi, the magnitude or the duration of the

FIGURE 4

EFFECT OF METHOD OF FEEDING ON THE pH OF CAT'S URINE[101]

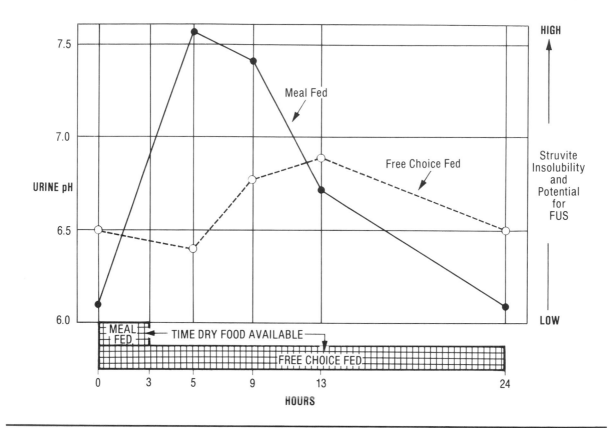

TABLE 7

PREFERRED METHOD OF FEEDING FOR FUS PREVENTION

| | Urine pH When | | |
Example Diet	Diet Always Available	Diet Meal Fed	Preferred Way to Feed that Diet*
A	≥ 6.8**	—	1–2 times/day
B	≤ 6.4	≥ 6.8	Always available
C	≤ 6.4	≤ 6.4	Doesn't matter

*Because the vast majority of feline uroliths are struvite (Table 2, page 9–7) which, when a low magnesium diet is not fed, are nearly always present in the cat's urine at a pH above 6.8, and are rarely present at a pH of 6.4 or less.[13]

**≥ means equal to or greater than and ≤ equal to or less than.

increase? And, therefore, which is better, meal-feeding or free-choice feeding? As shown in Table 7, the answer depends on the urine pH produced by a particular food.

As shown in Figure 5, different foods have greatly different effects on urine pH. When foods are meal fed some produce a much greater alkaline tide than others. Some cat foods fed free choice result in a urine pH that is always favorable for formation of struvite calculi (6.8 or more), whereas others result in a urine pH that is always unfavorable for struvite calculi formation (6.4 or less) no matter how they are fed. These differences are not related to the form of the food, i.e. whether it is canned or dry. Thus, **both the food and the method of feeding greatly alter the urine pH.**

SUMMARY OF CAUSES

Increasing both magnesium intake and urine pH increase the risk of struvite crystallization and formation of calculi in the cat's urinary tract. These

FIGURE 5

EFFECT OF DIFFERENT CAT FOODS ON URINE pH

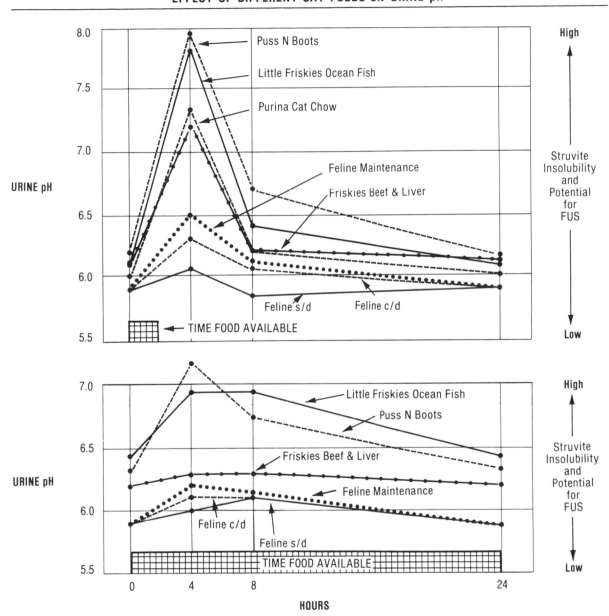

calculi are the main cause of cystitis and urethritis responsible for manifestations of the clinical signs referred to as FUS. Elevated urine concentration and reduced frequency of urination from confinement, inactivity, a dirty litter box, or unpalatable or inaccessible water also enhance calculi formation and therefore the occurrence of FUS. Bacteria or viruses in the urinary tract, or debris resulting from their presence, may also induce cystitis and urethritis and would enhance formation of calculi by more material available to serve as a nucleation center. However, there are neither bacteria nor viruses in the urinary tract of most cats with FUS[5,56] and, like an enlarged urachal diverticulum, when present appear to occur as a result and not as a cause of FUS.[5,57,76]

Thus, excess dietary magnesium and the resulting elevated urinary magnesium concentration (Figure 2, page 9-8) and urine pH appear to be the primary factors responsible for formation of struvite crystals

TABLE 8

DIET MAGNESIUM AND URINE pH INTERACTIONS ON FUS

Diet No.	Mg–% in Diet Dry Matter	Urine pH		No. of Cats	Effect
		Ad-Lib Fed	Post Prandial		
1	0.045	8.2	—	7	1 obstructed in 8 weeks, 6 hematuric by 20 weeks[11]
2	0.05	6.9	7.5	10	1 hematuric, 9 struvite crystalluric in 2 weeks[11]
3	0.37	5.9	—	12	2 developed uroliths in 11 months[102]
4	0.50	7.7	7.6	10	1 obstructed, 9 struvite crystalluric in 2 weeks[11]
5	0.50	5.7	6.4	10	No dysfunctions or crystalluria in 2 weeks[11]
6	0.37	7.0	—	12	7 obstructed twice and 2 had struvite uroliths by 11 months[102]
7	0.37	5.9	—	6	All had calculi when started on diet and all dissolved within 3 months[102]

and calculi and the occurrence of most cases of FUS. It can be determined from a nomogram for estimating the saturation of urine with the struvite constituents, magnesium, ammonium and phosphate, that a 10-fold increase in urine magnesium concentration causes the same increase in the factor that determines if struvite crystallization will occur (struvite activity product or AP) as does an increase in urine pH from 6.4 to 7.0.[64] Thus, an increase in either urine magnesium or urine pH enhances struvite calculi formation and a decrease in either inhibits it. Obviously, a change in both has the greatest effect. For example, the propensity for forming struvite crystals in the urine is from 30 to 5500 times greater* when the cat's food is the leading selling dry cat food (Cat Chow, Ralston Purina) than it is when the cat is consuming a low-magnesium, urine-acidifying cat food (Prescription Diet Feline c/d, Hill's). The effects of increases in dietary magnesium or urine pH, or both, on the determinent for struvite crystallization determined from this nomogram are confirmed in actual studies in the cat as shown in Table 8.

When urine pH was continually maintained at an extremely high 8.2, 1 of 7 cats became obstructed and the other 6 had hematuria, even though dietary magnesium was only 0.045% (Diet 1, Table 8). This urine pH is abnormally high for most diets. Rarely is the cat's urine pH greater than 7.0 for an extended time (Figures 4 & 5). Although an average urine pH of 8.2 has been reported for cats consuming free-choice the leading selling dry cat food (Cat Chow, Ralston Purina)[109] this pH is higher than others[101] have reported when this same brand of food is fed ad libitum. The cause may be differences in methodology or variations in different batches of this

particular brand of food. The ingredients of most regular commercial pet foods vary depending on their availability and cost. However, the high urine pH produced when diet 1 (Table 8) was fed does illustrate the point well: **FUS will occur if the urine pH is sufficiently high even when dietary magnesium is quite low.** Even when urine pH was only a moderately elevated 6.9 and post-prandially 7.5, and dietary magnesium was quite low (0.05%), hematuria developed in 1 of 10 cats and all of them had struvite crystalluria (Diet 2, Table 8).

Not only will FUS occur when dietary magnesium is quite low, if urine pH is sufficiently high, the reverse is also true. **FUS will occur even when urine pH is quite low if dietary magnesium is sufficiently high.** When dietary magnesium was 0.37%, struvite uroliths developed in 2 of 12 cats even though their diet contained 1.5% ammonium chloride, which maintained an average urine pH of 5.9 and never exceeded 6.4 in any of the cats at any time (Diet 3, Table 8). This high dietary level of magnesium, like the high urine pH produced by Diet 1, is abnormal, although commercial cat foods do contain up to 0.29% magnesium (Table 5).

As would be expected, **FUS is most likely to occur in the shortest period of time and be the most severe when both dietary magnesium and urine pH are high.** When dietary magnesium was 0.5% and urine pH was maintained at 7.7, 1 of 10 cats became obstructed and the others had crystalluria within two weeks (Diet 4, Table 8). No crystalluria occurred in 10 cats fed the same diet but with their urine pH maintained at 5.7 (Diet 5). When dietary magnesium was 0.37% and urine pH was 7.0, 7 of 12 cats became obstructed twice, and 2 others had struvite uroliths within 11 months (Diet 6), even though calculi dissolved in 6 cats fed this same diet containing 1.5% ammonium choloride, which maintained the urine pH at 5.9 (Diet 7).

*Based on urine magnesium concentration of 4.98 and 11.43 mg/dl when these two diets are fed,[27] and a urine pH of 6.0 (Figure 5) and 8.2[109] or 6.7[101] (5500 times greater using 8.2 and 30 times greater using 6.7).

FUS may be caused primarily by our domestication of the cat. This has resulted in: 1) more confinement, which reduces the amount of water consumed and the frequency of urination, and 2) feeding foods that are low in fat, high in calculi-forming constituents such as magnesium, and maintain a high urine pH. Low dietary fat lessens urine volume (page 9-14), which increases urine concentration[91,92] and reduces the frequency of urination, allowing more time for calculi to form.

In its natural state the cat is a predator, hunting, catching, and consuming small animals. The prey consists of birds and small mammals. The entire carcass of a small mammal, a rat for example, exceeds all nutrient levels recommended by the National Research Council (NRC) for the cat except selenium and vitamin E.[109] Selenium is close to the current recommendation (0.08 vs 0.1 ppm). The recommendation for vitamin E is 80 as compared to 33 IU/kg of food in the rat carcass. The amount of vitamin E in the rat carcass, however, is adequate in a fresh diet. Higher levels are recommended in prepared foods due to their occasional high content of unsaturated fatty acids, and as an attempt to decrease fatty acid oxidation during food storage. Of interest in regard to FUS is the fact that the entire rat carcass is high in fat and low in magnesium (37% and 0.085% in its dry matter, respectively). Even when rat carcasses were fed to cats ad libitum, and as a result they overate, an average urine pH of 7.0 resulted.[109] Always having food available, however, is abnormal for cats in the feral state. When a hunt is successful, the feral cat consumes its food in a relatively short time. The cat may not eat again for several days. During that time the urine pH would be at the fasting level of about 6.0 (Figures 4 & 5, pages 9-15 & 9-16).

CLINICAL SIGNS

The clinical signs in the majority of cats with FUS are caused by the presence and effects of crystals or calculi in the urinary tract. The calculi—single or multiple—may be several centimeters in diameter, but generally they are the size of a grain of sand or microscopic crystals. The calculi may cause no noticeable signs or may irritate the lining of the urinary tract, thus causing cystitis and/or urethritis. They may also occur in the kidney, or become lodged in the urethra or, rarely, the ureters, causing obstruction. Nephroliths occur less often in cats than dogs.[30] They generally cause no overt signs unless there is an upper urinary tract infection or enough damage to produce renal failure. Occasionally they may be associated with pyelonephritis; the result is hematuria, lumbar pain, and fever (see page 8-20). Obstruction of a ureter by a nephrolith can result in hydronephrosis and a loss of kidney function. Because more than two-thirds of total renal function must be lost before clinical signs appear, no observable effects occur unless both ureters are obstructed.

A house-trained animal dribbling urine or urinating in unusual locations signals the possibility of cystitis or urethritis, or the presence of a partial urethral obstruction. These signs are usually followed by frequent voiding of small quantities of urine (pollakiuria). The urine may be bloody and have a strong ammonia odor which, in conjunction with pyuria, suggests a urinary tract infection. A putrid odor may indicate severe tissue necrosis from cystitis. A lower urinary tract infection generally does not cause pain or fever. Although urine may flow freely, there may be signs of dysuria, such as continuance of squatting or straining when urination ends. These signs may be episodic, beginning abruptly and abating within a few days without treatment, only to recur again. They are generally the only signs in females, and may be the only signs in many affected males. However, obstruction commonly occurs in males because of their longer, narrower urethra; whereas urethral obstruction is uncommon in females.[23]

Urethral obstruction may occur suddenly or develop over a period of days or weeks. Initially attempts may be made to urinate, with only drops, a fine stream, or nothing being voided. Attempts to urinate are usually frequent. Affected cats may squat, strain and lick the penis excessively. Some owners mistake this for constipation.

If obstruction is sufficient, uremia occurs, resulting in anorexia, dehydration, lethargy, depression and occasionally vomiting and diarrhea. Untreated complete obstruction leads to coma and death within two to four days. However, the animal suffers pain from the time blockage occurs, and the pain increases until the animal is comatose. Increased back pressure of urine as a result of the obstruction may cause renal ischemia, resulting in renal damage. Reversible damage may occur within 24 hours, and irreversible renal damage within five days.[99] Hypertension, because of increased renin secretion, and hydronephrosis occur.[36,106] To prevent these effects and death, time is critical; treatment must begin shortly after obstruction occurs. If treatment is not started until the animal is comatose, its chances of survival are greatly reduced because the damage from uremia and renal cellular changes may be irreversible. The distended bladder may rupture. For a short time after it ruptures, the animal may appear improved due to relief of the pain caused by bladder distention. However, perito-

TABLE 9

CLINICAL SIGNS AND DIAGNOSIS OF FUS

Clinical Signs		Diagnostic Abnormalities
1. Urine dribbling 2. Urinating in unusual locations	Without Urethral Obstruction	1. Wet perineal hair 2. Palpate thickened bladder wall & grating

3. Pollakiuria
 	
4. ± Hematuria
 	
5. ± Continued squatting or
   straining after micturation
	With or Without
	Urethral Obstruction
		3. Inflamed penile epithelium
		4. Radiographic or sonographic
		   abnormalities
		      88% have detectable abnormalities
		         including[71]
		      24% have calculi
		      23% vesicourachal
		         diverticula
		      22% thickened bladder wall
		      10% urethral striclures,
		         and occasionally anomalies
		         or ureteral reflux

6. Anuria but frequent
   micturition attempts
 	
7. Squat, strain & lick penis
 	
8. Uremic induced signs:
   anorexia, depression ± vomiting
   & diarrhea, coma & death
	With Urethral Obstruction	5. Hypothermia, bradycardia &
		   tachypnea
		6. Increase capillary refill time
		7. Bladder distended, hard, painful
		   or occasionally ruptured
		8. Calculi or plug detected by
		   catheterization

nitis and absorption of waste products rapidly occur. This results in depression, abdominal distention, and death within 48-72 hours. Uremic animals seldom survive surgical repair of a ruptured bladder.

Owners, particularly of previously affected animals, should be made aware of these clinical signs so that treatment can be started early, thus preventing the permanent damage inflicted by prolonged obstruction. A summary of the major clinical signs due to FUS, and factors useful in its diagnosis are given in Table 9.

DIAGNOSIS

The owner may or may not have observed any clinical signs. In some cases the only signs are those described previously resulting from cystitis and urethritis. Nothing abnormal may be found on physical, laboratory, or radiographic examination. Wet hair in the perineal region and inflamed penile epithelium may be seen on physical examination. If the urethra is obstructed, hypothermia, bradycardia, tachypnea, and increased capillary refill time may be present. The bladder will be distended, hard, and painful and cannot be expressed. Care should be taken to avoid rupturing a distended bladder when it is palpated. Occasionally the bladder may be ruptured. The ruptured bladder cannot be palpated,

but there are large quantities of urine in the abdominal cavity. If suspected, this can be confirmed by paracentesis.

Abdominal palpation is often helpful in detecting cystitis, or cystic or urethral calculi. The bladder wall may be thickened and feel crepitus or impart a grating sensation when palpated. Even though a sufficiently large urolith can be palpated and multiple calculi can be recognized by their crepitation, palpation cannot be depended upon to reveal all cases of cystic calculi. Urethral calculi can be detected and their site located by passing a catheter (see page 9-22).

The clinical signs and physical examination findings summarized in Table 9 generally provide the only information necessary for diagnosing cystitis, urethritis or urethral obstruction. However, multiple calculi may be present throughout the urinary tract; therefore, a complete radiographic or sonographic examination of the entire urinary tract is indicated. With proper technique these examinations of cats with FUS will generally reveal any one or more of a variety of the abnormalities described in Table 9.

The diameter of the male cat's urethra is maximal at the ischiatic arch. It becomes progressively smaller toward the external urethral orifice, where uroliths may lodge.[51] In contrast, the female cat's urethra is uniform in diameter along its entire length

and its diameter is larger and its length shorter than the male's.[51] Lesions in the bladder and urethra can be detected by sonograms or a combination of positive contrast cystography, double contrast cystography and retrograde contrast urethrocystography.[69] Procedures for both radiographic examination and urine analysis are described on pages 10-11 and 10-12.

Although it is proper to recommend and conduct many diagnostic procedures, in actual practice few are required for the vast majority of cats with FUS because most of them can be successfully managed by feeding diets that dissolve and prevent the recurrence of struvite uroliths. Thus, a complete urinalysis, and diagnosis of urinary tract infection and the type of urolith present, is indicated only in nonresponsive or recurring cases of FUS when the recommended management is unsuccessful. The type of urolith present can be determined as described on page 10-13.

As shown in Table 2 (page 9-7), most calculi in cats with FUS are struvite. Struvite calculi are sometimes referred to as "double phosphate" or "triple phosphate" stones, depending on the number of cations present (Mg^{++}, NH_4^{++} and Ca^{++} if it also contains calcium phosphate). These calculi may resemble sand in the bladder or urethra, or both. Discrete uroliths, and uroliths in the kidney or ureters, are less common,[30] but radiographically visible calculi in 24% of cats with FUS have been reported.[71]

The gelatinous plugs present in 3.5% of cats with FUS (Table 2) differ from uroliths in that they contain a greater percentage of organic matrix; this gives them a toothpaste-like, compressible consistency. These plugs lodge in the urethra, most commonly near the urethral orifice. They are often cylindrical when forced out of the external urethral orifice of male cats, but they lack a definite internal structural organization.

TREATMENT AND PREVENTION

If urinary flow is completely obstructed, without treatment the animal will die within two to four days. Therefore, in case of obstruction, immediately obtain a blood sample for laboratory analysis, begin stabilizing the animal's condition, and relieve bladder distention. Severe bladder distention should be relieved immediately by cystocentesis. Urethral patency can be established after the animal's condition is stabilized. Above all, be gentle! The cat usually refuses to eat or drink when obstructed; therefore, it often is dehydrated and requires fluid therapy. In most cases fluid therapy is not needed unless the cat is obstructed. A summary of treatment and management recommendations is given on page 9-2.

FLUID THERAPY

Administration of fluids and electrolytes is extremely important if the animal is obstructed and visibly dehydrated. When no fluids were given 10 of 13 cats died after relief of obstruction.[28] In contrast, none of 23 severely dehydrated comatose cats died when proper fluid therapy was administered and obstruction was relieved.[12]

Obstructed animals are often depressed or comatose; some vomit, the majority are hypothermic, and the urine is turbid and contains glucose and blood.[12] The urine is usually acid because of metabolic acidosis, but it may be alkaline in some animals due to a urinary tract infection.[12] Therefore, the urine pH is an unreliable guide to the presence or severity of metabolic acidosis. Dehydration, uremia, hyperphosphatemia, hyperkalemia, and acidosis are routinely present in the obstructed cat. Because these abnormalities cause death of obstructed cats, they should be corrected quickly with proper fluid and electrolyte therapy. None of these conditions differs with the duration of obstruction[8,22] and therefore indicate only the degree of blockage. It has been reported that the longer the cat is obstructed, the lower the urine specific gravity, and that if the specific gravity is less than 1.020, that cat has been obstructed for at least 72 hours.[45]

TABLE 10

ESTIMATION OF FLUID AND BICARBONATE DEFICIT IN THE CAT OR DOG WITH URETHRAL OBSTRUCTION

	Mild	Moderate	Severe
Clinical Signs	Decreased skin pliability	Loss of skin pliability Dry or tacky membranes Scleral vessels prominent ▲Heart and respiratory rate ▼Temperature of extremities ▲Capillary refill time	Previous signs increase and coma present
% Dehydration	5–8	8–12	12–15
Fluid Deficit (ml/kg)	60	100	140
Bicarbonate Deficit (mEq/kg)	2.5	6	10

If the animal is alert and if little dehydration is evident, fluids may be given subcutaneously. However, if the animal is more severely dehydrated, fluids should be given via an intravenous catheter. The fluid should be warmed to 37-40°C just before it is administered. This can be achieved by letting it sit in hot tap water for 5 to 15 minutes, or in a microwave oven for a few minutes. Cold fluids given intravenously have a direct effect on the sinoatrial node and may result in arrythmia and death.[19] In addition, if the cat is hypothermic, it should be wrapped in a blanket or put on a heating pad or hot water bottle.

The animal's fluid and bicarbonate deficit can be estimated on the basis of clinical signs given in Table 10. A more accurate calculation of the amount of bicarbonate needed can be obtained by measuring the plasma total carbon dioxide content,* or the plasma bicarbonate concentration from the blood pH and carbon dioxide content, and then using the following formula.

$$\text{mEq of bicarbonate needed} =$$
$$(18 - \text{patient's } [HCO_3]_p) \times 2 \times 0.3 \times \text{kg body weight}$$

As extracellular acidosis is corrected, hydrogen ions move out of the cell, correcting the intracellular acidosis. As a result, the amount of bicarbonate needed to correct a metabolic acidosis is twice the bicarbonate deficit of the extracellular fluid (ECF). The ECF bicarbonate deficit is the bicarbonate deficit times the ECF volume, which is approximately 30% of the body wt ($0.3 \times$ kg body wt). The bicarbonate deficit that should be corrected is 18 minus the patient's plasma bicarbonate concentration. Care should be taken not to overcorrect acidosis or to give bicarbonate too rapidly. Either is very detrimental as they reduce cerebral blood flow and hemoglobin release of oxygen to the tissue, and depress respiratory drive—all of which may cause cerebral hypoxia and death.[60,61] To prevent these effects the patient's bicarbonate deficit should be added to the amount of fluid needed to correct the initial fluid deficit; this should be given intravenously over a three to six hour period. The animal's initial fluid deficit is the percent dehydration estimated from clinical signs times kilograms of body weight. For example, for a 5-kg cat 8% dehydrated the initial fluid deficit would be 5×0.08 or 0.4 liters.

The fluid recommended for correction of the initial fluid deficit is a one-half isotonic saline (0.45% sodium chloride) one-half isotonic dextrose (2.5% glucose) solution (a mixture of equal parts of 0.9% saline and 5% glucose) with the animal's bicarbonate deficit added. This fluid is preferred because:

1. It contains no potassium and the obstructed animal is generally hyperkalemic.
2. If rehydrated with an extracellular replacement fluid, such as Ringer's lactate, the plasma sodium and chloride concentrations are often increased.[12]
3. It provides glucose.

Administration of glucose is beneficial because it increases the movement of potassium into the cell, thus more rapidly correcting hyperkalemia. Although insulin also has this effect, it is not needed.[12,28] Hyperkalemia is rapidly corrected with fluid replacement and relief of bladder distention. After initiation of fluid therapy, urethral obstruction should be relieved.

After the obstruction is relieved, glomerular filtration rate is only 20-50% of normal and will remain abnormally low for as long as 7 days.[12] This reduction generally is self-limiting and diminishes spontaneously. However, diuresis and increased urinary loss of sodium and potassium, resulting in hypokalemia, commonly occur during this period.[12,28] For this reason additional fluids and electrolytes are often needed during the first several days after the obstruction has been relieved. Failure to provide adequate fluids after relief of obstruction is a common error.

If the cat is not eating and drinking well, following initial rehydration and relief of obstruction, give either intravenously or subcutaneously 60-80 ml/kg/day of an extracellular replacement fluid, such as Ringer's lactate or acetate. An extracellular replacement fluid is not recommended for initial rehydration because it contains 4-5 mEq/L of potassium. However, once initial rehydration and relief of obstruction are accomplished, potassium is needed. If the plasma potassium concentration is less than 3.5 mEq/L, add 10-20 mEq/L of potassium chloride to the fluid.

Oral administration of a nutrient electrolyte fluid, (Life-Guard, Norden Labs), instead of giving fluids parenterally, is effective in maintaining hydration, acid-base, and electrolyte balance when the initial fluid deficit has been corrected. The oral route may be preferred to the parenteral route because it is less costly and an easier treatment. Administration of fluids should continue until the animal is eating and drinking well. Palatable water and a calculolytic diet should always be available.

---

*Harleco Total CO_2 Kit, Harleco Division, American Hospital Supply Corp., Philadelphia, PA 19143. The plasma bicarbonate concentration is the total carbon dioxide in the plasma minus dissolved carbon dioxide, which is about 1 mEq/L.

RELIEVING URETHRAL OBSTRUCTION

If the bladder is severely distended it should be relieved by cystocentesis before an attempt is made to relieve urethral obstruction. This may be possible without sedation if the animal is particularly docile or lethargic. The minimum sedation needed for adequate restraint should be used. A low dose (3-5 mg/cat) of ketamine may be sufficient. However, some veterinarians recommend ketamine alone only when obstruction is acute. Ketamine and barbiturates are potentially toxic in patients with chronic obstruction or renal dysfunction.[77]

As a general rule anesthesia should not be induced if the animal is visibly dehydrated or the plasma potassium concentration is greater than 6 mEq/L. Inhalant anesthetics are preferable because variables associated with renal metabolism and excretion of drugs are eliminated.[77] The inhalants also have the advantage of permitting rapid change in depth of anesthesia and allowing rapid recovery after withdrawal. Halothane using chamber induction and maintenance with a mask, is effective and simple. Giving short acting barbiturates (e.g. thiamylal sodium) intravenously has also been recommended.[77] For dogs, narcotic agents such as oxymorphone (Numorphan, Endo Labs) or fentanyl-droperidol (Innovar Vet, Pitman Moore) have been recommended because their narcotic effects can be reversed. Regardless of the anesthetic used, it should be given cautiously since azotemic patients often require a reduced dosage.

Once restraint is satisfactory, relieve the urethral obstruction. Check the end of the penis for a gelatinous plug or calculus. These sometimes are lodged at the external urethral orifice and can be removed by gentle massage. Plugs in the abdominal or pelvic urethra can be dislodged by infusing a urethral lubricant and massaging the urethra per rectum or vagina. Before palpating the animal, a liberal quantity of a mixture consisting of equal parts sterile isotonic saline solution and sterile aqueous lubricant (Lubfax Surgical Lubricant, Burroughs Wellcome) should be injected through a catheter into the lumen of the urethra next to the urolith.

If the obstruction cannot be relieved by urethral massage, the urolith sometimes can be flushed out by dilating a portion of the urethra with fluid under pressure and then suddenly releasing it. The urolith can almost always be flushed back into the bladder. This is accomplished by using the largest catheter that can be passed easily to the obstruction. Infuse a solution of sterile saline and aqueous lubricant while firmly occluding the distal end of the urethral lumen around the catheter with a finger inserted in the rectum or vagina, or with digital pressure applied around the tip of the penis. The pressure produced by the solution dilates the urethra and flushes the urolith back into the bladder. Gentle digital manipulation may aid movement of the urolith. When treating a dog, it may help to have an assistant simultaneously insert a finger into the rectum and compress the urethra against the pelvic floor. If the urolith cannot be flushed back into the bladder, and bladder distention has not been relieved by cystocentesis, relieve bladder distention and try again. Hydropropulsion has been reported 100% effective in anesthetized dogs with urethral calculi.[73] After the obstruction has been relieved, flush the bladder repeatedly with isotonic saline or Ringer's lactate solution until the returning fluid is clear. Do not use an acid solution; it will remove the glycosoaminoglycans that line the urinary tract and, as a result, enhance adherence of bacteria and crystals to the mucosa.

Although urethral calculi may be pushed back into the bladder with the aid of a catheter, this technique if often unsuccessful and is associated with the greater risk of urethral trauma. Its use is justified only as a last resort. The catheter should be as large and rigid as consistent with atraumatic technique. Liberal amounts of sterile saline and aqueous lubricant solution should be constantly infused through the catheter as the urolith is being pushed toward the bladder. Caution must be used to avoid trauma; excessive force should never be applied.

Use of smooth muscle relaxants has been advocated as an aid in relief of urethral obstruction and to prevent reobstruction, but have not proven to be consistently effective.[77] Response may be inconsistent because both smooth and skeletal muscle surround the urethra.

In many cats obstruction recurs during the first few days after relief of obstruction and they may have temporary bladder atony from previous overdistention.[23,25] In one study 74% of obstructed cats reobstructed within one week.[6] Because of these problems the urethral catheter is sometimes left in place for several days after the obstruction is relieved. However, indwelling catheters in both cats and dogs commonly cause urethral damage and secondary bladder infection that may respond poorly to treatment.[3,56] The longer the catheter is left in, the greater the damage to the urinary tract and greater the risk of urinary tract infection. Urethral damage can lead to severe urethritis, urinary tract infection and, ultimately, stricture formation.[56] Therefore, if possible indwelling catheters should be avoided.

Indications for use of an indwelling urethral catheter are:[57]

1. An inability to restore a normal urine stream
2. An abundance of debris which cannot be lavaged or aspirated from the urinary tract
3. Evidence of bladder atony
4. In critically ill patients when urine formation is being monitored as a guide to fluid therapy

When an indwelling catheter is required:

1. Aseptic technique should be used.
2. The catheter should be as soft as possible and only as long as necessary to reach the preprostatic urethra (15 cm or less for most cats).
3. A closed rather than an open catheter should be used. Leave the catheter closed and aspirate urine every few hours. A closed catheter lessens the risk and delays the development of a urinary tract infection.
4. Antimicrobial drugs should be given while the catheter is in place and for several days afterwards. This delays the development of urinary tract infection, although it increases antibiotic resistant bacteria.[3]
5. It should be left in place for as short a time as possible, preferably not more than three days. In one study, even when all the procedures described above were followed, a urinary tract infection developed in 11 of 20 dogs.[3] In all but 1 of these dogs the catheter was left in for five days or longer as compared to three days or less in 7 of the 9 dogs in which a urinary tract infection did not develop.
6. While the catheter is in place cats may need an Elizabethan-type collar to prevent their removing the catheter.
7. Five to seven days after administration of antimicrobial therapy is discontinued a urine culture and antimicrobial sensitivity should be obtained on a sample taken by cystocentesis. If positive, the appropriate antimicrobial agent should be given.

SURGERY

In the unusual case that urethral obstruction cannot be relieved, surgery may be necessary. Initial rehydration should be completed and intermittent cystocentesis performed to correct dehydration, acid-base and electrolyte disorders, and azotemia, thus lessening anesthetic risk before surgery is performed. Procedures for both a urethrotomy and urethrostomy are described elsewhere.[8,9,92,115,116]

Urethrotomy is preferable to urethrostomy in most cases. However, a urethrotomy should be avoided, if possible, because of the many complications that can occur. These include:

1. Extravasation of urine, creating edema and inflammation
2. Hemorrhage for up to 10 days after surgery
3. Strictures at the surgical site

Urethrostomy to decrease or prevent strictures is preferred by some veterinarians. However, when a urethrostomy is performed, all of the complications of a urethrotomy may occur, including formation of a stricture, up to six months after surgery. Additional complications include rectal perforation during surgery, need for extensive care after surgery, atonic bladder, dehiscence, chronic cystitis routinely occurs, urine scalding, constipation due to nerve damage,[81] and chronically recurring urinary tract infection (Table 12, page 9-25). In addition, the animal may become incontinent, greatly reducing its desirability as a pet. Perineal urethrostomy has been described as a mutilating operation that few persons would choose for themselves and that with proper management is not needed in most clinical cases.[23,33] It is usually done to prevent recurrence of obstruction. However, it is partially or totally ineffective in some cats.[69] In one study, 20% of the cases recurred 1 to 36 months after surgery.[23] Although complications do not develop in all cases, some develop in many cases, even when the surgery is performed by a competent surgeon (Table 12, page 9-25). As stated by a prominent veterinary urology group: "We do not recommend surgical intervention to correct obstructive urethropathy in cats unless no reasonable alternative exists. **Amputation of the distal portion of the penis, or placing a longitudinal incision through a portion of the distal urethral wall, are outmoded techniques** once advocated for immediate relief of urethral obstruction."[78] "There is not one documented controlled prospective study of the effectiveness of feline urethral surgery in male cats with urethral obstruction. It is ironical that some form of proof of efficacy is not mandatory for surgical procedures, especially those that are irreversible."[79] For these reasons, in contrast to the management that has been used and advocated for many years, urethral surgery is not recommended for the vast majority of cases. It is unnecessary if the following dietary management is used.

INITIAL DIETARY MANAGEMENT

After relieving bladder distention and urethral obstruction, and stabilizing the animal's condition if these procedures are necessary, remove all crystals, microcalculi or uroliths from the urinary tract. As

FIGURE 6

RADIOGRAPHIC DEMONSTRATION OF DIETARY UROLITH DISSOLUTION

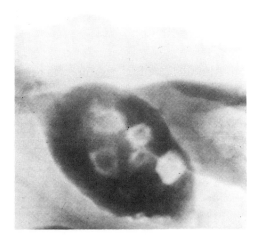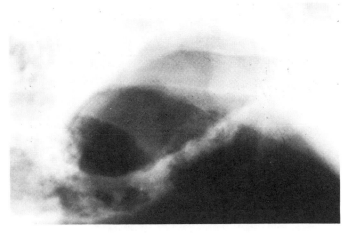

FIGURE 6: Pneumocystograms Demonstrating Dietary Dissolution of Uroliths. **Left**—Cat with 5 cystic struvite calculi. Cat switched to calculolytic diet. **Right**—All calculi dissolved.

shown in Figure 6, this can be accomplished by allowing them to dissolve in the cat. Dissolution is achieved by feeding the cat a calculolytic diet, which reduces urinary magnesium concentration and results in the maintenance of an acid urine. Dietary dissolution is recommended for all cats showing any of the signs of FUS (Table 9, page 9-19), regardless of whether uroliths, microcalculi or crystals can be detected. Uroliths may be too small to detect and no crystals may be present in the urine sediment if the urine is acidic (as it usually is if the cat has not

TABLE 11

CALCULOLYTIC DIET INDUCED DISSOLUTION OF NATURALLY OCCURRING, RADIOGRAPHICALLY VISIBLE UROLITHS IN CATS[76]

Number of Cats	Urinary Tract Bacteria	% of Cases	Results
14	None	64	Dissolved 31.9 days (range 14–36)
5	Urease –	23	Dissolved 23.2 days (range 15–48)
1	Urease +	4	Dissolved 82 days
2	None	9	Surgical removal of: —Ammonium urate after 112 days from one and —60% calcium phosphate + 20% calcium oxalate + 20% struvite after 61 days from the other

consumed a sufficient quantity of food within the last 12-18 hours). However, crystals, microcalculi or uroliths are responsible for causing the clinical signs of FUS in the majority of affected cats. Their dissolution is necessary to alleviate these signs.

As shown in Table 11, in one clinical study radiographically visible uroliths dissolved in 20 of 22 cats fed only the calculolytic diet (Prescription Diet Feline s/d, Hill's).[76,80] No other treatment was given. A urinary tract infection due to non-urease-producing bacteria did not slow the rate of urolith dissolution, whereas a urease-producing bacteria did. However, if there is a urinary tract infection, appropriate antimicrobial therapy should be instituted (page 9-30). In these 20 cats, neither during nor after consumption of the calculolytic diet was there any change in urine specific gravity, body weight, hematocrit or plasma concentrations of albumin, creatinine, calcium, phosphorus, sodium, potassium, chloride, magnesium, total bilirubin, alkaline phosphatase, or alanine aminotransferase.

The calculolytic diet for cats is severely restricted in magnesium (11 mg/100 kcal ME), maintains an acid urine pH (Figure 5, page 9-16) and is relatively high in sodium (0.79% in its dry matter). However, regular commercial canned cat foods contain this same amount of sodium (0.77%, see Table 8, page 11-30). Because of the calculolytic diet's high sodium content it should not be fed if edema, ascites, or congestion are present, or if liver disease or metabolic acidosis is present. Also, its use is not

recommended during growth or reproduction, although it has been successfully used to raise kittens. It is recommended for long-term maintenance only if FUS recurs when the diets recommended for preventing FUS are fed exclusively (Table 5, page 9-10). In contrast to the canine calculolytic diets (Prescription Diets Canine s/d, Hill's) the feline calculolytic diets are not restricted in protein (they contain 35 and 41% protein in their dry matter, Appendix Table A2-6). The calculolytic diets for dogs should not be fed to cats, nor should the one for cats be fed to dogs.

Surgical urolith removal has been used frequently in the past, but most clients greatly prefer dietary dissolution. This probably reflects the treatment they would prefer if they were affected. When surgical means are used the calculi are removed immediately. However, the aftercare required and the increased incidence of postsurgical complications (page 9-23) make surgery less desirable than dietary and medical dissolution. This was well demonstrated by the results of the study shown in Table 12. In this study, 30 cats with naturally occurring radiographically visible uroliths were randomly assigned to one of three treatments. All cats were examined 0.5, 1, 3, 6, and 12 months later. If a urinary tract infection (UTI) occurred, it was immediately and successfully treated. Thus, each UTI recorded is a new episode, not a continuation of a previously detected episode. As shown, there were 10 new episodes of UTI in the 10 cats in

TABLE 12

NUMBER OF EPISODES OF URINARY TRACT INFECTION OCCURRING IN NATURALLY OBSTRUCTED MALE CATS AFTER TREATMENT[74]

Time	Treatment (10 Cats/treatment group)		
	Perineal Urethrostomy Only (PU)*	PU and Dietary Management	Dietary Management Only**
Initial exam	0	0	0
By 12 months after initial treatment	10+	6	0

*By modified Wilson technique performed by a board certified surgeon.

**Fed a calculolytic diet (Prescription Diet Feline s/d, Hill's).

+One cat developed several radiodense uroliths 6 months after surgery and was withdrawn from the study. The uroliths in this cat dissolved when the calculolytic diet and Clavamox (Beecham Labs) were given. Two additional cats developed Staphylococcus spp induced urinary tract infection and radiographically visible uroliths, one at 12 months, and one at 17 months after surgery.

which the treatment consisted of only a perineal urethrostomy; no episodes in the 10 in which the treatment consisted of feeding the calculolytic diet only; and 6 episodes in the 10 in which both surgery and diet were used.

Perineal urethrostomy results in loss of periurethral striated muscle sphincter activity and urethral pressure.[34] This predisposes the urinary tract to more bacterial contamination and subsequent infection. Although urethral pressure was found to have returned to normal in some cats 36-96 months after surgery, a UTI still continued to occur in some of these cats.[34]

DIETARY MANAGEMENT FOR PREVENTION

Feeding a diet low in magnesium and that constantly maintains a urine pH of less than 6.4 is not only beneficial in dissolving uroliths; it is also helps in preventing the high rate of recurrence of FUS. This is well demonstrated by the results of several reports. In one, when a magnesium-restricted, urine-acidifying diet was not fed, FUS recurred in 72 of 101 cats from one week to six months later; 21% had a urethrostomy and 24% died.[6] In contrast, when a high caloric dense, restricted-magnesium, urine-acidifying diet (Prescription Diet Feline c/d, Hill's) was fed, the following results were noted:

1. Recurrence of FUS was prevented in 98% of all cases in one study.[33]

2. None of 91 male cats reobstructed during the three years that they were monitored in another study.[23]

In both of these studies clinical signs recurred repeatedly when the low-magnesium, urine-acidifying diet was discontinued; the signs were alleviated when feeding the diet was reinstituted. In another study, feeding low-magnesium food items (less than 0.10% magnesium in their dry matter) prevented recurrence in 12 of 14 known "stone-forming" cats during the one to three years they were monitored.[45] The urine pH of these cats was not reported. Similar results have also been demonstrated in other species. In 9 of 11 rats, cystic struvite calculi weighing 60 g completely dissolved in four weeks when the magnesium content in the diet dry matter was 0.07%; whereas, the calculi doubled in size when the diet contained 0.27% magnesium.[108] Again, urine pH was not reported. Thus, **not only does the consumption of high-magnesium, high-urine pH inducing diets result in FUS in most cats (page 9-17), low-magnesium, urine-acidifying diets greatly assist in preventing it.**

To prevent FUS the ration should:

1. Result in a urine pH of 6.4 or less and

2. Be sufficiently low in magnesium and high in caloric density so that the diet contains less than 20 mg of magnesium/100 kcal metabolizable energy (ME).

As the caloric density of the food increases, less of it will be consumed, and thus magnesium intake will be reduced. Increasing caloric density of the diet also decreases the quantity of feces and, therefore, the amount of fecal water excreted. As a result more water is excreted in the urine.[92] The greater urine volume and reduced magnesium consumption both lower the concentration of magnesium in the urine.[58,91] The lower this concentration, the less likely struvite crystals and uroliths will form and FUS will occur.

Neither of the two requirements recommended for preventing FUS is, by itself, sufficient to prevent FUS consistently. Struvite calculi formed in 17% of cats in which only urine acidification was employed (Diet 3, Table 8, page 9-17), and hematuria and/or struvite crystalluria occurred in all cats in which only magnesium restriction was used (Diet 2, Table 8). Table 5 (page 9-10) shows the cat foods found to consistently 1) meet the two requirements recommended for preventing FUS, 2) be nutritionally complete and adequate, and 3) have no nutritional imbalances, such as an inverse calcium:phosphorus ratio. It is emphasized that **all of these criteria— urine pH, magnesium content, caloric density, nutritional adequacy and consistency of nutrient content—should be evaluated in making diet recommendations for FUS management.**

The mineral contents of 55 other cat foods are also given in Table 5. The presence of an inverse calcium:phosphorus ratio, as well as their magnesium content, varied widely among different products produced by the same manufacturer and did not differ noticeably among: 1) national, regional, generic or private-label brands, 2) different flavors, or 3) different forms (dry, soft-moist or canned) of cat foods. Therefore, in regard to FUS, no general recommendation can be made for, or against, any specific category, flavor, form or manufacturer of cat food. Recommendations must be for a specific brand and flavor of cat food.

Management Costs

Costs are substantial for managing many clinical conditions. Fortunately such is **not** the case for preventing the occurrence or recurrence of FUS if the form of food remains the same and the recommendations contained herein are followed. Table 13 lists the magnesium content, urine pH, propensity for struvite crystallization, and feeding costs when different cat foods are fed.

It costs less to feed a restricted-magnesium, urine-acidifying dietary food that prevents FUS in the majority of cats than it does to feed either of the two largest selling brands of canned cat foods sold in grocery stores. This is primarily due to the high-water and low-fat contents of these cat foods, and the increased packaging cost of the 3, 6 and 6.5 oz cans. More than 75% of canned cat foods bought in grocery stores are packed in these small cans.[65]

Regardless of the diet, feeding a dry food costs much less. As compared to the annual cost of feeding a regular commercial dry cat food, the increase in cost to feed a restricted-magnesium, urine-acidifying dry food is less than most veterinary physical examinations. The cost is substantially less than treating one episode of FUS or the costs of antibiotics, urinary acidifiers, permanent surgical procedures, or changing from a dry to canned food with or without salt supplementation—all of which have been used in an attempt to prevent the recurrence of FUS. The cost to prevent FUS is less than that of most other preventive medical procedures, such as annual vaccinations. In summary, the cost to manage or prevent FUS it less than that of almost any other disease of the cat.

URINE ACIDIFICATION FOR TREATMENT OR PREVENTION

As discussed on page 9-24, maintaining an acid urine, together with restricting magnesium intake, greatly assists in dissolving and preventing the formation of struvite uroliths. In one study, lowering the urine pH from 6.8 to 6.1 reduced the amount of struvite crystals excreted from 65 to 8 mg/cat/day.[87] It has been shown that 5-g struvite uroliths dissolved in-vitro in four hours at a pH of 4.5, and that uroliths in the cat could be dissolved with no overt damage to the lining of the urinary tract using repeated lavage of a buffered solution having a pH of 4.5.[45] For these reasons, acidification of urine has commonly been attempted to treat or prevent struvite uroliths and FUS.

The two ways to attempt urine acidification are:

1. Feed a diet that metabolizes to form acid ions which are excreted in the urine.

2. Administer a urinary acidifying drug.

Different nutrients (protein, fat, carbohydrate, phospholipids, vitamins, and minerals) and food items have substantially different effects on secretion and buffering of gastric acid and, as a result, on urine

TABLE 13

COST, MAGNESIUM CONTENT, URINE pH AND PROPENSITY FOR STRUVITE FORMATION FOR DIFFERENT CAT FOODS

Cat Food	Pkg. Size	Cost[a] $/pkg.	kcal ME/ 100g	Intake[b] (g/cat /day)	Cost ($/day)	Cost ($/yr)	Magnesium (mg/100 kcal ME)	Urine pH[e]	Struvite Crystallization Propensity[f]
Canned:	oz.								
Regular Commercial[c]	6	0.43	100	240	0.61	223	38	6.7	55
Prescription Diets									
Feline s/d	15	1.163	151	159	0.43	d	11	5.9	1
Feline c/d	15	1.117	141	170	0.44	161	14	5.9	1.5
Science Diet									
Feline Maintenance	15	1.013	139	173	0.41	150	16	6.0	2
Friskies Beef & Liver Dinner	6.5	0.43	100	240	0.56	204	17	6.3	6
Fancy Feast Beef & Liver	3	0.38	102	199	0.89	325	14	NA	—
Homemade (Recipe 8, page A3-3)	26	2.40	207	116	0.38	139	7	NA	—
Dry:	lb.								
Regular Commercial[c]	7 or 10	6.40 or 7.70	352	68	0.13	47	45	6.7	60
Prescription Diets									
Feline s/d	10	NA	432	55	NA	NA	10	6.0	1
Feline c/d	10	14.90	426	56	0.18	66	16	6.0	2
Science Diet									
Feline Maintenance	10	11.95	414	58	0.15	55	17	6.1	3

[a]Grocery store cat foods—Safeway, Topeka, KS. Dietary foods—suggested retail (8/86). For homemade diet: Hamburger $1.30/lb, liver 82¢/lb, calcium carbonate (Tums—8 tabs) 22¢/tsp. and vitamin-mineral capsule 8¢/day. All costs may vary by area, discounts and local sales tax.

[b]Based on an 8 lb cat needing 240 kcal ME/day for maintenance. The amounts given have been confirmed by feeding tests.

[c]Cost and energy content for the largest selling canned cat food (9-Lives) and the average of the two largest selling dry cat foods (Purina Cat Chow and Meow Mix). Magnesium contents given are the mean of that product form (Table 5, page 9–10).

[d]Recommended only for 2–3 months after onset of clinical signs.

[e]Average pH of urine expressed from 12 cats at 7 a.m., noon and 4 p.m. on days 5, 6 and 7 when the diet was always available.

[f]Factor which determines the propensity or struvite crystal formation. It is arbitrarily set at 1 for the food with the lowest value. Thus, for example, the propensity for struvite crystal formation in the cat's urine is 55 times higher when a regular commercial canned food is consumed than when Prescription Diet Feline s/d is consumed. Struvite crystallization propensity determinations were made from a nomogram for the estimation of the saturation of urine with magnesium-ammonium-phosphate[64] using urine magnesium concentrations measured when that diet was fed (Fig. 2) and assuming the same urine ammonium and phosphate concentrations with all of the diets (since these concentrations were not available for all of the diets). However, these concentrations will be lower in the lower magnesium diets, because these diets are also lower in phosphorus. Thus, there is probably an even greater difference in struvite crystallization propensity than that shown.

NA = not available.

pH.[7] This is reflected in the substantially different urine pH that occurs when different cat foods are fed (Figure 5, page 9-16). Feeding a properly formulated diet assures a constantly acid urine pH, while successful use of a urinary acidifier depends on the selection of an effective acidifier, proper dosage, and proper administration by the owner.

Many substances have been used to attempt urine acidification. Tomato juice and garlic have been purported, primarily by folklore, to be urinary acidifiers. However, adding either or both to a canned cat food increased the urine pH from 6.7 to 7.1.[50] Three different brands of tomato juice were tested. The cats loved it, but in addition to elevating urine pH, it caused a marked microcrystalluria. Getting most of the cats to eat the garlic was difficult and, when they did, it resulted in a terrible odor in the cages.

The most commonly used urine acidifiers are:

1. Ethylenediamine dihydrochloride (Chlor-Etha-mine, Pittman Moore)
2. Dl-methionine
3. Ascorbic acid (vitamin C)
4. Ammonium chloride
5. The acid salts of phosphate, most often sodium hydrogen phosphate

Ethylenediamine dihydrochloride has been reported[77] and shown[6] to have no effect on the urine pH of the cat. At the dosages shown in Table 14, sodium acid phosphate, ascorbic acid (vitamin C), and 500-800 mg of methionine/cat/day are all ineffective as urine acidifiers. However, either 1000-1500 mg of methionine or 800 mg of ammonium chloride/cat/day, if properly administered, is quite effective and

TABLE 14

EFFICACY OF URINE ACIDIFIERS IN THE CAT*

Compound Administered	Dose (mg/cat/day)	Urine pH
None	—	6.6–7.2
Sodium acid phosphate[18]	3000	6.6–6.9
Ascorbic acid (Vit C)[18]	1860	6.3–6.9
Ammonium chloride[19,101]	800	5.5–6.2
	1000	6.0
Methionine[18,62,87]	500–800	6.4–6.9
	1000	6.1–6.2
	1500	6.0–6.1

*Compound given in the food, fed once daily. Urine pH measured 4–5 hrs later. A urine pH of 6.4 or less is recommended for FUS treatment.

FIGURE 7

EFFECT OF VARIOUS COMPOUNDS ON FELINE URINE pH WHEN ADDED TO DIET FED ONCE DAILY

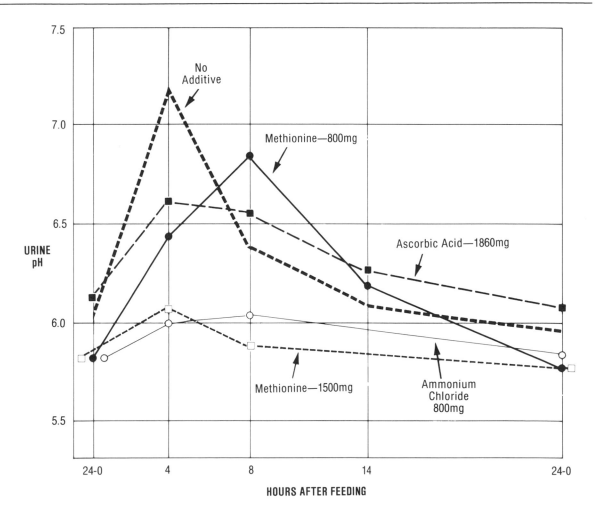

maintains a postprandial urine pH of 6.2 or less (Figure 7).

In the metabolism of the sulfate ($SO_4^=$) containing amino acid methionine, $SO_4^=$ is excreted in the urine as sulfuric acid (H_2SO_4), which in a sufficient amount acidifies the urine. The amount of hydrogen ions excreted in the urine relates directly to the amount of $SO_4^=$ excreted.[15] The hydrogen ions excreted with $SO_4^=$ reduce respiratory acid excretion so that no change in the body's acid-base status occurs unless too much methionine is consumed. Even at a dosage (500 mg/cat/day) less than that necessary for urine acidification, methionine affects struvite urolith formation. It significantly prolonged the interval before obstruction occurred when cats were fed a high-magnesium diet.[17] The effect of methionine on inhibiting calculi formation at this dosage may be because $SO_4^=$ displaced phosphate ($HPO_4^=$) from magnesium-ammonium-phosphate. Chloride (Cl^-) has been shown to have this mode of action in inhibiting formation of struvite uroliths in ruminants.[105] Thus, increased consumption of methionine in the diet is beneficial in dissolving and preventing feline uroliths because it may displace phosphate and, in sufficient amounts, acidifies the urine. A bonus benefit that might be obtained from increased dietary methionine is an improved protein quality of the diet since it is the most limiting essential amino acid in many diets. Excessive methionine consumption, however, is harmful (see item 4, that follows).

Ammonium chloride (NH_4Cl) is an effective urinary acidifier because its ammonia (NH_3) is used for protein synthesis or is excreted as urea. This leaves hydrochloric acid (HCl) which acidifies body fluids, resulting in an acid urine. In a study of 11 cats, ammonium chloride mixed in a dry ration (which resulted in an intake of 800 mg/cat/day) was fed free choice for 11 months. During that time the urine pH was constantly maintained in all 11 cats at 6.4 or less, with an average of 5.9 ± 0.3.[101] This is in contrast to previous undocumented reports that ammonium chloride loses its effectiveness as a urinary acidifier after five to six days.[39]

Methionine is readily available. Ammonium chloride is not available from most drug or veterinary supply companies or pharmacies, but is available from most chemical or laboratory supply companies. Both are present in a dried liver base (MEq, Vet-A-Mix, and Uroeze F.U.S., Daniels Pharmaceuticals). Enteric-coated tablets of ammonium chloride are available but are not recommended. Most enteric-coated tablets are excreted unchanged in the feces and therefore are ineffective.

Ammonium chloride and methionine, when properly administered, are effective urine acidifiers. But there are many reasons for not recommending that clients administer urinary acidifiers.

1. Urine acidifiers are ineffective unless they are consumed with all food eaten. The normal cat's urine pH is routinely about 6.0 except after a meal (Figures 4 and 5 page 9-15 and 16). Thus, the only purpose for a urinary acidifier is to eliminate the postprandial alkaline tide. To do this, the acidifier must be mixed in the cat's food or given each time food is consumed.

2. Urine acidifiers are ineffective if inadequate amounts are consumed (Table 14). This can happen because of either:
   a) Improper instructions to the client
   b) Inadequate compliance by either the client or the cat. In one study, even though proper instructions were given and the importance of following instructions was emphasized, 20-30% of the clients did not comply adequately.

3. Urine acidifiers may be unpalatable, or for some cats cause vomiting. This appears to be more common with ammonium chloride than with methionine.

4. Urine acidifiers may be toxic particularly to kittens that may consume other cats' food to which acidifiers have been added. They may decrease growth and in greater amounts result in death.[10] A dosage of 2 g/mature cat/day for 20 days induced anorexia, ataxia, cyanosis, methemoglobinemia, and Heinz body formation in erythrocytes resulting in hemolytic anemia.[63]

5. Urine acidifiers or a urine-acidifying diet should not be given if the cat has urate calculi, metabolic acidosis or hepatic failure. Urine acidifiers enhance the formation of urate calculi and tend to precipitate hepatic coma in the animal with hepatic failure.[38] However, urate uroliths are uncommon in cats (Table 2, page 9-7). If the animal is obstructed, or anuric, for any reason, until alleviated, acidifiers should not be given since acidosis is generally present.[12,28]

6. Urine acidifiers have been reported to be ineffective in preventing recurrence of urolithiasis when a magnesium restricted diet was not fed.[6,83] However, the prescribed acidifier, ethylenediamine dihydrochloride (Chlor-Ethamine, Pittman Moore) had no effect on urine pH.[6]

7. Urine acidification without restricting magnesium intake (0.37% magnesium in a dry diet) allowed the formation of struvite uroliths in 2 of 12 cats within 11 months even though urine pH was constantly maintained at 5.9.[102]

8. Urine acidifiers are unnecessary when feeding a diet that maintains a urine pH less than 6.4

(Table 13, page 9-27) and are potentially toxic when the calculolytic diet is fed.

9. Urine acidifiers unnecessarily increase the cost of FUS management.

The cat begins to develop metabolic acidosis when its urine pH is reduced to 5.7 or less. When the calculolytic diet is consumed the urine pH in some cats may be as low as 5.8. Thus, giving an acidifier when this diet is fed may induce metabolic acidosis.

Because of these disadvantages **urine acidifiers are not routinely recommended for treatment or prevention of FUS. Feeding a properly formulated diet is much more effective.**

DIURESIS
FOR TREATMENT OR PREVENTION

Inducing diuresis is often used to reduce urine concentration and increase the frequency of urination. Diuresis has been shown to prevent struvite urolith formation in rats.[35] Increased water intake and urine excretion can be induced by adding salt to the diet. From 0.25 to 1 g of salt/cat/day has been recommended.[77] Cats readily accept a high-salt diet,[37,43] and adding 4% salt to the ration dry matter lowered the incidence and severity of hematuria in cats.[43] However, adding 4% salt to the ration dry matter did not decrease the incidence or prolong the time until onset of obstruction in cats fed a diet high in magnesium.[37] In addition, diuresis is unnecessary if a low-magnesium, urine-acidifying diet is fed exclusively.

ANTIMICROBIAL THERAPY

A urinary tract infection (UTI) should be treated if present. However, most cats with FUS do not have a UTI. Therefore, antimicrobial therapy is of no benefit, as was demonstrated in a double-blind study of 20 clinical cases of FUS.[4] In that study, 10 cats were given chloramphenicol. Another 10 were given a placebo. No difference in response to therapy was noted.

A urine culture is necessary only in cases of FUS in which clinical signs are not alleviated within 10-14 days of feeding the calculolytic diet exclusively, or that recur when a low-magnesium, urine-acidifying diet is fed exclusively. If a positive culture is obtained in a urine sample taken by cystocentesis, antimicrobial drugs are indicated. They should be given for two to three weeks if no calculi are present or are no longer visible radiographically following their dietary dissolution or surgical removal. Generally UTI cannot be alleviated until the uroliths are eliminated. Wait five to seven days after the drug

was last given and obtain another urine culture and antimicrobial sensitivity. If the urine culture is positive, reinstitute appropriate therapy. See page 10-19 for a more comprehensive description of treatment for UTI.

CONCLUSIONS

The incidence of FUS is high and may be increasing (Table 1, page 9-3). Although many factors (Figure 1, page 9-5) may cause the array of clinical signs referred to as FUS (Table 9, page 9-19) by far the majority of cases appear to be caused by struvite crystals and calculi. These irritate the lining of the urinary tract, causing cystitis, urithritis, and excessive secretion of mucus. Mucoid plugs or calculi, particularly in males, may obstruct the urethra. Struvite calculi are caused by consuming diets low in caloric density, high in magnesium and that maintain a urine pH greater than 6.6.

If the bladder is severely distented, it should be relieved by cystocentesis and the cat's condition stabilized immediately by giving fluids and electrolytes. The obstruction should then be relieved. For all cats showing any of the clinical signs of FUS, regardless of whether obstruction occurs (and it does not in many cats), a calculolytic diet (Prescription Diet Feline s/d, Hill's) should be fed for two to three months. Urinary acidifiers, other foods, vitamins or minerals should **not** be given while the calculolytic diet is being fed. After two to three months a diet that consistently contains less than 20 mg of magnesium/100 kcal ME and that constantly maintains the urine at 6.4 or less (Table 5, page 9-10) should be fed indefinitely to prevent recurrence, as FUS recurs repeatedly in 50-70% of cats that have previously had the condition if they resume eating regular cat food.[6,29,83] If a low-magnesium, urine-acidifying diet is fed, recurrence is rare.[23,33,45] Urinary acidifiers should not be given if a low-magnesium, urine-acidifying diet is being fed. Crystallization inhibitors such as sodium tripolyphosphate (Curecal, Albion Labs) and tetrasodium ethylene diamine tetraacetate (EDTA), which chelates calcium and magnesium, appear to be of little benefit.[84]

Feeding a low-magnesium, urine-acidifying diet is unnecessary for cats that have never had FUS, but it is a relatively inexpensive means of protecting cats against this common disease ($8-19/yr - Table 13, page 9-27). Other aids in preventing FUS include encouraging exercise and frequent urination, preventing obesity, decreasing confinement, keeping the litter box clean and easily accessible, and always having palatable water easily available.

REFERENCES

1. Andre PG, Jackson OF: Lead foreign body in a cat's bladder. J Small Anim Pract 13:101-102 (1972).

2. Barker J, Povey RC: The feline urolithiasis syndrome: A review and an inquiry into the alleged role of dry cat foods on its aetiology. J Small Anim Pract 14:445-457 (1973).

3. Barsanti JA, Blue J, Edmunds J: Urinary tract infection due to indwelling bladder catheters in dogs and cats. J Amer Vet Med Assoc 187:384-388 (1985).

4. Barsanti JA, Finco DR, Shotts EB, Ross L: Feline urologic syndrome: Further investigation into therapy. J Amer Anim Hosp Assoc 18:387-390 (1982).

5. Bohonowych RO, Parks JL, Greene RW: Features of cystic calculi in cats in a hospital population. J Amer Vet Med Assoc 173:301-303 (1978).

6. Bovee KC, Reif JS, Maguire TG, et al: Recurrence of feline urethral obstruction. J Am Vet Med Assoc 174:93-96 (1979).

7. Brooks FP: Effect of diet on gastric secretion. Amer J Clin Nutr 42:1006-1019 (1985).

8. Brown SG: Surgery of the canine urethra. In Vet Clinics of North America 5(3):457-470 (1975).

9. Brown SG: Urethral surgery. In Current Techniques in Small Animal Surgery. Editor M Joseph Bojrab, Lea & Febiger, Philadelphia, PA pp 228-237 (1981).

10. Brown JE, Fox LM: Ammonium chloride/methionine toxicity in kittens. Feline Pract 14:16-19 (1984).

11. Buffinton CA, Rogers QA, Morris JG: Feline struvite urolithiasis: Magnesium effect depends on urinary pH. Feline Pract 15:29-33 (1985).

12. Burrows CF, Bovee KC: Characterization and treatment of acid-base and renal defects due to urethral obstruction in cats. J Amer Vet Med Assoc 172:802-805 (1978).

13. Carbone MG: Phosphocrystalluria and urethral obstruction in the cat. J Amer Vet Med Assoc 147:1195-1200 (1965).

14. Chan JCM: The influence of dietary intake on endogenous acid production. Nutr and Metab 16:1-9 (1974).

15. Chan JCM: Nutrition and acid-base metabolism. Fed Proc 40:2423-2428 (1981).

16. Chow FHC, Brase JL, Hamar DW, Udall RH: Effect of dietary supplements and methylene blue on urinary calculi. J Urol 104:315-319 (1970).

17. Chow FHC, Dysart I, Hamar DW, Lewis LD, Rich LJ: Effect of dietary additives on experimentally produced feline urolithiasis. Feline Pract 6(5):51-56 (1976).

18. Chow FHC, Taton GF, Lewis LD, Hamar DW: Effect of dietary ammonium chloride, dl-methionine, sodium phosphate and ascorbic acid on urinary pH and electrolyte concentrations of male cats. Feline Pract 8(4):29-34 (1978).

19. Copping JW Jr, Mather GG, Winkler JM: Physiological responses to the administration of cold, room temperature and warm balanced salt solutions in hemorrhagic shock in dogs. Surgery 71:206 (1972).

20. Dickinson CD, Scott PP: Failure to produce urinary calculi in kittens by the addition of mineral salts derived from bone meal in the diet. Vet Rec (Dec 8, 1956).

21. Duch DS, Chow FHC, Hamar DW, Lewis LD: The effect of castration and body weight on the occurrence of the feline urological syndrome. Feline Pract 8(6):35-40 (1978).

22. Dyer DV: Sales jump another 12%. Petfood Industry, pp 10-11 (Nov-Dec 1973).

23. Engle GC: A clinical report on 250 cases of feline urological syndrome. Feline Pract 7(4):24-27 (1977).

24. Eubank M, Fettman M, Hamar D: Dietary magnesium effects on urinary acidification in cats. Parenteral and Enteral Nutr 44(4):1147 Abstr 4308 (1985).

25. Fabricant CG: Feline urolithiasis. Chapter M-20 in Nutrition and Management of Dogs and Cats. Publisher Vet Services, Ralston Purina Co, St. Louis, MO (1980).

26. Finco DR, Barsanti JA: Role of diet in feline urologic syndrome. In Current Vet Therapy IX. Editor RW Kirk, WB Saunders Co. Philadelphia, PA, pp 1112-1114 (1984).

27. Finco DR, Barsanti JA, Crowell WA: Characterization of magnesium-induced urinary disease in the cat and comparison with feline urologic syndrome. Amer J Vet Res 46:391-400 (1985).

28. Finco DR, Cornelius LM: Characterization and treatment of water, electrolyte and acid-base imbalances of induced urethral obstruction in the cat. Amer J Vet Res 38:823 830 (1977)

29. Foster SJ: The "urolithiasis" syndrome in male cats: A statistical analysis of the problems, with clinical observations. J Small Anim Pract 8:207-214 (1967).

30. Gaskell CJ: Urolithiasis in the dog and cat. Vet Rec 102:546-547 (1978).

31. Gershoff SN, Andrus SB: Dietary magnesium, calcium, and vitamin B-6 and experimental nephropathies in rats: Calcium oxalate calculi, apatite nephrocalcinosis. J Nutr 73: 308-315 (1961).

32. Gershoff SN, Prien EL: Effects of daily MgO and vitamin B-6 administration to patients with recurring calcium oxalate kidney stones. Amer J Clin Nutr 20:393-399 (1967).

33. Gilbride AP: Practical approach to cystitis in the cat. Norden News 45(2):6-12 (1970).

34. Gregory CR, Vasseur PB: Electromyographic and urethral pressure profilometry: Long-term assessment of urethral function after perineal urethrostomy in cats. Amer J Vet Res 45:1318-1321 (1984).

35. Grove WJ, Vermeulen CW, Goetz CW, Ragens HD: Experimental urolithiasis II. J Urol 64:549 (1950).

36. Hall MA, Osborne CA, Stevens JB: Hydronephrosis with heteroplastic bone formation in a cat. J Amer Vet Med Assoc 160:857-860 (1972).

37. Hamar DW, Chow FHC, Dysart I, Rich LJ: Effect of sodium chloride in prevention of experimentally produced phosphate uroliths in male cats. J Amer Anim Hosp Assoc 12:514-517 (1976).

38. Hardy RM: Indications for acidifiers and antiseptics in urinary tract disorders. In Current Vet Therapy VI. Editor RW Kirk, WB Saunders Co. Philadelphia, PA pp 1176-1180 (1977).

39. Hardy RM, Osborne CA: The use and misuse of urinary acidifiers. Amer Anim Hosp Assoc Proc pp 276-296 (1973).

40. Hart BL: Feline behavior. Feline Pract 9(2):10-12 (1979).

41. Herron MA: The effect of prepubertal castration on the penile urethra of the cat. J Amer Vet Med Assoc 160:208-211 (1972).

42. Higgins CC: Experimental production of urinary calculi. J Amer Vet Med Assoc 118:81-85(1951).

43. Holme DW: Research into the feline urological syndrome. Proc Kal Kan Symp pp 40-45 (1977).

44. Jackson OF: PhD Thesis. University of London (1971).

45. Jackson OF: The treatment and subsequent prevention of struvite urolithiasis in cats. J Small Anim Pract 12: 555-568 (1971).

46. Jackson OF: Urolithiasis in laboratory and domestic cats. Vet Rec 91:292-293 (1972).

47. Jackson OF: The dry cat food controversy. Urolithiasis in laboratory and domestic cats. Vet Rec 91:292-293 (1972).

48. Jackson OF, as reported by Barker J, Povey RC: The feline urolithiasis syndrome: A review and an inquiry into the alleged role of dry cat foods on its aetiology. J Small Anim Pract 14: 445-457 (1973).

49. Jackson OF, Tovey JD: Water balance studies in cats. Feline Pract pp 30-33 (July 1977).

50. Jackson OF, Tovey JD: Tomato juice as a urinary acidifier. Feline Pract 8:33 (1978).

51. Johnston GR, Feeney DA, Osborne CA: Urethrography and cystography in cats Part I. Techniques, normal radiographic anatomy and artifacts. Comp Cont Ed 4:823-835 (1982).

52. Jorgensen FS: The urinary excretion and serum concentration of calcium, magnesium, sodium and phosphate in male patients with recurring renal stone formation. Scand J Nephrol 9:243-248 (1975).

53. Kallfelz FA, Bresset JD, Wallace RJ: Urethral obstruction in random source and SPF male cats induced by high levels of dietary magnesium or magnesium and phosphorus. Feline Pract 10:25-35 (1980).

54. Klausner JS, Osborne CA, O'Leary TP, et al: Experimental induction of struvite uroliths in miniature Schnauzer and Beagle Dogs. Invest Urol 18:127-132 (1980).

55. Lawler DF, Sjolin DW, Collins JE: Incidence rates of feline lower urinary tract disease in the United States. Feline Pract 15:13-16 (1985).

56. Lees GE, Osborne CA, Stevens JB, Ward GE: Adverse effects of open indwelling urethral catheterization in clinically normal male cats. Amer J Vet Res 42:825-833 (1981).

57. Lees GE: Feline urologic syndrome:Concepts and controversies. Amer Anim Hosp Assoc Proc pp 175-176 (1983).

58. Lewis LD, Chow FHC, Taton GF, Hamar DW: Effect of various dietary mineral concentrations on the occurrence of feline urolithiasis. J Amer Vet Med Assoc 172:559-563 (1978).

59. Lewis LD, Morris ML Jr: Feline urologic syndrome: Causes and clinical management. Vet Med, pp 323-337 (March 1984).

60. Lewis LD, Ponten U, Siesjo BK: Arterial acid-base changes in unanaesthetized rats in acute hypoxia. Resp Phys 19:312-321 (1973).

61. Lewis LD, Ponten U, Siesjo BK: Homeostatic regulation of brain energy metabolism in hypoxia. Acta Physiol Scand 88:284-286 (1973).

62. Lloyd WE, Sullivan DJ: Effects of orally administered ammonium chloride and methionine on feline urine acidity. Vet Med/Small Anim Clin 79:773-8 (1984).

63. Maede Y, et al: Methionie-induced hemolytic anemia with methemoglobinemia and Heinz body formation in erythrocytes in cats. J Japan Vet Med Assoc 38:568-571 (1985).

64. Marshall RW, Robertson WG: Nomograms for the estimation of the saturation of urine with calcium oxalate, calcium phosphate, magnesium ammonium phosphate, uric acid, sodium acid urate, ammonium acid urate and cystine. Clinica Chimica Acta 72:253-260 (1976).

65. Maxwell J: Pet food sales. As reported in Petfood Industry 28(1):23-25 (1986).

66. Morgan AF: Chronic irritation as a cause of bladder stones in cats. Feline Pract 9(4):41-42 (1979).

67. Morris Animal Foundation, 45 Inverness Dr East, Englewood, CO 80112 Survey of feline owners (1977).

68. Osborne CA: Symposium on polyuric renal disease in the dog, presented at Amer Vet Med Assoc Annual Meeting Washington DC, July 22 (1980).

69. Osborne CA: Feline uro-illogical syndrome. Amer Anim Hosp Assoc Proc pp 85-87 (1982).

70. Osborne CA: Feline urolithiasis: Urethral plugs differ from uroliths? DVM 14(7):47 (1983).

71. Osborne CA: personal communication (6/26/85).

72. Osborne CA: Clinical experience with medical dissolution of feline uroliths. DVM (June 1986).

73. Osborne CA, Abdullahi S, Klausner JS, et al: Nonsurgical removal of uroliths from the urethra of female dogs. J Amer Vet Med Assoc 182:47-50 (1983).

74. Osborne CA, Johnston GR, Caywood DC, et al: New insights into management of feline lower urinary tract disease. Proc Amer College Vet Int Med 1:4-7 to 4-10 (1986).

75. Osborne CA, Klausner JS: War on canine urolithiasis: Problems and solutions. Amer Anim Hosp Assoc Proc pp 569-620 (1978).

76. Osborne CA, Kruger JM, Polzin DJ, et al: Prospective clinical evaluation of feline struvite urolith dissolution. Proc Amer College Vet Int Med 1:4-11 to 4-16 (1986).

77. Osborne CA, Lees GE: Feline cystitis, urethritis, urethral obstruction syndrome: Part I, II, III and IV. Modern Vet Pract 59:173-180, 349-357, 513-520, 669-673 (1978).

78. Osborne CA, Lees GE, Polzin DJ, Kruger JM: Immediate relief of feline urethral obstruction. Proc Univ Minn Symposium (1984).

79. Osborne CA, Johnston GR, Polzin DJ, et al: Feline urologic syndrome: A heterogenous phenomenon. J Amer Anim Hosp Assoc 20:17-32 (1984).

80. Osborne CA, Kruger JM, Polzin DJ, et al: Medical dissolution of feline struvite uroliths. Minn Vet 24:22-32 (1984).

81. Parks JL: Complications of urogenital tract surgery. Amer Anim Hosp Assoc Proc pp 391-394 (1977).

82. Rawlings CA: Urethral reconstruction in dogs and cats. J Amer Anim Hosp Assoc 12:850-879 (1976).

83. Reif JS, Bovee K, Gaskell CJ, Batt RM: Feline urethral obstruction: A case control study. J Amer Vet Med Assoc 170:1320-1324 (1977).

84. Rich LJ: Urethral obstruction and urolithiasis in cats. In Current Vet Therapy IV. Editor RW Kirk. WB saunders Co, Philadelphia, PA pp 705-706 (1971).

85. Rich LJ, Dysart I, Chow FC, Hamar DW: Urethral obstruction in male cats: Experimental production by addition of magnesium and phosphate to the diet. Feline Pract 4:44-47 (1974).

86. Rich LJ, Fabricant CG, Gillespie JH: Virus induced urolithiasis in male cats. Cornell Vet 61:542 (1971).

87. Rich LJ, Kirk RW: Feline urethral obstruction: Mineral aspects. Amer J Vet Res 29:2149-2156 (1968).

88. Rich LJ, Kirk RW: The relationship of struvite crystals to urethral obstruction in cats. J Amer Vet Med Assoc 154:153-157 (1969).

89. Robertson WG, Peacock M, Nordin BEC: Activity products in stone-forming and non-stone-forming urine. Clinical Science 34:579-594 (1968).

90. Sadler M: Pet food sales hit $5.1 billion. Pet Food Industry 27:6-10 (1985).

91. Sauer SL, Hamar D, Lewis LD: Effect of dietary mineral composition on urine mineral concentration and excretion by the cat. Feline Pract 15:10-15 (1985).

92. Sauer SL, Hamar D, Lewis LD: Effect of diet composition on water intake and excretion by the cat. Feline Pract 15:16-21 (1985).

93. Schneck GW: Grass seed urinary calculi. Vet Rec 94:431 (1974).

94. Schneider HJ, Hesse A, Hensel K, Unger G, Berg W: Eifluss dur Nohrung auf die Zusammensetzung von Fremdkorpersteinen in Tierexperiment, II. Kalziumoxalat und Magnesiumtherapie, Zert Urol Nephrol 68:1-5 (1975).

95. Scott PP: Some aspects of the nutrition of the dog and cat, II, The cat. Vet Rec 72:5 (1960).

96. Scott PP: Nutritional requirements and deficiencies. In Feline Medicine and Surgery. Editor EJ Catcott, Amer Vet Publ Inc, Santa Barbara, CA (1964).

97. Seefeldt SL, Chapman TE: Body water content and turnover in cats fed dry and canned rations. Amer J Vet Res 40:183-185 (1979).

98. Sherding RG: The clinical manifestations and treatment of the feline urologic syndrome. In Proc Kal Kan Symp pp 32-35 (1977).

99. Stecker JF, Gillenwater JY: Experimental partial urethral obstruction, I. Alteration in renal function. Invest Urol 8:377(1971).

100. Stockman V: Treatment of urolithiasis in the male cat. Vet Rec 93:602-603 (1973).

101. Taton GF, Hamar D, Lewis LD: Evaluation of ammonium chloride as a urinary acidifier in the cat. J Amer Vet Med Assoc 184:433-436 (1984).

102. Taton GF, Hamar D, Lewis LD: Urine acidification in the prevention and treatment of feline struvite urolithiasis. J Amer Vet Med Assoc 184:137-143 (1984).

103. Thrall BE, Miller LG: Water turnover in cats fed dry rations. Feline Pract 6:10-17 (1976).

104. Tomey SL, Follis TB: Incidence rates of feline urologic syndrome (FUS) in the United States. Feline Pract 8:39-42 (1978).

105. Udall RH, Chow FHC: Studies on urolithiasis, VII. The effects of sodium, potassium, or chloride ions in the control of urinary calculi. Cornell Vet LV:538-544 (1965).

106. Vaughn ED, et al: Mechanism of acute hemodynamic response to urethral occlusion. Invest Urol 9:109(1971).

107. Vermeulen CW, Grove WJ, Goetz R, et al: Experimental urolithiasis I: Development of calculi upon foreign bodies surgically introduced into bladders of rats. J Urol 64:541 (1950).

108. Vermeulen CW, Goetz R, Ragens HD, Grove WJ: Experimental urolithiasis IV: Prevention of magnesium ammonium phosphate calculi by reducing the magnesium intake or by feeding an aluminum gel. J Urol 66:6-11 (1951).

109. VonDruska JF: The effect of a rat carcass diet on the urinary pH of the cat. Feline Practice (in press, 1986).

110. Walker AD, Weaver AD, Anderson RS, et al: An epidemiological survey of the feline urological syndrome. J Small Anim Pract 18: 283-301 (1977).

111. Willeberg P: A case-control study of some fundamental determinants in the epidemiology of the feline urological syndrome. Nord Vet Med 27:1-14 (1975).

112. Willeberg P: Diets and the feline urological syndrome: A retrospective case-control study. Nord Vet Med 27:15-19 (1975).

113. Willeberg P: Interaction effects of epidemiologic factors in the feline urologic syndrome. Nord Vet Med 28:193-200 (1976).

114. Willeberg P. Priester WA: Feline urologic syndrome: Associations with some time, space, and individual patient factors. Amer J Vet Res 37:975-978 (1976).

115. Wilson GP: Perineal urethrostomy in cats. J Amer Vet Med Assoc 159:1789-1793 (1971).

116. Wilson GP: Perineal urethrostomy in cats. In Current Techniques in Small Animal Surgery. Editor MJ Bojrab, Lea & Febiger, Philadelphia, PA pp 237-243 (1981).

117. Wilson GP, Dill LS, Goodman RZ: The relationship of urachal defects in the feline urinary bladder to feline urologic syndrome? Proc Kal Kan Symp pp 125-129 (1983).

CHAPTER 10

Canine Urolithiasis

CONTENTS

SUMMARY OF MANAGEMENT RECOMMENDATIONS

OBSTRUCTED CASES

1. **Stabilize the dog's condition.** If the bladder is severely distended, relieve it by cystocentesis. If the dog is visibly dehydrated, lethargic, or comatose, warm fluids to 37-40° and give intravenously over 3-6 hours a mixture of equal parts isotonic saline and isotonic dextrose (0.45% saline and 2.5% glucose) in the amount needed to replace the estimated fluid deficit (% dehydration × kg body weight). Based on the severity of clinical signs, add to this fluid 2.5-10 mEq of bicarbonate/kg body weight (Table 10, page 9-20). After initial rehydration give, either intravenously or subcutaneously, 60-80 ml/kg/day of an extracellular replacement fluid, such as Ringer's lactate. If the plasma potassium concentration is less than 3.5 mEq/L, add 10-20 mEq/L of potassium chloride. Palatable water and food should always be available. Continue giving fluids until the dog is drinking and eating well.

2. Following, if necessary, relief of bladder distention by cystocentesis and stabilization of the dog's condition, **relieve obstruction** by flushing the urolith or plug out of the urethra (as described on page 9-22). Be gentle and use the minimum anesthesia necessary. If a urethral catheter is passed, lubricate it well. Use aseptic techniques, and a catheter as soft and short as possible (page 9-23).

3. **Hospitalize** the dog for at least 5-7 days so that reobstruction can be managed, if it occurs. When the dog is sent home, instruct the client to monitor urination and watch for signs of dysuria during the first several weeks.

ALL CASES

1. **Treat urinary tract infection** (UTI) if present. Obtain a quantitative urine culture and identify bacterial pathogens and their sensitivity. The sample should be taken preferably by cystocentesis to prevent contamination. UTI caused by bacteria sensitive to ampicillin or Tribrissen (Burroughs Wellcome) (Table 4, page 10-12), or Clavamox (Beecham Labs) is present in most cases. If there is any delay in receiving culture results, one of these drugs may be given until the results are obtained. Give orally 25-35 mg/kg of ampicillin three times daily or 10 mg/kg of Tribrissen or Clavamox twice daily. To lengthen the time medicated urine remains in the bladder, allow opportunity for urination only just before the drug is administered. To maximize the rate of drug absorption, do not allow any food to be ingested for at least 30 minutes before or after drug administration. Obtain a urine culture 4-7 days after therapy begins. If the result is positive, therapy is ineffective and should be altered. If the result is negative, therapy is effective and should be continued for at least 2-3 weeks, or if uroliths are present, until 2-3 weeks after they are gone. Four to 7 days after the drug was last given, obtain another urine culture and sensitivity test. If the results are positive, reinstitute appropriate therapy (see page 10-20).

2. **Determine the type of urolith** most likely present in adult males (Figure 9, page 10-17) and treat accordingly to remove them and prevent their recurrence. A summary of the appearance, occurrence, and major factors useful in treating and preventing the different types of uroliths occurring in dogs are described in Table 1 (page 10-4). From 80-97% of uroliths present in males less than 1 year of age (except Dalmatians), and in all females are struvite. For this reason, determining the type of urolith present in these animals may not be warranted except in recurring cases. In contrast, the type of urolith in adult males should be determined, since only 23-60% of these uroliths are struvite.

3. **Urolith removal:**
   a. **Struvite** uroliths can be dissolved by feeding 2-3 times daily a struvite calculolytic diet (Prescription Diet Canine s/d, Hill's) exclusively (page 10-22). Nothing besides this diet

and water should be given (other than an antimicrobial drug if a urinary tract infection is present). This includes urine acidifiers, salt, vitamin or mineral supplements, or any other food. During pregnancy, lactation, heart failure, edema, ascites, or hypertension, the struvite calculolytic diet should not be fed; therefore, the uroliths should be removed surgically.

b. **Ammonium urate** uroliths can be dissolved by feeding 3 times daily a urate calculolytic diet (Prescription Diet u/d, Hill's) and administering 10 mg/kg of allopurinol (Zyloprim, Burroughs Wellcome) 3 times daily (page 10-28). If the urine pH is not maintained at 7-7.5, add to the diet **just enough** sodium bicarbonate (baking soda) to maintain this pH. Generally less than 1 g (1/4 tsp)/5 kg at every feeding will be needed.

c. As uroliths dissolve they may be excreted and obstruct the urethra. This occurs rarely with struvite uroliths but occasionally with urate uroliths. In these cases the uroliths can be easily returned to the bladder by hydropropulsion (page 9-22).

d. These calculolytic procedures should be continued until 4 weeks after the uroliths are no longer visible radiographically, except for immature dogs; they should be subject to the procedures only until the uroliths can no longer be seen radiographically. If the radiographic size or density of the uroliths has not decreased within 60 days, the procedures have been followed exactly as described, and a urinary tract infection, if present, is controlled (a negative urine culture is present), the uroliths are probably not struvite or ammonium urate. Therefore, they should be removed surgically and analyzed quantitatively.

e. Urolith dissolution, when possible, as compared to surgical removal:

   1) Is preferred by most informed clients
   2) Is less expensive
   3) Decreases the risk of recurrence because it assures that all uroliths are removed
   4) Alleviates the risk, time, and aftercare involved with surgery

4. **Prevention of recurrence:**

   a. In all cases, always ensure that a urinary tract infection is not present or is controlled (see page 10-20 for control procedures).

   b. If **any type of urolith** occurs more than once, prophylactic management is definitely warranted to prevent recurrence. In these cases, after dietary dissolution or surgical removal of the urolith the following procedures should be carried out.

   c. For **struvite** uroliths, feed a urine-acidifying, maintenance-type diet (Prescription Diet Canine c/d, Hill's). This diet is nutritionally adequate for adult maintenance and is lower in protein, calcium, phosphorus and magnesium than regular commercial dog foods (Table 9, page 10-24). It decreases urine concentration of the struvite constituents, magnesium, ammonium, and phosphate, and maintains a urine pH of 6.2. All of these effects greatly assist in preventing struvite urolith formation. Administration of urine acidifiers with this diet is not recommended. Salt supplementation is not usually required.

   d. For **ammonium urate, calcium oxalate, or cystine** uroliths feed a urine-alkalinizing, low-protein, low-purine, low-oxalate diet (Prescription Diet u/d, Hill's). This diet is nutritionally adequate for adult maintenance and is much lower in protein, urate precursors, calcium, phosphorus, magnesium, oxalate, and cystine than other dog foods (Table 9, 10-24). It decreases urine concentration of the constituents of all of these uroliths and maintains an alkaline urine. Although urine pH has no effect on calcium oxalate formation, an alkaline urine greatly assists in preventing ammonium urate and cystine uroliths.

   e. If **ammonium urate** uroliths recur when the procedures described are followed, allopurinol administration is indicated. If urine pH is not maintained at 7.0-7.5, adding sodium bicarbonate (baking soda) to the diet at each feeding is indicated. Generally less than 1 g (1/4 tsp)/5 kg will be needed. Allopurinol and sodium bicarbonate are recommended only if the uroliths recur in the absence of a urinary tract infection, and when u/d is the only food consumed. Neither salt supplementation nor administration of a diuretic is recommended.

   f. If **calcium oxalate** uroliths recur in the absence of a urinary tract infection and when Prescription Diet u/d (Hill's) is the only food consumed, the following procedures may be helpful.

      1) If hypercalcemia is not present, administer a thiazide diuretic.
      2) Give orally, potassium citrate (Polycitra-K syrup, Willen Drug or Uroeit tablets, Mis-

sion Pharmaceutical). Optimum canine dosage has not been established. Dosage for the human adult is 50-100 mg/kg/day. The pediatric dose is 5-15 ml of the syrup/day (page 10-31).

3) Salt supplementation, sodium bicarbonate, urine acidifiers, and vitamin C are contraindicated as they increase urine excretion of calcium or oxalate.

g. If **cystine** uroliths recur in the absence of a urinary tract infection and when Prescription Diet u/d (Hill's) is the only food consumed, administration of D-penicillamine (Cupri-

mine, Merck Sharpe & Dohme) is indicated. Give 5-15 mg/kg twice daily in the diet. If the urine pH is not maintained near 7.5, sodium bicarbonate (baking soda) supplementation may be helpful. Usually less than 1 g/5 kg of sodium bicarbonate at each feeding (2-3 times daily) is adequate. Urinary acidifiers, methionine, and possibly exess sodium are contraindicated as they enhance formation of cystine uroliths.

h. If **silicate** uroliths recur, prevent ingestion of dirt, avoid diets high in plant proteins or those that contain soybean hulls, and add salt to the diet (1g or 1/4 tsp/5 kg/day).

TABLE 1

APPEARANCE, OCCURRENCE TREATMENT AND PREVENTION OF CANINE UROLITHS

Urolith Type	Composition	Causitive or Predisposing Factors[a]	Distinguishing Features[b]	Occurrence	Treatment[c]	Prevention of Recurrence	
						Initially[c]	If Recurs[d]
Struvite	MgNH$_4$PO$_4$ ± small amounts Ca and urate	↑ intake Mg, P & protein & urease producing bacteria	Generally radiopaque	80–97% of uroliths in females & immature males, 50–75% of uroliths in adult males	Feed struvite calculolytic diet[e] only	Feed urine-acidifying maintenance diet only[f]	Add salt to diet, 1g (¼ tsp)/ 5 kg/day
Ammonium Urate	NH$_4$ Urate ± small amounts phosphate and/or oxalate	↑ protein, muscle & organ tissue intake. ↓ liver function & shunts	Often concentric laminations on cross section, ± radiolucent	Especially male Dalmatians & any breed with liver disease	Feed urate calculolytic diet[g] plus allopurinol[h]		Give allopurinol,[h] and if urine pH not 7-7.5 give sodium bicarbonate
Calcium Oxalate	Ca oxalate ± small amounts of phosphate	High Ca, Na, oxalate, vit. D & C intake. Ethylene glycol intake. ↑ PTH, osteolysis, renal dysfunction and acidosis	Smooth or sharp crystals on surface, & radiopaque	Often in acid urine. 10–20% of uroliths in adult males		Feed urine-alkalinizing, low-protein, low-purine, low-oxalate diet only[g]	Give thiazide diuretic and potassium citrate[i]
Cystine	Cystine	Inherited defect in cystine reabsorption	Moderate radiopacity	Adult males only, often in acid urine	Surgical removal		Give D-penicillamine.[j] If urine pH not near 7.5, give sodium bicarbonate
Silicate	Silicon dioxide	Probably high silicate intake	Spiculed or "jack stones"	Males, especially German Shepherds		Avoid diets high in plant proteins, ↓ dirt ingestion	Add salt to diet 1 g (¼ tsp)/ 5 kg/day

[a]Reduced urine volume and frequency of urination predisposes to all types of uroliths.

[b]See Fig. 3 (page 10–13) and Table 5 (page 10–13) for urine crystals that may be poresent with each type of urolith.

[c]In all cases eliminate or control urinary tract infection if present (page 10–20).

[d]Recommended only if there is recurrence when previous management is strictly followed.

[e]Prescription Diet Canine s/d (Hill's). Do not give acidifiers, salt, vitamin or mineral supplements or any other food item.

[f]Prescription Diet Canine c/d (Hill's). Do not give acidifiers, salt, vitamin or mineral supplements or any other food item.

[g]Prescription Diet u/d (Hill's).

[h]Zyloprim (Burroughs Wellcome) 10 mg/kg three times daily.

[i]Polycitrate-K syrup (Willen Drug) or Uroeit tablets (Mission Pharmaceutical) 50–100 mg/kg/day or 1 ml of syrup/kg/day.

[j]Cuprimine (Merck, Sharpe & Dohme) 5–15 mg/kg twice daily in the diet.

INTRODUCTION

Urolithiasis is a disease caused by the presence and effects of uroliths or excessive amounts of crystals in the urinary tract. Crystals or uroliths may irritate the mucosal lining, resulting in either or both the frequent voiding of oftentimes bloody urine, or obstructions of the urinary tract. The disease is referred to by many names, including cystitis, urethritis, urinary calculi, bladder stones, or kidney stones. A common disease affecting cats, dogs, humans, and ruminants, it is uncommon in horses and is rare in swine.

INCIDENCE

It is estimated that from 0.4-2.8% of all dogs develop urolithiasis.[10] In a closed colony of pure-bred Beagle dogs (Argonne National Laboratories) 2.6% (55 of 2125) developed struvite uroliths in 17 years.[33] This incidence is probably more accurate than others, at least for Beagles under this type of management, because the population at risk is defined. However, the incidence may be different for other breeds or even other lines of Beagles. Only 2.0% of the outbred line of these Beagles developed

TABLE 2

INCIDENCE OF DIFFERENT TYPES OF CANINE UROLITHS ANALYZED[a,11,78]

% of All Uroliths Analyzed[b]	Type of Urolith
64–69[c]	Struvite
7.4–10	Calcium oxalate
5.3–7	Urate[d]
2.4–3.5	Silicate
2.2–3.2	Cystine
1–2.4	Calcium phosphate
10.8	Nucleus and 1 or more layers of different types
4.6–6	Mixed (<70–80% of any one type)[e]
0.6	Matrix

[a]Based on quantitative analysis of 272 and 1147 canine uroliths in the two studies. Unless stated otherwise, the urolith consisted of 70-80% or more (in the majority 100%) of that substance with no nucleus or shell detected.

[b]The percentage obtained in the two studies.

[c]Since struvite uroliths are commonly dissolved by feeding a struvite calculolytic diet and therefore are not available for analysis, and because frequently the only uroliths analyzed are those that do not dissolve when this diet is fed, it is quite probable that **the actual percent of struvite uroliths occurring in the dog is higher than the percent obtained for analysis as shown here.**

[d]Of which 92% were ammonium acid urate, 4% sodium acid urate and 4% uric acid.

[e]82% have struvite as the main component.

struvite uroliths; whereas 10.7% of their inbred line were affected. The difference in the incidence between different breeds and different strains of the same breed suggests hereditary involvement in struvite urolith formation.

The breeds most commonly affected, listed in order of highest to lowest incidence (13- to 3-times greater incidence than other breeds) are Welsh Corgi, Miniature Schnauzer, Pug, Lhasa Apso, Pekingese, and Yorkshire Terrier.[11] Beagles, Dachshunds, Dalmatians, Pugs, Bulldogs, Basset Hounds, Cairn Terriers, and Scottish Terriers have also been reported to be more commonly affected, and German Shepherds and Boxers less commonly affected than other breeds.[10,11,16] Except for Dalmatians, small breeds are affected more frequently than large breeds.[10]

About 94% of all cases occurring in dogs less than 1 year old are in males.[29] However, in mature dogs urolithiasis appears to occur with equal frequency in adults of both sexes.[10] As expected, urethral obstruction is more prevalent among males than females because of the male's longer, narrower urethra. Eighty-one percent of all urolithiasis cases occur in dogs 2-10 years old, but it may occur in dogs less than 2 months old.[29] The mean age of occurrence is 5-8 years[10,29,70] except for carbonate uroliths, for which the mean is 12.3 years.[10]

CAUSES

Urolithiasis is caused by the presence and affect of uroliths or crystals in the urinary tract. In dogs they can be composed of any of the six substances shown in Table 2. Struvite is by far the most common, followed in decreasing order of incidence by, calcium oxalate, ammonium urate, silicate, cystine, and calcium phosphate. Among analyzed canine uroliths, 46% are composed entirely of, and 95% contain over 70% of, a single one of these 6 substances.[78] Only about 5% are a mixture of these constituents, although nearly 11% had one or more layers of more than one of these substances (Table 2). These six substances are dispersed as crystals in a characteristic and highly organized fashion. They are often, but not always, formed around a nucleation center or mucoprotein matrix. The organic matrix makes up less than 5% of the urolith.[66]

There are many theories for the initiation and growth of urine crystals and uroliths. However, an essential requirement is supersaturation of urine with urolith-forming constituents.[79] A crystal cannot be formed if urine is undersaturated with the crystal components. Thus, the formation of urine crystals and uroliths, and as a result urolithiasis, is caused by the following factors:

1. A sufficiently high urine concentration of urolith-forming constituents
2. Adequate time in the urinary tract
3. A urine pH favorable to crystallization
4. A nucleation center or nidus on which to form
5. A decrease in crystal or urolith formation inhibitors

The more conducive to urolith or crystal formation any one or more of these factors is, the less conducive the other factors need to be for urolith or crystal formation. However, uroliths cannot form without sufficient raw materials and time. The third factor, urine pH, affects struvite crystals, which form best in an alkaline urine, and cystine and urate crystals, which form best in an acid urine. Urine pH has little effect on calcium oxalate or silicate crystal formation. The fourth factor, a nucleation center or nidus, although not required, enhances urolith formation. This nidus may be foreign bodies,

bacteria, viruses (or damage or debris from their presence) or cells sloughed from the lining of the urinary tract. For example, in 2 dogs a grass seed and awn were found to have acted as a nidus, resulting in the formation of struvite uroliths around them.[61,99]

A **vitamin A** deficiency may result in increased debris available to serve as a nucleation center. Vitamin A is necessary for maintaining the integrity of epithelial and mucosal surfaces. A deficiency increases squamous metaplasia and sloughing of epithelial cells lining the urinary tract. Although a vitamin A deficiency has been associated with struvite uroliths in rats,[31] it has not been involved with uroliths in either cats or dogs, and is not considered to be a causative or predisposing factor in either of these two species. In addition, giving vitamin A has never been demonstrated to be of any benefit in treatment or prevention of urolithiasis in cats or dogs.

FIGURE 1

PATHOGENESIS OF UROLITH FORMATION

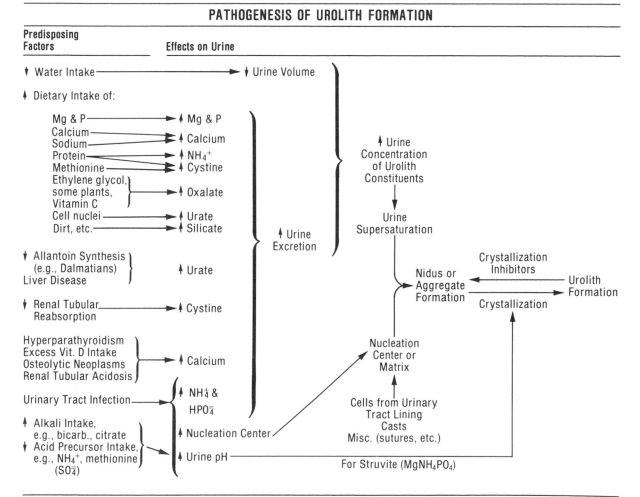

A decrease in **crystal-formation inhibitors** in the urine would enhance urolith formation. A glycoprotein that inhibits calcium oxalate crystallization has been found in human and rat urine and kidney.[62,63] In people who develop calcium oxalate nephroliths, this glycoprotein does not contain the gamma-carboxyglutamic acids needed to inhibit calcium oxalate formation.[64] Whether this occurs in animals, and if it does, what role it plays in them or in people in predisposing to calcium oxalate urolith formation is not known. Currently there is no evidence that urine contains other crystallization inhibitors.[96]

Anything that results in or increases any one or more of the five factors that enhance crystal and urolith formation will predispose to urolithiasis. Conversely, anything that lessens any of them assists in preventing urolithiasis. The first four factors are affected by urinary tract infection, diet, urine volume, frequency of urination, and genetics. The importance of each in causing or predisposing to urolithiasis or, conversely, in preventing it, differs in different species, and for different types of uroliths. Factors that contribute to urolith formation are summarized in Figure 1.

URINARY TRACT INFECTION (UTI)

A UTI is present in 50-97% of dogs with struvite urolithiasis and is a major factor causing the formation of these uroliths.[10,11] Although a UTI may be present in dogs with other types of uroliths, it is less common and occurs as a result, not as a cause, of nonstruvite uroliths.[72,74] Bacteria are commonly cultured from inside struvite uroliths, but rarely from nonstruvite uroliths.[6,72] This suggests that the bacteria were present when the struvite urolith formed.[74] In one study of normal dogs that had never had urolithiasis, struvite uroliths formed within 2-8 weeks after induction of a *Staphylococcus aureus* UTI.[34] Struvite uroliths are sometimes referred to as "infection stones" and nonstruvite uroliths as "metabolic stones." Both are poor terminology as UTI is not present in some dogs and most cats with struvite urolithiasis, and altered metabolism is not responsible for most nonstruvite uroliths.

A UTI enhances struvite urolith formation in the following ways:

1. It increases the material available to serve as a nucleation center on which the uroliths may form.

2. Because most of the bacteria responsible (*Staphylococcus* and *Proteus* spp.) produce urease, their presence increases the urine pH, and the amount of ammonium (NH_4^+) and phosphate (PO_4^{-3})

FIGURE 2

THE ROLE OF UREASE IN MAGNESIUM-AMMONIUM-PHOSPHATE (STRUVITE) UROLITH FORMATION*

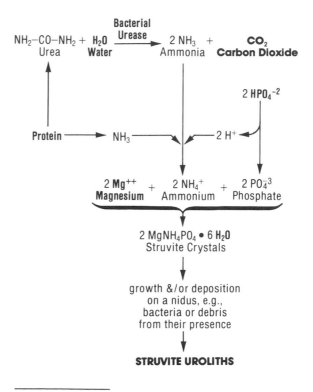

*Bold Print are substances needed, and **BOLDEST PRINT** are substances produced, by these reactions.

ions available for formation of struvite, which is magnesium-ammonium-phosphate-hexahydrate.

The mechanism of action of bacterial urease is shown in Figure 2. A persistent UTI not only may lead to struvite urolithiasis, but also pyelonephritis and eventual renal failure are major sequele.[46] Often there are no signs of a UTI until these consequences appear. Because of this, and because long-term corticosteroid therapy results in UTI in many dogs (39% of 71 in one study[21]), a urine culture should be obtained monthly from dogs being given corticosteroids for more than a brief period.

It is emphasized that UTI is only one factor that predisposes to, but is not needed for, struvite formation. A UTI cannot induce struvite formation if the urine lacks a sufficiently high concentrations of magnesium (Mg^{++}) and phosphate (HPO_4^{-2}), and if the struvite crystals formed are not sufficiently concentrated or retained in the urinary tract long

enough to allow them to grow or be deposited on a nucleation center. As shown in Figure 2, if bacterial urease is present, urea, magnesium, and phosphate at sufficiently high concentrations are all necessary for struvite urolith formation; whereas if bacterial urease is not present, ammonium ions (NH_4^+) rather than urea are necessary. A high protein intake results in an increased urinary concentration of both urea and ammonium and thus aids struvite urolith formation whether or not a UTI is present. Conversely, dietary protein restriction aids in prevention of struvite urolith formation by reducing urinary urea and ammonium concentrations.[67]

HIGH URINE CONCENTRATION OF UROLITH CONSTITUENTS

The greater the urine concentration of urolith constituents and the less often urination occurs, the greater the chance for urolith formation. Urine concentration increases and frequency of urination decreases with reduced water intake. Water intake decreases with lessened physical activity. Castration, obesity, cold weather, confinement and locomotion problems all lessen physical activity and thus water intake. Decreased water intake may also occur because water is not readily available, too cold or warm, or is of poor quality or palatability.

Consumption of water high in phosphate, carbonate, silicate, calcium, or magnesium (hard water) is generally thought to be of little or no consequence in clinical urolithiasis because the amounts of these minerals consumed in the water is much less than the amounts consumed in the diet. Water, even when it contains the upper safe level of hardness (200 ppm of calcium plus magnesium[65]), would supply only 1-8% of the total daily intake of calcium and magnesium. In addition, the greater the water intake, the greater the urine volume and lower the urine concentration, which is not the case when the urolith constituents are consumed in food. However, high amounts of calcium in drinking water (100 ppm) have been reported responsible for causing calcium oxalate nephroliths in people and boiling the water helps prevent their recurrence.[87] Boiling water decreases its calcium content (in this study 5-fold) as a result of calcium carbonate precipitation. However, diet plays a much more important role than water in causing or preventing the formation or dissolution of uroliths in the majority of cases. The role played by diet differs for the different types of uroliths.

Struvite Urolith Causes

Struvite uroliths are composed primarily or exclusively of magnesium-ammonium-phosphate hexa-hydrate crystals. They frequently contain small amounts (less than 10%) of calcium phosphate (apatite) and, less commonly, ammonium urate crystals.[11] Such uroliths are frequently referred to as "double" or "triple phosphate calculi," depending on the number of cations present (magnesium and ammonium, with or without calcium). In dogs, calcium phosphate also commonly occurs as a part of oxalate uroliths, but rarely occurs by itself. Pure calcium phosphate nephroliths have been induced experimentally in both cats[43] and rats,[100] but have not been induced in dogs, nor do they appear to occur clinically in dogs.

Magnesium, phosphate and calcium concentrations in the dog's urine have been shown to relate directly to the amount consumed.[59] Urine ammonium ion and urea concentration relate directly to the amount of protein in the diet.[59] Thus, the higher the intake of these minerals and protein, the more likely struvite uroliths are to form. In one study, cystic struvite calculi increased in size 5.5 times in 6 months in 6 dogs with a urinary tract infection (UTI) being fed a regular commercial dog food.[68] In contrast, the calculi dissolved within 6 months in 5 of 6 dogs with UTI, and 6 of 6 dogs without UTI, being fed a diet severely restricted in protein, phosphorus, and magnesium. Excess urinary excretion of these minerals as a result of renal, hormonal, or other dysfunctions would also be expected to enhance struvite urolith formation. However, this has not been demonstrated for struvite uroliths[74] but has been for other types of uroliths in dogs.

Ammonium Urate Urolith Causes

Urate uroliths in dogs are composed primarily of ammonium urate; in people they are composed primarily of uric acid. A sufficiently high urine concentration of both ammonium ions (NH_4^+) and urate is necessary for formation of ammonium urate uroliths.[88] A high urine concentration of either one without the other will not result in ammonium urate uroliths.

Urinary ammonium ion concentration increases with increased protein intake (and therefore NH_2 intake), decreased urine pH (acidity), decreased hepatic function and urinary tract infection with urease-producing organisms (Figure 2, page 10-7). Although a urinary tract infection has been reported present in from 3-80% of dogs with ammonium urate uroliths,[10] it is generally considered to be a sequela to, rather than a cause of, their formation.[74] Decreased hepatic function decreases ammonia (NH_3) conversion to urea, and urate conversion to allantoin, resulting in increased urinary excretion of both; thus, enhancing ammonium urate urolith formation. Ammonium urate crystals commonly

occur in dogs with portosystemic shunts.[52] Lymphoproliferative disorders also increase urine urate excretion by increasing endogenous urate production, and as a result predispose to urate urolith formation.[93]

Adult male Dalmatians and English Bulldogs appear to suffer a higher incidence of urate uroliths than other dogs.[75] The reason is well understood for Dalmatians. They, in contrast to all other dogs, normally excrete a high amount of urate in the urine because of minimal conversion of urate to allantoin in the hepatic cells[26] and reduced renal tubular reabsorption of urate.[107] Their decreased production of allantoin, and as a result increased plasma urate concentration, is also responsible for causing the **"bronzing syndrome."** This syndrome is characterized by patchy alopecia, giving a moth-eaten, motley appearance to the coat, reddish-brown discoloration of the white hair (bronzing), and predisposition to secondary skin infections.[91] Pruritus, urticaria, and erythema also may be present. The same dietary factors described for preventing urate urolith formation (page 10-29) result in marked clinical improvement of the "bronzing syndrome."

Urinary urate concentration is increased by the increased intake of purines. Purines, which are a major constituent of nucleic acids present in cell nuclei, are converted by the liver to urate. Cell nuclei are high in glandular organs and muscle tissues. These tissues are also high in protein. Therefore, a diet high in these tissues increases both urate and ammonium ion excretion. Although this is important for preventing recurrence of ammonium urate uroliths, it is probably of little concern in regard to animals never before affected.

Calcium Oxalate Urolith Causes

Anything that increases urinary calcium or oxalate excretion, or reduces urinary calcium oxalate inhibitors, predisposes to or causes calcium oxalate urolith formation. As shown in Table 3 many factors can cause these effects. The occurrence and relative importance of any of them as a cause of calcium oxalate urolithiasis in dogs or cats is unknown. Some, as indicated in the table, are not known to occur, or are not known to play a role in naturally occurring calcium oxalate formation in dogs or cats.

Silicate Urolith Causes

A high silicate intake is an important factor in predisposing to, or is the cause of, silicate urolith formation. They are the most common uroliths in grazing ruminants. During grazing, ruminants ingest sand (silicon dioxide). Silicate uroliths develop in people who consume large quantities of the antacid magnesium trisilicate used in treatment for peptic ulcers.[70,71] When the dog absorbs silica, it is rapidly excreted in the urine.[55] A diet containing 12% silicic acid and 3% magnesium silicate resulted in silicate uroliths in dogs within 4 months.[55] A high incidence of silicate nephroliths has been reported for wild native dogs, but not pet dogs, in Kenya (125 of 241 were affected).[7] It was suggested that the silicate content might be high in the corn consumed by these wild dogs. Silicate uroliths in several breeds of dogs have been reported, but occur most commonly in German Shepherds. It is not known whether this breed is more likely to consume dirt and therefore silica, or whether some other factor is involved in the breed's apparent increased susceptibility to this disease.

Cystine Urolith Causes

Cystine uroliths occur as a result of an inherited defect in renal tubular reabsorption of the amino acids cystine and lysine. The result is an increase in their excretion in the urine.[110] The only known clinical consequence of this defect is the formation of cystine uroliths, which are insoluble.[110] Although this defect occurs in both sexes in people, in dogs it is transmitted by a sex-linked inheritance that occurs only in males.[110]

The urine concentration of cystine or lysine can be measured as a screening test to identify dogs that have this defect and are therefore susceptible to cystine urolithiasis. The defect is present if the urine cystine/creatinine ratio is greater than 75 mg/g, or the lysine/creatinine ratio is greater than 25 mg/g in non-fasted dogs.[15,109] These values are normal, however, during fasting.

CLINICAL SIGNS

Clinical signs of urolithiasis depend on the degree and duration of either or both obstruction, or irritation of the mucosal lining of the urinary tract caused by uroliths, crystals, or urinary tract infection. The resulting signs, the same in both dogs and cats, are described on page 9-18.

DIAGNOSIS

Clinical signs and physical examination usually are all that is needed to accurately diagnose urolithiasis. If urethral obstruction is present, the bladder will be distended or, rarely, ruptured. If the bladder is ruptured, it cannot be palpated, but there are large amounts of urine in the abdominal cavity. If suspected, this condition can be confirmed by paracentesis. If the bladder is not ruptured and

TABLE 3

CALCIUM OXALATE UROLITH FORMATION — CAUSES AND PREDISPOSING FACTORS

Effect	Cause	Abnormality	Plasma Concentration[a]	
			Calcium	PTH
Hypercalciuria				
Absorptive	Excess intestinal calcium absorption	1. Unknown in most cases 2. Excess 1,25-vit D production[32,b] 3. High calcium intake	N N N	N to ↓ N to ↓ N to ↓
Renal-leak	Decreased renal tubular Ca reabsorption[85,106]	1. Renal dysfunction 2. High sodium intake 3. Furosemide administration	N to ↓ N N	↑ N N
Reabsorptive	Excess Ca resorption from bone	1. Primary hyperparathyroidism[c] 2. Pseudohyperparathyroidism 3. Excess vitamin D intake 4. Osteolytic neoplasms 5. Hyperthyroidism[39]	↑	N to ↑
Mixed	Renal-leak, resorptive and decreased plasma protein binding of Ca[106]	1. Metabolic acidosis, e.g. excess administration of urine acidifiers	Normal	Normal
Hyperoxaluria				
Absorptive	Excess intestinal oxalate absorption	1. Inherited defect in 79% of people with recurring Ca or oxalate calculi[2,b] 2. High oxalate intake[89]		
Productive	Excess endogenous oxalate production	1. Rare genetic disorder[116,b] 2. Excess vitamin C intake[4] 3. High galactose (e.g. milk lactose) intake[94,b] 4. Ethylene glycol (antifreeze) ingestion[19,25] 5. Vitamin B$_6$ (pyridoxine) deficiency[b]		
Reduced Urinary Calcium Oxalate Inhibitors				
Crystallization inhibitors	Abnormal urine glycoprotein[62,63]	Absences of gamma-carboxy-glutamic acids[64,b]		
Calcium binders	Increased renal tubular reabsorption of citrate[98]	Acidosis, hypomagnesemia, hypokalemia		
Oxalate binders	Decreased potassium excretion	Hypokalemia		

[a]PTH is parathyroid hormone, N normal, ↓ decreased and ↑ increased.

[b]Not known to occur or to play any role in calcium oxalate urolith formation in dogs or cats.

[c]Although uncommon in dogs, it is the only cause of resorptive hypercalciuria that has been associated with calcium-containing uroliths in dogs.[78] It should be considered when both hypercalcemia and hypercalciuria are present. In hyperparathyroidism from any cause, PTH increases renal calcium reabsorption; and therefore, initially urinary calcium excretion decreases, but later it increases. This increase occurs because of increased filtered calcium occurring as a result of PTH-induced hypercalcemia and PTH-induced renal damage (as described on page 8-34).

the urethra is obstructed, the bladder will be hard, distended, painful, and cannot be expressed. Urethral calculi may be detected and their site located by passing a catheter.

Abdominal palpation and, if necessary, simultaneous rectal or vaginal digital palpation, are often helpful in detecting the presence of cystitis, or cystic, or urethral calculi. The bladder wall may be thickened and give a grating sensation when palpated. Although a sufficiently large urolith may be palpated and multiple uroliths may be recognized by a grating sensation, palpation cannot be depended on to reveal all cases of cystic calculi. Multiple uroliths are often throughout the urinary tract; therefore, a complete radiographic or sonographic examination of the entire urinary tract is indicated.[57]

Urine pH, culture and sensitivity tests, and examination of the urine sediment to determine the presence and quantity of red and white blood cells, and type of crystals, are quite helpful. These tests are valuable in determining the number, location, and type of uroliths present so that optimal therapeutic and prophylactic measures can be instituted. The presence of a urinary tract infection has little effect on the hemogram. Varying degrees of azotemia may be present, depending on the degree and duration of obstruction of the urinary tract.

RADIOGRAPHIC EXAMINATION

Proper preparation of the patient is essential for optimal radiographic observation of urinary calculi and lesions. Small uroliths can be overlooked or misinterpreted in poorly prepared patients. An overnight fast and a cleansing enema are recommended prior to elective radiography. Pharmacologic restraint is usually needed to obtain good-quality radiographs and to minimize iatrogenic trauma. Survey mediolateral and ventrodorsal radiographs should be obtained. Renal calculi are best demonstrated by a ventrodorsal view; whereas, cystic and urethral calculi are both best seen in a mediolateral view. Two exposures may be needed. The correct exposure for the bladder may result in overexposure of the distal part of the urethra.[12]

Pneumocystography is often useful, since air is a satisfactory medium for outlining the bladder.[12] Air emboli are rare. The technique is easily performed as follows: Pass a urethral catheter into the bladder and gently inflate it with a large syringe. The catheter may be withdrawn and the air retained by the bladder sphincter. To outline the urethra, inject air as the catheter is withdrawn. The air is retained by clamping the end of the penis. The contrast in density produced by the presence of air allows even slightly radiographically dense uroliths to be seen and reveals thickening or irregularities in the bladder mucosa.[12]

Contrast media, such as diatrizoate meglumine (Hypaque, Winthrop or Cystografin, E. R. Squibb) may be used. Although they may mask the presence of small very radiopaque uroliths, most uroliths are less radiopaque than the contrast medium and will appear as a bubble or incomplete filling of the bladder lumen. Intravenous injection of contrast media is of limited value in revealing the presence of uroliths, but it gives a good outline of the renal pelves and ureters and may demonstrate other diseases such as dilation of the ureters. In addition to uroliths, radiographs of animals with urolithiasis may reveal bladder wall thickening, with or without mucosal erosion, and urethral strictures. A more

extensive description of radiographic techniques for visualizing the urinary tract is contained elsewhere.[76]

Approximately 97% of all uroliths in dogs are radiopaque.[10] Phosphate, oxalate, silicate, and carbonate calculi are quite dense and are visible radiographically when they are 3 mm or more in diameter. Ammonium urate uroliths may be radiolucent,[12] but are usually radiodense.[79] In addition, ammonium urate uroliths often contain 10-40% phosphate or oxalate or both.[88] The more phosphate and oxalate they contain, and the larger they are, the more visible they are radiographically. Cystine uroliths are generally radiopaque, although they are much less dense than either phosphate or oxalate, but generally are more dense than urate uroliths. In some cases they can be clearly seen; in others they are radiolucent.[10,12]

Uroliths are present in the kidney or ureter in approximately 2.5% of affected males and 7.5% of affected females.[10] Approximately 95% of all uroliths in dogs are in the bladder or urethra.[10,107,112] If obstruction occurs in the male, it is usually just behind the os penis, in the perineal urethra, or at strictures resulting from previous urethral surgery. Obstruction in the female, although uncommon, generally occurs in the perineal urethra, or at the junction of the bladder and urethra where, in addition to blocking the urethra, it may block both ureters.[69]

URINALYSIS

Urinalysis in dogs with urolithiasis is helpful in determining the type of uroliths responsible and should include culture, sensitivity, pH, and examination of the urine sediment. Hematuria, pyuria, and proteinuria may be present. Their presence and severity depend on the amount of irritation and damage caused by the uroliths and/or a urinary tract infection. Their presence and a stronger than normal urine ammonia odor often indicates the presence of a urinary tract infection.[6] A putrid odor suggests severe tissue necrosis from cystitis.[6]

Urine Culture

A quantitative urine culture and bacterial identification and sensitivity tests should be obtained from affected dogs, since a urinary tract infection (UTI) is present in most cases[10] and should be treated. The urine sample for culture preferably should be taken by cystocentesis. Samples obtained by any other method may be contaminated and thus give false results. A high number of organisms are often present in voided samples, even though UTI may not be present.[41] To minimize bacterial mul-

tiplication the urine sample should be cultured immediately, or refrigerated promptly after its collection and cultured within 6 hours. In over 90% of cases the presence of more than 3 white blood cells per high-powered field or bacteria indicate the presence of UTI. A UTI is confirmed by the presence of any organisms in a urine sample obtained by a properly conducted cystocentesis.[14,36,40,41] Although both false-negative and false-positive results may be obtained in urine samples taken by any other method, the presence of UTI is suggested if there are more than 10,000 organisms/ml in a midstream sample obtained aseptically or by catheterization, or more than 100,000 organisms/ml regardless of how the sample was taken.[14,36,40,41]

Microstix (Ames Co) is satisfactory for estimating bacterial concentration in urine. It works well unless gross hematuria is present.[35] However, the nitrite portion is not reliable in dogs or cats.[35] Screening tests are useful for rapid identification of patients with UTI; however, they are not a substitute for conventional laboratory techniques for identifying the organism and its drug susceptibility. Although antimicrobial susceptibility testing has been challenged,[115] if conducted correctly, it appears to be beneficial.[90] In one study, in vitro drug-susceptibility testing by a broth microdilution method correctly predicted response to administration of ampicillin or trimethoprin-sulfa in 84% of dogs with UTI, when proper dosage, treatment interval, and course of therapy were used.[49]

Canine UTI without urolithiasis is usually caused by gram-negative bacteria (*Escherichia coli, Proteus, Pseudomonas, Klebsiella,* and *Enterobacter* spp); whereas gram-positive bacteria (*Staphylococcus* or *Streptococcus* spp.) are the ones commonly found associated with uroliths (Table 4). Usually a single species of bacteria is responsible. The presence of more than one species in the culture is usually caused by contamination. UTI caused by two or more bacterial species occur in approximately 18% of affected dogs.[46]

Urine pH

In the normal, fasted dog the urine pH is near 6.0. However, it will routinely be greater than 7.0 if a urinary tract infection is present, or the urine is produced within 8 hours after eating most foods. Food ingestion stimulates gastric acid secretion. If this is not offset by the absorption of sufficient acid-producing ions, body fluids become alkaline, for which the kidney compensates by excreting alkaline ions. This is referred to as the "postprandial alkaline tide." As a result of this normal physiologic effect, the urine pH will increase for several hours

TABLE 4

CAUSE OF CANINE URINARY TRACT INFECTIONS (UTI) AND EFFICACY OF AMPICILLIN OR TRIBRISSEN IN THEIR TREATMENT

Bacteria	% of UTI Due to[10]	% Susceptible to[48,50*]	
		Ampicillin	Tribrissen
Staphylococcus spp.	50	100	100
Streptococcus spp.	20	100	56
Proteus spp.	20	80	73
Escherichia coli	4	80	82
Others	6	—	—
All	100	> 80**	> 72**

*Ampicillin 25-35 mg/kg three times daily orally, or Tribrissen 10-15 mg/kg twice daily orally. Allow opportunity for urination only just before drug administraton. Withhold food at least 30 min before and after administration.

**> indicates greater than. Sum of the % of UTI due to each of these four bacteria times the % of UTI caused by that bacteria that were effectively treated with that drug.

after a meal, then decrease to the fasting level by 8-14 hours after the meal.

Urine pH may change rapidly after voiding, particularly if the urine contains bacteria, which are frequently present in a voided sample.[41] Therefore, urine pH is of diagnostic benefit only if the following procedures are followed: 1) the bladder is emptied then, 2) the animal is fasted for at least 8-12 hours before the sample is obtained and 3) the pH is measured immediately after the sample is obtained. Paper accurate to within 0.2 pH units is available to measure urine pH (pHydrion, Microessential Labs and Nitrazine Paper, E. R. Squibb). However, if metabolic acidosis is present and renal function is sufficient, the urine will be acidic even though urinary tract infection is present. This applies regardless of when and how the sample was obtained. Metabolic acidosis routinely occurs in the obstructed animal, but its severity depends on the degree and duration of obstruction.

Urine Sediment

Urine sediment should be obtained by centrifuging at low speeds 10 ml of fresh urine, putting the sediment on a slide with a coverslip and viewing with a low-intensity microscope light.[3] The presence and identification of crystals may help suggest the type of urolith present. The major crystals involved with urolithiasis in dogs are described in Table 5 and shown in Figure 3.

The presence of cystine crystals in the urine sediment is abnormal; it is not abnormal for urine

TABLE 5

CHARACTERISTICS OF URINE CRYSTALS INVOLVED WITH CANINE UROLITHIASIS[3,79,82]

Crystal Type*	Description	pH Where Found*		
		Acid	Neu-tral	Alka-line
$MgNH_4PO_4$ (struvite)	3–6 sided colorless prisms with oblique ends ("coffin-lids")	±	+	+
$CaPO_4$ (apatite)	Amorphous or long thin prisms	±	+	+
Ammonium Urate	Yellow-brown spheres (thornapples) occasionally dumbbell or sheaves of needles	−	±	+
Calcium Oxalate	Small, clear octahedral envelopes (square maltese cross appearance), sometimes dumbbell and ring or hippurate (six-sided) forms	+	+	±
Cystine	Flat, clear, hexagonal	+	−	−
Calcium Carbonate	Tiny, clear spheres or dumbbells	−	+	+

*A few drops of acetic acid (vinegar) will cause cystine and calcium oxalate crystals to appear if they are in solution, and will dissolve struvite and ammonium urate crystals. Conversely, a few drops of hydrochloric acid will dissolve cystine and calcium oxalate crystals.

from dogs without urolithiasis to contain struvite, oxalate, or urate crystals.[3,82] Conversely, these crystals may not be present even in, dogs with urolithiasis. However, their presence in dogs known to have uroliths is indicative, although not confirmatory, of the urolith type. In order for urine crystals to be beneficial in determining the type of urolith present, the animal must be consuming its regular diet. Both the type and presence of crystals may differ when different diets are consumed.[83]

DETERMINATION OF UROLITH TYPE

Optimal therapeutic and prophylactic measures differ according to urolith type. Thus, it is important to determine the main type of urolith present. In addition, recurrence generally involves the same type of urolith that occurred previously,[10] unless urinary tract infection persists or develops; in which case a struvite urolith usually develops.

Urolith Analysis

The only way to confirm accurately the type of urolith present is to have it analyzed **quantitatively.** The urolith for analysis may be removed by hydropropulsion (see page 9-22) or surgery, or

FIGURE 3

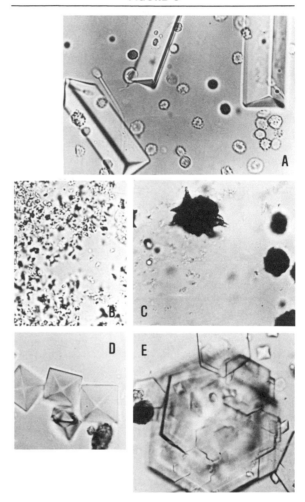

FIGURE 3: Urine Cyrstals involved with Canine Urolithiasis. A—Struvite, B—amorphous phosphate, C—ammonium urate, D—calcium oxalate and E—cystine with several smaller calcium oxalate crystals. A and E—100x, others 160x magnification. All unstained. The phosphate and cystine crystals were colorless; the urate crystals were dark yellow-brown; and the oxalate crystals were light clear-yellowish color. Reprinted from reference 82.

it may be passed, particularly by females. Urine sediment containing crystals may also be obtained for analysis by centrifuging 25-100 ml of urine in a conical-tipped tube. A calculi analysis kit is available.* However, it detects only the presence and not the quantity of calculi constituents and, therefore, is of no benefit in determining the major constituents in a mixed urolith. In addition, this kit does not detect the presence of silicate, has been reported unreliable in consistently detecting calcium, and may not correlate well to a quantitative analysis.[66]

* Oxford Labs, 107 N. Bayshore Blvd., San Mateo, CA 94401

In one study of 272 canine uroliths, qualitative analyses failed to detect 62% of calcium-containing uroliths and 83% of calcium phosphate uroliths.[11] Qualitative analyses gave false-positive results for urates in 55% of cystine uroliths, and agreed with less than 50% of calcium oxalate, urate, and cystine uroliths detected by quantitative analyses. Because of these factors, a quantitative analysis is recommended. It has been recommended that both the outer zone and the nucleus of the urolith be analyzed separately.[66] This is because they occasionally are composed of different materials (Table 2, page 10-5). Many laboratories do not conduct a quantitative analysis of uroliths.**

Urolith Appearance

Struvite uroliths range in color from yellow to tan to white. They may be relatively hard or soft and crumbly, with a smooth or roughened surface, but without spicules (Figure 4). Only one or many uroliths may be present varying in size from several centimeters in diameter, to sand and grit, to microscopic crystals.

Calcium Oxalate uroliths may contain small amounts of calcium phosphate. They are quite hard, brittle, usually small, and may be smooth or have sharp-edged crystals protruding from their surface. They are generally creamy or tan, but may be brownish-green because bile pigments are present (Figure 5).

Ammonium Urate uroliths are usually small, brittle, spherical, light yellow to brown to green, and on cross section often have concentric laminations (Figure 6).

Cystine uroliths tend to be small, brown to yellow-green, soft and smooth (Figure 7).

Silicate uroliths are tan, hard, rough stones with spicules. Because of these spicules they may resemble children's jacks and therefore are sometimes referred to as "jack-stones" (Figure 8). However, not all silicate uroliths have a jack-stone appearance and, conversely, all jack-stones are not silicate.[70] In dogs, in contrast to ruminants, silicate uroliths are generally multiple.

Calcium Carbonate uroliths, which are uncommon in dogs or cats, are smooth, light-colored, and hard.

**Several laboratories that conduct quantitative analyses are:
1) Urolithiasis Lab, Box 25375, Houston, TX 77005
2) Louis C Hering and Co, Orlando, FL 32802
3) Beck Analytical Services, Bloomington, IN 47401
4) Urinary Stone Analysis Lab, School of Veterinary Medicine, University of California, Davis, CA 95616

FIGURE 4

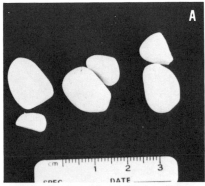

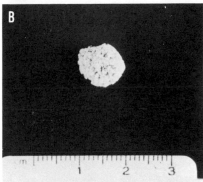

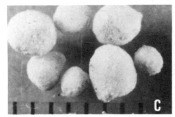

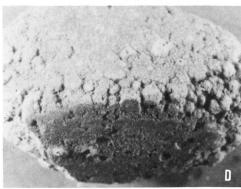

FIGURE 4: Struvite Cystic Uroliths. All were 100% magnesium-ammonium-phosphate hexahydrate except **D**, which was 20% ammonium urate. **A** and **B** were from adult male dogs, **C** an 8-week-old Beagle puppy whose littermates were unaffected, and **D** a 19-month-old female Beagle. **A** was smooth, white and hard. Others were rough and tan colored.

FIGURE 5

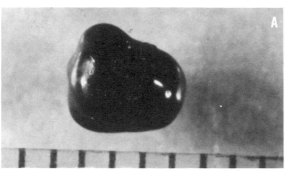

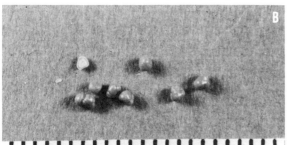

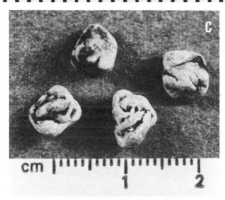

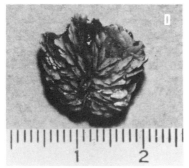

FIGURE 5: Calcium oxalate Uroliths. All were 100% calcium oxalate. **A** was dark green and removed from an adult male Pug. **B** was light green and from an adult male Yorkshire Terrier. **C** was tan-to-dark brown and from an adult female Dachshund. **D** was yellowish-tan and from an adult male Miniature Schnauzer.

FIGURE 6

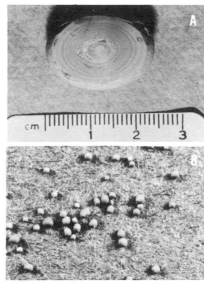

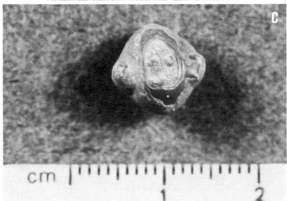

FIGURE 6: Ammonium Urate Uroliths. All were 100% ammonium urate, light yellowish-brown to tan and removed from males. **A** is from a Dalmatian, **B** a mixed breed dog and **C** a cat. Courtesy Dr. CA Osborne, University of Minnesota.

Clinical Indications of Urolith Type

If an analysis of the urolith or urine sediment crystals is not available, the factors given in Table 6 and diagramed in Figure 9 can be used to estimate the most probable type present. None of the factors given is conclusive by itself. The more factors that are present and that suggest a particular type of urolith, the more likely the dog is affected by that type. These factors correctly indicate the type of urolith present in the vast majority of cases and are often the only information available to the clinician for use in initiating therapeutic and prophylactic measures.

The presence of a urinary tract infection (UTI), alkaline urine, struvite crystals in the urine sedi-

FIGURE 7

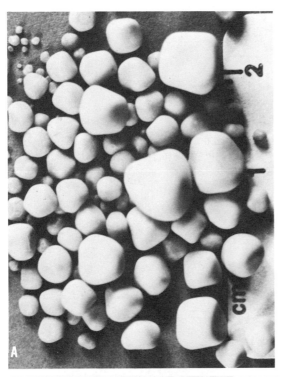

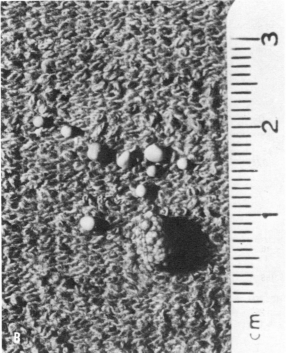

FIGURE 7: Cystine Uroliths. **A** are from a Bull Mastiff and **B** a Basset Hound. All were light tan. Courtesy Dr. CA Osborne, University of Minnesota.

FIGURE 8

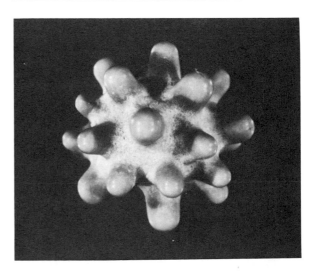

FIGURE 8: Silicate Urolith. Removed from an adult male German Shepherd. Courtesy Dr. AM Legendre, University of Tennessee.

ment, and quite dense uroliths radiographically all suggest that the uroliths are struvite. Struvite crystals are often present in the urine of dogs without urolithiasis and, conversely, may not be present in those that are affected. However, the presence of these crystals in the urine sediment of a dog with uroliths strongly suggests that the uroliths are composed of struvite. If UTI caused by *Staphylococcus* spp. is present, the uroliths invariably are struvite.[6,18,27,74] However, UTI with other organisms may occur secondarily to most other types of uroliths.

In dogs most uroliths, including calcium oxalate, are located in the bladder or urethra.[10,11,78,107,112] In contrast, in people calcium oxalate is the main type of urolith that occurs—most commonly in the renal pelvis and ureters. Three-fourths of canine nephroliths are struvite, less than one-fourth are calcium oxalate and, although rare, the occurrence of ammonium urate nephroliths in dogs has been reported (Table 6). If radiopaque calculi are present in the kidneys or ureters and UTI is present, the calculi usually are struvite; whereas, if no UTI is present, the calculi usually are oxalate.

Urolith Incidence by Breed, Age and Sex

Incidence of the different types of uroliths varies substantially among dogs of different breeds, ages, and sex, which aids in suggesting the type of urolith present.

FIGURE 9

DETERMINING CANINE UROLITH TYPES

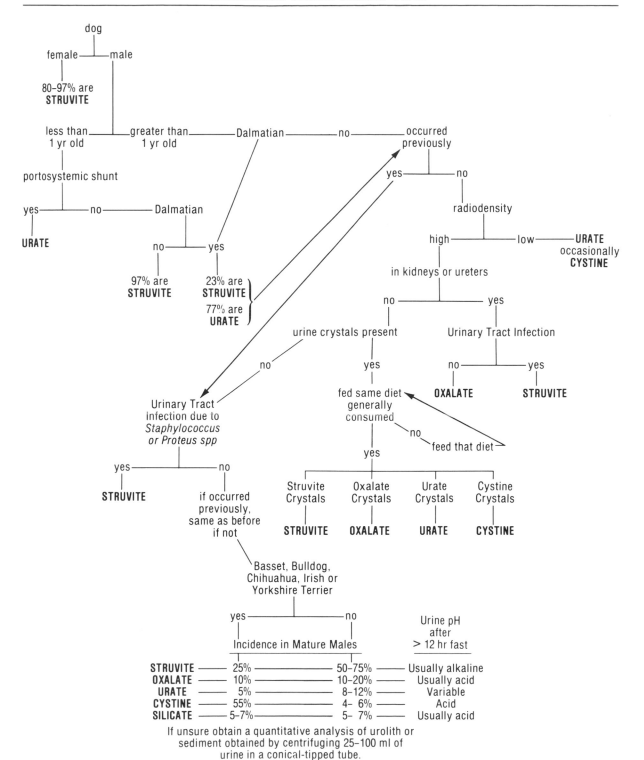

If unsure obtain a quantitative analysis of urolith or
sediment obtained by centrifuging 25–100 ml of
urine in a conical-tipped tube.

TABLE 6

FACTORS USEFUL IN SUGGESTING THE TYPE OF UROLITH PRESENT[a,6,10,11,13,18,67,72,107]

	UROLITH TYPE				
	Struvite	Oxalate	Urate	Cystine	Silicate
% in[b]:					
All Age Females—All Breeds	80–97	1–2	1–2	0	rare
All Age Male Dalmatians	23	uncommon	77	uncommon	uncommon
Immature Males—All Other Breeds[c]	97	1	1	1	rare
Mature Males—Basset, Bulldog,[d] Chihuahua, Irish and Yorkshire Terrier	25	10	5	55	5–7
Mature Males—All Other Breeds	50–75	10–20[d]	8–12[d]	4–6[d]	5–7
In Kidneys or Ureters[e]	74–78	20–22	0–4	uncommon	uncommon
Urinary Tract Infection Present[f]	majority	uncommon	——— occasionally ———		
Usual Urine pH[g]	alkaline	acid	varies	acid	acid
Urine Crystals[h]	phosphate	oxalate	urate	cystine	—
% Radiopaque	most	100	25–50[i]	75–95[i]	100

[a]None of these factors is pathognomonic. The more present, the more likely that type of urolith is present. A definitive diagnosis requires a quantitative analysis of the urolith or urine sediment. Carbonate uroliths account for less than 1% of all cases.

[b]Recurrence is generally caused by the same type of urolith that occurred previously. However, if a urinary tract infection persists or develops, a struvite urolith is generally responsible for recurrence.

[c]Except in those with portosystemic shunts, which usually have urate uroliths.[29,52]

[d]English Bulldogs appear to have an increased incidence of both urate[75] and cystine uroliths.

[e]Generally struvite if urine culture is positive, and oxalate if negative, in a sample obtained by cystocentesis.

[f]If the organisms involved are *Staphylococcus* spp, the uroliths are usually struvite.

[g]Alkaline, regardless of type of urolith if, 1) a urinary tract infection is present, 2) the urine sample is obtained within 4–8 hrs after eating, or 3) urine is retained in the bladder greater than 24 hrs. However, it may be acid, regardless of these factors if a sufficiently severe metabolic acidosis is present, as may occur with obstruction. Urine pH may also change with time after collection.

[h]With the exception of cystine these crystals may be present in dogs without uroliths and, conversely, they may be absent in those with uroliths. Thus, they are helpful in determining the type of urolith only if uroliths are present. See Table 5 and Figure 3 (page 10–13) for crystal identification.

[i]Pure urate uroliths are radiolucent. However, many contain varying amounts of phosphate or oxalate, which are radiopaque. The radiodensity of cystine uroliths is between struvite and urate uroliths.

Immature Dogs: Approximately 97% of all cases of urolithiasis in dogs of both sexes less than 1 year of age are caused by struvite uroliths. The two exceptions are males of any age with impaired hepatic function, such as portosystemic shunts, and male Dalmatians, both of which are most commonly affected by ammonium urate uroliths.[29,52]

Dalmatians and Dogs with Liver Disease: In affected male Dalmatians of any age, approximately 77% of urolithiasis cases are caused by ammonium urate and 23% by struvite uroliths (Table 6). Ammonium urate uroliths do occur in other breeds and in dogs with normal hepatic function. However, any dog with ammonium urate uroliths, except a Dalmatian, should be evaluated for liver disease.[29,52]

Females: From 80-97% of all uroliths obtained from females are struvite. With the exception of cystine, females produce the other types of uroliths. However, non-struvite uroliths are seldom found in females because they are readily excreted. Females have a much broader, shorter urethra than males and can excrete calculi up to 1 cm in diameter.[69] Usually, only struvite uroliths can attain sufficient size rapidly enough to be retained in the female's urinary tract. In addition, the female's shorter, broader urethra makes her more susceptible than males to an ascending infection. Urinary tract infection occurs twice as often in females as males and greatly enhances struvite urolith formation. Reproductive hormones may also be a factor. It has been postulated that the incidence of calcium oxalate uroliths in females is lower because estrogen increases urine citrate and decreases urine calcium concentration,[108] and because testosterone increases hepatic oxalate production.[102] In support

of the latter hypothesis, calcium oxalate uroliths are more common in intact than castrated male dogs.[77]

Adult Males: Struvite is the main urolith type affecting adult males other than Dalmatians, Basset Hounds, English Bulldogs, Chihuahuas, Irish Terriers, and Yorkshire Terriers (Table 6). With the exception of Dalmatians, adult males of these breeds are most often affected by cystine uroliths. English Bulldogs, like Dalmatians, have also been reported to have a higher than expected incidence of ammonium urate uroliths.[75]

Cystine uroliths occur in both men and women, but in dogs they occur only in males.[110] Affected dogs have an inherited sex-linked defect in renal tubular cystine reabsorption. This causes increased cystine excretion in the urine, which predisposes to urolith formation.[15,109] Cystine uroliths in dogs were first reported in 1935 in an Irish Terrier.[60] In one study cystine was the only type of urolith that occurred in 5 Bulldogs.[10] In contrast, cystine, and predominantly calcium phosphate, uroliths are the least common of the six major types of uroliths affecting other breeds (Table 2, page 10-5).

Silicate uroliths, which are the most common urolith occurring in ruminants consuming primarily pasture grass, are less common in other animals. Their presence in dogs was not reported in the United States until 1976.[42] Since that time they have been seen with increasing frequency.[70] They occur almost exclusively in adult males. They have been found in both sexes in wild, but not pet, dogs in Kenya.[7] In North American pet dogs only one case in a female has been reported.[72] Although their occurrence in many breeds has been reported, 40% of affected dogs in North America have been German Shepherds.[70,72]

Calcium carbonate is the most common urolith in horses but accounts for less than 1% of canine urolithiasis cases.[10,11,78] When such cases do occur, they tend to be in older dogs. In one study the mean age of affected dogs was 12.3 years as compared to 5-8 years for other uroliths.[10]

TREATMENT AND PREVENTION

Optimal procedures for removing all uroliths and preventing their recurrence differs for the different types of uroliths. Since 80-97% of all affected females and males less than 1 year of age (with the exception of Dalmatians) have struvite uroliths, determining the type of urolith present may be warranted only for those dogs in these categories that fail to respond to treatment for struvite uroliths, or that experience recurrence when proper management for prevention of struvite uroliths is followed. In contrast, in males over 1 year of age, only 50-75% of those affected have struvite uroliths (23% for Dalmatians), and the remainder may be any one of the four other types of uroliths (Table 6). Therefore, in all adult males it is important to determine the type, or at least the most probable type, of urolith. This is important not only for treatment but also for prevention because recurrence will generally be caused by the same type of urolith that occurred previously.[10,13]

Management of urolithiasis includes the following procedures instituted in the order given:
1. When necessary
   a. Relieve distention by cystocentesis if the bladder is severely distended.
   b. Stabilize the dog's condition with proper fluid and electrolyte therapy.
   c. Relieve urethral obstruction by hydropropulsion or other means if necessary.
2. Eliminate existing uroliths by surgery or, for struvite or ammonium urate uroliths, institute dietary dissolution.
3. Treat or manage causative factors such as a urinary tract infection.
4. Prevent recurrence with proper dietary and medical management (Table 1, page 10-4).

OBSTRUCTED CASES

If urinary excretion becomes completely obstructed, without treatment the animal will die within 2-4 days. In much less time renal damage from back pressure-induced renal ischemia occurs. Therefore, if obstruction is present, immediately stabilize the animal's condition, relieve bladder distention and, above all else, be gentle. The animal usually will not eat or drink when obstruction occurs and, therefore, is often dehydrated and requires fluid and electrolyte therapy. Fluid therapy and procedures for relieving obstruction are the same for both dogs and cats, and are described on pages 9-20 and 9-22, respectively. If obstruction is not present, neither procedure is needed.

URINARY TRACT INFECTION (UTI) TREATMENT

Once the animal's condition has been stabilized, the obstruction relieved, and the animal is eating normally, conduct the procedures described previously to determine if UTI is present (page 10-12). In all adult males determine the type of urolith responsible (page 10-13). As shown in Table 4 (page 10-12), UTI caused by bacteria sensitive to ampicillin and trimethoprim-sulfamethoxazole

TABLE 7

DRUGS MOST EFFECTIVE FOR TREATMENT OF CANINE URINARY TRACT INFECTION[*45,51,97]

| Organism | Antimicrobial Generally Most Effective | Oral Dosage | |
		mg/kg	times daily
Staphylococcus spp.	Ampicillin or Amoxicillin + Clavulanate	25-35	3
Strepococcus spp.		10	2
Proteus mirabilis			
Escherichia coli	Trimethoprin + Sulfa	10-15	2
Enterobacter spp.			
Pseudomonas spp.	Tetracycline	20	3
Klebsiella spp.	Cephalexin	10-20	3

*These drugs are recommended unless in vitro drug susceptibility tests indicate that others may be more effective. Gentamicin is also frequently effective against all of these organisms.[97] Combinations of antimicrobial agents are superior to a single drug in only a few instances, and are not generally recommended.[46]

(Tribrissen, Burroughs Wellcome) is present in most dogs with urolithiasis. If there is any delay in receiving results from the urine culture and sensitivity test, one of these drugs or amoxicillin with clavulanate (Clavamox, Beecham Labs) should be given until results are known. Clavulanate inhibits beta-lactamase (penicillinase), which is produced by numerous pathogens, particularly Staphylococcus spp. Clavulanate therefore potentiates the efficacy of penicillins against these organisms.

Antimicrobial drugs, and their dosages, which are usually the most effective against the organisms generally responsible for causing UTI in the dog, are shown in Table 7. Urinary antiseptics, such as methenamine and methylene blue, are less effective than specific antibacterial therapy. Irrigating the bladder with a solution containing an antimicrobial is of doubtful value.

Recommended therapy for a UTI is the following:

1. Allow opportunity for urination only just before drug administration. If time for urination is not restricted, there may be substantial periods when effective antimicrobial concentrations are not maintained in the urine.

2. Withhold food for at least 30 minutes before and after drug administration. Food in the stomach or duodenum interferes with antimicrobial drug absorption and substantially lowers urine concentration of the drug. Administration of subtherapeutic dosages and failure to follow these two recommendations are common causes of inability to correct UTI, and development of bacterial resistance.

3. Obtain a urine culture 4-7 days after therapy is begun.
   a. If it is positive, therapy is ineffective and should be altered.
   b. If it is negative, therapy is effective and should be continued.

4. Continue therapy for 2-3 weeks, or if uroliths are present, until 2-3 weeks after they are gone. A UTI will frequently recur if antimicrobial administration is stopped before all uroliths are eliminated.[81] This difficulty may be caused by bacteria in the urolith,[74] or because of urinary tract irritation by uroliths.

5. Obtain a urine culture and susceptibility test 4-7 days after therapy is stopped. If it is negative, treatment was successful. If it is positive, reinstitute appropriate therapy; the treatment was either unsuccessful or reinfection occurred. Bacteria colonizing the prepuce or vagina may sometimes reinfect the urinary tract after therapy is discontinued, particularly if the mucosa has been damaged.[48]

6. Recurrent UTI that does not respond to proper antimicrobial therapy indicates the presence of a predisposing cause such as uroliths, neoplasms, polyps, or diverticula. If the predisposing cause cannot be eliminated in these cases, it may be necessary to provide long-term, low-dose therapy with the appropriate antimicrobial agent as determined by results of susceptibility testing. For these cases, after the therapy described above to produce a negative urine culture, give one-third the normal daily dose once daily, usually at bedtime.[46] Drug administration at bedtime may increase the time the drug remains in the urinary tract because the frequency of urination is least during the night. Reculture the urine monthly; if it remains negative, continue therapy for 6 months. If reinfection occurs during this time, the appropriate drug based on susceptibility testing should be substituted at full dosage for 2 weeks. Nitrofurantoin, cephalexin, and Tribrissen are all good choices for long-term therapy if the organism responsible is gram-negative. Ampicillin or Clavamox are good choices for gram-positive bacteria.

STRUVITE UROLITHIASIS MANAGEMENT

Struvite uroliths can be removed surgically or dissolved by feeding a struvite calculolytic diet (Prescription Diet Canine s/d, Hill's).

Surgical Removal of Uroliths

Surgery is indicated in cases:

1. With obstruction to urine excretion that cannot be corrected by nonsurgical techniques
2. With unilateral nephroliths and/or ureteroliths that have caused obstruction and substantial impairment of kidney function
3. With surgically correctable anatomic defects of the urinary tract that predispose to a urinary tract infection or obstruction, such as strictures and neoplasms, but not urachal diverticulum

which, as described on page 9-5, usually respond to dietary urolith dissolution.

4. In which the density or size of the urolith increases or is not less within 60 days of feeding the calculolytic diet **exclusively** and successfully controlling a UTI
5. In which the calculolytic diet is contraindicated (during pregnancy, lactation, edema, ascites, heart failure, pleural effusions, or renal failure).

Surgery has the advantage that uroliths are removed immediately. It has the disadvantages inherent in all general anesthetic and surgical procedures: risk, aftercare, suture removal, more prolonged hospitalization, and more veterinary and staff time for both the surgery and the hospitalization.[8,9,86,92,105] Additional complications include postsurgical extravasation of urine, hematuria, or cystitis.

FIGURE 10

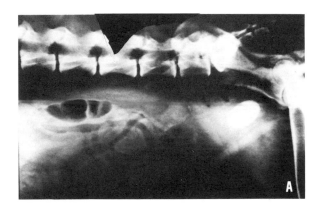
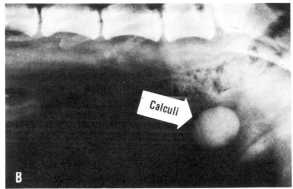
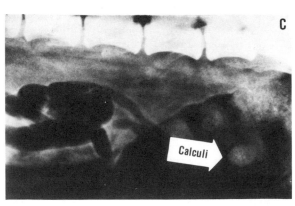
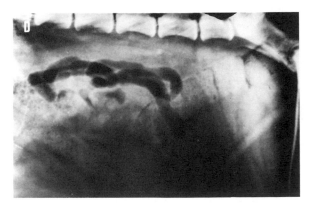

FIGURE 10: Dietary Urolith Dissolution in a Male Golden Retriever. **A**—at time of diagnosis. Dog was then fed a struvite calculolytic diet only. No medications were given. **B**—2 weeks later; calculi density is decreased. **C**—8 weeks later; both density and size of the calculi are decreased. **D**—10 weeks later; the urolith is completely dissolved. Courtesy Dr. CA Osborne, University of Minnesota.

Dissolution of Struvite Uroliths

Dietary dissolution avoids the disadvantages of surgery and, when feasible, is preferred by most informed clients. This preference probably reflects how they would prefer to be treated if they themselves were affected. Dietary dissolution also has the advantage of assurance that all uroliths, regardless of their size or location in the urinary tract, are dissolved. If surgery is used, failure to remove all uroliths is a common cause of recurrence.[74,81] This and a failure to change the urinary tract environment, which resulted in urolith formation initially, probably explains the apparently higher incidence and more rapid recurrence after surgical removal than after dietary dissolution.[79]

As shown in Figure 10 and 11, struvite uroliths can be dissolved by feeding a struvite calculolytic diet exclusively and treating a urinary tract infection (UTI) if present.[67,68,69,73] In one series of 20 clinical cases, the dogs had radiographically visible

FIGURE 11

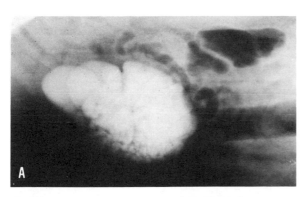

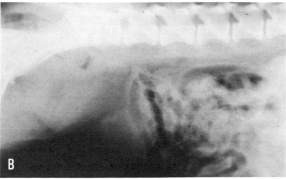

FIGURE 11: Dietary Dissolution of Multiple Cystic Calculi in a 12-year-old female Miniature Schnauzer with a urease-producing Staphylococcus urinary tract infection. **A—** bladder completely full of multiple calculi at the time of diagnosis. Struvite calculolytic diet and ampicillin were given. **B—**6 months later, at which time all calculi were gone. Courtesy Dr. CA Osborne, University of Minnesota.

uroliths believed to be struvite based on the criteria given in Table 6 (page 10-18) and Figure 9 (page 10-17). When the dogs were fed the struvite calculolytic diet (Prescription Diet Canine s/d, Hill's), all uroliths dissolved. The time for dissolution ranged from 0.5-7 months, with an average of 2.26 months.[81] Eleven of these dogs had UTI due to a urease-producing Staphylococcus spp. and were given amoxicillin (16 mg/kg/day).

Dissolution of large bilateral nephroliths in a dog with pyelonephritis and impaired ability to concentrate the urine, but not azotemia, has also been reported to occur when the struvite calculolytic diet was fed and an antimicrobial agent administered.[81] If renal azotemia is present, however, this diet should not be fed. Dogs with renal failure have an increased protein requirement (see page 8-40). Because of this increased requirement the struvite calculolytic diet may induce or aggravate protein malnutrition if fed to a dog with renal failure for a prolonged period. In addition, urolith dissolution in patients with poorly draining kidneys is unlikely to be effective because the uroliths will not be continually bathed with newly formed urine that will induce dissolution. Thus, unilateral nephroliths and/or ureteroliths that have caused obstruction and substantially impaired function of the associated kidney should be managed surgically.

In a controlled study, surgically implanted cystic struvite calculi dissolved in 8-20 weeks in 5 of 6 dogs with an untreated and persistent Staphylococcus aureus UTI when they were fed the struvite calculolytic diet (Table 8).[1] In 3 of these 5 dogs the UTI resolved without treatment following urolith dissolution. In the dog in which the urolith did not completely dissolve, the urolith decreased to one-fifth its original size by the end of the study. In contrast, in all 6 dogs fed a regular dog food the size of the uroliths greatly increased. The uroliths dissolved in 2-4 weeks in 6 of 6 dogs without a UTI when they were fed the struvite calculolytic diet. As this study demonstrates, **dissolution of struvite calculi is greatly prolonged and may not occur in some dogs unless a UTI is successfully treated.**

Although the struvite calculolytic diet had little effect on urine volume, the concentration of struvite-forming constituents ($Mg \times NH_3 \times P$) was decreased by 20 to 25-fold and the urine was acidified even when the UTI persisted (Table 8). Urine volume was greatest in dogs with a UTI, regardless of diet. Although the struvite calculolytic diet is relatively high in sodium (Table 9) and prolonged excessive sodium consumption may cause hypertension, blood pressure changed little during the 6 months the diet was fed (Table 8).

The high caloric density, digestibility, and palatability of the struvite calculolytic diet resulted in a 30% increase in the dog's body weight in the 6 months it was fed. Its low protein content, however, resulted in a slightly greater decrease (0.5-0.6 g/dl) in plasma albumin concentration than occurred in the dogs fed the regular diet, and resulted in a 4- to 5-fold increase in plasma alkaline phosphatase activity (liver isoenzyme) (Table 8). Both return to normal within 2-4 weeks when protein intake is increased. As a result of these effects, the protein content of the struvite calculolytic diet was increased by 36% from 5.6% to 7.6% in its dry matter. Clinical evaluation demonstrated that its calculolytic efficacy is comparable to the lower-protein diet and that it has less effect on plasma

alkaline phosphatase activity and plasma albumin concentration.[81]

As shown in Table 9, the canine struvite calculolytic diet is severely restricted in protein, calcium, phosphorus, and magnesium and relatively high in sodium as compared to non-dietary commercial dog foods. Protein restriction decreases the excretion of urea and ammonium ions and the mineral restrictions decrease their excretion. The high salt content stimulates thirst and promotes a diluted urine (specific gravity reduced from about 1.030 to 1.008, Table 8). When this diet is consumed, it produces a urine undersaturated in urea and the struvite constituents ammonium, magnesium, and phosphate. It is this undersaturation that brings about the dissolution of struvite uroliths when this

TABLE 8

DISSOLUTION OF STRUVITE UROLITHS IN DOGS[1]

Diet*	Calculolytic	Regular	Calculolytic	Regular
Urinary Tract Infection due to Urease-producing *Staphylococcus aureus*	yes and not treated	yes and not treated	no	no
Effect on Urolith	5 of 6 dissolved 1 decreased	6 of 6 were 5× larger & 14× heavier	6 of 6 dissolved	4 of 6 dissolved 2 decreased in size
Weeks for Effect— mean (range)	14.4 (8–20)	24	3.3 (2–4)	14 (8–20)
Urine Volume (ml/kg) Base line During study	45 54	24 42	42 39	31 32
Urine Specific Gravity+	1.008	1.028	1.009	1.031
Urine Conc: $[Mg \times NH_3 \times P \times 10^{-4}]$+ (all in mg/dl)	0.3	7.5	0.3	5.8
Urine pH+	6.2	7.6	6.5	7.6
Titratable Acidity (mM)+	+1.8	−11.7	+2.6	−11.0
Blood Press. change (mmHg/6 mo)+	+8	+7	+10	+2
Body Wt Change (kg/6 mo)	+2.3	−0.4	+2.7	+0.7
Plasma Albumin Change+ (mg/dl/6 mo)	−1.0	−0.5	−0.7	−0.1
Plasma Alk Phosphatase (mU/ml)+	148	32	183	25
Blood Urea Nitrogen (mg %/ml)+	3.5	27	2.2	24

*Calculolytic diet was canned Prescription Diet Canine s/d (Hill's), and regular diet was canned Ken-L-Ration (Quaker Oats).
+Initial values were similar in all groups.

TABLE 9

DIETARY FOODS: USE IN MANAGEMENT OF CANINE UROLITHIASIS, URINE pH AND NUTRIENT CONTENT (% in dry matter)

	Canine Prescription Diets				Regular Dog Foods
	s/d	c/d	u/d		
Use	Dissolution	Prevention	Dissolution	Prevention	
Urolith type	Struvite	Struvite	Urate	All Non-struvite	
Urine pH	6.2	6.0-6.3		7.6	6.7-8.3
Protein	7.6	22.2		9.5	24-55
Calcium	0.27	0.81		0.4	1-3
Phosphorus	0.12	0.52		0.13	1-2
Magnesium	0.017	0.10		0.04	0.17-0.25
Sodium	1.2	0.29		0.26	0.4-1.2

diet is fed. In one study, dogs with a urease-producing *Staphylococcus aureus* UTI and fed the struvite calculolytic diet, had a urinary relative supersaturation (RSS) of 0.5 as compared to 16 when a regular commercial dog food was fed, and 4 when either an antibiotic or a urease inhibitor was administered with the regular dog food.[101] A reduction in the RSS to less than 1 is necessary for urolith dissolution. When the struvite calculolytic diet was fed the RSS was reduced from 0.5 to 0.2 when an antibiotic was administered, and to 0.03 when the urease inhibitor flurofamide (Norwich-Eaton) was given with or without an antibiotic.

Procedures for and possible disadvantages and complications of dietary dissolution are the following:

1. Because of its high salt content, the struvite calculolytic diet should not be fed to dogs with heart failure, edema, ascites or pleural effusions from any cause.

2. The struvite calculolytic diet is not nutritionally adequate for dogs during pregnancy, lactation, or growth. It has been fed to puppies to dissolve cystic struvite uroliths. In all cases dissolution occurred within 2-4 weeks. No detrimental effects were observed during this short period.

3. The diet should be fed at least 2-3 times daily in whatever amount is necessary to maintain optimal body weight.

4. If a urinary tract infection (UTI) is present, appropriate antimicrobial drugs should be given during and for 2-3 weeks after urolith dissolution.

5. Giving **urinary acidifiers or additional salt is contraindicated** when the struvite calculolytic diet is being fed. The diet already contains additional salt and urine acidifying ability to

maintain a sufficiently dilute and acid urine for struvite dissolution (Table 9). More of either may be harmful. Giving a urine acidifier in conjunction with the struvite calculolytic diet could result in metabolic acidosis and/or excess urine acidification. These effects, and giving additional salt, may result in increased urinary calcium excretion (see page 10-30 for reasons) and the formation of calcium-containing uroliths.

6. Because the struvite calculolytic diet stimulates thirst and promotes diuresis, pollakiuria may increase for a variable period after dietary therapy is initiated. Pollakiuria, hematuria, and increased urine odor caused by bacterial degradation of urea, usually subside within 5-10 days as UTI is controlled and uroliths decrease in size.[81]

7. Dissolving uroliths may occasionally be excreted by females. Although sometimes these uroliths lodge in the urethra of a male, this is uncommon and they can be readily returned to the bladder lumen by hydropropulsion (see page 9-22). Complete obstruction of the urinary tract in patients with an uncontrolled UTI should be regarded as an emergency. If patency of the urinary tract cannot be rapidly restored by nonsurgical methods, surgical intervention should be considered. In this situation, rapid spread of infection and associated damage to the urinary tract, especially the kidneys, are likely to induce septicemia and peracute renal failure caused by a combination of obstruction and pyelonephritis.[81]

8. The size and density of the uroliths should be monitored by survey radiography, and the urine sediment should be evaluated periodically for crystals. There should be no struvite crys-

tals in fresh uncontaminated urine if therapy is effective in promoting urine that is undersaturated in magnesium, ammonium, and phosphate, as is necessary for struvite dissolution. If struvite crystals are present, something other than the calculolytic diet is being consumed, or possibly a UTI is not being successfully treated. The presence of crystals other than struvite suggests the urolith is not struvite and therefore, for success, the proper management for that type of urolith must be instituted. Crystals formed in urine stored at room or refrigeration temperatures may be in-vitro artifacts.[80]

9. It takes from 2 to 28 weeks, with an average of 9 weeks, for struvite uroliths to dissolve.[67] The time required for dissolution varies with the size, number, and site of the uroliths, and whether a UTI is present. The larger or more numerous the uroliths, the longer the time required for their dissolution. Nephroliths require more time than do cystic calculi. Sterile uroliths dissolve faster than infected ones, even when infected dogs receive concurrent antimicrobial therapy. The greater the calcium or urate and lower the struvite content of the urolith, the longer the time required for dissolution. A decrease in urolith size or density may not be evident for as long as 2 months. In other cases, the urolith may dissolve completely within 2 weeks.

10. Feeding the calculolytic diet should continue as long as the size or density of the uroliths continues to decrease. Because small uroliths may escape detection by survey radiography, the diet should be fed to mature dogs until 4 weeks after the uroliths are no longer palpable or visible radiographically. In growing dogs, as soon as the uroliths are no longer visible radiographically, the puppy should be returned to a diet designed for growth. If the struvite calculolytic diet is fed for an extended period, the growth rate will be reduced because of the restricted amounts of protein and minerals in the diet. Although mature dogs have been maintained on the diet for more than 18 months with no observable detrimental effects, the diet is not recommended for long-term feeding or for preventing recurrence after surgery (see page 10-26 for prevention). Its degree of protein restriction may slow wound healing and the rate of hair growth.

11. If the uroliths do not appear to be decreasing in size or density within 60 days there are three possible causes:

a. A UTI is present and is not being success-

fully treated. As shown in Table 8, dissolution may not occur in some cases and is greatly prolonged in all cases if a UTI is not successfully treated (see page 10-19 for UTI treatment). Sterilization of urine appears to be an important prerequisite for creating a state of struvite undersaturation that promotes urolith dissolution.[79]

b. The uroliths are not struvite (see page 10-13 for determination of urolith type).

c. Something besides the struvite calculolytic diet is being consumed. This is a common cause for dissolution failure. Success depends on proper instructions by the veterinarian and on compliance by the client. Consumption of anything other than the calculolytic diet and water (including vitamin-mineral supplements and urinary acidifiers), may slow or prevent urolith dissolution. This occurs because increased intake of minerals (from a vitamin-mineral supplement) or protein (from any other food) increases urine concentrations of minerals, urea, and ammonium ions. If the plasma urea nitrogen concentration (BUN) is 10 mg/dl or greater in dogs with normal renal function, or if struvite crystalluria is occurring, something in addition to the struvite calculolytic diet is being consumed. Because of the struvite calculolytic diet's low protein content (Table 9), when it is the only food consumed, dogs with normal renal function will have a BUN of 1-6 mg/dl (Table 8).

Urease Inhibitors

Administration of a urease inhibitor is of no benefit unless a urinary tract infection (UTI) due to a urease-producing bacteria is present, just as antibiotic administration is of no benefit unless a UTI is present. However, UTI is present in 50-97% of dogs with struvite urolithiasis and 70% of these are due to urease-producing bacteria (*Staphylococcus* and *Proteus* spp, Table 4). Thus, from one-third to two-thirds of dogs with struvite urothiasis may have a UTI due to a urease-producing bacterium. Giving a urease inhibitor to these animals would tend to retard urine alkalinization and ammonia production (Figure 2), and may inhibit bacterial growth; therefore, they would be expected to be beneficial.

In one study, oral administration of the urease inhibitor acetohydroxamic acid (Lithostat, Mission Pharmacal) at a dosage of 25 mg/kg twice daily, inhibited struvite urolith growth and lessened clinical signs of urolithiasis in dogs with a urease-producing *Staphylococcus aureus* UTI. These dogs were

being fed a regular dog food and were not given antibiotics.[38] Twelve dogs with urease-producing *Staphylococcus aureus* UTI were being fed the struvite calculolytic diet (Prescription Diet Canine s/d, Hill's) and given ampicillin (16 mg/kg/day orally). When acetohydroxamic acid was not given, struvite uroliths dissolved in 4 dogs and became smaller in 2 dogs in 5 months; whereas, when acetohydroxamic acid was given (25 mg/kg/day) the uroliths dissolved in all 6 dogs in 6 weeks.[81]

In another study, in which dogs with a urease-producing *Staphylococcus aureus* UTI were being fed a regular dog food, the effect of a more potent urease inhibitor, flurofamide (Norwich-Eaton, at a dosage of 5 mg/kg 3 times daily given orally) was equal to an antibiotic (amoxicillin with clavulanic acid, Clavamox, Beecham Labs, at a dosage of 10 mg/kg twice daily given orally) in decreasing the relative supersaturation of struvite in the urine (RSS).[101] The RSS determines the growth or dissolution rate of struvite uroliths. When the struvite calculolytic diet (Prescription Diet Canine s/d, Hill's) was fed, this urease inhibitor decreased the RSS 16-fold as compared to a 2-fold decrease when the antibiotic Clavamox was administered. However, the calculolytic diet by itself reduced the RSS 7- to 8-fold more than did either the urease inhibitor or the antibiotic. It was the only treatment or combination of treatments that reduced the RSS to less than 1, as is necessary for dissolution of struvite uroliths.

These studies indicate that when UTI due to a urease-producing bacterium is present in a dog with struvite uroliths, administration of a urease inhibitor:

1. Is more beneficial in enhancing urolith dissolution than is an antibiotic when the struvite calculolytic diet is fed, but is no more beneficial when a regular dog food is fed.

2. Will not result in dissolution when a calculolytic diet is not fed.

3. Shortens the time needed for struvite urolith dissolution when a struvite calculolytic diet is fed.

The urease inhibitor, acetohydroxamic acid should not be administered during pregnancy or at dosages exceeding 25-50 mg/kg/day. A daily dose of 25 mg/kg/day during pregnancy induced many anomalies and high mortality in the puppies.[81] A daily dose of 100 mg/kg/day, as is necessary to induce urolith dissolution when a regular diet is being fed, results in a reversible hemolytic anemia, blood dyscrasia, and abnormalities in bilirubin metabolism.[37]

Prevention of Struvite Urolithiasis

After the first episode of struvite urolithiasis, if a urinary tract infection is not present or is controlled, and other prophylactic measures are not employed, urolithiasis recurs in at least 20-30% of affected dogs.[10,13,22,33] Because of a lack of information on the present status of all dogs evaluated in reported clinical studies, the true incidence of recurrence is probably greater than these reported values.[10] The likelihood of recurrence greatly increases with each episode.

The younger the dog when first affected, the greater the incidence of recurrence.[10] Miniature Schnauzers, Poodles, and all males appear to have the highest incidence of recurrence.[10] These are also two of the breeds most commonly affected.[10,16] Most cases that recur will do so within 1 year, but the range is from 2-50 months.[10,107] As a result, a radiographic examination, 6-12 months after the initial episode has been recommended.[10] However, with proper management, this procedure is probably unnecessary in most of cases because the rate of recurrence can be greatly decreased.

Eradication or control of a urinary tract infection is the most important factor in preventing recurrence of struvite urothiasis in most affected dogs.[81] If recurrent urinary tract infection persists, therapy with a prophylactic dosage of an appropriate antimicrobial drug is indicated for a indefinite period of time (page 10-20).

In addition to eradicating or controlling a urinary tract infection, a diet should be fed that decreases the intake, and therefore the urine concentration of struvite constituents, and maintains an acid urine. The goal of preventive dietary management is a persistent state of undersaturation of urine with struvite.[73] Both urine acidification and protein and mineral restriction are necessary to best accomplish this objective. The degree of protein and mineral restriction needed to prevent struvite uroliths is not as severe as that required for dissolution. In addition, a salt-induced diuresis is unnecessary in most cases. The diet of choice for preventing recurrence of struvite urothiasis is Prescription Diet Canine c/d (Hill's). This diet is less restricted and does not contain the high salt content present in Canine s/d, but is restricted compared to non-dietary commercial dog foods (Table 9, page 10-24). In addition, Canine c/d maintains an acid urine (Table 9).

In the past, Prescription Diets Canine u/d and k/d (Hill's) have been recommended for preventing struvite urothiasis.[44,81] However, to compensate for the metabolic acidosis that develops as a result of decreased renal function, the alkalinizing ability of these diets was increased (see page 8-44). Because of

this change, these diets result in the production of an alkaline urine and therefore are not applicable for prevention of struvite uroliths for which an acid urine is important.

When a regular food is fed, giving salt (NaCl) to increase urine volume, and giving urinary acidifiers, are both beneficial in dissolving struvite uroliths and preventing their recurrence. Sodium (Na^+) may compete with and replace calcium (Ca^{++}) and magnesium (Mg^{++}), and chloride (Cl^-) may displace phosphate ($HPO_4^=$), thus helping prevent calcium phosphate and struvite urolith aggregation.[72] In ruminants, this mechanism has been demonstrated for chloride, and adding salt to the diet is beneficial in preventing struvite uroliths.[111] Salt-induced diuresis also prevents struvite urolith formation in rats.[111] For these reasons salt supplementation is often recommended for urolithiasis prevention in many species, including dogs.[72] Adding 1 g (1/4 tsp)/5 kg/day of salt to the dog's diet to keep the urine specific gravity less than 1.030 has been recommended.[72] Up to 3% salt in the diet has no adverse effect on its palatability for most dogs.

The addition of salt is contraindicated if Prescription Diet Canine s/d is the only food consumed; its salt content is already high enough to result in the production of a dilute urine (Table 8). Adding salt to Prescription Diet Canine c/d for preventing struvite urolithiasis is unnecessary in the majority of cases if this is the only food consumed. This diet's inducement of an acid urine and its restricted protein and mineral content (Table 9) reduce the urine saturation potential of struvite constituents without the need for increasing urine volume with salt-induced diuresis. Supplemental salt is recommended only if struvite uroliths recur when this diet is the only food consumed. If this occurs, a urinary tract infection is probably present. Therefore, the best means to prevent recurrence is to eradicate or control it, as previously described (page 10-19).

Urine acidification assists in dissolving and preventing struvite uroliths in many species of animals. It is often recommended for this purpose in dogs.[72] Although many substances have been recommended and used for urine acidification, few have been shown to be effective in controlled studies when the many pitfalls in obtaining a valid urine pH are avoided (page 10-12). One that has been shown effective is ammonium chloride. For 5 dogs that had a dry diet always available, giving 70 mg of ammonium chloride/kg 3 times daily decreased the average urine pH from 6.6 to 5.5 and maintained the urine pH at less than 6.0 in all dogs at all times.[103] A lower dosage resulted in a higher urine pH. When a UTI caused by *Proteus* spp. was present, giving ammonium chloride at this dosage

and frequency decreased the urine pH from 8.0 to 6.6.[103] Since struvite uroliths form best at a pH of 7.0 or greater, and since their solubility increases as the pH falls below 6.6,[95] this lower pH would be expected to be beneficial in dissolving or preventing their formation. However, the actual value of ammonium chloride in preventing recurrence of canine struvite urolithiasis is unknown.

Although ammonium chloride administered in the proper manner and in adequate amounts does reduce urine pH in dogs, its administration would be expected to increase urine ammonium ion concentration. What effect this would have on struvite urolith formation is unknown. If ammonium chloride is to be used to prevent recurrence of struvite uroliths, it should be mixed well in all food consumed or given just before feeding. The dose for urine acidification is 200 mg ammonium chloride/kg daily (1/2 tsp/10 kg).

As discussed on page 9-29, there are numerous disadvantages to the use of urinary acidifiers for cats. These same disadvantages apply to dogs. Urinary acidifiers are unnecessary when Prescription Diet Canine c/d (Hill's) is fed. This diet maintains a sufficiently acid urine (pH 6.2) without them. As previously described (page 10-24), giving a urine acidifier is contraindicated when the struvite calculolytic diet (Canine s/d) is being fed.

AMMONIUM URATE UROLITHIASIS MANAGEMENT

Ammonium urate uroliths can be removed surgically or dissolved by proper dietary and medical management. Dissolution of ammonium urate, though not as widely practiced as struvite dissolution, has been demonstrated in several clinical cases.[75] The indications for, and the advantages and disadvantages of both surgery and dissolution as discussed for struvite uroliths (pages 10-21 to 25) also apply to ammonium urate uroliths. Dissolution of canine ammonium urate uroliths is particularly important because the predisposing causes cannot be altered in Dalmatians and dogs with portovascular anomalies that cannot be surgically corrected. In addition, the tendency for ammonium urate uroliths to be multiple and radiolucent fosters recurrence after surgery.[75] Nonobstructing ammonium urate nephroliths in dogs that also have ammonium urate uroliths in the lower urinary tract may escape detection unless appropriate contrast radiographic or ultrasonographic studies of the kidneys are performed. Similarly, small uroliths inadvertently allowed to remain in the urinary tract after surgery to remove uroliths, may escape detection until they become symptomatic. These problems can be minimized by urolith dissolution rather than surgery.[75]

Dissolution of ammonium urate uroliths is induced by instituting all of the following procedures. Only the first two procedures are recommended for prevention.

1. Eradicate or control a urinary tract infection if present (see page 10-19). A UTI with a urease-producing organism induces urea hydrolysis, thus increasing urine ammonium ion concentration and, as a result, ammonium urate production.

2. Feed exclusively a diet that produces an alkaline urine, low in ammonium urate concentration (Prescription Diet u/d, Hill's).

3. Administer allopurinol (Zyloprim, Burroughs Wellcome) at 10 mg/kg 3 times daily to decrease endogenous urate production.

To decrease urine ammonium urate concentration there must be a low intake of ammonium, urate, or their precursors. A low intake of these substances can be accomplished by feeding a low-protein, low-purine diet that maintains an alkaline urine. A low-protein diet decreases ammonium ion production resulting from utilization of dietary protein. Urate production and excretion is greatly influenced by purine intake. In one study, dogs' plasma urate concentration increased from 32 μM/L when a purine-free diet was being consumed, to 150-200 μM/L when a high-purine diet was fed.[26]

The main source of purines is from ingested nucleic acids. Nucleic acids are the major constituent of cell nuclei. Thus, to dissolve or prevent urate urolith formation, foods high in cell nuclei, such as meat and glandular organs (common sources of protein in many dog foods), should be avoided.[17] In contrast protein derived from eggs and milk (casein) are extremely low in purines and are high in the best-quality protein available. A high-quality protein is necessary to meet an animal's essential amino acid requirement when protein intake is reduced. Thus, for ammonium urate dissolution or prevention, the diet should contain a low amount of protein provided primarily by egg or casein. This is the same type of diet needed for proper management of advanced severe renal failure. Thus, an advanced severe renal failure diet (Prescription Diet u/d, Hill's) should be fed for ammonium urate dissolution and prevention. In addition, the diet should maintain an alkaline urine.

In contrast to uric acid uroliths, which are more soluble in an acid urine, the solubility of ammonium urate uroliths is affected little by pH changes.[72,88] Urate uroliths in people are primarily uric acid, but in dogs they are primarily ammonium urate (Table 2, page 10-5). An alkaline urine, however, is beneficial in dissolving or preventing ammonium urate uroliths because a decrease in hydrogen ion concentration results in increased conversion of ammonium ions to ammonia ($NH_4^+ \rightarrow NH_3 + H^+$), thus decreasing urine ammonium ion concentration. Since a sufficiently high concentration of both ammonium ions and urate is necessary for ammonium urate formation, the resulting decrease in ammonium ion concentration helps dissolve ammonium urate or retard its formation. A high concentration of urate can be held in solution in the dog's urine when the ammonium ion concentration is low.[110] Giving sodium bicarbonate decreases both urine hydrogen ion concentration (i.e. increases the pH or alkalinity) and ammonium ion concentration, and assists in preventing ammonium urate crystal formation.[110] Thus, urine alkalinization may be helpful and is frequently recommended for preventing ammonium urate urolith formation.[110]

The struvite calculolytic diet (Prescription Diet Canine s/d, Hill's) has been used for canine ammonium urate urolith dissolution.[75,80] However, it maintains an acid, rather than an alkaline urine. If it is used, an alkalinizing agent should be added to it to maintain the urine pH at 7 to 7.5. Excessive alkalinization should be avoided as it may increase the risk of calcium phosphate urolith formation.[75] Urine alkalinization can be achieved by adding sodium bicarbonate (baking soda) to the diet. The amount needed should be individualized for each patient.[75] It has been reported that 1 g (1/4 tsp)/5 kg every 8 hours maintains the urine pH near 7.5 for most dogs.[110]

In contrast to the struvite calculolytic diet, an advanced severe renal failure diet (Prescription Diet u/d, Hill's) maintains an alkaline urine. It is an alkalinizing diet both to assist in dissolving and preventing ammonium urate uroliths, and to assist in preventing the metabolic acidosis that commonly occurs with advanced severe renal failure. Only if an alkaline urine is not maintained when this diet is fed 3 times daily is the addition of sodium bicarbonate recommended for ammonium urate dissolution.

In addition to decreasing urate intake by feeding a low-purine diet, urine urate concentration can be further reduced by decreasing endogenous urate production. This is done by administering allopurinol (Zyloprim, Burroughs Wellcome). Allopurinol interferes with conversion of xanthine to uric acid and decreases urine urate excretion by as much as 75% in Dalmatians.[91] For ammonium urate dissolution, administer orally 10 mg/kg of allopurinol 3 times daily. This amount has been given to nonazotemic dogs for up to 6 months without any detectable adverse effects.[75] In people, because allopurinol

and its metabolites depend on renal excretion, the dosage is commonly reduced in patients with renal dysfunction. Allopurinol has been reported to cause severe life-threatening erythematous desquamative skin rash, fever, hepatitis, eosinopenia, and further decline in renal function when given to people with renal insufficiency. Thus, caution should be used when considering use of allopurinol in dogs with decreased renal function.

During dissolution of ammonium urate uroliths the following should be monitored:

1. The patient, for clinical signs of urethral obstruction. Ammonium urate uroliths tend to move into the urethra.[75] They may be passed, or in males lodge behind the os penis. Owners should be informed of this likelihood and given a written summary of clinical signs associated with this problem. If obstruction occurs, the urolith can be easily returned to the bladder by hydropropulsion (see page 9-22).

2. Urine sediment, for crystalluria. Ammonium urate crystals should not be present in fresh urine if therapy is effective. Their presence suggests inadequate compliance by the client with instructions for dissolution (page 10-28). Crystals formed in urine stored at room or refrigeration temperatures may represent invitro artifacts.[80]

3. The size of the uroliths should be monitored by survey radiography and, if necessary, double-contrast radiography. It is more difficult to monitor changes in the size and number of uroliths that are radiolucent, as some urate uroliths may be. However, this can be accomplished using retrograde double-contrast urethrocystography.[75]

4. If an alkalinizing agent is being given, the urine pH should be maintained at 7.0-7.5.

To ensure dissolution of small uroliths that may escape detection, dissolution therapy should be continued as long as urolith size, density, or numbers are decreasing and for one month after the absence of detectable uroliths. The time required to induce ammonium urate urolith dissolution in the clinical studies reported to date has ranged from 8-11 weeks.[75] If uroliths enlarge during therapy, or do not begin to decrease in size after 8 weeks of proper dissolution therapy, alternate methods of management should be considered. The three causes of dissolution failure are discussed on page 10-25 (item no. 11).

If no prophylactic steps are taken following the first episode of ammonium urate urolithiasis in dogs without hepatic dysfunction, the disease recurs in 20-30% of affected dogs.[10,13,22,88] The likelihood of recurrence greatly increases with each episode and in the presence of hepatic dysfunction. To assist in preventing recurrence, continue to feed the low-protein, low-purine, urine-alkalinizing diet (Prescription Diet u/d, Hill's) and ensure that a urinary tract infection is not present or is controlled (see page 10-11). Allopurinol is not recommended unless there is recurrence when these procedures are followed. It has been recommended that allopurinol be given only if urine uric acid excretion exceeds 10 mg/kg/24 hours, and then only enough be given to decrease urine uric acid excretion to this amount.[47]

Increased urine volume, which would decrease urine concentration and increase the frequency of urination, theoretically should be beneficial for urolith dissolution or prevention. However, the administration of sodium chloride to healthy people did not alter urine uric acid concentration.[5] Long-term administration of hydrochlorothiazide to people with calcium-containing uroliths caused a rise in plasma and urine uric acid concentrations. For these reasons and a lack of any studies demonstrating benefit, neither salt supplementation nor diuretic administration is recommended for urate urolith dissolution or prevention.

A rice, oil, and vegetable puree diet referred to as the Dalmatian Research Foundation Diet is not recommended. It is quite deficient in calcium, potassium, and perhaps some vitamins. In addition, the urine pH when it is fed has not been reported.

CALCIUM OXALATE UROLITHIASIS MANAGEMENT

Dietary induced urolith dissolution is effective only when struvite or ammonium urate are the major urolith constituents present; therefore, other types require surgical removal. Various procedures (with and without surgery or catheterization) for pulverizing uroliths so they can be excreted are currently being used and investigated in humans. Such procedures are not currently available for clinical use for dogs.

After surgical removal, calcium oxalate uroliths will recur repeatedly in 20-30% of affected dogs if propylactic measures are not followed.[10,78] The reversal, treatment or prevention of the factors shown in Table 3 (page 10-10), which cause or predispose to calcium oxalate urolith formation, help prevent their recurrence. These include the following procedures:

1. Decrease urinary calcium excretion by:
   a. Decreasing calcium intake by feeding a low-calcium diet and, if the drinking water is particularly high in calcium, by giving dis-

tilled, deionized, or boiled, but not softened, water. Boiling decreases the calcium content of water due to calcium carbonate precipitation.[87] Do not give softened water. Although softened water is low in calcium, it is high in sodium, and increased sodium intake increases urinary calcium excretion.[106] Drinking water high in calcium (100 ppm) has been reported to be responsible for causing calcium oxalate nephroliths in people and boiling the water to prevent recurrence of the nephroliths.[87]

b. Decreasing intestinal calcium absorption by giving sodium cellulose phosphate or orthophosphates. These substances may also decrease intestinal oxalate absorption, and they have been shown to decrease calcium oxalate urolith formation in people with absorptive hypercalciuria or hyperoxaluria.[84,104,113] Their benefit for affected dogs is unknown. Increased magnesium intake may also decrease calcium absorption, and has been recommended and shown to be of some benefit in preventing experimentally induced calcium oxalate urolith formation.[24] However, in two randomized controlled clinical studies magnesium supplements were of no benefit.[20,114] In addition, increased magnesium intake enhances the formation of struvite uroliths (page 10-8).

c. Decreasing sodium intake by feeding a low-sodium diet and not supplementing with sodium chloride (salt) or sodium bicarbonate (baking soda). Changes in dietary sodium intake are accompanied by parallel changes in urinary sodium and calcium excretion.[106] Thus, salt supplementation, as is often recommended to assist in treating or preventing urolithiasis,[72] is contraindicated for calcium oxalate uroliths.

d. Administering thiazide diuretics. Thiazide diuretics dissociate renal sodium and calcium reabsorption, increasing sodium and decreasing urinary calcium excretion,[106] both of which help prevent calcium oxalate formation. Thiazide diuretics have been shown to be quite beneficial in preventing calcium oxalate urolith recurrence in people.[54] These diuretics should not be given, however, if hypercalcemia is present, as they may worsen it. Hypercalcemic hypercalciuria is uncommonly associated with calcium-containing uroliths in dogs,[78] but if it occurs, primary hyperparathyroidism should be considered. If primary hyperparathyroidism is present,

surgical correction may be possible. Thiazide diuretics, in addition to decreasing calcium, may also decrease urinary oxalate excretion. Both hydrochlorothiazide and amiloride administration corrected a cellular deficit that is present in the majority of people without primary hyperparathyroidism who had a history of calcium oxalate kidney stones.[2]

The benefit of thiazide diuretics in treatment and prevention of calcium oxalate uroliths in dogs or cats has not been reported; they appear to be indicated though, provided hypercalcemia is not present.[80] When thiazide diuretics are administered, plasma calcium concentration should be monitored and administration stopped if hypercalcemia occurs. In addition, potassium should be given to replace thiazide-induced potassium wasting and prevent hypokalemia. Hypokalemia decreases urinary citrate excretion,[98] which enhances calcium oxalate formation.

e. Urine acidifiers should not be given if calcium oxalate uroliths are present. Acidosis decreases renal tubular calcium reabsorption, increases bone calcium mobilization, and decreases plasma protein binding of calcium.[106] All of these effects increase urine calcium excretion. In addition, acidosis decreases urinary excretion of the calcium binder, citrate.[98] Both the increase in calcium and decrease in citrate excretion enhance calcium oxalate formation, which is unaffected by urine pH. Urine alkalinization has been recommended to prevent recurrence of calcium oxalate uroliths in dogs.[28] However, the solubility of calcium oxalate is unaffected by changes in pH from 4.5 to 8.[72] Urine alkalinization has not been shown and is unlikely to be of benefit.

2. Decrease urinary oxalate excretion by:

a. Decreasing oxalate intake by feeding a low-oxalate diet and avoiding foods high in oxalate, such as spinach, rhubarb, parsley, cocoa and tea, which are rarely fed to dogs. Because oxalate is not metabolized and is excreted exclusively by the kidneys, urinary excretion reflects absorption which, although quite low, varies with oxalate consumption.[89]

b. Giving thiazide diuretics which decrease both urine oxalate and calcium excretion as described previously.

c. Decreasing endogenous oxalate production by **not** giving vitamin C. An intake of greater than 4 g of vitamin C daily by people has caused hyperoxaluria and increases the risk of calcium oxalate urolith formation.[4] A vitamin

B-6 (pyridoxine) deficiency also increases urinary oxalate excretion.[23] However, neither a vitamin B-6 deficiency, nor administration of vitamin B-6 has ever been shown to be a factor in dogs or cats with clinically occurring urolithiasis caused by calcium oxalate or any other type of calculi.

3. Increase calcium oxalate inhibitors in the urine.

An increase in ions in the urine that bind calcium or oxalate, therefore making them less available for calcium oxalate formation, may help prevent its formation. The main ion that has this effect on oxalate is potassium, and the major ones having this effect on calcium are citrate, ketoacids, sulfate, and gluconate. Citrate, followed by potassium, has the major effect on decreasing urinary calcium oxalate supersaturation.[96] Thus, increased intake of potassium citrate may be beneficial in preventing calcium oxalate urolith formation and has been recommended.[80] Acidosis, hypokalemia, and hypomagnesemia, if present, should be corrected. They all increase renal tubular reabsorption of citrate and therefore decrease urinary citrate excretion.[87]

Thus, to assist in preventing calcium oxalate urolith formation, a diet low in sodium, calcium, and oxalate should be fed (Prescription Diet u/d, Hill's). This diet contains 25-50% as much sodium, 15-30% as much calcium, and 30-35% as much oxalate as in regular commercial dog foods. Feeding u/d resulted in a urine oxalate concentration of only 30% of that which occurred when either canned or dry regular commercial dog foods were fed.[59] Administration of thiazide diuretics and potassium citrate (Polycitra-K syrup, Willen Drug or Uroeit tablets, Mission Pharmaceutical) may be beneficial. Optimum potassium citrate dosage for the dog has not been established. The human adult dosage is 50-100 mg/kg/day; the pediatric dosage is 5-15 ml of the syrup/day. Do not give salt, sodium bicarbonate, urine acidifiers, or vitamin C.

SILICATE UROLITHIASIS MANAGEMENT

After surgical removal, to assist in preventing the recurrence of silicate uroliths, decrease urine silicate concentration by decreasing silicate intake and increasing urine volume. Since increased silicate intake induces silicate urolith formation (page 10-9), it seems probable that decreasing silicate intake will assist in preventing their formation. Silicate intake can be reduced by preventing dirt consumption and avoiding diets that may be high in silicate. Diets highest in silicate are generally those high in plant proteins and those containing soybean hulls. Urine volume can be increased by adding salt to the diet. A dosage of 1 g (1/4 tsp)/5 kg/day has been recommended.[72] Altering urine pH is of no benefit.

CYSTINE UROLITHIASIS MANAGEMENT

Cystine uroliths should be removed surgically. Following the first episode after cystine urolith removal, if no prophylactic measures are instituted, uroliths recur in 50-75% of affected dogs.[10,13,22] The likelihood of recurrence increases with each episode. To assist in preventing recurrence, feed a low-protein, urine-alkalinizing diet (Prescription Diet u/d, Hill's). This diet is adequate for long-term maintenance while greatly decreasing urine cystine excretion. Diets low in protein are low in the sulfur-containing amino acids, cystine, cysteine, and methionine. Urinary excretion of cystine decreases markedly with the decreased intake of protein or any of the sulfur-containing amino acids.[30]

Urine cystine and hydrogen ion concentrations (above a pH of 7) have fairly equal and similar effects on cystine urolith formation, e.g. a 10-fold decrease in hydrogen ion concentration (such as an increase in pH from 7 to 8) has about the same effect on cystine urolith formation as a 10-fold decrease in urine cystine concentration.[53] Thus, urine alkalinization is beneficial and is often recommended for preventing cystine urolith formation.[28,72,110] Urine alkalinization has dissolved cystine uroliths and prevented their recurrence in people.[56] Cystine uroliths in dogs' urine are twice as soluble at a pH of 8.0, and are 30% more soluble at a pH of 7.5 than at 7.0.[110] A change in urine pH below 7.0 has minimal effect on their solubility.[53] Thus, to prevent cystine uroliths optimally, the urine pH should be maintained near 7.5 or greater. If the diet does not maintain a urine pH near 7.5, sufficient sodium bicarbonate (baking soda) may be added to the diet to accomplish this objective. Urinary acidifiers and methionine are contraindicated; they decrease the urine pH, and methionine may be converted to cystine and increase urinary cystine concentration.[30]

As with all other types of uroliths, ensure that a urinary tract infection is not present or is controlled (see page 10-20). Adding salt to the dog's diet, although often recommended, may be harmful. Increased sodium intake has recently been reported to increase urine cystine excretion in people.

Administration of D-penicillamine (Cuprimine, Merck Sharpe & Dohme) also may help prevent recurrence of cystine uroliths. D-penicillamine forms a soluble disulfide compound with cystine and thus

decreases cystine excretion in the urine. This compound is 50 times more soluble than cystine in the urine.[72] The daily dose of 10-30 mg/kg should be divided and given at least twice a day with the food to prevent vomiting.[72] If vomiting still occurs, use a lower dosage and gradually increase it, or give an antiemetic first. D-penicillamine may also be given, at a dose of 10 mg/kg, only in the evening. The drug should not be used for 3 weeks postoperatively because it adversely affects wound healing by interfering with collagen cross-linking.[58] In addition, its efficacy in preventing cystine uroliths in dogs is questionable. Cystine uroliths were reported to have recurred in 9 dogs being given this drug.[10] For these reasons, it is recommended only in recurring cases when salt is being added to the low-protein, urine-alkalinizing diet (Prescription Diet u/d, Hill's) and urinary tract infection is eliminated or controlled.

Since the potential to develop cystine urolithiasis is caused by a genetic defect in renal tubular cystine reabsorption, affected dogs should not be used for breeding.

REFERENCES

1. Abdullahi SU, Osborne CA, Leininger JR, et al: Evaluation of a calculolytic diet in female dogs with induced struvite uroithiasis. Amer J Vet Res 45:1508-1519 (1984).

2. Baggio B. Gambaro G, Marchini F, et al: An inheritable anomaly of red-cell oxalate transport in "primary" calcium nephrolithiasis correctable with diuretics. New Engl J Med 314:599-604 (1986).

3. Benjamin MM: Outline of Veterinary Clinical Pathology, 3rd Ed, publisher Iowa State Univ Press, Ames, IA pp 180-212 (1978).

4. Bleich HL, Boro ES: Metabolic basis of renal stone disease. New Engl J Med 300:839-845 (1979).

5. Breslaw NA, Pak CYC: Lack of effect of salt intake on urinary acid excretion. J Urol 129:531-532 (1983).

6. Brodey RS: Canine urolithiasis: A survey and discussion of 52 clinical cases. J Amer Vet Med Assoc 126:1-9 (1955).

7. Brodey RS, Thomson R, et al: Silica renal calculi in Kenyan dogs. J Small Anim Pract 18:523-528 (1977).

8. Brown SG: Surgery of the canine urethra. In Vet Clinics of North America 5(3): 457-470 (1975).

9. Brown SG: Urethral surgery. In Current Techniques in Small Animal Surgery, Editor MJ Bojrab, Lea & Febiger, Philadelphia, PA 228-237 (1981).

10. Brown NO, Parks JL, Greene RW: Canine urolithiasis. Retrospective study of 438 cases, and recurrence of canine urolithiasis. J Amer Vet Med Assoc 170:414-422 (1977).

11. Bovee KC, McGuire T: Oualitative and quantitative analysis of uroliths in dogs: Definitive determination of chemical type. J Amer Vet Med Assoc 185:983-987 (1984).

12. Clark WT: Urolithiasis in the dog IV. Diagnosis. J Small Anim Pract 7:553-556 (1966).

13. Clark WT: Urinary calculi in the dog and their recurrence following treatment. J Small Anim Pract 15:437 (1974).

14. Comer KM, Ling GV: Results of urinalysis and bacterial culture of canine urine obtained by antepubic cystocentesis, catheterization, and the midstream voided methods. J Amer Vet Med Assoc 179:891-895 (1981).

15. Cornelius CE, Bishop JA, Schaffer MH: A quantitative study of amino aciduria in Dachshunds with a history of cystine urolithiasis. Cornell Vet 57:177-183 (1981).

16. DiBartola SP, Chew DJ: Canine urolithiasis. Comp Cont Ed 3:226-236 (1981).

17. Finco DR: Current status of canine urolithiasis. J Amer Vet Med Assoc 158:327-335 (1977).

18. Finco DR, Rosin E, Johnson KM: Canine urolithiasis: A review of 133 clinical and 23 necropsy cases. J Amer Med Assoc 157:1225-1228 (1970).

19. Foit FF, Cowell RL, Brobst DF, et al: X-ray powder diffraction and microscopic analysis of crystalluria in dogs with ethylene glycol poisoning. Amer J Vet Res 46:2404-2408 (1985).

20. Ettinger B, Citron J, Tang A: Controlled studies in stone prophylaxis: Comparison of placebo versus allopurinol, chlorthalidone, magnesium hydroxide. Urol Res 12:49 abstr (1984).

21. Ihrke PJ, Norton AL, Ling GV, Stannard AA: Urinary tract infection associated with long-term corticosteroid administration in dogs with chronic skin diseases. J Amer Vet Med Assoc 186:43-46 (1985).

22. Gaskell CJ: Urolithiasis in the dog and cat. Vet Rec 102:546-547 (1978).

23. Gershoff SN, Prien EL: Effect of daily MgO and vitamin B-6 administration to patients with recurring calcium oxalate kidney stones. Amer J Clin Nutr 20:393-399 (1967).

24. Gershoff SN: Treatment of type I primary hyperoxaluria. New Engl J Med 313:959 (1985).

25. Gessner PK, Parke DV, Williams, RT: The metabolism of ¹⁴C-labelled ethylene glycol. Biochem J 79:482-489 (1961).

26. Giesecke D, Kraft W. Tiemeyer W: The reason for uric acid excretion in the Dalmatian dog. Causes and consequences of a classical metabolic disorder. Tierarztl Prox 13:331-341 (1985).

27. Goulden BE: Clinical observations on the role of urinary infection in the etiology of canine urolithiasis. Vet Rec 83:509-514 (1968).

28. Greene RW, Scott RS: Diseases of the bladder and urethra. Chapt 76 in Textbook of Veterinary Internal Medicine, Editor SJ Ettinger, WB Saunders Co. Philadelphia, PA 1890-1936 (1983).

29. Hardy RM, Osborne CA, Cassidy FC, Johnson KH: Urolithiasis in immature dogs. VM/SAC 67:1205-1211 (1972).

30. Hess WC, Sullivan MX: Canine cystinuria. The effect of feeding cystine, cysteine and methionine at different dietary protein levels. J Biol Chem 143:545-550 (1942).

31. Higgins CC: Experimental production of urinary calculi. J Amer Vet Med Assoc 118:81-85 (1951).

32. Kaplan RA, Haussier JR, Deftos LJ, et al: The role of 1-alpha, 25-dihydroxy vitamin D in the mediation of the intenstinal hyperabsorption of calcium in primary hyperparathyroidism and absorptive hypercalciuria. J Clin Invest 59:756-760 (1977).

33. Kaspar LV, Poole CM, Norris WP: Incidence of struvite urinary calculi in two ancestral lines of Beagles. Lab Anim Sci 28:545-550 (1978).

34. Klausner JS, Osborne CA, O'Leary TP, et al: Experimental induction of struvite uroliths in Miniature Schnauzer and Beagle dogs. Invest Urol 18:127-132 (1980).

35. Klausner JS, Osborne CA, Stevens JB: Clinical evaluation of microstix for detection of significant bacteriuria in the dog and cat. Amer J Vet Res 37:719 (1976).

36. Klausner JS, Osborne CA, Stevens JB: Screening tests for the detection of significant bacteriuria. In Current Vet Therapy VIII, Editor RW Kirk, WB Saunders Co, Philadelphia, PA, pp 1154-1157 (1980).

37. Krawiec DR, Osborne CA, Leininger JR, Griffith DP: Effects of acetohydroxamic acid on dissolutin of canine struvite uroliths. Amer J Vet Res 45:1266-1275 (1984).

38. Krawiec DR, Osborne CA, Leininger JR, Griffith DP: Effect of acetohydroxamic acid on prevention of canine struvite uroliths. Amer J Vet Res 45:1276-1282 (1984).

39. Kruger JM, Osborne CA, Polzin DJ: Treatment of hypercalcemia. In Current Vet Therapy IX, Editor RW Kirk, WB Saunders, Philadelphia, PA (1986).

40. Lees GE, Simpson RB, Green RA: Results of analysis of bacterial cultures of urine specimens obtained from clinically normal cats by three methods. J Amer Vet Med Assoc 184:449-454 (1984).

41. Lees GE: Canine urological disorders. Amer Anim Hosp Assoc Proc 479-485 (1983).

42. Legendre AM: Silica urolithiasis in a dog. J Amer Vet Med Assoc 168:418-419 (1976).

43. Lewis LD, Chow FHC, Taton GF, Hamar DW: Effect of various dietary mineral concentrations on the occurrence of feline urolithiasis. J Amer Vet Med Assoc 172:559-563 (1978).

44. Lewis LD, Morris ML, Jr: Canine uroithiasis. In Small Animal Clinical Nutrition, publisher Mark Morris Assoc, Topeka, KS, 2nd edition, pp 10-1 to 10-39 (1984).

45. Ling GV: Treatment of urinary tract infections with antimicrobial agents. In Current Vet Therapy VIII, Editor RW Kirk, WB Saunders, Philadelphia, PA, pp 1051-1055 (1983).

46. Ling GV: Therapeutic strategies involving antimicrobial treatment of the canine urinary tract. J Amer Vet Med Assoc 185:1162-1164 (1984).

47. Ling, GV: Diagnosis and management of urinary calculi in dogs. Proc Amer Anim Hosp Assoc, pp 469-470 (1984).

48. Ling GV, Gilmore CF: Penicillin G or ampicillin for oral treatment of canine urinary tract infections. J Amer Vet Med Assoc 171:358-361 (1977).

49. Ling GV, Rohrich PJ, Ruby AL, et al: Canine urinary tract infections: A comparison of in vitro antimicrobial susceptibility test results and response to oral therapy with ampicillin or with trimethoprim-sulfa. J Amer Vet Med Assoc 185:277-281 (1984).

50. Ling GV, Ruby AL: Trimethoprim in combination with a sulfonamide for oral treatment of canine urinary tract infections. J Amer Vet Med Assoc 174:1003-1005 (1979).

51. Ling GV, Ruby AL: Cephalexin for oral treatment of canine urinary tract infection caused by Klebsiella pneumoniae. J Amer Vet Med Assoc 182:1346-1347 (1983).

52. Marretta SM, Park AJ, Greene RW, Liu S: Urinary calculi associated with portosystemic shunts in six dogs. J Amer Vet Med Assoc 178:133-137 (1981).

53. Marshall RW, Robertson WG: Nomograms for the estimation of the saturation of urine with calcium oxalate, calcium phosphate, magnesium ammonium phosphate, uric acid, sodium acid urate, ammonium acid urate and cystine. Clinica Chimica Acta 72:253-260 (1976).

54. Mathew T: Treatment of renal calculi. Drugs 8:62-69 (1974).

55. McCullagh KG, Ehrhart LA: Silica urolithiasis in laboratory dogs fed semisynthetic diets. J Amer Vet Med Assoc 164:713-714 (1974).

56. McDonald JE, Henneman PH: Stone dissolution in vivo and control of cystinuria with D-penicillamine. New Engl J Med 272:578-583 (1965).

57. Morgan RV: Urogenital emergencies - Part II. Comp Cont Ed 5:43-53 (1983).

58. Morris JJ, Seifter E, et al: Effect of penicillamine upon healing wounds. J Surg Res 9:143-149 (1969).

59. Morris ML, Doering GG: Diet and canine urolithiasis. Canine Pract 5:53-58 (1978).

60. Morris ML, Green DF, Dinkel JH, Brand E: Canine cystinuria. N Amer Vet 16(10):16 (1935).

61. Morshead D: Submucosal urethral calculus secondary to foxtail awn migration in a dog. J Amer Vet Med Assoc 182:1247-1248 (1983).

62. Nakagawa Y, Abram V, Kezdy FJ, et al: Purification and characterization of the principle inhibitor of calcium oxalate monohydrate crystal growth in human urine. J Biol Chem 258:12954-12600 (1983).

63. Nakagawa Y, Abram V, Coe FL: Isolation of calcium oxalate crystal growth inhibitor from rat kidney and urine. Amer J Physiol 247 (Renal Fluid Electrolyte Physiol 16):F765-F772 (1984).

64. Nakagawa Y, et al: Kidney stones caused by defective protein not defective diet. J Amer Diet Assoc 85:1493 (1985).

65. National Academy of Sciences, Washington DC: Nutrients and Toxic Substances in Water for Livestock and Poultry, pp 1-93 (1974).

66. Osborne CA: Diagnosis of urolithiasis. DVM, pp 44-46 (May 1982).

67. Osborne CA, Abdullahi SU, Leininger JR, et al: Medical dissolution of canine struvite uroliths. Minn Vet 22:14-17 (1982).

68. Osborne, CA, Abdullahi SU, Krawiec D, et al: Strategy for nonsurgical removal of canine struvite uroliths. Amer Anim Hosp Assoc Proc 211-214 (1982).

69. Osborne CA, Abdullahi SU, Klausner JS, et al: Nonsurgical removal of uroliths from the urethra of female dogs. J Amer Vet Med Assoc 182:47-50 (1983).

70. Osborne CA, Hammer RF, Klausner JS: An emerging disease: Canine silica urolithiasis. DVM, pp 38 (June 1978).

71. Osborne CA, Hammer RF, Klausner JS: Canine silica urolithiasis. In Current Vet Therapy VII, Editor RW Kirk, WB Saunders Co, Philadelphia, PA 1184-1186 (1980).

72. Osborne CA, Klausner JS: War on canine urolithiasis. Problems and solutions. Amer Anim Hosp Assoc Proc 569-620 (1978).

73. Osborne CA, Klausner JS, Abdullahi S, Krawiec DR: Medical dissolution and prevention of canine struvite uroliths. In Current Vet Therapy IX, Editor RW Kirk, WB Saunders, Philadelphia, PA, pp 1066-1072 (1986).

74. Osborne CA, Klausner JS, Krawiec DR, Griffith DP: Canine struvite urolithiasis: Problems and their dissolution. J Amer Vet Med Assoc 1791:239-244 (1981).

75. Osborne CA, Kruger JM, Johnston GR, Polzin DJ: Dissolution of canine ammonium urate uroliths. Vet Clinics N Amer Sm Anim Pract 16:375-387 (1986).

76. Osborne CA, Low DL, Finco DR: Chapter 8 In Canine and Feline Urology. WB Saunders Co. Philadelphia, PA (1972).

77. Osborne CA, Poffenbarger EM, Bamman LR, et al: Prevalence of canine uroithiasis: Minnesota urolith center. Vet Clin N Amer 16:27-44 (1986).

78. Osborne CA, Poffenbarger EM, Klausner JS, et al: Canine calcium oxalate urolithiasis. Proc Amer College Vet Int Med 1:4-23 to 4-37 (1986).

79. Osborne CA, Polzin DJ, Abdullahi SU, et al: Struvite uroithiasis in animals and man: Formation detection and dissolution. Ad in Vet Sci and Comp Med 29:1-101 (1985).

80. Osborne CA, Polzin DJ, Kruger J, et al: Current status of medical dissolution of canine uroliths. Proc Amer College Int Med 1:4-39 to 4-45 (1986).

81. Osborne CA, Polzin DJ. Kruger JM, et al: Medical dissolution of canine struvite uroliths. Vet Clinics of N Amer Sm Anim Pract 16:349-372 (1986).

82. Osborne CA, Stevens JB: Digest of canine and feline urine sediments. Vet Services Ralston Purina Co, St. Louis, MO (1978).

83. Osborne CA, Stevens JB: The significance of crystaluria. Mod Vet Pract pp 885-888 (Nov 1983).

84. Pak CYC: New drug for kidney stone prevention. The NIH Rec (Dec 7, 1982).

85. Pak CYC: Pathophysiology of calcium nephrolithiasis. In the Kidney: Physiology and Pathophysiology, Vol 2, Editors PW Seldin, G Glebisch. Raven Press, New York, NY pp 1365-1379 (1985).

86. Parks JL: Complications of urogenital tract surgery. Amer Anim Hosp Assoc 391-394 (1977).

87. Popovtzer MM, Stein P, Rubinger D, et al: Kidney stones and drinking water. New Engl J Med 310:721 (1984).

88. Porter P: Urinary calculi in the dog. II. Urate stones and purine metabolism. J Comp Path 73:119-135 (1963).

89. Prenen JAC, Boer P, Dorhout Mees EJ: Absorption kinetics of oxalate from oxalate-rich food in man. Amer J Clin Nutr 40:1007-1010 (1984).

90. Prescott JF, Baggot JD: Antimicrobial susceptibility testing and antimicrobial drug dosage. J Amer Vet Med Assoc 187:363-368 (1985).

91. Pukay BP: Dalmatian bronzing syndrome. Modern Vet Pract:641-643 (Aug 1982).

92. Rawlings CA: Urethral reconstruction in dogs and cats. J Amer Anim Hosp Assoc 12:850-879(1976).

93. Reif MC, Constantiner J, Levitt MF: Chronic gouty nephropathy: A vanishing syndrome? New Engl J Med 304:535-536 (1981).

94. Ribaya-Mercado J, Gershoff SN: Effects of sugars and vitamin B-6 deficiency on oxalate synthesis in rats. J Nutr 114:1447-1453 (1984).

95. Rich LJ, Kirk RW: The relationship of struvite crystals to urethral obstruction in cats. J Amer Vet Med Assoc 154:153-157 (1969).

96. Robertson WG, Peacok M, Norden BEC: Activity products in stone-forming and non-stone-forming urine. Clinical Science 34:579-594 (1968).

97. Rohrich PJ, Ling GV, Ruby AL, et al: In vitro susceptibilies of canine urinary bacteria to selected antimicrobial agents. J Amer Vet Med Assoc 183:863-867 (1983).

98. Rudman D, Dedonis JL, Fountain MT, et al: Hypocitraturia in patients with gastrointestinal malabsorption. New Engl J Med 303:657-661 (1980).

99. Schneck GW: Grass seed urinary calculi. Vet Rec 94:431 (1974).

100. Schneider HJ, Hesse A, Hensel K, et al: Einfluss dur nohrung auf die zusammensetzung von fremdkorpersteinen in tierexperiment. II. Kalziumoxalat und magnesiumtherapie. Zert Urol Nephrol 68:1-5 (1975).

101. Senior DF, Thomas WC Jr, Gaskin JM, Finlayson B: Relative merit of various nonsurgical treatments of infection stones in dogs. Proc V International Symposium on Urolithiasis and Related Clinical Research. West Germany (1984).

102. Sherms V, Murthy MSR, Thind SK, Nath R: Regulation of oxalate synthesizing enzymes by sex hormones in weanling rats. Urol Res 12:75 (1984).

103. Short EC, Hammond PB: Ammonium chloride as a urinary acidifer in the dog. J Amer Vet Med Assoc 144:864-866 (1964).

104. Smith LH: The effects of orthophosphates and ion binders. In Urolithiasis and Related Research, Editors PO Schwille, et al, Plenum Press, 483-489 (1985).

105. Stone EA: Surgical management of urolithiasis. Comp Cont Ed 3:627-635 (1981).

106. Sutton RAL, Dirks JH: Renal handling of calcium. Feder Proc 37:2112-2119 (1978).

107. Takahashi M: Canine urolithiasis: Incidence in 126 cases. J Japan Vet Med Assoc 35:504-509 (1982).

108. Tawashi R, Cousineau M, Dennis G: Calcium oxalate crystal growth in normal urine: Role of concentration of hormones. Urol Res 12:7-9 (1984).

109. Tasn MF, Jones TC, Thornton GW, et al: Canine cystinuria: Its urinary amino acid pattern and genetic analysis. Amer J Vet Res 33:2455-2461 (1972).

110. Treacher RJ: Urolithiasis in the dog. II. Biochemical aspects. J Small Anim Pract 7:537-547 (1966).

111. Udall RH, Chow FHC: Studies on urolithiasis. VII. The effects of sodium, potassium, or chloride ions in the control of urinary calculi. Cornell Vet LV:538-544 (1965).

112. White EG: Symposium on urolithiasis in the dog. I. Introduction and incidence. J Small Anim Pract 7:529-535 (1966).

113. Williams HE, Smith LH Jr: Disorders of oxalate metaolism. Amer J Med 45:715-735 (1968).

114. Wilson DR, Strauss AL, Manuel MA: Comparison of medical treatments for the prevention of recurrent calcium nephrolithiasis. Urol Res 12:40 abstr (1984).

115. Woolcock JB, Mutimer MD: Antibiotic susceptibility testing: caeci caecos ducentes. Vet Rec 113:125-128 (1983).

116. Yendt ER, Cohanim M: Response to physiologic dose of pyridoxine in type I primary hyperoxaluria. N Engl J Med 312:953-957 (1985).

117. Yu TF, Berger L, Kupfer S, Gutman AB: Tubular secretion of urate in the dog. Amer J Physiol 199:1199 (1960).

CHAPTER 11

Heart Failure*

CONTENTS

---

*Written by **James N. Ross, Jr.,** DVM, PhD, Professor and Chairman Dept. of Medicine, School of Veterinary Medicine, Tufts University, North Grafton, MA 01536

SUMMARY OF MANAGEMENT RECOMMENDATIONS

Drugs and nutrients useful in the management of heart disease are given in Table 1 (page 11-3).

ACUTE FAILURE

Acute congestive heart failure with pulmonary edema is an emergency and requires rapid aggressive therapy.

1. Place patient in an environmentally controlled cage at 18° (64°F) in 40-50% oxygen nebulized through 40% ethanol.
2. Give morphine sulfate to dogs that are restless, anxious, and dyspneic with pulmonary edema (Table 1).
3. Give furosemide intravenously (Table 1).
4. Evaluate arrhythmias and if severe treat with appropriate agents given intravenously. Use lidocaine initially in a 2-4 mg/kg bolus in dogs with ventricular tachycardia. Give propranolol to cats by slow intravenous injection. For severe bradyarrhythmias, use an isoproterenol drip to effect (Table 1).
5. Administer dobutamine (Table 1) in a continuous intravenous drip beginning at $5\mu g/kg/min$ to patients with poor myocardial function. Adjust the drip to improve contractility without increasing heart rate.
6. Give theophylline parenterally to patients with bronchoconstriction (Table 1).
7. Administer a vasodilator such as captopril or hydralazine to patients in severe congestive heart failure and pulmonary edema (Table 1). Alternatively, using gloves, nitroglycerin ointment (Table 1) can be applied to hairless areas of the skin. If blood pressure monitoring is available, use sodium nitroprusside in an intravenous drip (Table 1).
8. Remove pericardial fluid as soon as possible to improve ventricular performance. Remove thoracic fluid and some abdominal fluid as soon as possible if they are contributing to respiratory distress.

CHRONIC FAILURE

Therapy should be individualized and varied depending on underlying condition, rate of disease progression, associated illnesses, animal's age and family setting, owner's ability and motivation to cooperate, and response to treatment. The general approach is to remove underlying or precipitating causes of heart failure and to control the congestive state. Congestion is controlled by reducing the cardiac workload, controlling salt and water retention, and improving the heart's pumping ability. All cases benefit from these approaches.

1. Restrict sodium intake appropriate to the severity of the disease. Moderate restriction (Prescription Diets k/d or Feline k/d, Hill's, or Recipes 2 or 8) in Phase 2, and severe restriction (Prescription Diets h/d or Feline h/d, Hill's, or Recipes 5 or 8—Appendix Table 3) in Phases 3 and 4.

TABLE 1

DRUGS USEFUL IN MANAGEMENT OF HEART DISEASE

Chemical Name (Product Name)	Source	Indications	Common Adverse Effects	Approximate Dosage
Atropine Sulfate USP (0.4 mg/ml)	Many	Sinus bradycardia, sinoatrial arrest, incomplete AV block	Sinus tachycardia, ectopic complexes, ocular, gastrointestinal, and pulmonary side effects, paradoxic vagomimetic effects	0.01–0.02 mg/kg IV, IM 0.02–0.04 mg/kg SQ (Dog and cat)
Captopril (Capoten)	Squibb	Arterial vasodilator, venodilator, angiotensin-converting enzyme inhibitor (decreases aldosterone)	Same as hydralazine	1–2 mg/kg *tid*
Digoxin (Lanoxin, Cardoxin)	Burroughs Wellcome, Evsco	Increases myocardial contractility, decreases heart rate, treats supraventricular tachyarrhythmias	Anorexia, depression, vomiting, diarrhea, AV block, ectopia, junctional tachycardia	Dogs: Oral maintenance: 0.01–0.02 mg/kg divided *bid* Cats: Oral maintenance: 0.007–0.015 mg/kg/day
Dobutamine (Dobutrex)	Eli Lilly	Increases myocardial contractility	Sinus tachycardia at high doses, ectopia	2–15 μg/kg/minute, constant-rate infusion*
Furosemide (Lasix)	Hoescht-Roussel	Reduces blood volume, venous pressure, edema, and ascites	Dehydration, azotemia electrolyte imbalance, loss of compensatory increases in ventricular preload	Dogs: 2–4 mg/kg Cats: 0.5–2 mg/kg (IV, IM, SQ, oral) repeat *bid* or *tid* if needed
Hydralazine (Apresoline)	Ciba	Arterial-vasodilator, decreases regurgitant fraction, increases cardiac output, reduces myocardial tension and preload	Weakness, depression, hypotension, fainting, emesis, sinus tachycardia	0.5–2 mg/kg *bid* to *tid*
Hydrochlorothiazide (Hydrodiuril) (combined with 25 mg spironolactone as Aldactazide)	Merck	Same as furosemide, potassium sparing with spironolactone	Same as furosemide	2–4 mg/kg *bid* 2 mg/kg *bid* (Aldactazide)
Isoproterenol (Isuprel, Proternol)	Breon	Sinoatrial arrest, sinus bradycardia, complete AV block	CNS stimulation, tachycardia, emesis	0.4 mg in 250 ml of 5% glucose, drip slowly to effect Proternol—10–20 mg q4–6 hours, Isuprel glossets—5–10 mg sublingual or per rectum q4–6 hours
Lidocaine HCL (Xylocaine 2% without epinephrine)	Astra	Ventricular premature complexes, ventricular tachycardia	CNS excitation, seizures, tremors, emesis, (Rx with diazepam), other rhythm disturbances	2–4 mg/kg IV slowly, repeat to maximum of 8 mg/kg. Constant rate infusion* for the dog: 25–75 μg/kg min. For the cat: up to 0.5 mg/kg over 5–10 min.

(Continued next page)

TABLE 1—Continued

DRUGS USEFUL IN MANAGEMENT OF HEART DISEASE

Chemical Name (Product Name)	Source	Indications	Common Adverse Effects	Approximate Dosage
Morphine (Morphine Sulfate)	Wyeth, Elkins-Sinn	Pulmonary edema, relieve anxiety	Respiratory depression, diarrhea	0.1–0.25 mg/kg IV or SQ; repeat to desired effect
Nitroglycerine Ointment 2% (Nitrol, Nitro-bid)	Kremers-Urban, Marion	Vasodilator-primarily venous, reduces venous pressure, decreases myocardial oxygen consumption	Hypotension, weakness, depression, sinus tachycardia	¼" to ¾" cutaneously every 4–8 hours
Potassium Chloride (Salt Substitute)	Grocery Stores	Lethargy, anorexia, weakness, replace diuretic losses	Hyperkalemia	2–5 g (0.5–1 t)/day mixed in food
Prazosin (Minipress)	Pfizer	Arterial and venodilator, reduces afterload and preload, other effects as per hydralazine	Same as hydralazine	1–2 mg *bid* to *tid*
Procainamide (Pronestyl, Procan)	Squibb, Parke-Davis	Ventricular premature complexes, ventricular tachycardia	Weakness, hypotension, decreased contractility, gastrointestinal side effects, widening of QRS-T complex	6–8 mg/kg IV over 5 min., 8–20 mg/kg IM q4–6h, tablets—8–20 mg/kg q6h
Propranolol (inderal)	Ayerst	Beta-adrenergic blocker, antiarrhythmic, slows response to atrial fibrillation, decreases myocardial oxygen consumption	Reduces myocardial contractility, bronchial constriction, hypotension, loss of compensatory mechanisms	Dogs: 0.1–1.0 mg/kg (oral) *bid* or *tid* 0.04–0.06 mg/kg IV slowly Cats: 2.5–5.0 mg/kg (oral) *bid*
Quinidine (Quinaglute, Cardioquin)	Many, Berlex	Ventricular premature complexes, ventricular tachycardia, acute atrial fibrillation, refractory supraventricular tachycardias	As per procainamide, drug interaction with digoxin	6–20 mg/kg IV, q6h 6–16 mg/kg orally q6h (sulfate) 8–20 mg/kg orally q6–8h dogs only
Sodium Nitroprusside (Nipride)	Roche	Ultra short acting vasodilator	Reduces blood pressure, reflex tachycardia	5–10 µg/min infusion with monitoring of heart rate and blood pressure
Theophylline (Aminophylline, Elixophylline)	Searle, Berlex	Bronchodilation, mild increase in myocardial contractility	Emesis, Excitement, Urticaria	Aminophylline: 6–10 mg/kg (IV, SQ, oral), repeat q6–12h. Elixophylline: 0.3–0.4 ml/kg *bid-tid*

*Formula for CRI: Bodyweight (in kg) × dose (in µg/kg/min) × .36 = total dose in mg to administer IV over 6 hours. Example of unitless formula: For a 10 kg dog, an infusion of 50 µg/kg/min (10) × (50) × (.36) = 180 mg infused over 6 hours.

2. Restrict exercise and activity as necessary to prevent dyspnea.

3. Ensure free access to clean fresh water that is low in sodium (non-softened or distilled).

4. Use diuretics as necessary to relieve signs of congestion and to reduce preload. Give furose-mide orally as needed (Table 1). It may be given three times daily but should not be given this frequently unless signs so dictate. Hydrochlorothiazide with spironolactone for potassium-sparing effects may be given (Table 1).

5. Potassium and B-vitamin supplementation aren't

necessary when the prepared low-sodium diets are being fed. (These diets already contain increased levels of these nutrients.) However, if the homemade diets are being fed or the plasma potassium concentration falls below 4.5 mEq/L when non-potassium sparing diuretics are being given, add potassium chloride to the ration (Table 1).

6. Digitalize dogs and cats having poor myocardial performance, supraventricular tachyarrhythmias, or both. Decompensated chronic valvular heart disease and congestive (dilatative) cardiomyopathies require digitalis, whereas hypertrophic cardiomyopathies and animals with pericardial disease should generally **not** receive digitalis glycosides. Digoxin is preferred and should be given at home whenever possible. Begin with maintenance dosages (Table 1), and adjust the dosage as necessary to achieve the desired effect. Withdraw the drug if toxic signs such as vomiting, diarrhea or anorexia appear, and resume at a lower dosage when signs of toxicity subside.

7. Give a vasodilator to dogs or cats with congestive heart failure if they have mitral regurgitation or hypertension. Captopril or hydralazine are vasodilators of choice in these conditions (Table 1).

8. Use appropriate antiarrhythmic therapy to correct arrhythmias unresponsive to the medications cited above. Propranolol is preferred for most tachyarrhythmias in cats (Table 1). Propranolol is recommended for all cats with hypertrophic cardiomyopathy. Orally administered quinidine sulfate and/or propranolol may be used to control tachyarrhythmias in dogs. Dogs with symptomatic bradyarrhythmias such as complete heart block or sick sinus syndrome usually require pacemaker therapy.

INTRODUCTION

Heart failure is the disease in which an abnormality of cardiac function causes a cardiac output inadequate to meet the body's needs. It is often caused by myocardial failure and characterized by defects in myocardial contraction. Heart failure can also result from constrictive pericarditis, pericardial effusion and valvular regurgitation and/or stenosis with myocardial function minimally impaired or normal.[25] Thus, diseases known to cause heart failure may involve the heart's valves, myocardium, endocardium, cardiac innervation, pericardium or the blood vessels. In addition, abnormalities in preload, afterload, contractility and heart rate, as well as distensibility and synergy of ventricular contraction, may also contribute to heart failure.[128]

Congestive heart failure is a clinical syndrome characterized by: 1) exercise intolerance, 2) pulmonary and/or systemic venous congestion, 3) low cardiac output initiated by myocardial dysfunction or cardiac failure, and 4) retention of sodium and water resulting from the body's attempt to compensate for an inadequate cardiac output. The heart is generally enlarged and filling pressure is elevated.

INCIDENCE

Heart disease is a common cause of morbidity and mortality in dogs and cats. The precise incidence is unknown, but studies conducted nearly 20 years ago indicated an incidence of approximately 11% of all dogs presented to veterinary clinics (Table 2). Congenital heart defects occur in 0.5%-1.0% of all dogs, accounting for 5-10% of all heart disease seen in dogs.[124]

Congenital heart disease seems less prevalent in

TABLE 2
INCIDENCE OF CANINE CARDIOVASCULAR DISEASE[34,40,43,44,48,111,114]

Condition (Breed Predilection)	Incidence/1000
Congenital (purebred dogs)	5.5
Patent ductus arteriosus (Min. & Toy Poodle, Collie, Pomeranian, Shetland Sheep Dog)	
Pulmonic stenosis (Beagle, Schnauzer, others)	
Aortic stenosis (German Shepherd, Boxer, Newfoundland, Golden Retriever, Pointer)	
Interventricular septal defect (English Bulldog, others)	
Tetralogy of Fallot (Keeshond, Wire-Haired Fox Terrier)	
Persistent right aortic arch (German Shepherd, others)	
Atrial septal defect (German Shepherd, others)	
Mitral (dysplasia) insufficiency (Large and Giant Breeds)	
Acquired	107.2
Chronic valvular disease, mitral esp. (Small and Toy Breeds)	
Myocardial disease (Large Breeds)	
CVD and myocardial disease (Small Breeds, aged)	
Heartworm, pericardial disease and other	
Total	112.7

cats than in dogs. Acquired heart diseases account for more than 90% of the heart disease seen in veterinary medicine. The frequency of acquired heart disease increases with age.

The incidence and causes of heart diseases vary by geographic location. In endemic areas heartworms account for the majority of heart disease. Feline cardiomyopathies appear to be much more prevalent on both the east and the west coasts. Veterinarians who see a preponderance of geriatric cases see a higher incidence of valvular and myocardial heart disease, whereas veterinarians seeing a lot of young animals see a higher incidence of congenital heart disease.

Heart disease is not synonymous with heart failure. Although heart failure can result from any of the heart diseases, only about 10-15% of heart disease cases exhibit heart failure. The most common cause of heart failure in dogs is mitral insufficiency. The incidence of mitral insufficiency in dogs has been reported to vary from 8% of dogs presented to veterinary clinics to 42% presented to necropsy.[54] Feline cardiomyopathy is by far the most common cause of congestive heart failure in cats.[78,143]

Acquired diseases of the myocardium and of the atrio-ventricular valves account for the vast majority of heart failure cases. In many instances, especially in dogs, mitral insufficiency and arteriosclerosis of intramural coronary vessels resulting in microscopic intramural myocardial infarction (MIMI) leads to left heart failure. Systemic arterial thromboemboli are found in a high percentage of feline cardiomyopathy cases.[97,98,99]

Heartworm disease has been estimated to account for 11% of congestive heart failure cases;[40,43] although, in endemic areas the incidence is undoubtedly greater. Heartworm disease causes chronic cor pulmonale with elevated pulmonary arterial pressure leading to right heart failure.

The most common congenital anomalies responsible for congestive heart failure in dogs in order of their relative clinical frequency are: patent ductus arteriosus, pulmonic stenosis, aortic stenosis, ventricular septal defect, tetralogy of Fallot, persistent right aortic arch, atrial septal defect, and mitral insufficiency (Table 2).[124] These conditions occur more commonly in purebred animals, and several forms have been shown to be inherited in certain breeds of dogs (Table 2).[109-114] There is substantial experimental evidence for suspecting a genetic problem in congenital heart disease in dogs and cats, but it is also known that some of these defects can originate from non-genetic causes during gestation.

Pericardial disease occurs in about 1% of all dogs with cardiovascular disease, but the percentage rises to 5% or more if congestive heart failure is present.[48,142] Pericardial disease is one of the more common causes of right heart failure in dogs after heartworm disease.[142] There are several congenital pericardial defects. Peritoneopericardial diaphragmatic hernia is a rare cause of congestive heart failure in young dogs and cats.[48] Pericardial disease is most commonly due to pericardial effusion, constrictive pericardial disease, and pericardial mass lesions. All of these conditions may decrease diastolic ventricular compliance, impair ventricular filling, and therefore limit cardiac output.[88,142] Neoplastic conditions may be associated with some forms of pericardial disease. Predominant tumors causing congestive heart failure in dogs are hemangiosarcoma (generally right atrium) and heartbase tumors.[89,92,107,142]

PATHOPHYSIOLOGY

NORMAL CARDIOVASCULAR FUNCTION

The circulatory system is controlled by a number of neurohumoral regulatory systems which:
1. Change the caliber of arterioles and other resistance vessels,
2. Vary the rate and stroke volume of the heart,
3. Increase or decrease blood storage in capacitive venous vessels, and
4. Under certain circumstances alter the caliber and permeability of capillaries.

With cardiac disease these functions are impaired. As a result, multiple organs are affected. The signs of heart failure occur because of derangements of these organs brought on by inadequate cardiac output or through compensatory functions that attempt to maintain homeostasis.[128]

Cardiac performance is determined by six major factors: 1) preload, 2) afterload, 3) contractility, 4) heart rate, 5) distensibility, and 6) synergy or correlated action of ventricular contraction. Some of the interactions between these factors are shown in Figure 1.[128] Abnormalities in any of these factors may contribute to heart failure.

Preload (ventricular end-diastolic volume) determines the length-tension relationship and thus cardiac performance by the well-known Frank-Starling mechanism. This relationship states that as the end-diastolic (pre-contraction) length of the myocardial fibers of the heart increase (i.e., the more the heart fills), the strength of contraction increases, resulting in a larger heart stroke volume. Up to the point of heart failure, increases in preload

FIGURE 1

INTERACTIONS BETWEEN COMPONENTS THAT DETERMINE CARDIAC PERFORMANCE[128]

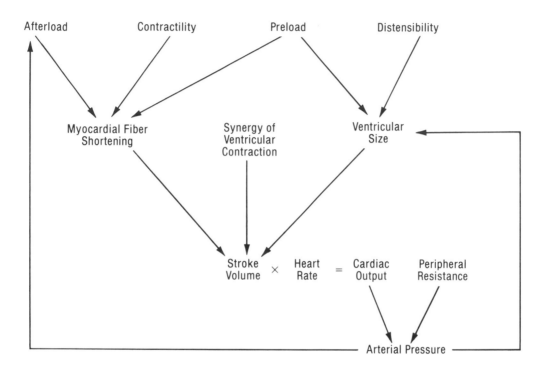

cause increases both in myocardial fiber shortening when contracted and in ventricular size. The factors determining preload include:

1. Blood volume,
2. Venous tone,
3. Intrapericardial and intrathoracic pressures,
4. Body position,
5. Atrial systole, and
6. Muscular activity,

Preload is estimated clinically by judging the distention of the venous system, especially the jugular veins. Radiographic assessment of vascular and cardiac distention are also helpful in estimating preload. Accurate determination of preload requires echocardiography, or invasive techniques such as angiocardiography.

Afterload is the impedence to ventricular emptying and is frequently estimated by aortic and pulmonary arterial pressures for the left and right ventricles respectively. Afterload is inversely related to cardiac performance and output. Thus, as afterload increases, cardiac output decreases. This is opposite to preload because, within limits, as preload increases, cardiac output increases. Afterload

is estimated clinically by judging the intensity of the second heart sound. As afterload increases, the volume of the second heart sound increases. However, the second heart sound is also affected by many other properties of the heart, lungs, and thoracic wall.

Contractility (the inotropic state of the myocardium) is determined by the rate of myocardial reaction at contractile sites. Thus contractility determines myocardial fiber shortening independent of preload or afterload. Clinically, intensity of the left ventricular apical impulse and the rise in the rate of the arterial pressure pulse can be grossly related to contractility. Numerous other indices of contractility can be determined both by invasive and non-invasive parameters, including systolic time intervals, echocardiograms, angiocardiograms, and measurements derived from intraventricular pressure.

Distensibility relates to ventricular diastolic properties and the heart's ability to fill and accommodate the volume of blood presented to it. Factors affecting distensibility include the pericardium, intrapericardial pressure, cardiac hypertrophy, cardiac fibrosis, ventricular interdependence, and any dis-

ease that affects myocardial metabolism, composition, or fiber orientation. Abnormalities in distensibility may be suggested by the presence of pathologic gallop rhythms. Third heart sound gallops are commonly associated with dilated heart failure. Fourth heart sound gallops are typically associated with cardiac hypertrophy. Simultaneously derived pressure and volume measurements are necessary for the most accurate estimates of distensibility and ventricular compliance.

Complete synergy of ventricular contraction is necessary for maximal cardiac performance. Asynergy reduces the efficiency of ventricular ejection and thus lowers stroke volume and cardiac output. Arrhythmias and splitting of heart sounds detected on auscultation may indicate a problem with synergy of ventricular contraction. Angiocardiography, radioangiocardiography, and/or cross-sectional echocardiography are used to quantitate the abnormalities present.

Heart rate is directly related to cardiac performance since heart rate times stroke volume equals cardiac output. Increasing the heart rate up to approximately 2.5 times the normal resting rate is an effective means of increasing cardiac output.[125] At faster rates the heart has insufficient time to fill, and the efficiency of ventricular contraction decreases, causing stroke volume and cardiac output to begin falling. In addition, tachycardia reduces coronary blood flow and, therefore, myocardial oxygen supply. At the same time the demand for myocardial oxygen is increased.

COMPENSATION TO REDUCED CARDIAC FUNCTION

With reduced cardiac function, cardiovascular reserves are used at rest, and exercise tolerance is reduced. However, the animal can live a fairly normal life provided physical exertion is reduced and cardiovascular reserve is not exceeded at rest.[130] Circulatory manifestations of heart failure may be stalled for years by the intervention of a number of compensatory mechanisms such as increased heart rate, cardiac enlargement through dilatation, and myocardial hypertrophy. Although various types of cardiac disease deplete the total cardiovascular reserve in different ways, the result is always some reduction in the delivery of total oxygen to tissues. Therefore, diminished exercise tolerance is a common denominator of heart disease.[32]

In the presence of an increased work load, the heart attempts to compensate in the following ways:[23]

1. Increased preload improves cardiac performance by the Frank-Starling mechanism.

2. Increased sympathoadrenal activity increases heart rate and myocardial contractility through the release of catecholamines.

3. Myocardial dilatation and hypertrophy augment contractile tissue. Cardiac dilatation and hypertrophy enable the heart to adapt to increased work loads. Both pressure and volume overload lead to cardiac dilatation and increased end-diastolic myocardial fiber length. This dilatation induces myocardial hypertrophy.[95,132,149]

Each of these mechanisms has a limited potential and may ultimately fail, resulting in heart failure.

Cardiac dilatation may be caused by either an increased volume load or an increased pressure load. Diseases causing an increased volume load on one or more of the cardiac chambers include all forms of valvular insufficiency, left to right shunts, chronic anemia, and hyperthyroidism.[136] Chronic pressure loads are imposed on the heart by such diseases as aortic or pulmonic stenosis and systemic or pulmonary arterial hypertension.

With chronic increased volume loads, myocardial hypertrophy occurs in an eccentric fashion with the volume of the chamber increasing in conjunction with the increase in muscle mass. In contrast, chronic increased pressure loads tend to produce concentric myocardial hypertrophy. This condition is characterized by an increase in muscle mass with the chamber volume remaining normal or even being reduced. Both increased wall tension from dilatation and increased muscle mass with hypertrophy increase demands for myocardial oxygen and energy and the need for improved coronary blood flow. Coronary insufficiency seems to be the limiting factor in chronic hypertrophy. The ultimate lack of sufficient coronary blood flow and myocardial oxygenation lead to the compensated ventricle becoming the failing ventricle.[130]

Expansion of blood volume constitutes an important compensatory mechanism that tends to maintain cardiac output by increasing preload. The augmented ventricular end-diastolic volume helps maintain cardiac output, except in the terminal stages of heart failure. This is of course self-limiting because elevated end-diastolic volumes and pressures not only improve cardiac performance but also promote pulmonary or systemic venous congestion and edema.

Sympathoadrenal activity occurs whenever cardiac output is insufficient to maintain normal blood pressure and tissue perfusion. This increase in sympathoadrenal activity increases myocardial contractility and heart rate and causes a redistribution of cardiac output to and within a number of organs.[3,47,102] Vasoconstriction, induced largely by

the adrenergic nervous system, tends to maintain perfusion of the heart and brain by reducing blood flow to the kidneys, viscera, and skin. In animals with mild to moderate heart failure, these changes occur primarily during exercise; but in those with more severe heart failure, they are present at rest.[133] Vasoconstriction increases peripheral resistance (afterload) which may prevent cardiac output from rising normally to meet new demands. The reduced renal blood flow leads to activation of the renin-angiotensin-aldosterone system, resulting in sodium and water retention and increased vascular volume. Fluid retention is an important compensatory mechanism but is also responsible for many of the clinical manifestations of heart failure.

FLUID RETENTION

Sodium intake in excess of that excreted is a cardinal feature of congestive heart failure. Failure to excrete a sodium load has been used for decades as an index to the presence of heart failure.[24,83,134] The abnormal accumulation of sodium and water in heart disease is due to a complex sequence of adjustments which vary with the type, severity, and time of the disease present. Any decrease in cardiac performance impairs the kidney's ability to excrete salt and water. The general mechanism for the renal sodium and water retention is a decrease in the amount filtered and an increase in the amount reabsorbed.

Numerous neuroendocrine alterations have been reported to play a role in causing sodium retention in congestive heart failure. These include:

1. Increased activity of the renin-angiotensin-aldosterone system,[7,11,28,33,35,58,87,103,145]

2. Increased plasma levels of norepinephrine and epinephrine,[30,104]

3. Depletion of myocardial norepinephrine,[123]

4. Decreased plasma dopamine-beta-hydroxylase activity,[82,104]

5. Increased antidiuretic hormone (ADH) secretion,[126,139]

6. Alteration and resetting of arterial stretch (pressure) receptors,[61,153,154]

7. Attenuation of arterial baroreceptor (afferent and efferent),[60,81,127,148] and

8. A deficiency in atrial natriuretic and diuretic factors.[31]

Decreases in either cardiac output, or blood pressure, or both, cause reduction in renal blood flow both directly and via activation of the sympathetic nervous system. The result is renal vasoconstriction and a redistribution of blood flow within the kidney so that renal cortical blood flow is reduced while a relatively normal renal medullary flow is maintained.[8,9,10] There is a proportionately greater fall in renal blood flow than glomerular filtration, thus the fraction filtered rises. This results in elevated protein concentration in the peritubular renal capillaries and a decline in the post-glomerular capillary hydrostatic pressure. Both of these factors are thought to increase sodium reabsorption.

Decreased renal perfusion activates the juxta-glomerular apparatus to enhance release of renin. Renin acts on angiotensinogen to produce angiotensin I. Converting enzyme converts angiotensin I to angiotensin II which then stimulates aldosterone secretion. Aldosterone further augments retention of sodium by the kidneys (Figure 2). Angiotensin II is also a potent vasoconstrictor that contributes to maintenance of an increased afterload and, as a result, a further decrease in cardiac output and further renal vasoconstriction.

Renal fluid retention expands the extracellular fluid volume and tends to return the renin-angiotensin-aldosterone system toward normal. Plasma renin activity and aldosterone concentration in heart failure are correlated with the stage and clinical status of the patient.[36,46,57,105,147] The system appears to be activated early in heart disease, especially with acute cardiac decompensation. In chronic "compensated" heart failure, the system is self-limiting or reflexly reduced. Stimulation of cardiac receptors as the heart distends may cause a reflex inhibition of the renin-angiotensin-aldosterone system, as well as ADH and sympathetic activity at this stage.[1,25] However, late in heart failure the cardiac receptors become "desensitized" or are reset; thus, the inhibition may be removed and the activity of the renin-angiotensin system, as well as the sympathetic systems, again increase.[1,25,93,96] At this stage there is again severe sodium retention, tachycardia, and vasoconstriction leading to progressive deterioration characteristic of end-stage heart failure.

Increased sodium retention results in the release of antidiuretic hormone (ADH) from the posterior pituitary. Antidiuretic hormone permits more water to be reabsorbed by the kidneys. Increased water ingestion is stimulated by angiotensin II.[55,56]

Atrial peptides may also contribute to compensation and homeostasis in early cardiac disease and heart failure.[31] These substances, present in atrial granules, cause both a natriuresis and a diuresis. It is possible that their depletion in heart disease may enhance retention of sodium and water.

As a result of fluid retention, the extracellular fluid volume and blood volume are increased,

FIGURE 2

EXTRAMURAL COMPENSATION OF HEART FAILURE

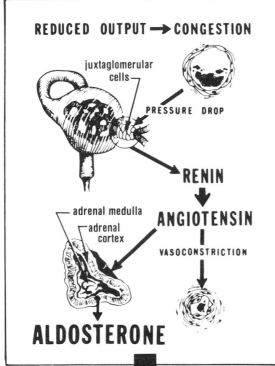

REDUCED OUTPUT → CONGESTION

juxtaglomerular cells

PRESSURE DROP

RENIN

ANGIOTENSIN

adrenal medulla

adrenal cortex

VASOCONSTRICTION

ALDOSTERONE

Upper left: Reduced cardiac output decreases renal blood flow and increases venous congestion which stimulate renin secretion, which induces angiotensin activation. Angiotensin causes vasoconstriction and aldosterone secretion.

Lower left: Aldosterone increases sodium (Na+) retention which results in increased ADH secretion.

Lower right: ADH permits increased water reabsorption which increases the extracellular fluid volume resulting in edema and ascites.

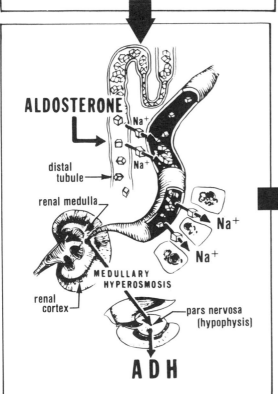

ALDOSTERONE

Na+

distal tubule

Na+

renal medulla

Na+

Na+

MEDULLARY HYPEROSMOSIS

renal cortex

pars nervosa (hypophysis)

ADH

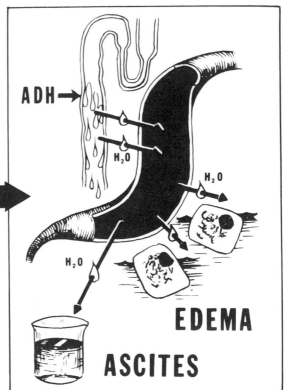

ADH →

H_2O

H_2O

H_2O

EDEMA

ASCITES

FIGURE 3

MECHANISMS FOR DEVELOPMENT OF EDEMA IN HEART FAILURE

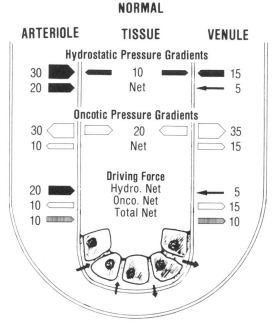

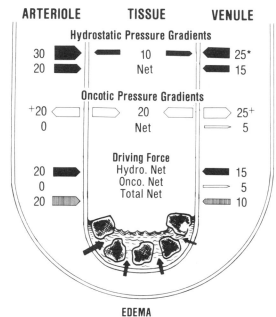

FLUID BALANCE

Total net driving force in arteriole of 10mm Hg into and in venule of 10mm Hg out of the tissue results in fluid movement through but no accumulation in tissues.

EDEMA

Total net driving force in arteriole of 20mm Hg into and in venule of 10mm Hg into the tissue results in fluid movement into and accumulation in tissues.

*Increased as a result of venous congestion.
+Decreased as a result of water retention.

which increases cardiac preload. The increased extracellular fluid causes a relative decrease in plasma protein concentration. This reduces plasma oncotic pressure, resulting in a loss of fluid from the plasma to the interstitial fluid compartment (Figure 3). The increase in blood volume and increased venous pressure from the inability of the heart to pump the blood presented to it also increase the interstitial accumulation of fluid (Figure 3). Consequently, interstitial fluid may increase from a normal of 15% to as much as 30% of the body weight.[116] Intraperitoneal fluid may increase dramatically, especially in right heart failure. The resulting edema and ascites are responsible for the signs occurring in heart failure. However, it is increased sodium retention that is responsible for the presence of the excess fluid.

HEART FAILURE

The heart can fail acutely due to:

1. Toxins or infectious agents causing acute myocardial damage,
2. Acute hemodynamic volume or pressure overloads,
3. Acute arrhythmias, or
4. Acute restrictions in cardiac filling.

However, the most common forms of heart disease in dogs and cats are chronic heart disease and chronic cardiac disability, both of which ultimately lead to congestive heart failure.[53] As depicted in Figure 4, the most common form of acquired cardiovascular disease in dogs appears to follow a protracted time course.[42] The onset of valvular lesions may occur early in the dog's life and slowly progress. Mitral insufficiency may not appear until the middle years and may be tolerated well into late life. Clinical signs of left ventricular failure may not develop until the last years of life when small intramural coronary arteriosclerosis creates focal myocardial necrosis and fibrosis, and myocardial

FIGURE 4

DEVELOPMENT OF CONGESTIVE HEART FAILURE IN A DOG WITH ACQUIRED CARDIOVASCULAR DISEASE[42]

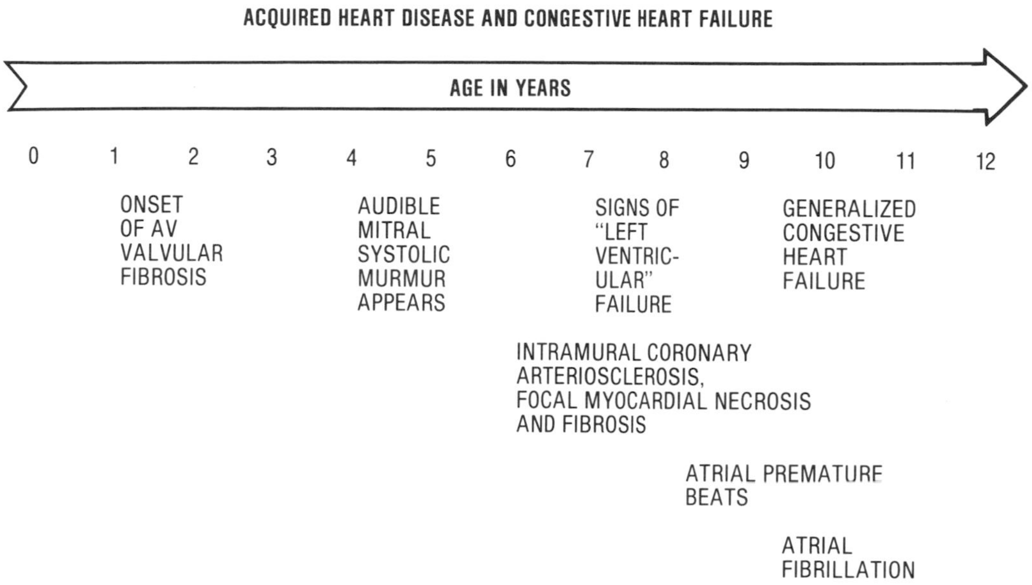

ACQUIRED HEART DISEASE AND CONGESTIVE HEART FAILURE

AGE IN YEARS

0	1	2	3	4	5	6	7	8	9	10	11	12

ONSET
OF AV
VALVULAR
FIBROSIS

AUDIBLE
MITRAL
SYSTOLIC
MURMUR
APPEARS

SIGNS OF
"LEFT
VENTRIC-
ULAR"
FAILURE

GENERALIZED
CONGESTIVE
HEART
FAILURE

INTRAMURAL CORONARY
ARTERIOSCLEROSIS,
FOCAL MYOCARDIAL NECROSIS
AND FIBROSIS

ATRIAL PREMATURE
BEATS

ATRIAL
FIBRILLATION

depression along with mitral regurgitation, resulting in progressive cardiac deterioration and congestive heart failure. At any time, however, acute events such as ruptured chordae tendineae, cardiac arrhythmias, or the development of pericardial effusion or tamponade may result in acute heart failure. In heart disease when the heart reaches a point where it can no longer compensate sufficiently and the cardiac output falls below reserves, exercise tolerance is reduced. As cardiac output continues to fall, the patient may be unable to maintain even household activity.

Many heart diseases affect predominantly one side of the heart. It is convenient to separate the signs of congestive heart failure into those referable to left or right ventricular failure. Involvement of both sides is referred to as generalized heart failure.

Left Heart Failure

Left heart failure is caused by diseases that affect primarily the left ventricle, aortic valve, or the mitral valve. Common causes in dogs are mitral insufficiency, myocardial disease or cardiomyopathy, and aortic stenosis. In cats hypertrophic and/or dilatative cardiomyopathy manifest principally as left heart failure. Signs associated with left heart failure are mainly attributable to pulmonary congestion. Signs include dyspnea upon exertion, cough,

orthopnea, paroxysmal (nocturnal) dyspnea or cardiac asthma, hemoptysis, and sometimes cyanosis. Pulmonary edema may occur in varying degrees and when severe may cause bubbling and frothing from the mouth or nose.

In left heart failure, left ventricular end-diastolic volume and pressure increase, resulting in increases in left atrial and pulmonary venous pressures and volumes. When pulmonary capillary pressure exceeds colloid osmotic pressure, fluid filters out of capillaries and into the interstitial spaces and alveoli. The result is pulmonary edema (Figure 3).

Anything that increases pulmonary engorgement in the face of a decompensated left ventricle may result in pulmonary signs. Thus, dyspnea upon exertion occurs as the right ventricle continues to pump the increased venous return of exercise, but the left ventricle cannot respond sufficiently. Respiratory distress may develop in animals with left ventricular failure when they lie down. When the animal reclines, blood volume is redistributed from the peripheral to the central circulation and it accumulates in the pulmonary tree. This respiratory distress is termed orthopnea and may be responsible for waking the animal or causing restlessness at night. In normal animals, the shift of blood into the lungs produces no problem, but in the animal with pulmonary congestion due to left ventricular failure, the added load induces dyspnea. Paroxysmal

dyspnea (cardiac asthma) may also occur and is frequently associated with coughing or choking in dogs. Cats seem to cough less frequently with heart failure, but they often exhibit dyspnea.

Right Heart Failure

Diseases affecting primarily the right heart are pulmonic stenosis, tricuspid insufficiency, heartworm disease,[108] or other primary lung diseases, resulting in cor pulmonale. Right heart failure may also occur secondary to left heart failure. With right heart failure, right ventricular end-diastolic pressure and volume increase, which leads to increases in right atrial pressure and volume with parallel rises in the vena cavae and veins. Signs of right heart failure typically are manifestations of generalized systemic venous congestion. In addition, total cardiac output is reduced. Sodium and water retention occurs which increases blood volume and further aggravates venous distention and pressure elevation (Figure 3). Characteristic signs of right heart failure include distention of the jugular and other superficial veins, hepatic and splenic enlargement and diffusion of fluid into serous cavities, appearing particularly as ascites in dogs. Dependent subcutaneous edema can occur but is relatively rare in dogs and cats, whereas effusion of fluid into the pleural or peritoneal cavity is relatively common.

The engorged liver may be tender to abdominal palpation, and hepatic function tests, though not specific for heart failure, often show some abnormality. The extent of effusion into the peritoneal cavity tends to correlate with the elevated pressures in the portal circulation rather than with the overall cardiac status.[130]

Generalized Heart Failure

Usually when one side of the heart fails, the ensuing sequence of events results in the ultimate failure of the opposite side as well. For example, in dogs with left ventricular failure as a result of chronic mitral valvular fibrosis and mitral insufficiency, left atrial and ventricular pressure and volume are increased. This results in pulmonary venous congestion, pulmonary arteriolar constriction,[86] elevation of pulmonary hydrostatic pressure, and ultimately a rise in pulmonary arterial pressure. The resulting additional pressure load on the right ventricle, in conjunction with the compensatory increase in fluid volume from fluid retention, may cause right ventricular failure. Conversely, when the primary failure is in the right ventricle, this failure may reduce the overall cardiac output so that coronary blood flow is reduced, which weakens the left ventricle.

Frequently, generalized heart failure does not occur for several months to several years after the onset of failure of either side of the heart. However, occasionally it occurs spontaneously, or it may be the primary condition when it is caused by generalized myocardial disease, pericardial disease, or certain congenital heart diseases.

Obvious malnutrition and emaciation may accompany chronic congestive heart failure. This condition, referred to as "cardiac cachexia,"[121] occurs as a result of:

1. Reduced blood flow to skeletal muscle and cellular hypoxia which result in generalized weakness,
2. A poor appetite, and
3. A variety of gastrointestinal disturbances including malabsorption of nutrients due to pooling and stasis of visceral blood.

Ascites is usually present in animals with generalized heart failure. Its presence may mask cardiac cachexia and weight loss.

DIAGNOSIS

The diagnosis of heart failure, as with any other disease, requires a consideration of the animal's history and owner's observations, a thorough physical examination, and recognition of clinical signs the animal exhibits. Electrocardiography and thoracic radiographs are important parts of a cardiovascular evaluation. A number of laboratory examinations are an important part of the data base for animals suspected of having cardiac disease. Echocardiography, angiocardiography and/or cardiac catheterization may be needed to diagnose the specific heart disease present and to define the degree of functional cardiac impairment.

Early detection of heart disease is important so that the most effective therapy can be instituted. Ideally, heart disease is detected before heart failure becomes clinically apparent to the animal's owner. Nevertheless, animals with heart disease are presented in virtually any stage of the syndrome. Observant clients with working animals may detect a subtle reduction in exercise tolerance in the early stages of the condition. Other animal owners may not be aware of the animal's illness until the animal is obviously wasting away or its abdomen is so enlarged that it is presented for a sudden weight problem or an inability to rise.

SIGNS AND OWNER COMPLAINTS

The more common presenting manifestations and signs suggesting heart disease in dogs and cats, not necessarily listed in order of frequency or

severity, include:
1. Weakness,
2. Easy fatigability or reduced exercise tolerance,
3. Cough, particularly after exertion or excitement,
4. Dyspnea,
5. Restlessness when lying down or sleeping,
6. Syncope, fainting, or similar "spells,"
7. Abdominal enlargement or distention,
8. Sudden "weight problem" due to ascites,
9. Emaciation or cachexia,
10. Reduced appetite,
11. Cyanosis,
12. Ventral or peripheral edema, and
13. Polyuria and polydypsia, especially at night.

None of these signs is pathognomonic for heart failure and can be produced by many other diseases.[67]

A cough is a prominent feature of chronic left-sided heart failure in dogs,[117] and animals with heart disease are often presented for this reason. Coughing, like dyspnea, is a prominent feature of many other pulmonary diseases of non-cardiac origin. In addition, some dogs and cats with severe congestive heart failure and markedly enlarged hearts with fluid retention rarely cough. Thus, additional clinical evidence of cardiac disease must be present before a diagnosis of heart failure can be made. Such additional evidence may include arrhythmias, heart murmurs, prolonged circulation time or capillary refill, or radiographic demonstration of cardiac enlargement. The finding of cardiac enlargement coupled with evidence of increased filling pressures is highly suggestive of heart disease and heart failure.[128] Although heart murmurs and electrocardiographic abnormalities are highly suggestive of heart disease as well, they do not specifically indicate heart failure.

HISTORY

In addition to recording such routine historical facts such as age, sex, weight, diet, immunization record, etc., a number of other items in the patient's history are helpful in establishing a diagnosis of heart disease and heart failure. Specific attention should be given to:[48,117]

1. Past coughing experience including its frequency, duration, timing, and associated events that might exacerbate these signs. The typical cardiac cough is low-pitched, resonant, and often manifested in paroxysms after sleeping. Coughing may end with gagging which is sometimes mistaken for an attempt to vomit.

2. The pattern of water consumption and urination.
3. Exercise—amount and tolerance. Significant heart disease is always accompanied by a reduction in exercise tolerance, but many pets simply do not exercise sufficiently to make this readily apparent. The animal's activity must be related to signs in order to characterize the phase of heart disease and thus assist in diagnosis and prognosis.
4. Any history of previous heart disease and its treatment.
5. Weight gain or loss and whether it is due to changes in the amount of body fluid or mass.
6. Diet and environment. Knowledge of these are important for both diagnostic and therapeutic reasons. It may be evident that certain snacks high in sodium seem to bring on signs of congestion. Animals kept in the heat or those having to go up and down stairs may have difficulty and show signs of respiratory problems.

PHASE AND SEVERITY OF HEART DISEASE

In addition to establishing the etiologic diagnosis for heart failure, it is important to recognize the severity of the animal's disease by phase, status, and prognosis.[48,49] An outline of the various phases and terminology of heart failure are given in Table 3, and the factors useful in determining the severity of heart failure are given in Table 4. The severity of any sign will depend on the phase of failure to which the animal has progressed when examined. Determining the animal's cardiac status is important in instituting optimal management and determining the prognosis. Thus, a thorough history and physical examination to establish the phase of heart disease is as important as diagnosing the presence of congestive heart failure. The success of therapy and prognosis depends largely on how well the history of the heart disease for a given patient is known and developed.

PHYSICAL EXAMINATION

In addition to recording body temperature, body weight, and condition of musculature, skin, and coat, other aspects of the physical examination such as inspection, palpation, auscultation, and percussion may be particularly revealing in patients with heart disease. Note particularly the pattern of respiration and its character in the animal at rest and after exercise. Inspection of skin and mucous membranes may reveal cyanosis either in the oral, ocular, or abdominal regions. Abdominal enlarge-

TABLE 3

PHASES OF CARDIAC DISEASE — DIAGNOSIS AND PROGNOSIS*

Phase	Description
I	Normal activity does not produce undue fatigue, dyspnea or coughing. Physical activity need not be limited in animals in this phase of cardiac disease.
II	The animal is comfortable at rest, but ordinary physical activity causes fatigue, dyspnea or coughing. In these animals, exercise should be limited moderately, such activities as hunting and long periods of strenuous exercise should be avoided.
III	The animal is comfortable at rest; but minimal exercise may produce fatigue, dyspnea or coughing. Signs may also develop while the animal is in a recumbent position (orthopnea). Physical activity must be limited, free running and stair climbing should be strictly avoided. Exercise should be limited to short walks and moderate house activity.
IV	Congestive heart failure, dyspnea and coughing are present even when the animal is at rest. Signs are exaggerated by any physical activity. Total exercise restriction, i.e., absolute cage rest, is essential.

Phase	Cardiac Status**
I	Uncompromised
II	Slightly compromised
III	Moderately compromised
IV	Severely compromised

Phase	Prognosis**
I	Good
II	Good with therapy
III	Fair with therapy
IV	Guarded despite therapy

*Ettinger, S. J., and Suter, P. F.: *Canine Cardiology.* W. B. Saunders Co., Philadelphia, 1970. *Current Veterinary Therapy VI.* Edited by Robert W. Kirk, DVM, 1977, p. 314.

**Criteria Committee, New York Heart Association, 1974. *Current Veterinary Therapy VI.* Edited by Robert W. Kirk, DVM, 1977, p. 314.

TABLE 4

FACTORS USEFUL IN THE DIAGNOSIS OF HEART DISEASE AND ITS SEVERITY

	Sub-Clinical	Moderate Clinical	Severe Clinical	Acute (Emergency)
Heart Rate	Elevated	Elevated	Tachycardia	Up to 280
Systolic Murmur (L)	Mitral, Grade 3	Same-Grade 3	Same-Grade 4-5	Same-Grade 4-5
Cardiac Enlargement (L) (R)	Present	Present	Present	Present
Arrhythmias (L) (R)	Occasional	Occasional	Present	Frequent
Pulmonary Edema (L)	Absent	After exercise	Moderate	Constant
Dyspnea (L)	After exercise	Increased by exercise	Constant	Constant
Cough (L)	Exercise may precipitate	Sporadic after exercise	Constant	Constant
Rales (L)	Absent	Occasional	Frequent	Constant
Ascites (R)	Absent	Rare	Constant	Constant
Hepatomegaly (R)	Rare	Occasional	Frequent	Constant
Venous Engorgement (R)	Absent	Absent	Occasional	Frequent
Orthopnea (L)	Absent	Absent	Apparent	Exaggerated
Cyanosis (L) (R)	Absent	Absent	Occasional	Occasional
Body Weight (R)	Normal	Elevated (excess fluids)	Below normal (emaciation)	Variable
Circulation Time (L) (R)	May be increased	Usually increased	Increased	Increased
BUN (L) (R)	20-40	20-40	20-40	20-Up

(L) = Left side failure.
(R) = Right side failure.

ment, peripheral edema, or other swellings may be suggestive, and capillary refill time may be prolonged. Of particular importance is examination of the jugular veins with the animal sitting with its head elevated. The finding of bilateral jugular venous distention frequently indicates elevated right heart filling pressures due to heart disease. Jugular pulsations may also be present and correlate with tricuspid insufficiency or stenosis or reduced ventricular distensibility or compliance.

Palpation

By placing both hands on the thorax with the forefingers in the axilla and the fingertips slightly below the costochondral junction, the examiner can identify the character and location of the cardiac impulse. In fact, both heart sounds and their location can often be felt. Loud heart murmurs are perceived as thrills. Posterior displacement of the cardiac apex suggests left ventricular enlargement. A prominent right ventricular lift felt with the right hand may indicate right ventricular enlargement. Displacement of the heart due to intrathoracic masses may be determined by these techniques. The cardiac rhythm should also be readily discernible in most animals. Thoracic palpation may give the first clue to cardiac arrhythmias.

Arterial pulses, which are usually most discernible in the femoral arteries, should be characterized as to rhythm and character. Bounding arterial

pulses characteristic of increased pulse pressures are typical of patent ductus arteriosus, aortic insufficiency, and peripheral arteriovenous fistulas. Pulses that are weak and short-lived typically indicate a reduced stroke volume.

Abdominal palpation can reveal hepatic and/or splenic enlargement or ascites, which may indicate right heart failure. With the animal standing, elevate its anterior abdomen while viewing the jugular vein to check for the hepatojugular reflux associated with hepatic congestion and right heart failure. Elevating the abdomen while ausculting may also help reveal the presence of gallop rhythms brought on by the enhanced venous return.

Tracheal palpation can often be revealing in animals showing respiratory signs. Identification of cervical tracheal collapse is particularly important, and coughing due to tracheal-bronchial disease may be elicited by tracheal palpation.

Auscultation

Auscultation is a most practical method for screening animals clinically for evidence of heart disease.[44,65]

The auscultatory examination should be conducted in a quiet environment. Each auscultatory examination should be made in a prescribed manner. It is helpful to move the stethoscope slowly from one auscultatory area to the other. The standard areas for auscultating the various cardiac

---

FIGURE 5

AREAS FOR AUSCULTATING CARDIAC VALVES

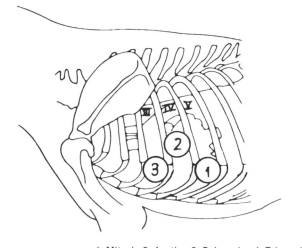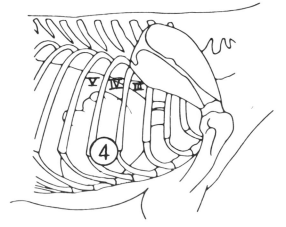

1. Mitral, 2. Aortic, 3. Pulmonic, 4. Tricuspid areas. III, IV and V Intercostal Spaces

valves are shown in Figure 5. Using the bell of the stethoscope with light pressure is best for hearing the first heart sound and gallop rhythms due to a third or fourth heart sound, all of which are typically low in frequency. The diaphragm of the stethoscope is best for detecting and characterizing sounds of higher frequency such as the second heart sound and many cardiac murmurs.

During auscultation, it is helpful to use one hand to control the animal's breathing and to alter venous return by elevating the abdomen. Techniques to alter venous return, arterial blood pressure, or both, are helpful in identifying the site or cause of particular abnormalities. When a rapid heart rate is present, it is helpful to massage the carotid sinus or gently press on the eyeballs, which should elicit cardiac slowing by enhanced efferent vagal activity.

Auscultatory examination of the heart should reveal the presence of any cardiac arrhythmias, cardiac murmurs, or gallop rhythms. All sounds (both normal and abnormal) should be characterized as to intensity, location, character, frequency, duration, quality, and direction of transmission.[41,135] Sources of recorded heart sounds occurring with cardiac dysfunctions are given in Table 5.

Arrhythmias are detected as a change in the rate or rhythm of the heart sounds. A normal dog has a respiratory sinus arrhythmia characterized as an increase in heart rate during inspiration and a decrease during expiration. Premature atrial or ventricular contractions can be detected by an interruption of the regular heart beat by premature heart sounds. A compensatory pause typically occurs after the premature beat before the next normal heart beat is heard.

Although atrial fibrillation may occur in giant breeds of dogs without heart disease, its presence in any breed of dog or cat usually indicates that heart disease is present. It is a common sequella to many diseases that cause atrial enlargement, including mitral insufficiency and cardiomyopathies in dogs.[29,51,86] It is characterized by a rapid

TABLE 5

SOURCE OF RECORDED HEART SOUNDS

1. Geckeler GD: Heart recordings. Columbia LP No. ML-4936, Columbia Records, Inc., Terre Haute, IN (33 1/3 rpm disc).

2. Geckeler GD: Gitaligin Audiovisual Heart Atlas. White Laboratories, Inc., Kenilworth, NY (1957) (78 rpm disc).

3. Detweiler DK, Patterson DF: Heart recordings of the dog. American Animal Hospital Association, South Bend, IN.

4. Ettinger SJ: Heart sounds. EVSCO Pharm. Co., Oceanside, NY (33 1/3 rpm).

irregular heart rate, a varying intensity of the first heart sound, and a pulse deficit. A holosystolic murmur of varying intensity, typical of mitral insufficiency is often detected as well. The overall heart rate often exceeds 180 beats per minute and may be much faster. Whenever arrhythmia are detected by auscultation, electrocardiography should be performed to confirm and define the type of arrhythmia present.[51,52]

Gallop rhythms may be due to loud third heart sounds, loud fourth heart sounds, or both (summation gallop). The presence of a protodiastolic gallop or accentuated third heart sound is associated with cardiac dilatation and failure in small animals. Pre-systolic gallops due to accentuated fourth heart sounds are associated with reduced ventricular distensibility and reduced ventricular compliance associated with myocardial hypertrophy. The fourth heart sound is associated with atrial systole, whereas the third heart sound is associated with the period of rapid ventricular filling in early diastole.

Auscultatory clues of cardiac dysfunction may also be indicated by the intensity and character of the first and second heart sounds. Splitting of the first heart sound may occur with asynchronous ventricular contraction due to various intraventricular conduction blocks. The intensity of the first heart sound is grossly related to the intensity of ventricular contraction, although a number of other factors are involved in its perception. The second heart sound is related to semilunar valve closure. Loud tambour-like second heart sounds may indicate aortic and/or pulmonary hypertension. Splitting of the second heart sound, especially when wide and fixed splitting occurs, indicates delayed or prolonged ejection of one ventricle or the other. Splitting of heart sounds should prompt further exploration for the presence of heart disease.

Cardiac Murmurs

Murmurs are due to turbulent blood flow. Turbulence, in turn, depends on a number of factors, including the velocity of blood flow, blood viscosity, and diameter of the blood vessel involved. Turbulence is favored by high velocity, low viscosity, and large blood vessels. Murmurs frequently give clues to the presence of heart disease or faulty heart valves, but the presence of a heart murmur does not always indicate cardiac pathology. When a heart murmur is detected, its location within the cardiac cycle should be determined along with its location of maximal intensity and direction of transmission on the wall of the thorax. Characterization of murmurs in this fashion in conjunction with their intensity, frequency, duration, and quality is

most helpful in identifying the underlying lesions responsible for their generation.

Systolic murmurs by definition occur during systole, which is identified on auscultation as between the first heart sound (S_1) and the second heart sound (S_2) as shown in Figure 6. Systolic murmurs are the most common murmurs detected in small animals but are not always indicative of cardiac lesions.[41,48,135] When murmurs are not due to lesions, they are termed "physiologic" or "functional" murmurs. Most functional murmurs occur in early systole during rapid ventricular ejection. They rarely are greater than grade 2 in intensity. Grade 1 murmurs are the softest murmurs that can possibly be detected, and grade 6 are those that can both be felt and heard without a stethoscope. Grade 3 to 6 murmurs are generally associated with significant cardiac lesions. The intensity of the murmur does not always correlate with the severity of the underlying lesion.

Clinically significant systolic murmurs occur with mitral insufficiency, tricuspid insufficiency, aortic stenosis, pulmonic stenosis, tetralogy of Fallot, ventricular septal defect, and atrial septal defect. Pansystolic or holosystolic murmurs characterize insufficiency of the atrioventricular valves and ventricular septal defects (Figure 6). These murmurs tend to mask both the first and second heart sounds. A murmur of mitral insufficiency is in the mitral area of auscultation on the left side of the chest (Figure 5, page 11-16). The murmurs of tricuspid insufficiency and of ventricular septal defect are typically loudest on the right side of the chest.

Aortic stenosis, pulmonic stenosis, and tetralogy of Fallot all produce systolic ejection murmurs. With such murmurs, the first and second heart sounds can be heard on either side of the crescendo-decrescendo murmur, which is loudest in mid-systole (Figure 6). Differentiation of these types of murmurs depends on whether the sound is more intense over the aortic or pulmonic areas and the direction of transmission. The murmur of aortic stenosis is sometimes heard with maximal intensity on the right side of the chest and is often detected in the neck when auscultating over the carotid arteries. The murmur of pulmonic stenosis is maximal on the left side of the chest in the pulmonary area of auscultation.

Diastolic murmurs occur, by definition, during the period of diastole after the second heart sound and before the next first heart sound. Diastolic murmurs are due to semilunar valve regurgitation as occurs with aortic insufficiency and/or pulmonic insufficiency. In dogs and cats, these murmurs are not as common as systolic murmurs. Aortic insufficiency in dogs is often due to bacterial endocarditis involving the aortic valve.[51] Aortic insufficiency also typically produces a widened pulse pressure and can be detected as a bounding arterial pulse.

A continuous murmur is a murmur that never ends but may vary in intensity throughout systole and diastole. It is sometimes referred to as a machinery murmur. Continuous murmurs are associated with arteriovenous fistula and fistula between the aorta and pulmonary artery. Patent ductus arteriosus is the most common cause of a continuous murmur in dogs and cats.

RADIOGRAPHY

Thoracic radiographs should be obtained of any animal suspected of having heart disease that is not dyspneic or orthopneic. They are a required part of any cardiovascular examination.[48,66,74,75,76] Both lateral and dorsoventral views should be obtained and used to determine if there is:

1. Cardiac enlargement (as shown in Figure 7) and, if so, which chambers or great vessels are involved.
2. Pulmonary venous engorgement along with left atrial enlargement,
3. Evidence of pulmonary congestion or edema. Particular attention should be paid to the pulmonary vascular markings which are increased in all left to right shunts and decreased in all right-to-left shunts.
4. Evidence of pulmonary hypertension as manifested by enlarged tortuous pulmonary vessels, and
5. Any evidence of pulmonary and/or thoracic or mediastinal lesions.

By correlating auscultatory with clinical and radiographic findings, it is often possible to arrive at a definitive anatomic or morphologic diagnosis of the type of heart disease present, as indicated in Table 6.

ELECTROCARDIOGRAPHY

The electrocardiogram, like the thoracic radiograph, is an important part of a complete cardiovascular examination.[48,49,51] Irregularities or abnormal rhythms detected on auscultation require electrocardiographic confirmation. The EKG serves as the definitive diagnostic tool for cardiac arrhythmias and is helpful in identifying cardiac enlargement. Changes in the EKG may also give clues as to the presence of myocardial hypoxia or eletrolyte imbalances such as hyperkalemia, hypokalemia, hypercalcemia or hypocalcemia. The EKG changes

FIGURE 6

NORMAL AND ABNORMAL CARDIAC CYCLE, EKG, HEART PRESSURES, AND HEART SOUNDS

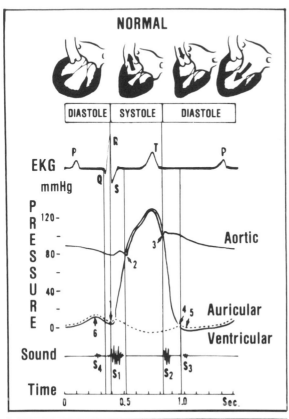

NORMAL

DIASTOLE | SYSTOLE | DIASTOLE

EKG

mmHg

PRESSURE

120 —

80 —

40 —

0 —

Aortic

Auricular

Ventricular

Sound

S₄ S₁   S₂ S₃

Time

0   0.5   1.0   Sec.

1. AV valve closure
2. semilunar valve opening
3. semilunar valve closure
4. AV valve opening
5. end of rapid filling
6. atrial contraction

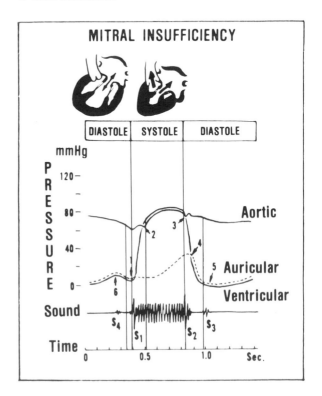

AORTIC STENOSIS

DIASTOLE | SYSTOLE | DIASTOLE

mmHg

PRESSURE

120 —

80 —

40 —

0 —

Aortic

Auricular

Ventricular

Sound

S₄ S₁   S₂ S₃

Time

0   0.5   1.0   Sec.

MITRAL INSUFFICIENCY

DIASTOLE | SYSTOLE | DIASTOLE

mmHg

PRESSURE

120 —

80 —

40 —

0 —

Aortic

Auricular

Ventricular

Sound

S₄   S₁   S₂   S₃

Time

0   0.5   1.0   Sec.

FIGURE 7
RADIOGRAPH OF NORMAL AND ABNORMAL HEARTS

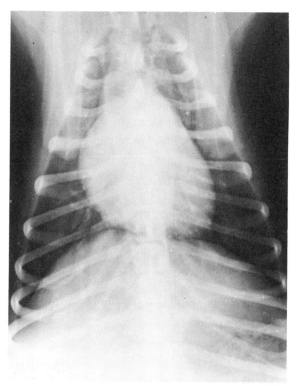

NORMAL

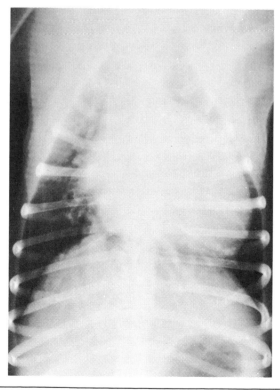

LEFT VENTRICULAR
ENLARGEMENT

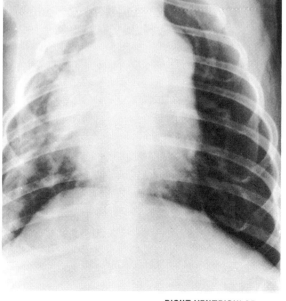

RIGHT VENTRICULAR
ENLARGEMENT

may also suggest the presence of pericardial effusion and/or pericarditis. Serial EKGs are useful in monitoring response to therapy and they improve diagnosis and prognosis. Continuous electrocardiographic monitoring is often useful and frequently necessary in dealing with acutely ill animals and those to which intravenous vasoactive or cardiotonic drugs are being administered. However, electrocardiographic changes, by themselves, do not constitute a diagnosis of heart failure.

Some of the more common EKG findings or diagnoses and their associations are:

1. P mitrale is a P wave which is prolonged in duration and indicates left atrial enlargement. Left atrial enlargement, in turn, usually accompanies mitral insufficiency and/or cardiomyopathy in dogs and cats. Left atrial enlargement does not always indicate left ventricular failure, but left atrial enlargement always ultimately results when left ventricular failure is chronically present.

2. P pulmonale is indicated by tall, peaked P waves. P pulmonale usually indicates right atrial enlargement and is often associated with cor pulmonale.

3. Sinus tachycardia is an increase in heart rate of normal sinus origin. It is a normal response to fever, excitement, and exercise; it may also be a compensatory response to heart disease.

4. Atrial premature beats are commonly associated with atrioventricular valvular insufficiency, atrial enlargement, and chronic valvular or myocardial disease.

5. Atrial fibrillation in dogs and cats is almost always associated with severe atrial enlargement and significant cardiac disease. It can be a sequela to valvular heart disease, and it is often present in large breeds of dogs with cardiomyopathy.

6. Ventricular premature beats are indicated by wide bizarre QRS complexes without associated P waves occurring prematurely in the sequence. While they are frequently associated with myocardial lesions,[51] isolated ventricular premature beats occurring infrequently can occur in the absence of significant heart disease. They also occur in many anesthetized animals, especially those receiving short-acting barbiturates, and may be a reflection of autonomic imbalance.

7. Ventricular tachycardia occurring paroxysmally or continuously is a severe arrhythmia requiring immediate attention. Ventricular tachyarrhythmias predispose to ventricular fibrillation, which is incompatible with life.

8. First-degree atrioventricular (A-V) block is an abnormal prolongation of the P-R interval. It may occur with increased efferent vagal activity, with myocardial disease, and with administration of digitalis and other drugs.

9. Second degree A-V block indicates that a P wave occurs without a following QRS complex. This may be caused by increased efferent vagal activity, digitalis intoxication, and a variety of other antiarrhythmic drugs. It has been identified in clinically normal dogs as well as in dogs with myocardial disease. By itself, however, it is not diagnostic of severe heart disease.

TABLE 6

COMPARISON OF RADIOGRAPHIC AND AUSCULTATORY FINDINGS ASSOCIATED WITH HEART DISEASE IN DOGS[76]

	Radiographic Findings			Auscultatory Findings	
Lesion	Left Ventricle	Right Ventricle	Pulmonary Artery	Murmur	Location of Greatest Intensity
Mitral insufficiency	Enlarged	Normal, slightly enlarged in later stages	Normal to slightly enlarged	Systolic	Left 5th to 7th intercostal space
Tricuspid insufficiency	Normal	Enlarged	Normal to small	Systolic	Right 4th intercostal space
Combined A-V insufficiency	Enlarged	Enlarged	Normal to slightly enlarged	Systolic	Left and right 4th to 7th intercostal space (usually left)
Pulmonic stenosis	Normal	Enlarged	Markedly enlarged	Systolic (thrill)	Left 2nd to 3rd intercostal space
Patent ductus arteriosus	Markedly enlarged	Normal, slightly enlarged in later stages	Normal to slightly enlarged	Systolic diastolic (thrill)	Left 3rd intercostal space

10. Complete heart block or third-degree heart block is indicated when no relation exists between P waves and QRS complexes. When no atrial impulse is passed through to the ventricles, complete heart block is diagnosed and is generally indicative of severe myocardial disease requiring pacemaker therapy.

For a more thorough review of canine and feline electrocardiography, consult other texts.[12,48,51,115,129]

LABORATORY EXAMINATION

Heart disease is generally diagnosed on the basis of clinical signs, history and physical, and radiographic and electrocardiographic examinations rather than by laboratory examinations. However, specific laboratory tests may provide adjunctive information useful in confirming heart disease. The finding of microfilariae of Dirofilaria immitis is definitive of heartworm disease. Since heart failure results in dysfunction of other organs as well, it is not unusual, indeed it is expected, that abnormalities in laboratory tests, indicative of liver, renal and circulatory dysfunctions and/or altered serum eletrolyte concentrations will be present.

Prerenal azotemia is commonly present in congestive heart failure.[84] The principal mechanism involves a reduction in the glomerular filtration rate.[26] The BUN is generally elevated prior to an increase in serum creatinine, which may remain normal until severe heart failure is present with markedly reduced renal blood flow and glomerular filtration rate. Thus, an elevation of serum creatinine is usually a sign of advanced heart failure.[26] If concurrent renal failure is present, the BUN and creatinine will be elevated accordingly and may reach remarkably high levels.

With inadequate hepatic circulation, cellular hypoxia or necrosis may occur. Mild elevations in liver enzymes occur with heart failure; and as heart failure progresses, liver function tests such as BSP retention may be prolonged (see page 7-53).

Circulation time may be useful in diagnosing heart disease, as significant heart disease always prolongs circulation time, which can be detected after injection of appropriate substances.[85]

Measurements of serum electrolyte concentrations, particularly sodium and potassium, may be useful in determining prognosis and treatment of animals with heart disease and suspected concomitant renal disease. Hyponatremia in the presence of heart failure is generally a grave prognostic sign. Hypokalemia precipitates digitalis intoxication and can result from the use of diuretics. If present, it should be corrected by administering potassium, preferably by mixing it in the food.

The examination of blood for microfilariae of Dirofilaria immitus is part of a complete cardiovascular examination and should be conducted on all animals in most areas.[90,94,108] The modified Knott technique and microfiltration are both accurate concentration procedures. Animals with negative microfilaria examinations but with other signs suggesting heartworm disease should be tested for occult dirofilariasis with immunofluorescence or ELISA techniques. These techniques detect either the presence of the heartworm antibodies or antigens.[45,94]

Additional aids to the diagnosis, prognosis, and therapy of congestive heart failure are obtained from the complete blood count and the examination of any fluids accumulating abnormally in the thorax, abdomen, or pericardium. Anemia stresses the heart. Both anemia and heart disease impair tissue oxygenation, greatly increasing the risk of severity of damage to numerous organs. Therapy to correct the anemia is, therefore, important in animals with heart disease. Hypoproteinemia is common in severe congestive heart failure. Correcting it reduces or helps prevent edema and ascites. An elevated white blood cell count in the presence of an undulating fever suggests the need to obtain blood cultures as bacterial endocarditis would be suspected.

Specific gravity, protein content, and cytology should be determined on any fluid detected in the thorax, abdomen, or pericardium. Fluid due to congestive heart failure initially is a transudate with a specific gravity less than 1.018. With chronicity, however, the fluid may become blood tinged and the specific gravity may rise. Typically, the fluid is clear and contains small numbers of mesothelial cells and macrophages.

ECHOCARDIOGRAPHY

Echocardiography provides a non-invasive method of cardiac imaging using ultrasound. Its use is rapidly growing in veterinary medicine. Although the equipment is expensive, the use of echocardiography in diagnosing heart disease in small animals is becoming a routine part of the cardiologist's armamentarium. The combined use of quantitative M-mode echocardiography and two-dimensional echocardiography permits identification of malformations of cardiac structures, their continuity, motion, and dimensions; and with intracardiac contrast techniques allows for identification of most congenital cardiac defects in small animals.[16] Aortic stenosis, pulmonic stenosis, intra-ventricular shunts, and dysplasia or malformed atrioventricular valves can be identified.

The echocardiogram is useful in acquired heart disease as well. The echocardiographic features of pericardial effusion and intra- and extra-pericardial masses have been described.[19,20] The echocardiogram is also useful in identifying ventricular dilatation and hypertrophy, ventricular wall motion, regional dysfunction, and as an aid to diagnosing heartworm disease.[100,152] It is most useful in identifying the type and severity of cardiomyopathy in cats and dogs. Whenever available, echocardiography should be considered as an aid to the diagnosis of heart disease.

Echocardiography has proved to be most helpful in identifying the degree of ventricular and functional impairment in valvular heart disease and as an aid to therapy. Many dogs with mitral insufficiency and congestive heart failure have had relatively normal ventricular contractility.[91] The need for digitalis glycosides in such animals, therefore, has been questioned. There are numerous publications providing additional information on echocardiography. [2,14,16,18,21,22,38,100,101,120,122,138,150,152]

CARDIAC CATHETERIZATION AND ANGIOCARDIOGRAPHY

Cardiac catheterization and angiocardiography are necessary in some cases of heart disease. In suspected congenital heart disease they are particularly indicated for making a definitive diagnosis if surgery is contemplated. Echocardiography has alleviated the need for some of the application of these techniques in diagnosing and quantifying heart disease in dogs and cats. Radionuclides or other contrast media may be used for angiocardiography. They are equally beneficial except that the use of radionuclides allows for a quantitative evaluation. Measurement of intracardiac pressures by cardiac catheterization is necessary, however, in a number of diseases. In cats suspected of having cardiomyopathy non-selective angiography has been used to define whether it is hypertrophic, dilatative, or restrictive. Echocardiography, however, is of great benefit for this purpose.

THERAPY

While certain generalizations concerning the treatment of congestive heart failure are warranted, each case must be individually evaluated and managed.[48,128] Management depends on a knowledge and appreciation of the underlying condition, the rapidity of its progression, the presence of associated conditions, the patient's age, the family setting, the owner's ability and motivation to provide treatment, and the response to therapeutic measures.

GENERAL APPROACHES IN THE TREATMENT OF HEART FAILURE

There are three general approaches to treating heart failure.[137]

1. Remove the primary cause. Although this is desirable, it cannot always be accomplished. It includes surgical correction of structural abnormalities responsible for heart failure. Surgery is particularly applicable for patent ductus arteriosus, pulmonic stenosis, and other congenital heart diseases. Medical treatment of such conditions as infectious endocarditis, primary hypertension, or the medical/surgical treatment of idiopathic pericardial effusion may also be useful in removing the cause of heart failure.

2. Remove the precipitating cause. This involves the recognition and treatment or prevention of specific causes or incidents that produce or exacerbate heart failure. A few of these are arrhythmias, infections, anemia, hyperthyroidism, acid-base or eletrolyte disturbances, and pulmonary emboli. The prompt treatment or prevention of these alterations is critical to the successful management of the patient with heart failure.

3. Control of congestive heart failure to:
    a. improve the heart's pumping performance. This may involve the use of digitalis glycosides, sympathomimetic agents, other positive inotropic agents, or a cardiac pacemaker.
    b. reduce the heart's workload. This may involve restricted activity, treatment for obesity, vasodilator therapy and reduction of fluid retention.
    c. control of excessive salt and water retention. This is accomplished primarily by restricting sodium intake. Diuretics may also be used, or fluid may be removed by thoracentesis, paracentesis, pericardiocentesis or, in an extreme case, phlebotomy.

Many agents and techniques are available for use in accomplishing these objectives. Which ones are best varies with the patient, myocardial performance, and previous therapy. Myocardial demand is reduced by agents or techniques that decrease heart rate and wall tension. Heart rate may be reduced by cardiac glycosides, rest, or antiarrhythmic drugs. Wall tension is reduced by making the heart smaller. This is accomplished through sodium restriction, and in the case of preload, with the use of diuretics and venodilators; in the case of afterload, with arteriodilators . Myocardial size may also be reduced by improving ejection fraction with

positive inotropic agents. Congestive heart failure may also be affected by a reduction in exercise, sedation, mechanical removal of accumulated fluid, bronchodilatation, proper nutrition, and administration of oxygen.

The best approach to treatment for heart failure involves prevention whenever possible, and early detection and removal of all underlying causes. Client education in a manner that motivates compliance by the client is of paramount importance and may initially be time-consuming. This time taken early in the course of heart disease may, however, act as prophylaxis for the frequently unrewarding heroics necessary to save the animal with end-stage heart disease.

PROPHYLAXIS OF HEART FAILURE

Dogs and cats with heart disease begin to retain sodium before exhibiting clinical signs of congestive heart failure. Indeed, inability to excrete a sodium load is an index to the presence of heart failure.[24,83] An early diagnosis of heart disease permits institution of sodium restriction (though it may need be only moderate) as a prophylactic measure to deter acute congestive heart failure.[69,70] Dogs in early heart failure stop retaining sodium when sodium restriction is initiated. Evaluation of body weight is important. If any obesity is present, weight reduction should be initiated to further delay onset of heart failure. Properly approached, clients welcome this means of deterring active congestive heart failure and allowing their pets to remain more comfortable and free of signs for a longer time. The time when daily medication must be given may also be delayed. Correcting other factors in the animal's environment or daily activity such as avoiding excessive heat or forced hard play or work, may also be prophylactic. Client education regarding their animal's disease process, as well as "training them" to obtain the animal's resting heart rate and to be careful observers, also assist in prophylaxis and therapy.

ACUTE CONGESTIVE FAILURE— EMERGENCY PROCEDURES

An emergency exists when a patient is presented showing acute congestive heart failure with obvious severe respiratory distress, cyanosis and/or severe tachyarrhythmias with pulmonary edema. Such animals require rapid evaluation of their condition without undue stress, and rapid institution of emergency therapy according to the following guidelines.[13,15,128,146]

1. Place the patient in a cool (18°C or 64°F), well-ventilated, oxygen-enriched (40-50%) environ-

ment. This is best achieved using a controlled environmental cage with the oxygen introduced via a nebulization unit through 35-40% ethanol, a surfactant that reduces airway foaming in the presence of pulmonary edema. The importance of making the animal comfortable at strict cage rest without stress cannot be overemphasized.

2. Give morphine sulfate subcutaneously, to dogs with acute congestive heart failure and to dogs being placed in the controlled environment that are restless, anxious, and dyspneic with pulmonary edema (Table 1). This treatment not only has a sedative effect, which makes the animal more comfortable, it also may increase cardiac output while decreasing pulmonary edema. Morphine can be repeated as needed, but overdosing should be avoided because it markedly depresses the respiratory center. Other undesirable side effects may include vomiting or defecation. Acepromazine should not be used for this purpose in dogs, but it has been advocated for use in cats to reduce stress. It should be administered in low doses and may have the additional effect of afterload reduction. Overdoses of acepromazine cause marked hypotension and hypothermia and should be avoided.

3. Give furosemide intravenously to enhance diuresis (Table 1). This should be done at the same time the animal is placed in the controlled environment.

4. Evaluate arrhythmias. If severe ventricular tachyarrhythmias, heart block, or exceptionally slow bradyarrhythmias are present, institute appropriate intravenous antiarrhythmic therapy. Lidocaine may be used for ventricular tachyarrhythmias. Initially it is given slowly in an intravenous bolus. The bolus may be repeated (Table 1). If a positive effect is obtained, continue giving lidocaine at a constant infusion rate of 25-75 μg/kg per minute. Lidocaine must be used much more cautiously in cats because of its neurotoxicity in this species. The intravenous dose should not exceed 0.5 mg/kg over a period of 5-10 minutes. Propranolol may be given intravenously to cats at a dosage of 0.06 mg/kg over 5-10 minutes.[14,17] To improve severe bradyarrhythmias or heart block, 0.4 mg isoproterenol may be given in 250 ml of 5% dextrose and water (Table 1). Administration is by slow intravenous infusion to effect.[17,50]

5. Give dobutamine to patients requiring positive inotropic therapy (Table 1). It is particularly useful in patients with congestive cardiomyopathies and acute heart failure with large dilated hearts. Contraindications may include ruptured

chordae tendineae in the presence of good myocardial function and/or the presence of ventricular tachyarrhythmias. Dobutamine is given by constant intravenous infusion.[17,128] The rate of administration is adjusted to produce minimal changes in heart rate, rhythm, or arterial pressure. Begin at the low infusion rate. Increase as necessary for the desired inotropic effect without producing an increase in heart rate. Dobutamine is the preferred drug for short-term therapy to provide cardiac support in critical situations requiring increased contractility, increased stroke volume, and cardiac output.

6. Give theophylline as a bronchodilator (Table 1). It is beneficial in animals with cardiac asthma, wheezing, or concomitant bronchial disease with bronchial constriction.[13]

7. Administer a vasodilator to patients in severe congestive heart failure with pulmonary edema. Vasodilators are particularly useful in almost every state of congestive failure, particularly when severe mitral regurgitation is present. If blood pressure can be monitored, sodium nitroprusside should be given intravenously (Table 1). Slow the rate of administration if the blood pressure falls below 90/50 mmHg or a tachycardia greater than 170 beats/min occurs. If blood pressure cannot be monitored, using gloves, nitroglycerin ointment may be applied to hairless regions of the skin every 4-8 hours (Table 1).[17] Other orally administered vasodilators such as hydralazine, prazosin, or captopril may also be beneficial. If oral medication is chosen, give captopril. It is not only a vasodilator; because it inhibits formation of angiotensin II, it reduces aldosterone levels and, therefore, may also have useful diuretic properties in animals with congestive heart failure. It also slows heart rate. All vasodilator drugs should be carefully monitored, especially after their initial administration, for toxic effects which are generally manifested as

hypotension with a corresponding increase in heart rate.[17,128]

8. Remove fluid from the thoracic or abdominal cavities only if it is contributing to respiratory distress; then remove only enough to relieve distress. This should be done as soon as possible once the patient is stable. However, avoid removing excessive quantities of abdominal fluid as it may intensify hypoproteinemia. Excess pericardial fluid, if present, should be removed to improve cardiac filling and output.

CHRONIC HEART FAILURE THERAPY

General approaches to therapy were discussed previously (page 11-23). The course of the disease in any given patient is rarely smoothly progressive, but rather is characterized by abrupt changes due to acute decompensation, which is frequently due to some precipitating cause. Once the precipitating cause has been removed and treatment is further intensified, the patient's previous status may be restored or improved.

Other than feeding a low sodium diet, treatment for heart failure is generally not begun until signs of diminished cardiac reserve are evident. It is important to determine the animal's underlying disease and its rate of progression in order to properly apply the principles of restricted activity, dietary sodium restriction, and use of such pharmacologic agents as digitalis, diuretics, and vasodilators. Many animals with heart failure are not seen by a veterinarian until they are in Phase 3 (Table 3, page 11-15) and demonstrating considerable signs in response to minimal exertion. Pharmacologic therapy is always indicated in Phases 3 and 4 and often in Phase 2. Although proper therapy depends on the underlying cause of heart disease, a number of factors are useful in monitoring the animal's response to therapy and its prognosis, regardless of what that

TABLE 7

FACTORS USEFUL IN MONITORING RESPONSE TO THERAPY AND PROGNOSIS

	Favorable	Fair	Poor
Heart Rate	Decreases	Static	Increases
Systolic Murmur	Decrease in grade	Static	Increases in grade
Cardiac Enlargement	Reduces	Static	Increases
Arrhythmias	Disappears	Improves	Static
Dyspnea	Subsides	Decreases	Increases
Cough	Disappears	Static or decrease	Static or increase
Rales	Disappear	Disappear	Static or increase
Ascites	Disappears	Disappears	Static or increase
Body Weight	Normal	Approaches normal	Weight loss
Circ. Time	Decreases below 13	Decreases	Static or increase

therapy is. These factors are given in Table 7.

With the exception of acute emergency and severe clinical cases which should be hospitalized for therapy, whenever possible it is best to bring heart failure under control slowly at home with the animal in its natural environment. This requires owner participation, often leading to better communication between veterinarian and owner as the owner should be in frequent contact with the veterinarian after therapy is instituted. Education of the client in the factors used in monitoring this response to therapy, as indicated in Table 7, is necessary. Each drug, therapeutic agent, or technique prescribed should be explained. The owner should be taught how to measure the animal's heart rate and observe for signs of favorable or unfavorable response. Side effects or undesirable effects of drugs should be thoroughly explained, along with what to do if they occur.

Digitalis Glycosides

The digitalis glycosides (digoxin and digitoxin) are used widely in veterinary medicine for improving myocardial contractile performance in congestive heart failure. Their beneficial effects, in addition to improved contractility, include antiarrhythmic properties and decreases in ventricular rate, venous pressure, cardiac size, circulating blood volume, and the signs of dyspnea.[71,73] Increases occur in cardiac output and urine flow when digitalis is used properly. Electrocardiographic changes include ST-T changes and prolongation of the P-R interval.[63]

Digitalis appears to produce increased contractility by inhibiting the cardiac receptor sodium-potassium-ATPase. This results in greater availability of intracellular calcium ions during excitation. In addition, digitalis slows the heart rate both by increasing vagal efferent activity and by prolonging atrioventricular conduction time.[62,63]

Indications for using digitalis glycosides include decompensated chronic valvular heart disease, congestive cardiomyopathy, right heart failure, congestive heart failure from congenital heart disease or heartworm disease, and supraventricular tachyarrhythmias. Since digitalis suppresses atrial arrhythmias and slows ventricular response, it is particularly useful for the latter effect in atrial fibrillation. However, digitalis must be used very cautiously in animals with preexistent ventricular premature beats because arrhythmias may worsen after its administration. When ventricular arrhythmias are due to ventricular dilatation and poor cardiac output, digitalis may improve them, but it must always be used with caution.

Digitalis glycosides are not indicated in patients with heart disease unless they have impaired myocardial contractility or supraventricular tachycardias. Therefore, digitalization is not indicated in the absence of signs of heart disease or in animals with pericardial disease or hypertrophic cardiomyopathy. Myocardial contractility is generally not greatly depressed in these animals. It has also been shown that myocardial function may be only minimally depressed in many patients with heart failure caused by mitral insufficiency.[91]

Of all the cardiac glycosides available, digoxin and digitoxin are most commonly used in veterinary medicine. Of the two, digoxin is more commonly used, and has been more thoroughly studied. Also, there is more concurrence about its efficacy, dosage, and method of administration.[39,48,64,80] Digitoxin is more completely absorbed from the gastrointestinal tract than is digoxin; but it is also more highly protein-bound. Therefore, for its therapeutic effects, digitoxin requires higher blood levels than digoxin.[27] Digitoxin is eliminated by the liver, whereas digoxin requires renal elimination. Thus, digitoxin may be beneficial in dogs with concurrent advanced renal disease. Because digitoxin requires higher doses to achieve therapeutic blood levels, it may have to be given more often to dogs. It seems to offer no advantage over digoxin except perhaps to patients with renal failure. Digitoxin is given in oral maintenance doses ranging from 0.04 to 0.1 mg/kg/day divided into two to three doses daily. Therapeutic blood levels are reported to range from 15 to 35 ng/ml.

When digoxin is used in either dogs or cats, slow oral digitalization is recommended. This requires a maintenance dose of 0.01-0.02 mg/kg/day divided into two doses for dogs and of 0.007-0.015 mg/kg daily for cats.[17] Because the half-life of digoxin in dogs is 20-36 hours,[27] the low oral maintenance dose will produce a near steady-state blood level within three to five days. However, the narrow range between clinical efficacy and toxicity dictates establishment of the appropriate dose for each individual animal.

The dose should be based on lean body mass; therefore, body weight should be corrected for ascitic fluid and fat. However, the correct dosage is probably more affected by internal factors than by body weight.[128] Cats are more sensitive to digoxin than are dogs. Thyroid and renal function and numerous other factors have a marked influence on digitalis intoxication. One of the main factors is eletrolyte status, especially potassium. Hypokalemia, which may be caused by vomiting, anorexia, and particularly diuretic therapy, predisposes to digitalis intoxication. Quinidine, furosemide, and

verapamil administered concurrently with digoxin may increase its effect.[17]

Therapeutic blood levels of digoxin in dogs and cats range from 1.0-2.5 ng/ml.[17,27,39] These values may help in the clinical management of digitalized patients, particularly giant breeds of dogs or hypothyroid animals that require a considerably lower dose of digoxin on a body-weight basis. However, some animals may show clinical signs of toxicity even when plasma concentrations are within this range.[39,64,140]

Serum digoxin level submitted for radioimmunoassay measurement should be obtained eight to ten hours after the previous dose. Obviously, if signs of digitalis intoxication occur, the drug should be withheld until these signs abate. Then it is advisable to reduce the dosage. Nearly any arrhythmia can be caused by digitalis intoxication.

Even when digitalization has been effective, clients should be cautioned that changes in a variety of factors, including renal function, thyroid function, and eletrolyte imbalances, may precipitate signs of digitalis intoxication. The client should be instructed to stop giving digoxin whenever the animal exhibits anorexia, vomiting, or diarrhea. These signs could be due to other diseases or problems, but digitalis intoxication must be suspected if the drug is being given. If the animal does not resume eating within 12 hours, the client should be instructed to return the animal for evaluation. Clients should also be warned of the toxicity hazard to children and adults, and childproof containers should always be used.[37]

Diuretics

Diuretics may be useful either alone or in conjunction with digoxin and other measures in the therapy of congestive heart failure. Because the clinical manifestations of heart failure result largely from renal retention of sodium and water, diuretics may relieve the congestion and thus the signs associated with the disease.[77] By promoting renal loss of water and sodium, diuretics may decrease vascular resistance and cardiac size. This also decreases both systolic and diastolic wall tension. **Even though diuretics are frequently useful in many forms of heart disease and generally in heart failure, they are not a substitute for dietary sodium restriction. Diuretics do not eliminate the cause, only the signs.** In addition, because of adverse effects that may occur, particularly with long-term usage, diuretics are recommended only for initial management to stabilize the animal more rapidly, and in Phase 4 heart disease when all available methods are required to minimize clinical signs.

Many diuretics are available. Their precise mechanism of action varies, but most of those commonly used act on the renal tubules and/or loop of Henle to inhibit the reabsorption of sodium and water. The diuretics recommended because of their proven efficacy in dogs and cats include furosemide, the thiazides including hydrochlorothiazide and spironolactone an aldosterone antagonist which is used frequently in conjunction with the thiazides.[17,128]

Furosemide is especially potent and is the diuretic of choice in treating for severe congestive heart failure in dogs and cats. Intravenous administration, in addition to causing a diuresis, shifts blood from the pulmonary to the systemic circulation. The diuretic response to furosemide is dose-dependent. Unlike many other diuretics, it is often effective in producing a diuresis even when glomerular filtration is severely reduced. Diuresis is initiated within minutes after intravenous administration; it generally persists for two hours. Intravenous administration of 2-4 mg/kg is indicated in all cases of life threatening pulmonary edema. The same dosage is recommended orally for dogs; whereas the oral dosage for cats is 0.5-2mg/kg (Table 1). Diuresis begins within an hour after oral administration of furosemide, and generally peaks within two hours, with a diuretic effect noted six to eight hours later. Oral administration can be repeated two to three times daily if necessary.

Thiazide diuretics act on the distal tubule and ascending loop of Henle to prevent reabsorption of sodium and chloride. They are generally well-tolerated and their duration of action is relatively long. Thus they can be given orally once or twice a day. Hydrochlorothiazide is given to dogs in doses of 2-4 mg/kg with spironolactone. Spironolactone is a competitive antagonist of aldosterone; therefore, it is effective as a diuretic only when aldosterone is present. It is used because of its potassium-sparing qualities but is rarely used alone as a primary diuretic in dogs and cats. When combined with a thiazide, it is effective as a potassium-sparing diuretic. Whenever possible, the daily dosage of any diuretic should be reduced, and diuretics should be used intermittently and for a short time.[128]

Diuretics are tolerated well by most dogs and cats with heart failure. There are complications with their use, but adverse side effects can be minimized by intermittent administration. Side effects include alterations in electrolyte balance - especially hypokalemia, dehydration, and plasma volume contraction, thus reducing ventricular filling and cardiac output. At all times, but particularly when receiving diuretics, animals should have free access to water. Animals receiving diuretics, especially animals that are anorectic, may become dehydrated, with pre-

renal azotemia and hypokalemic hypochloremic metabolic alkalosis.

Hypokalemia is particularly common with prolonged administration of diuretics. If the plasma potassium concentration is less than 3.8 mEq/L or if it is less than 4.5 mEq/L when nonpotassium-sparing diuretics are being given, add potassium chloride to the daily ration (Table 1). Do not give supplemental potassium if the prepared restricted sodium diet (Prescription Diet h/d) is being fed, as its potassium level is already increased (1-1.2% in diet dry matter).

Another potential hazard of diuretic therapy is the depletion of water-soluble vitamins. Accordingly, prepared diets (such as Prescription Diets k/d or h/d) containing additional quantities of B-vitamins to compensate for these losses, or a B-complex vitamin supplement are advocated for patients with congestive heart failure receiving diuretic therapy.[128] The supplement is not required if the prepared diet is being fed.

Vasodilators

Compensatory reactions elicited in heart failure tend to cause peripheral vasoconstriction and, therefore, increase afterload, which tends to reduce cardiac output. The use of arterial and venous vasodilators such as hydralazine and/or captopril (Table 1) has proved to be remarkably beneficial in many forms of congestive heart failure.[17,72] Combined arterial-venous vasodilators, such as prazosin or the various nitrates such as nitroglycerin ointment (Table 1), also reduce preload and thus may offer considerable benefit in the large dilated overfilled heart. These vasodilators appear to hold the most promise for use in veterinary medicine. All can be used in conjunction with digoxin, diuretics, and restricted sodium diets. A tolerance, and thus reduced efficacy, may develop to both hydralazine and prazosin.

At the present time there is no uniformity of opinion as to precisely when in the course of heart failure vasodilator treatment should be started. Although the efficacy of using vasodilators seems unquestioned, especially in acute congestive heart failure or in the presence of mitral insufficiency, long-term benefits from chronic oral use of vasodilators in animals has not been proven. In the future vasodilators may prove to be beneficial early in the course of mitral insufficiency, but at the present time vasodilators are advocated for use in patients with large dilated ventricles, mitral regurgitation, and elevated venous pressures. Therefore, they should be used in severe congestive heart failure with pulmonary edema, in right ventricular

failure, and in moderate-to-severe mitral regurgitation.[91]

Arterial vasodilators reduce afterload and the mitral regurgitant fraction, causing an increase in forward stroke volume and cardiac output.

Captopril blocks the enzymatic conversion of angiotensin I to angiotensin II, thus preventing the stimulation of aldosterone secretion by angiotensin II and resulting vasoconstriction. In addition, it is a potent dilator of those arterioles that are highly sensitive to angiotensin II, such as the renal vascular bed. Captopril also causes dilation of the venous bed and reduces filling pressures.[137] Captopril has been used with considerable benefit in dogs and cats with congestive cardiomyopathy.[17] Prazosin, like captopril, is both an arterial and a venous vasodilator.

Nitrates are primarily venous vasodilators. Nitroglycerin ointment has been used in both dogs and cats.[17] For acute congestive heart failure, sodium nitroprusside given intravenously is advocated as an ultra-short-acting vascular smooth muscle dilator of both arterioles and veins. Sodium nitroprusside is used only for the acute stabilization of patients in severe acute congestive heart failure. It is infused at a rate of 5-10 μg/minute with continuous monitoring of heart rate and blood pressure (Table 1). The rate of administration is reduced if arterial pressure falls below 90/50 mmHg and/or causes a reflex tachycardia. Stabilization is usually achieved within a few hours. The patient is then switched to oral vasodilator therapy.

Side effects of all of the vasodilators are tachycardia, weakness, depression, and hypotension. Clients should be advised of these side effects, and the first doses of vasodilator drugs should be carefully monitored and assessed for effects and toxicity.

Antiarrhythmics

The control and suppression of arrhythmia is important to the overall management of patients with heart failure. There are many antiarrhythmic drugs. Their proper use depends on the underlying pathophysiology as well as clinical response and experience. The established drugs used in veterinary medicine include propranolol, lidocaine, procainamide, and quinidine.[14,17,52] Arrhythmias often originate from eletrolyte imbalance and/or hypoxia. Clearly these problems should be identified and corrected before antiarrhythmic drug therapy is started.

Digoxin is useful in treatment for supraventricular arrhythmias such as atrial premature complexes, atrial fibrillation, and atrial tachycardia (see page

11-26. Propranolol is an unusually useful anti-arrhythmic drug. Its effects include:

1. Depression of AV nodal conduction, thus decreasing ventricular response to supraventricular tachyarrhythmias,
2. Beta-adrenergic blockade,
3. Slowing of the sinus rate, thus increasing the time for ventricular filling,
4. Reduction of myocardial oxygen consumption and, therefore, arrhythmias due to myocardial hypoxia,
5. Reduction of left ventricular outflow-tract gradient and improvement of ventricular relaxation,
6. Negative inotropic effect, and
7. Bronchoconstriction.

Because of these effects, propranolol is contraindicated in animals with:

1. Dilatative congestive heart failure unless a positive inotropic drug is given,
2. Preexistent diseases causing bronchoconstriction, and
3. Diabetes mellitus.

It must be used with extreme caution in patients with early congestive heart failure and reduced myocardial contractility, in which it may precipitate severe congestive heart failure.

Propranolol is most useful in heart diseases characterized by ventricular hypertrophy, such as hypertrophic cardiomyopathy in either dogs or cats, and in the control of tachyarrhythmias, especially those due to excessive catecholamines (Table 1).

The use of lidocaine has been described for emergency control of ventricular tachyarrhythmias (Table 1). Procainamide may be used in dogs to control ventricular premature beats or ventricular tachycardia (Table 1).

Quinidine closely resembles procainamide in its electrophysiologic actions. It has been used as an antiarrhythmic agent to treat for atrial fibrillation and to suppress atrial, junctional, and ventricular premature complexes, as well as to control ventricular tachycardia. Quinidine potentiates the action of digoxin, frequently necessitating a smaller dose of digoxin. It can be given either intravenously or orally to dogs. When given to convert atrial fibrillation to sinus rhythm, it may cause an increase in ventricular rate due to anticholinergic or sympathomimetic effects. Due to side effects, all antiarrhythmic drugs must be given cautiously and with careful frequent monitoring (Table 1).

Exercise Restriction

Many signs of congestive heart failure are precipitated by exercise. For this reason, reduction of physical activity reduces demands for additional cardiac output and helps alleviate the aggravation of signs. One of the most effective procedures for controlling the effects of heart failure, especially when the effects are severe, is cage rest. However, most properly instructed owners can adequately reduce their pet's activity at home. Any activity that causes dyspnea should be avoided. In the early stages of heart disease, avoiding forced play and stressful situations may be the only restrictions necessary. As the disease progresses, step-climbing and other similar activities should be avoided. Keeping the animals in a cool place, particularly in the summer, also helps. Restriction of exercise appropriate to the severity of the condition is an integral part of the therapy in animals with heart disease.

Dietary Management

Dietary management is an important part of therapy for all animals with heart disease. Clinical evidence of heart failure need not be present for animals to benefit from proper dietary management (see Chapter 3). The goal of dietary management of congestive heart failure is to reduce the workload on the heart while meeting nutritional needs of the body. This goal is accomplished by:

1. Reducing the sodium intake enough to prevent its accumulation,
2. Preventing or correcting hypoproteinemia,
3. Preventing a total-body potassium deficit, which is often induced by administrating diuretics,
4. Reducing the metabolic stress on a congested or cirrhotic liver by providing calories from carbohydrates and fats, and reducing the need for gluconeogenesis,
5. Reducing the need for renal function by reducing the level of catabolic waste products of protein metabolism,
6. Providing calories at a level that prevents excessive weight gain or loss,
7. Providing additional B-complex vitamins, especially during diuresis when their loss is increased, and
8. Providing an acid ash diet to aid in sodium excretion.

Sodium Restriction—One of the major goals in the dietary management of heart disease is to restrict sodium intake. Dogs with heart disease have been shown to excrete sodium at a rate much less than

normal, even before heart failure is evident.[68,69] Indeed, a decreased rate of excretion of a sodium load is characteristic of all states of heart failure. This reduced rate of excretion becomes progressively worse as congestive failure worsens. To be effective, sodium restriction must apply to all potential sources of sodium within the pet's environment. These sources include food, water, treats, and neighbors' handouts. The main source of sodium for most pets is ingested food. For example, one pretzel supplies five times the daily sodium needed by a toy or miniature dog.[48]

Sodium restriction has long been used in managing congestive heart failure. The American Heart Association has divided sodium restriction into three levels: severe, moderate, and mild, with sodium intakes of 7, 13, and 30 mg/kg body weight/day respectively. An average diet for human subjects provides about 65 mg/kg body weight/day or more than ten times the requirement. A similar relationship exists with dogs and cats if commercial pet foods are being consumed.[4]

The degree of sodium restriction required in each case depends on the severity of the lesions and the state of congestion present. Many states of congestive heart failure are not discovered until well-advanced. The kidneys of dogs and cats retain sodium more efficiently than do those of man, as

TABLE 8

SODIUM CONTENT OF PET FOODS

The veterinarian faced with treating a patient with congestive heart failure needs to know the sodium level of the food the animal has been consuming before prescribing treatment. Several nationally distributed pet foods were analyzed for sodium content and the results are listed below. Because the water content of these foods varies widely, the figures are expressed as milligrams of sodium per 100 grams of diet dry matter in order to make a valid comparison.

DOG FOODS

Class of Food	mg/100 g dry matter	Class of Food	mg/100 g dry matter
CANNED		DRY	
Ken-L-Ration	1140	Cycle 2	740
Friskies Dog Food	1036	Ken-L-Ration Biskit	600
Kal Kan Chunks of Beef By-Products	894	Gravy Train	563
Alpo Beef Chunks Dinner	868	Iams Chunks	540
Mighty Dog	583	Purina Dog Chow	508
Average	904	Gaines Meal	340
		Average	548
SEMI-MOIST		DIETARY	
Gainesburgers	950	Prescription Diet k/d	230
Top Choice	812	Prescription Diet h/d (canned)	90
Prime	809	(dry)	55
Average	857	Recipe 5 (Appendix Table 3)	52

CAT FOODS

Class of Food	mg/100 g dry matter	Class of Food	mg/100 g dry matter
CANNED		DRY	
Purina 100 Tuna	3790*	Friskies Ocean Fish	877
Fancy Feast Seafood	890	Special Dinner Tuna & Herring	615
Friskies Fish Flavor	857	Crave	600
Puss-N-Boots Fish	830	Fish Ahoy	590
Kal Kan Mealtime	790	Kitten Chow	570
9-Lives Tuna	730	Iams	500
Friskies Buffet Seafood Supper	690	Tamiami	485
Bright Eyes Seafood Supper	590	Cat Chow Original Blend	470
Average (*excluded)	768	9-Lives Tuna	370
		Average	564
SEMI-MOIST		DIETARY	
9-Lives	737	Prescription Diet Feline c/d	460
Happy Cat	647	Prescription Diet Feline k/d (canned)	400
Tender Vittles	535	(dry)	250
Average	640	Prescription Diet Feline h/d	240
		Recipe 8 (Appendix Table 3)	160

evidenced by the fact that man develops hypo-natremia on levels of salt intake which do not lead to hyponatremia in dogs. A single diet at the severe sodium restriction level is satisfactory and practical in managing most cases of Phase 3 or 4 canine congestive heart failure.[131,141] To achieve this level of sodium restriction (13 mg sodium/kg/day) the diet must contain about 0.025% sodium in a canned food (70% moisture) or 90 mg/100g of dry food; i.e., for either about 100 mg/100g of diet dry matter (Prescription Diet h/d).

Dogs with mild lesions of heart disease and in precongestive and early congestive states require only moderate sodium restriction. Such restriction can be accomplished with an intake of approxi-mately 30 mg/kg/day. To accomplish this level of sodium restriction, the diet must contain about .065% sodium in a canned food (70% moisture) or 210 mg/100g of dry food, i.e., for either about 240 mg/100g of diet dry matter (Prescription Diet k/d).

In initiating dietary sodium restriction, first feed a moderately restricted sodium diet. The magnitude of change in sodium intake is reduced and it allows the pet to become accustomed to a reduced sodium intake. After the animal is consuming the moder-ately restricted sodium diet well, a change to a severely restricted diet, if required to prevent clinical signs, is accomplished with much greater ease than a change directly from a high-sodium pet food to a severely-restricted sodium diet. The initiation of dietary sodium restriction by using this stepwise method can be accomplished readily in the home by most owners, thereby eliminating hospi-talization.

Table 8 shows the sodium content of several commercially available pet foods. Dogs and cats eating these foods consume an average of 130 mg sodium/kg/day. This is twice the average amount a human subject eats in an average diet and 30 times the amount shown to be adequate for growth in the dog.

The reason commercial pet foods contain such high amounts of sodium is so that they will meet or exceed the amount deemed by the National Research Council to be "an appropriate allowance that probably exceeds the dog's requirements."[5]

The principle of sodium restriction in the man-agement of congestive heart failure is visually sum-marized in Figures 8 and 9. In dogs with edema and ascites, when sodium intake is reduced sufficiently, retention of sodium and water ceases and body excesses are excreted. Just as water follows sodium into the body, water follows sodium out, and spontaneous diuresis occurs. This response is often seen in animals with congestive heart failure when they are given cage rest and a low-sodium diet without any other treatment.

Chronic dilutional hyponatremia in pets with congestive heart failure is rare. When it does occur, it is because of the animal's impaired ability to excrete water rather than to inadequate sodium intake. Even when hyponatremia exists, the animal with congestive heart failure has an excess of total-body exchangeable sodium. In cases where chronic hyponatremia occurs, it is quite difficult to manage and, therefore, indicates a very poor prog-nosis.

Sodium restriction is contraindicated in cases of dehydration, debilitation, cachexia, chronic diar-rhea, hyponatremia, and during reproduction. Preg-nant females confined to severely restricted sodium diets (less than .03% of dry matter) experience problems during the last two weeks of pregnancy. These include abortion, fetal death, and resorption resulting in toxemia or still births.

Other Dietary Considerations—Other elec-trolytes in addition to sodium are important in animals with congestive heart failure. Calcium, potassium, and magnesium all have important functions in the myocardium. Presence or absence of potassium deficiency materially effects the tox-icity of cardiac glycosides and their action on the heart. Cardiac glycosides and diuretics, with the exception of spironolactone (see page 11-27), enhance potassium excretion; therefore, when cardiac glycosides and diuretics are given, potas-sium intake must be increased to prevent a total-body potassium deficit or hypokalemia.

The provision of adequate quantities and ratios of other mineral elements in a sodium-restricted diet is essential to maintain the patient's eletrolyte balance and homeostasis. These are taken into considera-tion in the formulation of the prepared sodium-restricted diets (Prescription Diets h/d and Feline h/d and Recipe 5 and 8—Appendix Table 3). When these diets are fed to animals with heart disease, supplements (other than those called for in the recipes for the homemade diets) are contraindi-cated.

The availability of water to the pet with conges-tive heart failure should never be limited. Restricted access to water only worsens cellular dehydration and eletrolyte imbalance.[146] However, drinking water must be considered a source of ingested sodium. Some city and home water softeners utilize sodium cation exchangers. In these circumstances, non-softened water should be given. In severely congested patients requiring maximum sodium restriction, distilled water should be used during

FIGURE 8

SODIUM BALANCE — NORMAL AND DURING HEART FAILURE

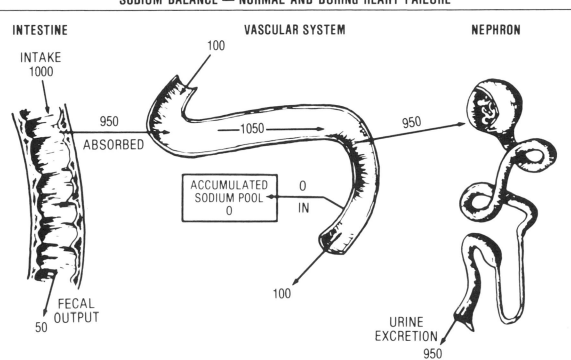

Normal (above): Most of the sodium intake is absorbed (with suitable amounts of water to maintain isotonicity of the blood), filtered through the glomerulus and excreted in the urine. To maintain proper levels of total exchangeable body sodium and to prevent hemodilution, an amount equal to that absorbed must be excreted.

During Heart Failure (below): Most of the sodium intake is absorbed and filtered through the glomerulus. The appearance of the aldosterone and ADH, however, results in sodium being reabsorbed in the distal tubules of the nephron (again with suitable water to maintain isotonicity).This causes a hemodilution and the sodium (with its water) moves into the intercellular spaces (refer to Fig. 3 for this mechanism). Less sodium is excreted than absorbed, and sodium and water accumulate in the body.

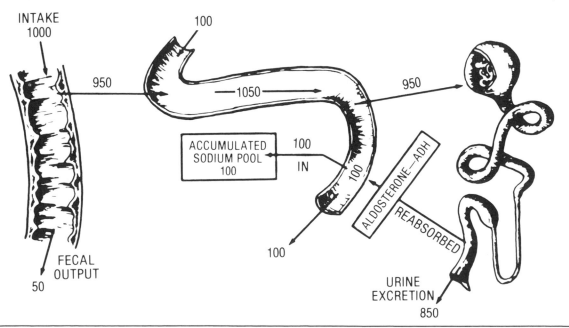

FIGURE 9

EFFECT OF SODIUM RESTRICTION ON SODIUM BALANCE IN HEART FAILURE

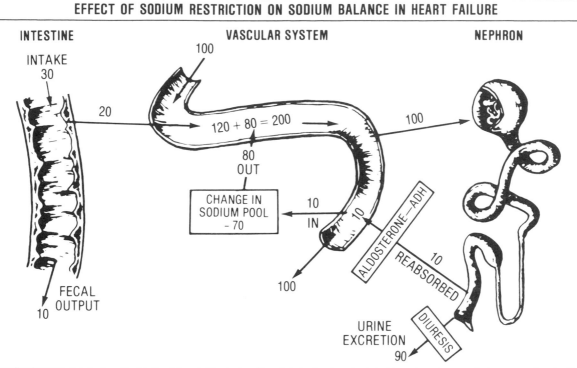

Immediately Following Sodium Restriction (above): Most of sodium intake is absorbed, but in reduced amounts because of reduction in intake. Because the kidney is excreting salt at a high rate, the excess total exchangeable sodium accumulated in the inter-cellular spaces moves back into the vascular system to replace that being excreted by the kidney. The aldosterone—ADH complex accounts for less and less reabsorption as the edema and congestion is reduced and cardiac output improves.

During Compensation (below): With the restriction of salt intake, the amount absorbed remains low. The aldosterone—ADH complex, while still active, reabsorbs greatly reduced amounts of sodium (and its accompanying water for isotonicity). The dilutional effects are minimal, and most of the reabsorbed sodium is refiltered and excreted as rapidly as it is absorbed. (The effect of sodium restriction during compensation explains why salt restriction in pre-congestive states is effective in delaying the onset of congestion.)

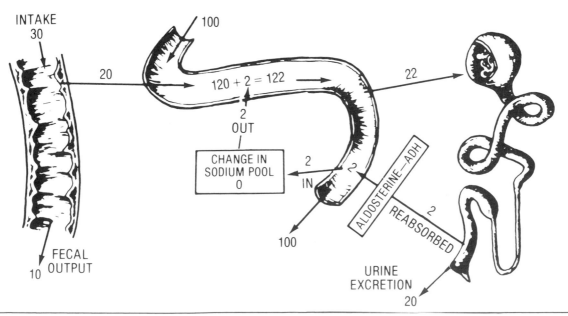

the early stages of therapy until ascites and edema are eliminated. Municipal water departments will make available the sodium content of their water on request.* If the water supply contains 150 ppm sodium or more, distilled water should be used until congestion is relieved.

Many cats and dogs with congestive heart failure are hypoproteinemic because of faulty protein absorption, transportation, and metabolism. Hypoproteinemia may be exacerbated if excessive quantities of abdominal fluids are removed by paracentesis. Hypoproteinemia accentuates more retention in the extracellular spaces (Figure 3, page 11-11). However, excess protein intake should be avoided because the incidence of chronic renal failure is greater in older dogs and cats with heart disease. In dogs, renal failure is often concurrent with heart failure. Therefore, dogs in congestive heart failure should be fed a diet with a protein level from 14-18% in diet dry matter. Renal failure is less common in cats with heart failure. Thus, cats with heart failure can be fed diets containing more protein. A level of 35-45% in the diet dry matter enhances the palatability of feline restricted sodium diets and aids voluntary consumption.**

The proteins fed to dogs should be of high biologic value in order to meet the protein requirement at the reduced level, thus reducing the quantity of nitrogenous waste products to be excreted by the kidneys. The reduced blood supply to the kidneys with heart failure (see page 11-22) increases the necessity of reducing the requirement for renal function. Protein restriction will help prevent the azotemia, which commonly occurs with heart failure.

Congestive heart failure may be accompanied by chronic liver congestion, which reduces liver function. Therefore, nutrients should be supplied in a form that minimizes the need for liver function. Proteins of high biologic value, which reduce the need for transamination of amino acids, are indicated. Simple sugars and emulsified fats are the best sources of energy for both the heart and the liver.

In heart failure, the gastrointestinal tract also suffers from a lack of adequate arterial circulation and from venous congestion. This contributes to nutritional inadequacies as a result of poor intestinal absorption. Foods administered to patients in congestive heart failure, therefore, should be highly digestible and fed in small frequent feedings to allow the maximal quantities of nutrients to be absorbed.

The patient in congestive heart failure who is given diuretics loses large quantities of sodium, water, and water-soluble B-complex vitamins.[59] Therefore, the dietary intake of the B-vitamins should be increased to five times normal. This is accomplished by adding 1 g of brewer's yeast/kg/day or by using a B-complex vitamin preparation. Prepared restricted sodium diets (Prescription Diets k/d or h/d) contain increased amounts of B-complex vitamins, thus vitamin supplements or yeast should not be added if they are being fed.

Diets restricted in sodium should metabolize to an acid ash. It is beneficial to increase formation of metabolic acids, which combine with sodium and are excreted in the urine. Excretion of sodium with metabolic acids results in a reduction of extracellular sodium and fluid, thus enhancing diuresis. While most foods commonly fed to pets metabolize to an acid ash, many foods eaten by man produce an alkaline ash. Adding foods for human beings to a prepared pet food to reduce its sodium level may result in a deleterious alkaline ash diet.

Palatability—Palatability is often a problem with low-sodium diets for man. Salt enhances the palatability of food for many people. This is not the case, however, for most dogs and cats. The most common reason why dogs and cats refuse a low-sodium diet is a sudden dietary change or the change from a higher protein diet to a lower protein diet, not the fact that the diet contains less sodium.

Many heart failure patients are older and may have somewhat fixed and fussy eating habits. The veterinarian must emphasize to the client the importance of feeding a sodium-restricted diet, and that the success or failure of treatment depends to a large extent on strict adherence to the diet.[106,118,119]

Changing the fixed **eating** habits of most dogs is relatively easy, but changing the fixed **feeding** habits and preconceived ideas of the owner as to what the pet prefers is often much more difficult. Results of feeding studies with hospitalized dogs have shown that most dogs will readily accept a severely restricted sodium diet and that by the third day less than 5% will continue refusing it. The most practical solution for this problem 5% is to make the change more gradually. Begin by feeding the dog a moderately restricted sodium diet such as Prescription Diet k/d or Feline h/d. The prepared restricted sodium diet for cats contains the same sodium content as the moderately restricted diet for dogs. Due to its higher protein content it is readily eaten by dogs and is a good diet to use for initia-

---

*This information is usually supplied in parts per million (ppm). To convert this figure to mg/100 ml, divide it by 10.

**The % of a nutrient in the diet dry matter equals the % in the diet as fed ÷ by the diet's dry matter content. For example, a canned food containing 5% protein and 75% moisture would contain 20% protein in its dry matter [5% ÷ (1 − 0.75) = 5% ÷ 0.25 = 20%].

tion of sodium restriction. Once the animal is accustomed to this less restricted diet, switch to the severely restricted sodium diet (Prescription Diet h/d) if required to control clinical signs. Another approach is to spread the change over a longer period of time, gradually decreasing the amount of the previous diet fed while increasing the amount of the low-sodium diet fed. Using this approach, begin by feeding one part h/d to three parts of the previous diet, mixing them thoroughly. The animal's sodium intake is reduced about 20%. When this mixture is being consumed readily (which may take anywhere from one to five days), mix equal parts of each diet and again allow the pet to become thoroughly accustomed to this mixture, which reduces its sodium intake about 50%. Continue this procedure until the animal is eating only the low-sodium diet.

This method has proven highly successful in converting those few pampered pets who initially refused to accept the new dietary regimen. If continued problems with palatability are encountered, even though these procedures are used, the diet should be individualized by adding low-sodium foods which the pet enjoys. Table 9 lists foods commonly found in the home. Both foods that can be used and those that should not be used are listed.

Other techniques that have been used with success when animals are being converted to a low-sodium diet are: 1) warming the food, particularly if the animal is accustomed to having its food warmed, 2) sprinkling a salt substitute (potassium chloride) on the food, and 3) giving B-complex vitamins.

In initiating any dietary change for medical purposes, always assume the pet will make the change voluntarily, as the vast majority will do so. Statements such as "Your dog may not eat this low-salt food" or "Some dogs don't like low-salt diets" almost assures that the owner will have trouble converting the pet to the new diet. A statement such as "It is extremely important that your pet eat this new diet, if it is to live" greatly enhances the probability that the conversion will be accomplished, as the owner becomes dedicated to the task. As a last resort, if the owner cannot, or will not, accomplish the dietary change at home, the veterinarian may suggest the dog be hospitalized to "adjust the drug dosages." During a 3-4 day hospitalization over 95% of dogs can be converted to a restricted-salt diet, eliminating the need to accomplish this task in the home, as the dog is already consuming the restricted-sodium diet when released from the hospital.

TABLE 9

SODIUM CONTENT OF HUMAN FOODS[4]

Foods Permitted	mg/100 g dry matter	Foods to Omit	mg/100 g dry matter
Beans, Dried	23	Beef Kidney	730
Beans, Lima	Trace	Beef Liver	453
Beef	143	Beef Stew, Canned	2,349
Chicken (dark meat)	255	Beets	473
Chicken (light meat)	190	Bologna	2,968
Corn	Trace	Bread, White	786
Corn Grits	1	Carrots, Canned	2,730
Egg Yolks	106	Cheese, Cottage	1,055
Farina (Cream of Wheat)	2	Cheese, Processed	1,890
Fish, Fresh Water	265	Cookies, Retail, Average	375
Horsemeat	210	Crackers, Saltine	1,100
Lamb	192	Corn Flakes	1,045
Meat Baby Foods, Average	294	Egg, Fried	1,046
Milk, Whole	397	Frankfurters	2,477
Oatmeal	2	Margarine and Butter	1,168
Peas, Blackeyed	40	Pancakes	978
Potatoes, Sweet	28	Peanut Butter	616
Rabbit, Domestic	143	Popcorn, Salted	2,002
Rice	6	Potato Chips	600
Squash	10	Pretzels	1,361
		Roll, Plain	738
Foods to Omit	mg/100 g dry matter	Wheat Flakes	1,036
Bacon	1,111		
Beef Heart	382		

Values for vegetables are for fresh items, boiled and drained without added salt. Values for unprocessed meats are for fresh, uncured, raw items.

REFERENCES

1. Abboud FM, Thames MC, Mark AL: Role of cardiac afferent nerves in regulation of circulation during coronary occlusion and heart failure. In: Disturbances in Neurogenic Control of the Circulation. Editors Abboud FM, Fozzard HA, Gilmore JP, Reis DJ. Bethesda, MD Amer Physiol Soc pp 65, (1981).

2. Allen DG: Echocardiographic study of the anesthetized cat. Can J Comp Med 46:115-122 (1982).

3. Amorim DS, Heer K, Jenner D, et al: Is there autonomic impairment in congestive (dilated) cardiomyopathy? Lancet I:525 (1981).

4. Anonymous: Composition of foods, Agriculture Handbook, No. 8. United States Department of Agriculture, Washington, DC.

5. Anonymous: Nutrient requirements of domestic animals, No.8. Nutrient requirements of dogs, National Academy of Sciences, Washington, DC (1974).

6. Anonymous: Nutrient requirements of domestic animals, No. 13. Nutrient requirements of cats, National Academy of Sciences, Washington, DC (1978).

7. Ayers CR, Bowden RE, Schrank JP: Mechanisms of sodium retention in congestive heart failure. Adv Exp Med Biol 17:227 (1972).

8. Barger AC, Herd A, Sparks HV: The kidney in congestive heart failure. American Heart Association Monograph. No. 1, 2nd ed., (1966).

9. Barger AC, Yates FF, Rudolph AM: Renal hemodynamics and sodium excretion in dogs with graded valvular damage, and in congestive failure. Amer J Physiol 200:601 (1961).

10. Barger AC, Muldowner FP, Lubowitz MR: Role of the kidney in the pathogenesis of congestive heart failure. Circ 20:273 (1959).

11. Belleau L, Mion H, Simard S, et al: Studies on the mechanism of experimental congestive heart failure in dogs. Can J Physiol Pharmacol 48·450 (1970).

12. Bolton GR: Handbook of canine electrocardiography. WB Saunders Co, Philadelphia, PA (1975).

13. Bonagura JD: Acute heart failure. In Current Veterinary Therapy VII, Editor RW Kirk, WB Saunders Co, Philadelphia, PA (1980).

14. Bonagura JD, Muir WW: Antiarrhythmic therapy. In Essentials of Canine and Feline Electrocardiography, Editor LP Tilley, 2nd edition (1984).

15. Bonagura JD: Cardiovascular emergencies. Proc Amer Anim Hosp Assoc (1979).

16. Bonagura JD: Clinical applications of echocardiography. Amer College Vet Int Med Proc, pp 210-219

17. Bonagura JD: Current concepts in the therapy of heart disease. Amer Anim Hosp Assoc pp 13-22 (1984).

18. Bonagura JD, Pipers FS: Diagnosis of cardiac lesions by contrast echocardiography. J Amer Vet Med Assoc 182:396-402 (1983).

19. Bonagura JD, Pipers FS: Echocardiographic features of pericardial effusion in dogs. J Amer Vet Med Assoc 179:49-56 (1981).

20. Bonagura JD: Electrical alternans associated with pericardial effusion in the dog. J Amer Vet Med Assoc 178:574-579 (1981).

21. Bonagura JD: M-mode echocardiography. Vet Clin N Amer I3: 299-319 (1983).

22. Boon J, Wingfield WE, Miller CW: Echocardiographic indices in the normal dog. Vet Radiol J 24:214-221 (1983).

23. Braunwald E: Heart Disease: A Textbook of Cardiovascular Medicine, 2nd edition. WB Saunders Co, Philadelphia, PA (1984).

24. Braunwald E, Plauth WH, Morrow AG: A method for detection and quantification of impaired sodium excretion. Circ 32:223-231 (1965).

25. Braunwald E: Pathophysiology of heart failure, Chapter 13 in Heart Disease, 2nd edition, WB Saunders Co, Philadelphia, PA (1984).

26. Braunwald E: Renal disorders and heart disease, Chapter 52 in Heart Disease, 2nd edition, WB Saunders Co, Philadelphia, PA (1984).

27. Breznock EM: Application of canine plasma kinetics of digoxin and digitoxin to therapeutic digitalization in the dog. Amer J Vet Res 34:993-999 (1973).

28. Brown JJ, Davies DL, Johnson VW, et al: Renin relationship in congestive cardiac failure, treated and untreated. Amer Heart J 80:329 (1970).

29. Buchanan JW: Atrioventricular insufficiency and sequelae. In Current Veterinary Therapy III, Editor RW Kirk, WB Saunders Co, Philadelphia, PA (1968).

30. Chidsey CA, Sonnenblock EH, Morrow AG, Braunwald E: Norepinephrine stores and contractile force of papillary muscle from the failing human heart. Circ 33:43 (1960).

31. Chimoskey JE, Spielman WS, Brandt MA, Heidimann SR: Cardiac atria of bio 14.6 hamsters are deficient in natriuretic factor. Science 223:820-821 (1984).

32. Conn RD: Ventricular volumes and myocardial mass in patients with heart disease. In Cardiovascular Dynamics, Editor RF Rushmer, 3rd edition, WB Saunders Co, Philadelphia, PA (1970).

33. Curtiss C, Cohn JN, Vrobel T, Franciosa JA: Role of the renin-angiotensin system in the systemic vasoconstriction of chronic congestive heart failure. Circ 58:763-770 (1978).

34. Das KM, Tashjian RJ: Chronic mitral valve disease in the dog. VM/SAC 60:1209 (1965).

35. Davis JO: Adrenocortical and renal hormonal function in experimental cardiac failure. Circulation 25:1002 (1962).

36. Davis JO: Adrenocortical and renal hormonal function in experimental heart failure. Circ 25: 1007 (1962).

37. Davis LE: Pharmacodynamics of digitalis, diuretics and antiarrhythmic drugs. In Current Veterinary Therapy VII, Editor RW Kirk, WB Saunders Co, Philadelphia, PA (1980).

38. Dennis MO, Nealeigh RC, Pyle RL, et al: Echocardiographic assessment of normal and abnormal valvular function in Beagle dogs. Amer J Vet Res 39:1591-1598 (1978).

39. DeRick A, Belpaire FM, Bogaert MG, Mattheeuws D: Plasma concentrations of digoxin and digitoxin during digitalization of healthy dogs and dogs with cardiac failure. Amer J Vet Res 39:811 (1978).

40. Detweiler DK, Patterson DF, et al: Diseases of the cardiovascular system. In Canine Medicine, 1st Catcott Edition, Amer Vet Publ, Inc, Santa Barbara, CA (1968).

41. Detweiler DK: Heart sounds and murmurs. In Canine Medicine, 2nd edition, Amer Vet Publ, Inc, Santa Barbara, CA (1959).

42. Detweiler DK, et al: The natural history of cardiac disability of the dog. J Amer Anim Hosp Assoc 5:1 (1969).

43. Detweiler DK, Patterson DF: The prevalence and types of cardiovascular disease in dogs. Ann NY Acad Sci 127:481 (1965).

44. Detweiler DK, et al: Survey of cardiovascular disease in dogs— Preliminary report on the first 1,000 dogs screened. Amer J Vet Res 21:329 (1960).

45. Dillon R: Canine heartworm disease. Amer Anim Hosp Assoc Proc (1984).

46. Dzau VJ, Colucci WS, Hollenberg NK, William GH: Relation of the renin-angiotensin-aldosterone system to clinical state in congestive heart failure. Circ 63:645-651 (1981).

47. Eckberg DL, Drabinsky M, Braunwald E: Defective cardiac parasympathetic control in patients with heart disease. New Engl J Med 285:877 (1971).

48. Ettinger SJ, Suter PF: Canine Cardiology. WB Saunders Co, Philadelphia, PA (1970).

49. Ettinger SJ: Introduction to the diagnosis and management of heart disease. In Current Veterinary Therapy VI, Editor RW Kirk, WB Saunders Co, Philadelphia, PA (1977).

50. Ettinger S: Isoproterenol treatment of atrioventricular block in the dog. J Amer Vet Med Assoc 154:398 (1969).

51. Ettinger SJ: In Textbook of Veterinary Internal Medicine. 2nd edition, WB Saunders Co, Philadelphia, PA (1983).

52. Ettinger SJ: Cardiac Arrhythmias. In Textbook of Veterinary Internal Medicine, 2nd edition, WB Saunders Co, Philadelphia, PA (1983).

53. Ettinger SJ: Therapeutic digitalization of the dog in congestive heart failure. J Amer Vet Med Assoc 148:525 (1966.

54. Ettinger SJ: Valvular heart disease. In Textbook of Veterinary Internal Medicine, 2nd edition, WB Saunders Co, Philadelphia, PA (1983).

55. Fitzsimmons JT, Simons BJ: The effect on drinking in the rat of intravenous infusion of angiotensin given alone or in combination with other stimuli of thirst. J Physiol (Lond) 203:45 (1969).

56. Fitzsimmons JT: Thirst. Physiol Rev 52: 468 (1972).

57. Freeman RH, Davis JO, Williams GM, et al: Effects of oral converting enzyme inhibitor, SQ14225, in a model of low cardiac output in dogs. Circ Res 45:540 (1979).

58. Genest J, Granger P, DeChamplain J, Boucher R: Endocrine factors in congestive heart failure. Amer J Cardiol 22:35 (1968).

59. Gertler MM, Rusk HA: Rehabilitation principles in congestive heart failure. American Heart Association Monograph No. 1, 2nd ed (1966).

60. Goldstein RE, Beiser GD, Stempfer M, Epstein SE: Impairment of autonomically mediated heart rate control in patients with cardiac dysfunction. Circ Res 36:571 (1975).

61. Greenberg TT, Richmond WH, Stocking RA, et al: Impaired arterial stretch receptor responses in dogs with heart failure due to tricuspid insufficiency and pulmonary artery stenosis. Circ Res 32:424 (1973).

62. Gross DR, Pipers FS, Hamlin RL: Normal systolic time intervals in awake dogs and their response to digitalis glycosides. Am J Vet Res 35:15-21 (1974).

63. Gross DR, Hamlin RL, Pipers FS:Response of P-Q intervals to digitalis glycosides in the dog. J Amer Vet Med Assoc 162:888-890 (1973).

64. Hahn AW: Digitalis glycosides in canine medicine. In Current Veterinary Therapy VI, Editor RW Kirk, WB Saunders Co, Philadelphia, PA (1977).

65. Hahn AW: Auscultation of the canine heart, parts I, II, III, and IV. Sm Anim Clin I:320, I:348, I:377, 2:13 (1961-62).

66. Hamlin RL: Analysis of the cardiac silhouette in dorsoventral radiographs from dogs with heart disease. J Amer Vet Med Assoc 153:1446 (1968).

67. Hamlin RL: Congestive heart failure. In Current Veterinary Therapy III, Editor RW Kirk, WB Saunders Co, Philadelphia, PA (1968).

68. Hamlin RL, Smith CR, Ross JN Jr: Detection and quantitation of subclinical heart failure in dogs. J Amer Vet Med Assoc 150:1513 (1966).

69. Hamlin RL, et al: Detection and quantitation of subclinical heart failure in dogs. Proc Am Physiol Soc (1966).

70. Hamlin RL, et al: Effects of a controlled electrolyte diet, low in sodium, on healthy dogs. VM/SAC 59:743 (1964).

71. Hamlin RL, Dutta S, Smith CR: Effects of digoxin and digitoxin on ventricular function in normal dogs and dogs with heart failure. Amer J Vet Res 32:1391-1398 (1971).

72. Hamlin RL: New ideas in the management of heart failure in dogs. J Amer Vet Med Assoc 171:114-118 (1977).

73. Hamlin RL, Pipers FS, Carter K: Preference of veterinarians for drugs used to treat heart failure in dogs. J Amer Vet Med Assoc 161:504-506 (1972).

74. Hamlin RL: Prognostic value of changes in the cardiac silhouette in dogs with mitral insufficiency. J Amer Vet Med Assoc 153:1446 (1968).

75. Hamlin RL, Smetter DL, Smith CR: Radiographic anatomy of the normal cat heart. J Amer Vet Med Assoc 143:957 (1963).

76. Hamlin RL: Radiographic diagnosis of heart disease in dogs. J Amer Vet Med Assoc 137:458 (1960).

77. Hamlin RL, Piper FS, Carter K: Treatment of heart failure in dogs without use of digitalis glycosides. VM/SAC 68:349-356 (1973).

78. Harpster NK: Feline cardiomyopathy. Vet Clin of N Amer 7:355 (1977).

79. Harris SG, Ogburn PN: The cardiovascular system. In Feline Medicine and Surgery, 2nd edition. Editor EJ Catcott. Am Vet Publ, Santa Barbara, CA (1975).

80. Harris SG: Digitalis glycosides. In Current Veterinary Therapy V, Editor RW Kirk, WB Saunders Co, Philadelphia, PA (1974).

81. Higgins CB, Vatner SF, Eckberg DL, Braunwald E: Alterations in the baroreceptor reflex in conscious dogs with heart failure. J Clin Invest 51:715 (1972).

82. Horowitz LD, Travis VL: Low serum dopamine-B-hydroxylase activity: A marker of congestive heart failure. J Clin Invest 62:899 (1978).

83. Hostetter TH, Pfeffer JM, Pfeffer MA, et al: Cardiorenal hemodynamics and sodium excretion in rats with myocardial infarction. Amer J physiol 245 (Heart Circ Physiol 14):H98-H103 (1983).

84. Hricik DE, Kassirer JP: Azotemia in cardiac failure. J Cardiovasc Med 8:397 (1983).

85. Jackson WF: Circulation time in heartworm disease. Sm Anim Clin 2:336 (1962).

86. Jameson AG: Pathologic physiol in mitral valve disease. Ann of NY Acad of Sci 118:486 (1965).

87. Johnson CI, Davis JO, Robb CA, Mackenzie JW: Plasma renin in chronic experimental heart failure and during renal sodium "escape" from mineralocorticoids. Circ Res 22:113 (1968).

88. Johnson CL: Pericardial effusion in the dog. Compend Cont Educ I:680 (1979).

89. Jubb KVF, Kennedy PC: Pathology of Domestic Animals. 2nd ed, Academic Press, NY (1974).

90. Kelly ID: Canine heartworm disease. In Current Veterinary Therapy VIII, Editor RW Kirk, WB Saunders Co, Philadelphia, PA (1980).

91. Kittleson MD, Eyster GE, Knowlen GG, et al: Myocardial function in small dogs with chronic mitral regurgitation and severe congestive heart failure. J Amer Vet Med Assoc 184:455-459 (1984).

92. Kleine JL, Zook BC, Munson TO: Primary cardian hemangiosarcomas in dogs. J Amer Vet Med Assoc 157:326 (1970).

93. Kluger J, Cody RJ, Laragh JH: The contributions of sympathetic tone and the renin-angiotensin system to severe chronic congestive heart failure: Response to specific inhibitors (prazosin and captopril). Amer J Cardiol 49:1667 (1982).

94. Knight DH: Heartworm disease. In Textbook of Veterinary Internal Medicine, 2nd edition, Edited by SJ Ettinger, WB Saunders Co, Philadelphia, PA (1983).

95. Laks MM, Morady F, Garner D, Swan HJC: Temporal changes in canine right ventricular column, mass, cell size, and sarcomere length after banding the pulmonary artery. Cardiovasc Res 8:106 (1974).

96. Levine TB, Francis GS, Goldsmith SR, et al: Activity of the sympathetic nervous system and renin-angiotensin system assessed by plasma hormone levels and their relation to hemodynamic abnormalities in congestive heart failure. Amer J Cardiol 49:1659 (1982).

97. Liu SK: Acquired cardiac lesions leading to congestive heart failure in the cat. Amer J Vet Res 31:2071 (1970).

98. Liu SK, Tashjian RJ, Patnaik AK: Congestive heart failure in the cat. J Amer Vet Med Assoc 156:1319 (1970).

99. Liu SK: Pathology of feline heart disease. In Current Veterinary Therapy V, Editor RW Kirk, WB Saunders Co, Philadelphia, PA (1974).

100. Lombard CW, Buergelt CD: Echocardiographic and clinical findings in dogs with heart-worm-induced cor pulmonale. Comp Cont Educ 5:971-979 (1983).

101. Lombard CW, Buergelt CD: Vegetative bacterial endocarditis in dogs; echocardiographic diagnosis and clinical signs. J Amer An Pract 24:325-329 (1983).

102. Mark AL, Mayer HE, Schmid PG, et al: Adrenergic control of the peripheral circulation in cardiomyopathic hamsters with heart failure. Circ Res 33:74 (1973).

103. Merrill AJ, Morrison JL, Brannon ES: Concentration of renin in renal venous blood in patients with chronic heart failure. Amer J Med I:468 (1946).

104. Minami M, Yasuda H, Yamazaki N, et al: Plasma norepinephrine concentration and plasma dopamine-beta-hydroxylase activity in patients with congestive heart failure. Circ 67:1324-1329 (1983).

105. Morris BJ, Davis JO, Zatzman ML, Williams GM: The renin-angiotensin-aldosterone system in rabbits with congestive heart failure produced by aortic constriction. Circ Res 40:275 (1977).

106. Morris ML, Jr, et al: Sodium, how low is low? VM/SAC 71:1225-1227 (1976).

107. Nilsson T: Heart-base tumors in the dog. Acta Pathol 37:385 (1955).

108. Otto GF, Jackson RF: Heartworm disease. In Textbook of Veterinary Internal Medicine, Editor SJ Ettinger, WB Saunders Co, Philadelphia, PA (1975).

109. Patterson DF: Canine congenital heart disease:Epidemiology and etiological hypotheses. J Small Anim Prac 12:263 (1971).

110. Patterson DF: Congenital defects of the cardiovascular system of dogs:Studies in comparative cardiology. Adv Vet Sci Comp Med 20:(1976).

111. Patterson DF: Epidemiologic and genetic studies of congenital heart disease in the dog. Circ Res 23:171 (1968).

112. Patterson DF, Pyle RL, Buchanan JW: Hereditary cardiovascular malformation of the dog. The Clinical Delineation of Birth Defects. Birth Defects 8:160 (1972). Williams and Wilkins Co, Baltimore.

113. Patterson DF, Pyle RL, van Mierop LHS, et al: Hereditary defects of the conotruncal septum in keeshond dogs:Pathologic and genetic studies. Amer J Cardiol 34:187 (1974).

114. Patterson DF, Pyle RL, Buchanan JW, et al: Hereditary patent ductus arteriosus and its sequelae in the dog. Circ Res 29:1 (1971).

115. Patterson DF, et al: Spontaneous abnormal cardiac arrhythmias and conduction disturbances in the dog. Amer J Vet Res 22:355 (1961).

116. Pensinger RR: Clinical and physiological aspects of congestive heart failure in the dog. Amer Anim Hosp Assoc Proc (1968).

117. Pensinger RR: Congestive heart failure patho-physiology in dogs. In Cardiology II Independent Study Course, Amer Anim Hosp Assoc Proc (1978).

118. Pensinger RR: Dietary control of sodium intake in spontaneous heart failure in dogs. VM/SAC 59:743 (1964).

119. Pensinger RR: Nutritional management of heart disease. In Current Veterinary Therapy III, Editor RW Kirk, WB Saunders Co, Philadelphia, PA (1968).

120. Pipers FS, Reef V, Hamlin RL: Echocardiography in the domestic cat. Amer J Vet Res 40:882-886 (1979).

121. Pittman JG, Cohen P: The pathogenesis of cardiac cachexia. New Engl J Med 271:403 (1964).

122. Pohosst GM, Dinsmore RE, Rubenstein JJ, et al: The echocardiogram of the anterior leaflet of the mitral valve. Correlation with hemodynamic and cineroentgenographic studies in dogs. Circ 51:88-97 (1975).

123. Pool PE, Covell JW, Levitt M, et al: Reduction of cardiac tyrosinehydroxylase activity in experimental congestive heart failure: Its role in depletion of cardiac norepinephrine stores. Circ Res 20:249 (1967).

124. Pyle RL: Congenital heart disease. In Textbook of Veterinary Internal Medicine, Edited by SJ Ettinger, WB Saunders Co, Philadelphia, PA (1983).

125. Remington JW: Relation between length of diastole and stroke index in intact dog. Amer J Physiol 162:273 (1950).

126. Riegger GAJ, Liebau G, Kochsiek K: Antidiuretic hormone in congestive heart failure. Amer J Med 7249 (1982).

127. Roskoski R, Jr, Schmid PG, Mayer HE, Abboud FM: In vitro acetylcholine biosynthesis in normal and failing guinea pig hearts. Circ Res 36:547 (1975).

128. Ross JN, Jr: Heart failure. In Textbook of Veterinary Internal Medicine, 2nd edition, Editor SJ Ettinger, WB Saunders Co, Philadelphia, PA (1983).

129. Rubin JG: Applications and electrocardiology in canine medicine. J Amer Vet Med Assoc 153:17 (1968).

130. Rushmer RF: Cardiovascular Dynamics. WB Saunders Co, Philadelphia, PA (1970).

131. Schuchman SM: Low sodium diet. In Current Veterinary Therapy V, Editor RW Kirk, WB Saunders Co, Philadelphia, PA (1974).

132. Scheuer J, Bhan AK: Cardiac contractile proteins. Adenosine triphosphatase activity and physiological functions. Circ Res 45:1 (1979).

133. Schmid PG, Lund DD, Roskoski R, Jr: Efferent autonomic dysfunction in heart failure. In Disturbances in Neurogenic Control of the Circulation, Editors Abboud FM, Fozzard Ha, Gilmore JB, Reis DJ, American Physiological Society (1981).

134. Schroeder HA: Studies on congestive heart failure. I. The importance of restriction of salt as compared to water. Amer Heart J 22:141 (1971).

135. Smetter DL, Hamlin RL, Smith CR: Cardiovascular sounds. In Duke's Physiology of Domestic Animals, 9th ed. Editor MJ Swenson, Comstock Publishing Associates, Ithaca, NY (1977).

136. Smith RC, Hamlin RL: Circulation to skeletal muscle circulatory adjustments during exercise and cardiac enlargement. In Duke's Physiology of Domestic Animals, 8th ed, Editor MJ Swenson, Cornell University Press, Ithaca, NY, (1970).

137. Smith TW, Braunwald E: The management of heart failure. In Heart Disease, 2nd ed, Editor E Braunwald, WB Saunders Co, Philadelphia, PA (1984).

138. Soderberg SF, Boon JA, Wingfield WE, Miller CW: M-mode echocardiography as a diagnostic aid for feline cardiomyopathy. Vet Radiol J 24:66-73 (1983).

139. Szatalowicz VL, Arnold PE, Chaimovitz C, et al: Radioimmunoassay of plasma arginine vasopressin in hyponatremic patients with congestive heart failure. New Engl J Med 305: 263 (1981).

140. Teske RH, Bishop SP, Righter HF, et al: Subacute digoxin toxicosis in the Beagle dog. Toxicol Appl Pharmacol 35:283 (1976).

141. Thomas WP: Low sodium diets. In Current Veterinary Therapy VI, Editor RW Kirk, WB Saunders Co, Philadelphia, PA (1977).

142. Thomas WP: Pericardial disease. In Textbook of Veterinary Internal Medicine, 2nd edition, Editor SJ Ettinger, WB Saunders Co, Philadelphia, PA (1983).

143. Tilley LP: Feline cardiomyopathy. In Current Veterinary Therapy VI, Editor RW Kirk, WB Saunders Co, Philadelphia, PA (1977).

144. Tilley LP, Weitz J: Pharmacologic and other therapy in cardiac disease. Vet Clin of N Amer 7:415-428 (1977).

145. Vandongen R, Gorden RD: Plasma renin in congestive heart failure in man. Med J Aust I:215 (1970).

146. Wallace, CR: Chronic congestive heart failure, In Current Veterinary Therapy II, Editor RW Kirk, WB Saunders Co, Philadelphia, PA (1966).

147. Watkins L, Burton JA, Haber E, et al: The renin-angiotensin-aldosterone system in congestive failure in conscious dogs. J Clin Invest 57:1601 (1976).

148. White CW: Reversibility of abnormal arterial baroflex control of heart rate in heart failure. Amer J Physiol 241 (Heart Circ Physiol 10):H778 (1981).

149. Wikman-Coffelt J, Parmley WW, Mason DT: The cardiac hypertrophy process:Analyses of factors determining pathological vs. physiological development. In Brief Review from Circ Res 1980. Amer Hosp Assoc Monograph, 69:51 (1980).

150. Wingfield WE, Boon J, Miller CW: Echocardiographic assessment of mitral valve motion, cardiac structures, and ventricular function in dogs with atrial fibrillation. J Amer Vet Med Assoc 181:46-49 (1982).

151. Yamaguchi RA, Pipers FS, Gamble DA: Echocardiographic evaluation of a cat with bacterial vegetative endocarditis. J Amer Vet Med Assoc 183:118-120 (1983).

152. Yamahara H, et al: Echocardiography in ten dogs with mitral insufficiency. J Japan Vet Med Assoc 31:641-647 (1978).

153. Zucker IH, Earle AM, Gilmore JP: The mechanism of adaptation of left atrial stretch receptors in dogs with chronic heart failure. J Clin Invest 60:323 (1977).

154. Zucker IH, Share L, Gilmore JP: Renal effects of left atrial distention in dogs wth chronic congestive heart failure. Amer J Physiol 236:H554 (1979).

CHAPTER 12

Skeletal and Neuromuscular Diseases*

CONTENTS

---

*Written by **Francis A. Kallfelz,** DVM, Ph.D., Prof. of Clinical Nutrition, Dept. of Clinical Sciences, N.Y.S. College of Veterinary Medicine, Cornell University, Ithaca, NY 14853.

SUMMARY OF MANAGEMENT RECOMMENDATIONS

SKELETAL DISEASES

1. If possible, determine if a nutritional imbalance is causing the skeletal disease observed. The diet history, clinical signs, radiographic changes, and alterations from normal in plasma calcium, phosphorus and alkaline phosphatase values given in Table 2 (page 12-7) may be helpful.
2. For either deficiencies or excesses feed a nutritionally adequate commercially prepared growth diet (see pages 3-12 and 4-10) in amounts that prevent excessive growth rate (see page 3-13). Do not feed animals free choice that are experiencing diet related skeletal diseases.
3. If a well balanced growth diet is being fed, and skeletal diseases occur, reduce food intake by 25%.
4. Do not give vitamin or mineral supplements, particularly calcium, phosphorus, vitamin D, or vitamin A. If a nutritionally adequate growth diet is being fed, supplementation is contraindicated.
5. Provide appropriate therapy for specific problems, such as pathologic fractures. If bone demineralization has occurred, remineralization will require several weeks or months, so fracture repair will occur more slowly than in a normal adult animal.

NEUROMUSCULAR DISEASES

1. Puerperal Tetany
   a) Generally occurs in small breeds of dogs two to three weeks after parturition.
   b) Clinical signs are restlessness, nervousness, and panting progressing to ataxia, trembling, muscle tetany, convulsions, and fever.
   c) Give a calcium solution such as 20% calcium borogluconate intravenously to effect over 10-15 minutes. About 1 ml/kg is usually required. Apply cold water or ice to combat fever.
   d) Remove young for at least 24 hours. Feed them solid food and wean entirely, if possible.
   e) Be prepared to wean subsequent litters early. During lactation in bitches having a history of eclampsia, feed a diet containing at least 1.4% calcium in the dry matter. Calcium supplementation during gestation is contraindicated.

2. Steatitis or Yellow Fat Disease in Cats
   a) Generally associated with consumption of a diet high in fish content.
   b) Clinical signs are anorexia, pyrexia, pain over the thorax and abdomen, neutrophilia and subcutaneous nodules.
   c) Give orally 10-20 mg of vitamin E twice daily for five to seven days.
   d) Feed a nutritionally balanced commercially prepared diet.

3. Thiamine Deficiency
   a) Generally occurs in cats. The causes are heat destruction of thiamine in the diet, eating raw fish containing thiaminase or raw meat low in thiamine.
   b) Clinical signs are anorexia and ataxia. Ataxia progresses to clonic convulsions and recumbency with ventral flexion of the head when the animal is suspended by the rear legs.
   c) Give parenterally 100-250 mg of thiamine twice daily for several days.
   d) Feed a nutritionally balanced commercially prepared ration.

INTRODUCTION

Diseases related to the skeletal and the neuromuscular systems are relatively common in veterinary medicine. Many such diseases are not related to nutrition. Included are such abnormalities as traumatic fractures and dislocations, primary and metastatic bone tumors, neuritis, encephalitis, and others. However, nutritionally related diseases are still common even though the basic nutritional requirements for minerals and vitamins are well known.[1,2] Many diseases of the skeleton and neuromuscular systems related to nutrition are more common in growing animals, but adults are by no means without risk from these disorders.

In order to assure optimum conditions for skeletal and neuromuscular growth and maintenance, the ration must contain appropriate amounts and ratios of many nutrients, including those providing energy, protein, calcium phosphorus, copper, iodine, vitamins D and A, thiamine, and others. Maximum safe levels as well as minimum requirements must be considered for these nutrients.

The mineral portion of the diet is only a small fraction (5-8%) of the diet dry matter. However, it is extremely important, as a lack of any essential mineral can lead to death of the animal. The mineral fraction of the diet is divided into macrominerals, required in amounts of approximately 0.1-1.0% of diet dry matter each, and trace minerals, which are required in amounts of approximately 0.1-100 ppm

each. For a summary of the requirements and clinical signs of deficiency or excess of minerals, see Table 8, Chapter 1.

CALCIUM AND PHOSPHORUS METABOLISM

CALCIUM METABOLISM

Of the minerals, calcium is required in the greatest amount. The amounts needed in the diets of dogs and cats are shown in Table 1. Calcium is essential in the body for many functions, including bone formation, blood coagulation, muscle contraction, nerve impulse transmission, secretory activity, and membrane activity. The concentration of calcium differs dramatically in various tissues of the body, ranging from 11,000 mEq/kg in bone to 0.001 mEq/L in the cytoplasmic fluid of most cells.

The calcium content of food ingredients vary widely (Appendix Table 4). Bone, dairy products, and leguminous plants contain large amounts of calcium, whereas most cereal grains, meat, and organ tissues contain small amounts. Many foods that are low in calcium content contain significant amounts of phosphorus; most food ingredients containing significant amounts of calcium also have high amounts of phosphorus. Thus, providing the desired Ca:P ratio of 1:1 to 2:1 in the diet can be a problem unless the proper minerals are added.

Calcium is absorbed almost entirely in the small intestine by a combination of active transport and diffusion processes.[49] Although the efficiency of absorption is greatest in the duodenum, most of the calcium is absorbed from the ileum where the ingesta resides for a longer time due to its longer length.[44] Several factors control calcium absorption. The most important of these factors is the circulatory level of 1,25 dihydroxycholecalciferol [1,25(OH)$_2$D], the active metabolite of vitamin D.[17] This metabolite increases calcium absorption by a number of mechanisms including stimulation of intestinal synthesis of a calcium binding protein which is involved in the transport mechanism for calcium.[48] It may also alter membrane structure in a way that increases calcium absorption.[33]

Other factors, such as increased acidity of the ingesta, which increases absorption, and the presence of binding agents such as phytate and oxalate, which reduce absorption, also affect calcium absorption. The calcium requirements given in Table 1 take into consideration the variability in availability and absorption of calcium.

After calcium is absorbed it enters the blood. There it exists in three different forms: ionized, complexed (primarily to phosphate), and protein-bound. Unless specified otherwise, the plasma calcium concentration routinely reported by the laboratory includes all three forms. Because of the protein-bound calcium, plasma calcium concentration rises and falls with changes in the plasma protein concentration. Normally about half the plasma calcium is in the ionized form, which is the

FIGURE 1

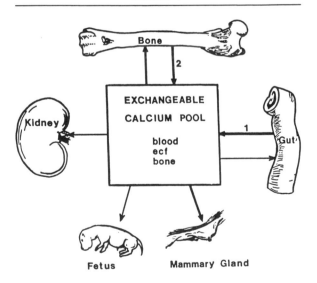

FIG. 1: Pathways of calcium influx to and efflux from the exchangeable calcium pool. Bone contains both exchangeable and unexchangeable (deposited) calcium. Maintenance of normal calcium concentration in the exchangeable calcium pool depends on intestinal absorption (1) and resorption of mineralized bone (2). Magnitude of outflow to the urine, fetus or milk depends on species and physiological state (age, pregnancy, lactation).

TABLE 1

CALCIUM AND PHOSPHORUS REQUIREMENTS OF DOGS AND CATS

	% in Food (DM)*	
	Ca**	P**
Peak Growth and Lactation	1.0–1.8	0.8–1.6
Half-grown and Last Trimester of Pregnancy	0.8–1.5	0.6–1.2
Adult Non-reproducing	0.5–0.9	0.4–0.8

*Assumes 4 kcal/g dry matter (DM).

**Calcium should equal or exceed phosphorus. To convert to an as-fed basis multiply these values times 0.9 for dry food, 0.7 for soft-moist food and 0.25 for canned food.

only biologically active form. The plasma calcium concentration will rise or fall in a way that maintains a normal ionized calcium concentration.[30] Plasma calcium is a major fraction of the exchangeable calcium pool of the body (Figure 1). Inputs to this pool include intestinal absorption and bone resorption. Outputs include bone deposition (accretion), fetal growth, milk production, urinary calcium loss, and small losses back to the intestine from pancreatic and biliary secretions and sloughing of intestinal cells. These various mechanisms of calcium inflow and outflow are closely controlled in order to maintain a normal plasma calcium level. In pathologic states, this control mechanism may fail, resulting in serious disease problems.

PHOSPHORUS METABOLISM

Phosphorus is the other dietary mineral besides calcium required in a relatively high amount in the diet. This element is required at levels only slightly less than those of calcium (Table 1). Phosphorus deficiency is a significant problem in herbivores and is probably the most prevalent mineral nutrition abnormality in animals on a global basis. However, phosphorus deficiency occurs infrequently in dogs and cats, as most of the ingredients used in pet foods contain high amounts of phosphorus (Appendix Table 4). In fact, excessive dietary phosphorus which accelerates the progression of renal failure in dogs and cats by exacerbating osteodystrophy or renal secondary hyperparathyroidism, is a major defect in many commercially prepared canine and feline maintenance diets (see Renal Failure page 8-10).

Phosphorus, like calcium, is involved in many functions in the body. These functions include bone formation, energy metabolism (high energy phosphate bonds), membrane integrity (phosphoproteins and phospholipids), nucleic acid metabolism, and phosphate buffering. However, metabolism of phosphate is not as carefully controlled as is that of calcium; therefore, the concentration of phosphorus in the plasma varies more than that of calcium.

Like calcium, phosphorus is absorbed mainly from the small intestine and is influenced by vitamin D.[50] The chemical form of phosphorus and binding agents in the ingesta can affect its availability. For example, the phytate phosphorus, prevalent in cereals, is poorly available.

Plasma phosphorus exists in both ionized and organic forms. Normally the plasma phosphorus concentration in dogs and cats ranges from 3.5-7.5 mg/dl, being highest following weaning and declining slowly during growth until it reaches the normal adult level. The plasma phosphorus concentration varies slightly with dietary intake, whereas the plasma calcium concentration does not. Plasma phosphorus is a major component of the exchangeable phosphorus pool, and the inflows and outflows for the pool are similar to those of calcium (Figure 1).

CONTROL OF CALCIUM AND PHOSPHORUS METABOLISM

The body has intricate and sophisticated systems for controlling calcium (and secondarily phosphorus) metabolism. Body Ca balance and the maintenance of plasma levels are controlled by interactions between vitamin D, parathyroid hormone and calcitonin. The entire regulatory system is designed first and foremost to maintain the plasma Ca levels which are critical for the life and function of the animal on a moment to moment basis. This regulatory system is shown in Figure 2.

Parathyroid Hormone

Parathyroid hormone is a polypeptide hormone containing 84 amino acids. The n-terminal 33 amino acid peptide is the active metabolite.[21] It is synthesized in the four parathyroid glands. In dogs and cats they occur in two pairs, one of which is associated with each thyroid lobe. The secretion of PTH is controlled by, and is inversely related to, the ionized plasma calcium concentration ($[Ca++]p$). Thus, secretion of PTH is maximal at low $[Ca++]p$ and minimal (but still present) at high $[Ca++]p$.[4] The major effects of PTH are on calcium metabolism by bone and kidney, but it also secondarily affects intestinal calcium absorption.

Parathyroid hormone increases the activity and numbers of osteoclasts. The result is increased bone resorption and the release of calcium, phosphorus, and magnesium into the circulation. Thus, when the $[Ca++]p$ falls slightly, PTH secretion increases. This results in bone resorption, a return of the $[Ca++]p$ to normal, and a subsequent reduction in PTH secretion.

Parathyroid hormone exerts several effects on the kidney tubule. A primary response is inhibition of renal tubular phosphate resorption, resulting in greater loss of urinary phosphate.[11] This lessens or prevents an increase in the plasma phosphorus concentration which would otherwise occur as a result of PTH-induced bone resorption and, therefore, allows a specific rise in the $[Ca++]p$. Parathyroid hormone also increases tubular reabsorption of calcium to aid in normalizing $[Ca++]p$. However, since very little calcium is excreted in the urine of dogs and cats under normal circumstances, this

FIGURE 2

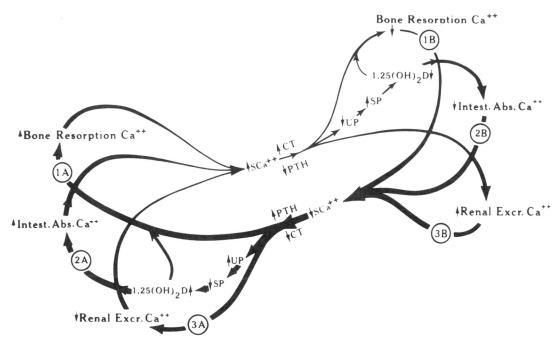

FIG. 2: The model consists of three overlapping control loops (negative feedback) that interlock and relate to one another through the level of blood concentrations of ionic calcium, parathyroid hormone, and calcitonin. The loops are numbered 1, 2, and 3; the limbs of the three loops that describe physiological events that increase blood concentrations of calcium are designated "A" (left) and the limbs that describe events that decrease blood concentrations of calcium are designated "B" (right). Thus, loop 1 represents bone resorption; limb 1A increased bone resorption; and limb 1B decreased bone resorption. Loop 2 represents intestinal absorption of calcium; limb 2A increased; and limb 2B decreased absorption. And loop 3 represents renal excretion of calcium; limb 3A decreased; and limb 3B increased excretion.

Abbreviations used: SCa^{++} = serum ionized Ca concentration; CT = calcitonin; UP = Urine P excretion; SP = serum phosphorus concentration. Reprinted courtesy of Arnaud, C.D., Fed. Proc., *37*, 2557–2560, 1978.

action of PTH has little effect in these species.

A third action of PTH on the kidney is to stimulate the formation of 1,25-dihydroxy chole-calciferol [1,25(OH)$_2$D], the most active metabolite of vitamin D. It is required for the calcium mobilizing action of PTH on bone and is responsible for increasing intestinal absorption of calcium. Thus, PTH indirectly stimulates intestinal absorption of calcium.

Vitamin D

Vitamin D is a steroid derived from cholesterol. The plant form of vitamin D, ergocalciferol or vitamin D$_2$, is truly a vitamin since it is found in foodstuffs and has biologic activity in animals. In contrast, the animal form cholecalciferol or vitamin D$_3$, is actually a hormone because it is produced in the skin by the action of ultraviolet light on 7-dehydrocholesterol.

Vitamin D$_3$ is generally more effective in mammals than is D$_2$. After being formed in the skin,

vitamin D$_3$ is transported to the liver bound to a plasma transport protein. In the liver, a microsomal hydroxylase enzyme converts cholecalciferol to 25-hydroxycholecalciferol [25(OH)D]. The 25(OH)D leaves the liver, again bound to the plasma transport protein. It is carried to the kidney where another hydroxylase converts this intermediate metabolite to the most active metabolite of vitamin D, 1,25(OH)$_2$D. There are many other metabolites of vitamin D, some of which may also have biologic activity.[10]

Several mechanisms control the formation and thus the circulating levels of 1,25(OH)$_2$D. A primary stimulator of renal synthesis is PTH.[43] A low [Ca++]p stimulates PTH secretion which in turn stimulates 1,25(OH)$_2$D production leading to a rise in [Ca++]p via increased intestinal absorption of calcium and increased mobilization of calcium from bone. Hypophosphatemia also stimulates renal synthesis of 1,25(OH)$_2$D.[41] In contrast, when [Ca++]p is normal, PTH level is lowered leading to a

reduction in $1,25(OH)_2D$ production.[18] Elevated $1,25(OH)_2D$ levels stimulate another renal hydroxylase, leading to the formation of $24,25(OH)_2D$ from $25(OH)D$ and thus decreasing $1,25(OH)_2D$ level.[42]

A primary site of action of $1,25(OH)_2D$ is the intestinal mucosal cells where it stimulates calcium absorption by several mechanisms. The second important site of action of $1,25(OH)_2D$ is bone, where it functions in concert with PTH to stimulate mobilization of calcium through bone resorption.[19] The increased blood calcium and phosphorus levels that occur as a result of vitamin D allow mineralization of osteoid to continue, thus preventing or curing rickets. Although $1,25(OH)_2D$ has been isolated from several other tissues in addition to intestine, kidney, and bone, its function in these other tissues is unknown.[40]

Calcitonin

Calcitonin (CT) is a polypeptide hormone containing 32 amino acids. It is produced in the parafollicular cells of the thyroid gland. The function of CT is to reduce $[Ca++]p$. Hypercalcemia is the primary stimulus for CT secretion, but hormones such as gastrin also stimulate CT secretion.

The primary effect of CT is on bone, where it reduces osteoclastic activity, thus decreasing calcium mobilization and $[Ca++]p$.[16] It also has minor effects on the intestine and kidney, where it influences calcium absorption and excretion, but does not directly affect vitamin D metabolism. Under normal circumstances, the actions of PTH and $1,25(OH)_2D$ adequately control $[Ca++]p$. CT may, however, play a physiologic role during growth, pregnancy, and lactation.

Thus, calcium homeostasis is under tight control. While $1,25(OH)_2D$ is the primary "effector" in this system, PTH is the primary "controller." CT is of lesser importance. Of course, for adequate control of calcium and phosphorus metabolism, adequate amounts of all elements in the system must be present. This includes calcium, phosphorus, vitamin D, PTH, and CT. When deficiencies or excesses of any of these substances occur, abnormal metabolism (disease) may result.

BONE TURNOVER

Mature bone contains 25% water, 45% ash, and 30% organic material. Approximately 96% of the organic matrix of bone is collagen, a fibrillar-type protein. The collagen microfibrils become chemically cross-linked to form collagen fibers. This cross-linking, which requires copper, provides the strength of collagen.

There are three types of bone cells: osteoblasts, osteocytes, and osteoclasts. Osteoblasts are located in areas where bone is being formed (periosteum, epiphyseal plate, etc.). Their main function is to produce collagen or bone matrix (osteoid). Under appropriate conditions, which include adequate calcium and phosphorus concentrations in the fluid phase, the matrix becomes calcified producing bone.[12] The actual mineralization process does not directly require vitamin D or PTH; however, their action is needed to ensure that the circulating concentrations of calcium and phosphorus are sufficient to allow mineralization.

As bone matrix is formed and becomes calcified, the osteoblasts become trapped and change their functional characteristics. These altered osteoblasts become the osteocytes which are responsible for maintaining bone.[32] Although there have been suggestions that osteocytes also can be involved in bone resorption (osteocytic osteolysis),[6] their significance in bone turnover is probably limited.[31]

Osteoclasts, which arise from the mononuclear-phagocytic cell system, are the main cells involved in bone resorption. They develop a modified cell membrane in areas of bone contact called a "ruffled border." This border enlarges under PTH stimulation and is thought to be intimately involved in bone resorption, including removal of both the mineral and organic phases.[9] The presence of both PTH and $1,25(OH)_2D$ is needed for bone resorption.

SKELETAL DISEASES

Nutritional abnormalities can be responsible for skeletal disease involving either the mineral or organic phases of bone, or both. Usually both phases are involved, as bone resorption requires simultaneous removal of both mineral and organic components. A classic example of nutritional bone disease is "rickets." Rickets is a general term for the epiphyseal enlargement and bending of long bones (humerus, femur, ribs). It can result from vitamin D, calcium, or phosphorus deficiency. Histologically, rickets is characterized by the presence of unmineralized osteoid in regions of bone formation, i.e. insufficient mineralization.

For convenience, metabolic bone disease may be classified in the following manner:

1. Too little bone due to
    a. inadequate matrix production, resulting in osteoporosis,
    b. insufficient osteoid mineralization, which produces
        1) rickets in growing animals, and
        2) osteomalacia in adults.

TABLE 2

DIET INDUCED SKELETAL DISEASES — CAUSES AND EFFECTS

Nutritional Imbalance	Diet History	Plasma*			Radiographic Changes	Clinical Signs
		Ca	P	AP		
Ca deficiency	Meat or organ tissues.	N	N	↑	Fractures, bone demineralization, loss of lamina dura dentes.	Sudden paralysis, can't rise, alert and eating normally.
Vit D deficiency	Homemade or poor, high-cereal prepared ration.	↓	N	↑	Same as Ca def. but less severe; fibrous osteodystrophy.	Same as Ca deficiency.
P deficiency	Homemade or poor commercial ration high in vegetables.	N	↓	↓	Decreased bone density, but lamina dura dentes not lost.	Same as Ca def. but slower developing.
Ca excess	Overfeeding a prepared diet high in Ca, or oversupplementation.	N	N	↓	Increased cortical bone density.	Hip dysplasia, OCD, wobblers or hypertrophic osteodystrophy.
Vit D toxicity	Oversupplementation.	↑**	N	N	Dystrophic calcification of soft tissues.	Weakness, joint pain, stiffness.
Vit A toxicity	Liver diet or vit A supplementation.	N	N	N	Exostosis, esp. of cervical vertebrae and ends of long bones.	Lameness, esp. posterior, cutaneous hyper- or hyposensitivity.

*Plasma calcium and phosphorus concentrations or alkaline phosphatase activity. N = normal, ↑ = increased, and ↓ decreased.

**Reduced several days following administration of 5–10 mg/day of prednisone, whereas it is not reduced with other causes of hypercalcemia.

c. excessive mineral resorption, resulting in fibrous osteodystrophy.

2. Too much bone, termed osteopetrosis, is due to excessive mineralization with insufficient resorption.[25]

The major nutritional imbalances responsible for causing skeletal diseases, the diets responsible, clinical signs, and factors useful in their diagnosis are given in Table 2.

SKELETAL DISEASES DUE TO NUTRITIONAL DEFICIENCIES

Calcium Deficiency

Historically, one of the more common nutritional deficiencies in young dogs and cats is calcium deficiency or nutritional secondary hyperparathyroidism (NSHP). This syndrome, still seen clinically, is usually caused by feeding a high meat or organ tissue diet. Meat and organ tissues contain an insufficient amount of calcium but an adequate amount of phosphorus (Appendix Table 4).

The lack of available calcium reduces the plasma calcium concentration enough that the ion-product of calcium and phosphorus is reduced to the point that bone mineralization ceases. If nutrition otherwise is normal, bone matrix continues to form but is not mineralized. Concurrently, the hypocalcemia results in release of PTH. The elevated levels of PTH cause increased production of 1,25(OH)$_2$D, which stimulates intestinal calcium and phosphorus absorption, and in association with PTH, induces resorption of bone. Both of these actions tend to raise the plasma calcium concentration. Because of the continuing lack of dietary calcium, however, bone resorption is the major factor in restoring the concentration of calcium in the plasma. Since bone mineralization is compromised, the resorbed bone is replaced by fibrous connective tissue, resulting in fibrous osteodystrophy.[26]

Clinically, the animal appears normal until the bone is weakened to the point that pathologic fractures occur. These most often are compression fractures of the vertebrae or folding fractures of the femur. The patient suddenly shows signs of paralysis, is down and unable to rise but continues to be alert and to eat (Figure 3).

Radiographs reveal thin and poorly mineralized (radiolucent) cortical bone (Figure 4) and a loss of the lamina dura dentes. Plasma calcium and phosphorus concentrations are usually normal, but

FIGURE 3

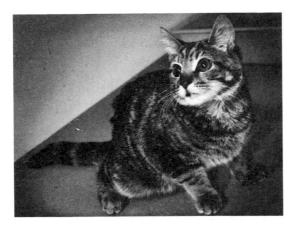

FIG. 3: Young cat with calcium deficiency induced nutritional secondary hyperparathyroidism. This patient had been fed from weaning a diet of hamburger and egg. It was presented because of inability to stand on the rear legs.

FIGURE 4

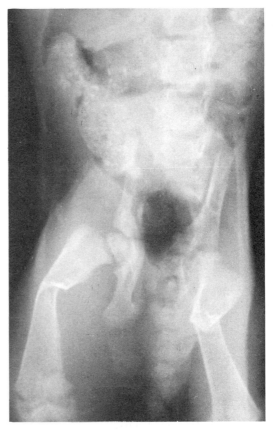

FIG. 4: Radiography of patient shown in Fig. 3. Note radiolucency of bones, thinness of cortices and folding fractures of femurs with lack of callous formation.

the alkaline phosphatase is elevated. Serum immunoreactive PTH (iPTH) is significantly elevated. This assay is not readily available, but it is not required for the routine diagnosis of NSHP, which is based on clinical and radiographic changes and diet history. Treatment is the feeding of a nutritionally balanced, commercially prepared growth ration (pages 3-12 and 4-10). Calcium and vitamin D supplementation should be avoided, thereby preventing improper dietary mineral ratios and delaying bone mineralization. Fractures should be repaired using techniques that provide full support, because the bones will remain weakened for several weeks.[27] Fractures have been shown to heal and bone to remineralize when the patient is provided a balanced-growth diet, thus the prognosis is good.[27] However, severe neurologic damage secondary to pathologic fractures may occur and dramatically worsen the prognosis.

Vitamin D Deficiency

Vitamin D deficiency in dogs and cats is rare. Almost all commercially prepared pet foods and foods for human beings contain adequate levels. The pathogenesis and clinical signs of vitamin D deficiency are almost identical to those of calcium deficiency; both result in an initial hypocalcemia. However, since $1,25(OH)_2D$ is needed for both intestinal calcium absorption and bone resorption, a detectable hypocalcemia can persist in vitamin D deficiency. In contrast, with calcium deficiency, resorption tends to maintain a normal plasma calcium concentration. Also, since $1,25(OH)_2D$ needed for bone resorption is lacking, fibrous osteodystrophy is not as dramatic in vitamin D deficiency as it is in calcium deficiency. Diagnosis of vitamin D deficiency requires a careful diet history in addition to clinical findings. Treatment consists of feeding a balanced growth diet (see pages 3-12 and 4-10) without vitamin D supplementation, or vitamin D supplementation at not more than 500 IU/kg of diet or 10-20 IU/kg of body weight daily.[1] Additional amounts may result in vitamin D toxicity. The prognosis in vitamin D deficiency is similar to that in calcium deficiency.

Phosphorus Deficiency

Phosphorus deficiency is a significant problem in herbivores, but it is rare in dogs and cats because the ingredients used in pet foods contain adequate or even excessive amounts of phosphorus. The usual circumstance leading to phosphorus deficiency is

when a large quantity of a calcium supplement not containing phosphorus, such as calcium carbonate or limestone, is added to a high cereal diet that contains a high percentage of its phosphorus in the form of phytin. The resulting Ca:P ratio may exceed 10:1. Under such circumstances the large amount of calcium present can prevent intestinal absorption of the small amount of available phosphorus. The clinical signs observed are similar to those with calcium or vitamin D deficiency, but the progression of the changes is much slower. Plasma calcium concentration remains normal, so PTH secretion is not stimulated, thus excessive bone resorption and fibrous osteodystrophy do not occur. The primary histologic abnormality is unmineralized osteoid (rickets). Phosphorus deficiency is, in fact, the only condition in which pure rickets is observed.

There is no homeostatic mechanism to restore normality as there is with calcium, thus hypophosphatemia occurs. Radiographically, bone density lessens due to normal resorption but reduced mineralization. However, the lamina dura dentes do not disappear as they do with a calcium or vitamin D deficiency. Diagnosis is based on these findings and dietary history. Treatment consists of feeding a balanced, commercially prepared growth diet (see pages 3-12 and 4-10) without supplementation of any type, and to provide supportive therapy for any secondary problems. The prognosis is good.

Other Deficiency Induced Skeletal Diseases

Calcium, phosphorus, and vitamin D are the major nutritional deficiencies that cause skeletal disease. However, deficiencies of several other nutrients have either been shown to cause, or are suspected of causing, skeletal disease. These nutrients include vitamins A and C, copper, iodine and protein.

Vitamin A deficiency results in significant abnormalities of reproduction, epithelial surfaces, vision, and skeletal development in growing animals. The skeletal abnormalities are related to a retardation of bone growth and perhaps a reduction in endosteal bone resorption.[22] The result is a shortening and thickening of the long bones and abnormal development of the skull. Primary manifestations are neurologic in character due to pinching of cranial and spinal nerves as they pass through foramina and to herniation of the brain.

Almost all commercially prepared pet foods are supplemented with adequate levels of vitamin A. Additionally, most animal species can produce vitamin A from its precursor, beta-carotene, which is present in corn and is a very common ingredient in pet foods. The cat is the exception and has an absolute dietary requirement for vitamin A.

Vitamin C (ascorbic acid) is an essential dietary nutrient for normal skeletal growth and metabolism in several species including guinea pigs, human beings, and other primates. Dogs and cats synthesize adequate amounts of ascorbic acid in the liver, therefore, it is not required in their diets.[24] Vitamin C deficiency has been suggested as a causative factor in canine hypertrophic osteodystrophy (HOD) and hip dysplasia.[7,29] However, there have been no controlled studies that confirm a role for vitamin C in the cause or treatment of these conditions, and evidence derived from experiments suggests that vitamin C supplementation is of no value prophylactically and may, in fact, increase the probability of skeletal disease development.[45]

Copper is an essential nutrient affecting bone. It is an essential cofactor for activity of the enzyme lysyl oxidase. This enzyme is essential for normal cross-linking of collagen fibers in forming of bone matrix or osteoid. Copper deficiency is thus associated with abnormalities of osteoid formation which results in deformities of the ends of long bones and pathologic fractures.

Iodine deficiency can result in bony changes due to its involvement with thyroxine, which is required for normal growth of the skeleton. The lesions produced are related to retarded growth at epiphyseal plates and delayed closure of plates and sutures. Protein and energy deficiencies can also produce similar lesions.

SKELETAL DISEASES DUE TO NUTRITIONAL EXCESSES

Historically, the science of nutrition has been concerned with ascertaining the number of essential nutrients and the minimum daily intake of these nutrients needed to prevent deficiency disease. Only recently have veterinary nutritionists realized that excessive intake of essential nutrients may also result in disease. Therefore, the concept of "recommended daily allowance" or "optimal dietary level" is gradually replacing the older idea of "minimum daily requirement."

Calcium Excess

Overfeeding of calcium has been implicated as a cause of skeletal disease in growing dogs of large breeds.[23] The diets of such dogs are often supplemented with calcium because pet owners are concerned that the basic diet may not contain enough calcium to support the rapid growth of these big dogs. This is done despite the fact that most commercially prepared pet foods, especially dry dog

foods, contain several times the required amount of calcium.

In this situation it has been hypothesized that a chronic excessive level of circulating calcitonin, secreted in response to a persistent relative hypercalcemia, results in altered bone turnover and initiation of skeletal disease.[23] The main action of calcitonin is to decrease bone resorption and thus reduce the blood calcium level. Chronic suppression of bone resorption, both at endosteal surfaces and in resorption cavities, results in a gradual thickening and increased density of cortical bone (osteopetrosis) (Figure 5). In growing animals, retarded resorption interferes with normal structural remodeling and may lead to abnormal morphology of bony structures such as the acetabulum, femoral head and neck, vertebral canal, etc. This sequence of events has been hypothesized to be involved in such conditions as hip dysplasia and the wobbler syndrome.

There is also evidence that excessive calcium intake and subsequent hypercalcitoninism may result in retarded maturation of articular cartilage,

with subsequent detachment resulting in osteochondrosis dissecans[23] (Figure 6). Similarly, it has been suggested that hypercalcitoninism may result in excessive sub-periosteal bone deposition causing clinical signs of hypertrophic osteodystrophy.[23]

Unlike calcium deficiency, calcium excess presents clinical signs that may be quite variable. Hip dysplasia, osteochondrosis dissecans, wobbler syndrome or hypertrophic osteodystrophy may occur. Diagnosis of dietary calcium excess is based on clinical signs of one of the suspected related problems and a diet history revealing feeding of a diet high in calcium or chronic calcium supplementation. In calcium excess, the plasma calcium concentration is normal but the alkaline phosphatase value may be low suggesting decreased bone turnover. Unfortunately, no valid assay is available for measuring calcitonin concentration in dogs.

Treatment of these conditions requires reduction of the calcium intake and initiation of recommended therapy for specific individual problems. Calcium excess may be a major factor, but the diets used in experimental studies as well as those frequently used as growth diets by breeders, often contain much higher than recommended levels of many other nutrients such as energy, protein, vitamins A and D, and phosphorus. Therefore, it is recommended that the entire feeding program be evaluated to be sure that the diet provides, but does not greatly exceed, the recommended nutrient requirements for growth (see pages 3-12 or 4-10 and that it is fed properly (page 3-13).

The prognosis is poor because the skeletal changes associated with overfeeding of calcium usually are

FIGURE 5

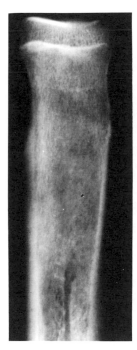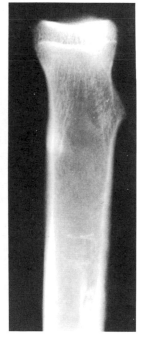

FIG. 5: Radiograph of proximal radius from a growing Great Dane that was overfed (left) compared to a control dog (right). Note thickness of cortices, roughness of periosteal and endosteal surfaces and persistence of trabeculae in affected dog compared to control. (Reproduced courtesy of The Cornell Veterinarian)

FIGURE 6

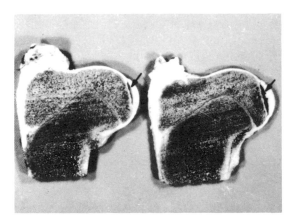

FIG. 6: Osteochondrosis dissecans on heads of left and right humerus from a growing Great Dane puppy that suffered from excessive calcium intake. (Reproduced courtesy of The Cornell Veterinarian)

irreversible. Because of the poor prognosis, the goal should be prevention. This can be accomplished by feeding the growing dog as described beginning on page 3-13. Only good quality nutritionally balanced diets, which have been biologically tested and proven to be adequate for growth, should be fed. Diets high in protein, fat, and minerals should be avoided. Mineral and vitamin supplements are contraindicated unless a diet made from individual food ingredients is being fed and specific needs for these supplements have been demonstrated.

Vitamin D Toxicity

In addition to supplementation with minerals, many owners and breeders supplement the diets of growing animals with vitamin D. Although normal levels of vitamin D can be controlled physiologically, a large amount of this vitamin/hormone can overwhelm the regulatory mechanisms. There is no control of 25(OH)D production, and this metabolite, which can be present at high levels with excessive vitamin D intake, has actions similar to those of 1,25(OH)$_2$D, described previously. The margin of safety for water-soluble vitamins, where excesses are excreted in the urine, is very large. Such is not the case with fat-soluble vitamins, particularly A and D. Dosages of 50-100 times the minimum daily requirement may do harm when given daily for several weeks or months. These dosages may, at first glance, appear to have a wide margin of safety. However, the amount of vitamin D in some nutritional supplements can result in doses of several thousand units per day, as compared to the minimum daily requirement of only 10-20 IU/kg of body weight.

The clinical signs of vitamin D toxicity are related to the hypercalcemia it induces. These signs include weakness, joint pain, and stiffness. Prolonged hypercalcemia results in dystrophic calcification of soft tissues particularly the kidney, lungs, large blood vessels, joints, and intestinal tract. This calcification can lead to dysfunction in these tissues and organ systems.

Diagnosis of vitamin D toxicity is based on the clinical signs, a history of long-term ingestion of a large amount of vitamin D, and differentiation from other causes of hypercalcemia such as hyperparathyroidism and pseudohyperparathyroidism. The cortisone suppression test may help in this regard. Daily administration of 5-10 mg of prednisone (or equivalent) for several days will usually significantly reduce hypercalcemia due to vitamin D toxicity, but will not affect hypercalcemia resulting from the hyperparathyroid states.

Treatment of vitamin D toxicity requires removal of the source of the excessive vitamin. Because vitamin D is stored in the liver, complete removal of vitamin D from the diet may be required until the amount in the liver is reduced. Cortisone therapy during this time may help control the hypercalcemia. The prognosis is guarded, the resolution of soft-tissue calcification will be slow and probably incomplete.

Vitamin A Toxicity

Excessive supplementation with vitamin A can also cause skeletal abnormalities. The classical syndrome occurring as a result of vitamin A toxicity is deforming cervical spondylosis of the adult cat.[36,46] The disease most often is associated with feeding large amounts of liver, but can occur with vitamin A supplementation such as daily administration of cod liver oil (which can contain more than 5000 IU of vitamin A/tsp). In cats administration of 100,000 IU of vitamin A/day for six months induces the disease.[36] This dosage is about 100 times the recommended daily requirement.[2]

The clinical signs of vitamin A toxicosis include postural changes (affected cats assume a marsupial-like position while sitting with the front feet raised), lameness, and cutaneous hyper- and/or hyposensitivity. Radiographs reveal new bone formation in association with cervical vertebrae and possible new periosteal bone formation in the long bones of the forelegs. Large amounts of vitamin A inhibit both intramembranous and endochondral ossification, resulting in dystrophic calcification without measurable hypercalcemia.[37]

Treatment consists of removing the source of the excessive vitamin A from the diet, and supportive therapy. As with vitamin D toxicity, the prognosis is guarded because complete resolution of the pathologic changes is doubtful.

NEUROMUSCULAR DISEASES

PUERPERAL TETANY (ECLAMPSIA)

In addition to effects on the skeleton, abnormalities in mineral nutrition may also be involved in neuromuscular and other diseases. Calcium stabilizes nerve and muscle cell membranes against continuous depolarization. In the absence of adequate extracellular calcium and magnesium, these membranes become hyperexcitable, and tetany can occur.

A primary example of this phenomenon is puerperal tetany or "eclampsia."[3,8] This disease affects both bitches and queens of all breeds, but occurs

primarily in small breeds of dogs two to three weeks after parturition. The cause is an inability of the calcium regulatory system to compensate for the loss of calcium in the milk. As a result, the plasma calcium and (frequently) magnesium concentrations fall, and tetany occurs.

Before tetany develops, restlessness, nervousness, and panting occur. If the problem is not recognized at this time, signs become more severe, progressing to ataxia, trembling, muscular tetany, and within 8-12 hours, convulsive seizures. As a result of the uncontrolled and continuous muscular activity, affected patients become hyperthermic. The body temperature can rise to as high as 41°C (106°F) or more. To survive, patients in advanced stages of the syndrome must be treated promptly.

The plasma calcium concentration of affected bitches or queens will be less than 7 mg/dl. Treatment is intravenous administration of calcium to effect. Generally it requires about 1 ml/kg of a 20% solution of calcium borogluconate which must be given slowly to prevent cardiac arrest. With calcium administration the amplitude of the heart sounds increase and the heart rate decreases. If the heart rate begins to increase or arrhythmias occur, calcium administration must stop immediately. Clinical signs of eclampsia usually cease within 15-30 minutes. Nursing puppies or kittens should be removed from the dam for at least 24 hours after clinical signs appear. The infants may be gradually returned to the dam thereafter; if possible, weaning or supplementation of the young with a milk replacer or solid food is recommended (see page 3-18). For bitches with a history of eclampsia, plan to wean subsequent litters early and make certain the diet fed during lactation contains at least 1.4% calcium in the dry matter. Checking the calcium content of the diet fed the bitch during lactation is particularly important if the animal is consuming a diet composed of foods for human consumption, a diet heavily supplemented with meat or organ tissues or a meat-type canned dog food.

A similar parturient hypocalcemic syndrome called "milk fever" occurs in cows. In the bovine species large amounts of dietary calcium during late pregnancy **increase** the incidence of this disorder. The relative hypercalcemia caused by excessive calcium intake during gestation alters the calcium-regulating system in a way that bone and intestine cannot adapt to the sudden drain of calcium into milk when lactation begins. Specific corollaries have not been demonstrated in puerperal tetany in bitches or queens. However, based on information derived from cattle, it is reasonable to recommend avoiding high levels of dietary calcium during pregnancy. Feeding a commercially prepared diet,

FIGURE 7

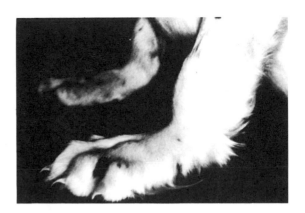

FIG. 7: Photograph of front feet of a growing puppy on a magnesium deficient diet. Note overextension of carpo-metacarpal joint. (Reproduced courtesy of Ralston Purina)

proven to be nutritionally adequate for reproduction (page 2-20) and fed in sufficient amounts (see pages 3-7 and 4-7), will adequately support nutrient needs of the bitch or queen during gestation. Prophylactic supplementation with minerals and vitamins should be avoided; instead, the young should be encouraged to begin eating solid food at the youngest age possible (see pages 3-12 and 4-10).

MAGNESIUM DEFICIENCY

Magnesium deficiency results in neuromuscular abnormalities. Although this deficiency is exceptionally rare, it may occur when homemade diets are fed.

Initial signs of magnesium deficiency are anorexia and weight loss followed by muscular weakness. The muscular weakness progresses to a laxity in tone, particularly in the legs. The result is such overextension that the affected animal rests on the carpus with the foot extended (Figure 7).[13] With prolonged magnesium deficiency, animals may exhibit convulsive behavior similar to that seen in puerperal tetany if serum levels are less than 1 mg/dl.

The condition can be reversed rapidly by changing the diet to a nutritionally complete, growth ration. Tetanic seizures can be treated with calcium borogluconate as in puerperal tetany (see page 12-12). It will not recur after magnesium status has been normalized.

SELENIUM/VITAMIN E DEFICIENCY

Neuromuscular diseases resulting from selenium deficiency, vitamin E deficiency, or both, are well known in veterinary medicine. They occur often in many food animals.[35] Such problems are uncommon in dogs and cats; however, there are a few circumstances in which they may occur. The most familiar of these is steatitis or "yellow fat disease" in cats.[15] Although not specifically a disorder of the neuromuscular system, this disease is associated with clinical signs that resemble those of a neuromuscular disorder.

Steatitis was first seen as a clinical problem in cats fed commercially prepared diets containing large quantities of fish.[14] The clinical signs include anorexia, lethargy, pyrexia, and evidence of tenderness and pain in the thorax and abdomen when palpated. Palpation often reveals many small nodules (ceroid deposits) in the subcutaneous tissues. The subcutaneous tissues of the thorax and abdomen may appear mottled on radiographs.

Affected animals usually have a significantly elevated neutrophil count with a left shift. Diagnosis can be confirmed with a biopsy of subcutaneous fat, which is yellow and may contain small brownish nodules. Histologically, fat-cell necrosis and significant neutrophilic infiltration are evident.[20]

This disease has been shown to be caused by vitamin E deficiency. The natural vitamin E in fish-based rations may be scant or destroyed by oxidation of unsaturated fats. Ingestion of large amounts of unsaturated fat without sufficient dietary antioxidant leads to peroxidation of depot fat with subsequent fat necrosis.[20]

Most commercially prepared cat foods contain added vitamin E or other antioxidants. Thus, the incidence of the condition has dropped dramatically. However, it still occurs occasionally, particularly when home-prepared diets incorporating a high proportion of tuna fish are fed.

Treatment of steatitis includes an oral dose of 10-20 mg of alpha tocopherol acetate twice daily for five to seven days. Corticosteroids may be valuable in reducing inflammation and pain. Fish products should be removed from the diet and replaced by a nutritionally complete cat food. The prognosis is good, but recovery may be slow.

Selenium deficiency has long been recognized as a cause of muscle necrosis (white muscle disease) in young calves and lambs.[35] There are few reports of similar problems in puppies that can be prevented or treated with selenium supplementation.[47] It has been suggested that selenium supplementation may be valuable in the prevention and treatment of hip dysplasia. There is no theoretical reason to explain why selenium supplementation should be beneficial in prophylaxis or therapy of hip dysplasia, and there is no objective evidence to support the use of selenium supplementation for such purposes. Theoretically, selenium deficiency could cause muscle necrosis in dogs as it does in other species. However, based on commonly used ingredients, it is doubtful that any commercially prepared diet would be selenium deficient.

THIAMINE DEFICIENCY

Thiamine (vitamin B-1) is a necessary dietary nutrient for most vertebrates. It functions in the energy metabolism pathway. In the form of thiamine pyrophosphate (formerly known as cocarboxylase), this vitamin is essential for the decarboxylation of alpha keto acids. A primary transformation requiring thiamine is the conversion of pyruvate to acetyl CoA for entry into the Krebs cycle. In thiamine-deficient animals, this reaction is compromised, and blood levels of pyruvate and lactate rise. Energy metabolism is seriously reduced. Because nervous tissue has a high metabolic rate, central nervous system signs occur.

Central nervous system disorders due to thiamine deficiency occur in many animals, including horses and ruminants. In herbivores, it results from consumption of certain plants which contain thiaminase, or secondary to clinical or subclinical gastrointestinal acidosis. The acidosis is induced by a high grain ration due to production of thiaminase by abnormal ruminal flora. In small animals, thiamine deficiency occurs most commonly in cats, but also in dogs.[28,34] It is sometimes referred to as "Chastek paralysis."

Clinical cases of thiamine deficiency in cats have been associated with the feeding of either canned commercial cat foods or raw fish.[28,38] The overprocessing of canned foods destroys a considerable amount of thiamine. This may result in deficiencies in the final product if sufficient thiamine had not been added before canning. Certain fresh fish, particularly carp and herring, have been shown to contain a heat-labile thiaminase.

Anorexia is a prominent initial clinical sign in both cats and dogs. After a few days ataxia with vomiting may occur. The ataxia progresses to clonic convulsions of short duration. Affected animals remain recumbent between convulsive episodes. At

this stage, when suspended by the hind legs the cat shows a characteristic ventro-flexion of the head. Severe mydriasis is also present. Patients who have reached the convulsive stage will usually die within 24 hours if not treated.

Thiamine deficiency leads to hemorrhages in the periventricular gray matter of the brain. Lesions may be found in the inferior colliculi, medial vestibular nuclei, lateral geniculate bodies, and elsewhere. Microscopically, hemorrhage and edema are prominent.

Diagnosis is based primarily on history and clinical signs and, if measured, elevated plasma pyruvate and lactate concentrations. Reduced activity of erythrocyte trans-ketolase (a thiamine-requiring enzyme) is used to confirm the diagnosis, but is not readily available. Treatment with thiamine (100-250 mg by intravenous or subcutaneous administration, twice daily) usually brings about gradual regression of clinical signs, with complete recovery in a few days. Animals with severe neurologic damage may not recover. Therefore, rapid diagnosis and therapy are desirable.

In order to prevent the development of this problem, pet owners should be cautioned to avoid feeding raw fish to cats and should be encouraged to feed only cat foods that have been shown in actual feeding trials (page 2-20) to be nutritionally adequate.

RIBOFLAVIN AND NIACIN DEFICIENCIES

Riboflavin (vitamin B-2) deficiency can result in neurologic signs. Frequently, animals deficient in this vitamin are also deficient in niacin. These two vitamins are important in energy metabolism by functioning as co-factors in the electron transport system as well as in other biosynthetic pathways. Because of the diverse functions of these vitamins, deficiencies result in several abnormalities, including dermatitis, conjunctivitis, enteritis, stomatitis, as well as central nervous system disorders.

In dogs, riboflavin deficiency causes an initial conjunctivitis followed by corneal vascularization (pannus). A flaky dermatitis then ensues. This is accompanied by marked erythema of the hind legs, abdomen, and thorax. In the final stages of the disease, muscular weakness develops and progresses within a few days to ataxia, followed by collapse, coma, and death.[5]

Niacin deficiency alone does not cause as severe central nervous system disorders in dogs as it does in man. Rather, the disease is characterized by severe stomatitis and enteritis. Because of the stomatitis and necrosis the disease was named blacktongue Of historical interest, a veterinarian first reported that blacktongue was indeed the canine form of pellagra.[39] This report led to the use of blacktongue in dogs as a model for the disease in man, resulting in the eventual discovery of niacin deficiency as the cause.

Large amounts of riboflavin and niacin are found in meat and dairy products. Lesser quantities are present in vegetables and fruits. Most animal species except the cat can synthesize sufficient niacin from the amino acid tryptophan. Because ingredients from animal sources are used in almost all commercially prepared pet foods, and most prepared products are also supplemented with riboflavin and niacin, the chance of these deficiencies occurring clinically is very small. The exception is where a nonsupplemented homemade vegetarian diet is being fed, for example, to Dalmatian dogs to prevent urate calculi or "bronzing syndrome" (Chapter 10). If such deficiencies are suspected, therapeutic amounts of B-complex vitamins should be given.

To determine requirements and clinical signs of deficiency or excess of vitamins or minerals, see Tables 11 and 13, Chapter 1.

REFERENCES

1. Anonymous: Nutrient Requirements of Dogs. Publication no. 0-309-03496-5, National Academy of Sciences, National Academy Press, Washington, D.C. (1985).

2. Anonymous: Nutrient Requirements of Cats. Publication no. 0-309-03682-8, National Academy of Sciences, National Academy Press, Washington, D.C. (1986).

3. Austad R, Bjerkas E: Eclampsia in the bitch. J Small An Pract 17:793-798 (1976).

4. Avioli LV, Raisz LG: Bone metabolism and disease. In Metabolic Control and Disease, Bondy PK and Rosenberg LE eds. WB Saunders Co. Philadelphia, PA; pp 1709-1814 (1980).

5. Axelrod AE, Tipton MA, Elvehjem CA: The production of uncomplicated riboflavin deficiency in the dog. Am J Physiol 108:703-708 (1940).

6. Belanger LF, Robichon J: Parathormone-induced osteolysis in dogs. A microradiographic and alpha radiographic survey. J Bone Joint Surg 46A:1008-1012 (1964).

7. Belfield WO: Chronic subclinical scurvy and canine hip dysplasia. VM/SAC 71:1399-1403 (1976).

8. Bjerkas E: Eclampsia in the cat. J Small An Pract 15:411-414 (1974).

9. Bonucci E: New knowledge on the origin, function and fate of osteoclasts. Clin Orthoped 158:252-269 (1981).

10. Boris A, Hurley JF, Trmal T: Relative activities of some metabolites and analogs of cholecalciferol in stimulation of tibia ash weight in chicks otherwise deprived of vitamin D. J Nutr 107:194-198 (1977).

11. Borle AB: Calcium and phosphate metabolism. Ann Rev Physiol 36:361-390 (1974).

12. Boskey AL: Current concepts of the physiology and biochemistry of calcification. Clin Orthop 159:225-257 (1981).

13. Bunce GE, Jenkins KJ, Phillips PH: The mineral requirements of the dog III. The magnesium requirement. J Nutr 76:17-22 (1962).

14. Cordy DR, Stillinger CJ: Steatitis ("yellow fat disease") in kittens. North Am Vet 34:714-718 (1953).

15. Cordy DR: Experimental production of steatitis (yellow fat disease) in kittens fed a commercial canned cat food and prevention of the condition by vitamin E. Cornell Vet 44:310-318 (1954).

16. Deftos LJ: Calcitonin secretion. In Disorders of Mineral Metabolism, Vol. II. Bronner F and Coburn JW eds. Academic Press, New York, NY; pp 433-479 (1982).

17. DeLuca HF, Schnoes HK: Vitamin D: Recent advances. Ann Rev Biochem 52:411-439 (1983).

18. Garabedian M, Holick MF, Deluca HF, Boyle IT: Control of 25-Hydroxycholecalciferol metabolism by parathyroid glands. Proc Nat Acad Sci USA 69:1673-1676 (1972).

19. Garabedian M, Tanaka Y, Holick MF, DeLuca HF: Response of intestinal calcium transport and bone calcium mobilization to 1,25 dihydroxyvitamin D3 in thyroparathyroidectomized rats. Endocrin 94:1022-1027 (1974).

20. Gaskell CJ, Leedale AH, Douglas SW: Pansteatitis in the cat: A report of four cases. J Small An Pract 16:117-121 (1975).

21. Habener JF: Regulation of parathyroid hormone secretion and biosynthesis. Ann Rev Physiol 43:211-223 (1981).

22. Hayes KC: On the pathophysiology of vitamin A deficiency. Nutr Rev 29:3-6 (1971).

23. Hedhammar A, Wu F, Krook L, Schryver HF, deLahunta A, Whalen JP, Kallfelz FA, Nunez EA, Hintz HF, Sheffy BE, Ryan GD: Overnutrition and skeletal disease: An experimental study in growing Great Dane dogs. Cornell Vet 64:Supp 5 (1974).

24. Innes JRM: Vitamin C requirements of dogs: Attempts to produce experimental scurvy. 2nd Rep Dir Camp Inst Anim Pathol pp 143-150 (1931).

25. Krook L: Metabolic bone diseases in dogs and cats. Proc 38th Ann Mtng AAHA, pp 350-354 (1971).

26. Krook L, Barrett RB, Usui K, Wolke RE: Nutritional secondary hyperparathyroidism in the cat. Cornell Vet 53:224-240 (1963).

27. Krook L, Lutwak L, Henrikson P, Kallfelz F, Hirsch C, Romanus B, Belnager LF, Marier JF, Sheffy BE: Reversibility of nutritional osteoporosis: Physiocochemical data on bones from an experimental study in dogs. J Nutr 101:233-246 (1971).

28. Loew FM, Martin CL, Dunlop RH, Mapletoft RJ, Smith SI: Naturally-occurring and experimental thiamine deficiency in cats receiving commercial cat food. Can Vet J II:109-113 (1970).

29. Meier H, Clark ST, Schnelle GB, Will DH: Hypertrophic osteodystrophy associated with disturbance of vitamin C synthesis in dogs. JAVMA 130:483-491 (1957).

30. Meuten DJ, Chew DP, Capen CC, Kociba GJ: Relationship of serum total calcium to albumin and total protein in dogs. JAVMA 180:63-67 (1982).

31. Parfitt AM: The cellular basis of bone turnover and bone loss: A rebuttal of the osteocytic resorption-bone flow theory. Clin Orthop 127:236-247 (1977).

32. Raisz LG: Bone metabolism and calcium regulation. In Metabolic Bone Disease Vol. I, Alvioli LV and Krane SM eds. Academic Press, New York, NY; pp 1-58 (1977).

33. Rasmussen H, Matsumoto T, Fontaine O, Goodman DBP: Role of changes in membrane lipid structure in the action of 1,25-dihydroxyvitamin D3. Fed Proc 41:72-77 (1982).

34. Read DH, Jolly RD, Alley MR: Polio-encephalomalacia of dogs with thiamine deficiency. Vet Pathol 14:103-112 (1977).

35. Scott ML: Advances in our understanding of vitamin E. Fed Proc 39:2736-2739 (1980).

36. Seawright AA, English PB, Gartner RJW: Hypervitaminosis A and deforming cervical spondylosis of the cat. J Comp Path 77:29-39 (1967).

37. Seawright AA, Hrdlicka J: Severe retardation of growth with retention and displacement of incisors in young cats fed a diet of raw sheep liver high in vitamin A. Aust Vet J 50:306-315 (1974).

38. Smith DC, Proutt LM: Development of thiamine deficiency in the cat on a diet of raw fish. PSEBM 56:1-2 (1944).

39. Spencer TN: Is "black-tongue" in dogs pellagra? JAVMA II:325 (1916).

40. Stumpf WE, Sar M, Reid FA, Tanaka Y, DeLuca HF: Target cells for 1,25-dihydroxyvitamin D3 in intestinal tract, stomach, kidney, skin, pituitary and parathyroid. Science 206:1188-1190 (1979).

41. Tanaka Y, DeLuca HF: The control of 25-dihydroxyvitamin D metabolism by inorganic phosphorus. Arch Biochem Biophys 154:566-574 (1973).

42. Tanaka Y, Lorenc RS, DeLuca HF: The role of 1,25-dihydroxyvitamin D3 and parathyroid hormone in the regulation of chick renal 25-dihydroxyvitamin D3-24-hydroxylase. Arch Biochem Biophys 171:620-626 (1975).

43. Tanaka Y, Deluca HF: Measurement of mammalian 25-dihydroxyvitamin D3 24R-and 1α-hydroxylase. Proc Nat Acad Sci USA 78:196-199 (1981).

44. Taylor AN, Wasserman RH: Vitamin D3 induced calcium-binding protein: Partial purification, electrophoretic visualization and tissue distribution. Arch Biochem Biophys 119:536-540 (1967).

45. Teare JA, Krook L, Kallfelz FA, Hintz HF: Ascorbic acid deficiency and hypertrophic osteodystrophy: A rebuttal. Cornell Vet 69:384-401 (1979).

46. Vanderlip SL: What is your diagnosis? Hypervitaminosis A in the cat. JAVMA 183:1472-1473 (1983).

47. Van Vleet JF: Experimentally induced vitamin E-selenium deficiency in the growing dog. JAVMA 166:769-774 (1975).

48. Wasserman RH, Corradino RA, Taylor AN: Vitamin D-dependent calcium binding protein. Purification and some properties. J Biol Chem 243:3978-3986 (1968).

49. Wasserman RH, Taylor AN: Some aspects of the intestinal absorption of calcium with special reference to vitamin D. In Mineral Metabolism Vol. III, Comar CL and Brunner F, eds. Academic Press, New York, NY; pp 321-403 (1969).

50. Wasserman RH, Taylor AN: Intestinal absorption of phosphate in the chick: Effect of vitamin D3 and other parameters. J Nutr 103:586-599 (1973).

Index of Dietary Management

CONTENTS

INTRODUCTION

The Index of Dietary Management is composed of a list of conditions in which proper dietary management plays an important role in therapy, health maintenance, or performance. The clinical conditions discussed may be a specific disease syndrome, or merely clinical signs for which treatment includes the application of dietary management. For each condition, the aim of dietary management, the management necessary to accomplish that aim, and the diets of choice which most closely implement that management, are presented. Specific considerations which necessitate dietary alteration also are presented. These are areas where

the clinician must use judgment based on the conditions which may exist in individual cases.

A list of the diet types useful in dietary management of clinical conditions is given in Appendix Table 1. These diets can be purchased as commercially prepared dietary animal foods, or prepared from human foods. A description and the nutrient contents of the prepared dietary foods are given in Appendix Table 2. Recipes for, and the nutrient contents of, homemade dietary foods are given in Appendix Table 3. The nutrient contents of human foods used to make homemade diets, or commonly fed to dogs and cats are given in Appendix Table 4.

ALLERGY, FOOD-INDUCED
(See page 7-32)

Aim—To identify and eliminate foods from the diet that produce an allergic response.

Management

1. Treat any secondary skin complications present.
2. Hospitalize, fast for 48 hours, give 3 enemas at 12-hour intervals, and allow free access to distilled water.
3. Feed a diet composed of as few ingredients as possible and ones not present in the previous diet. Feed at least twice daily. Restrict intake to the amount needed for maintenance.
4. Send patient home with instructions to maintain this feeding regimen. Eliminate access to all other food and water.
5. When improvement occurs (usually by second or third week) give regular drinking water rather than distilled.
6. If signs do not recur within 7 days, the animal may be maintained on the hypoallergic diet or provocative testing can be initiated by adding a small amount of one of the ingredients in the original diet. If there is no recurrence of signs within 7 days, try a different ingredient until the offending ingredient is identified. Life-long avoidance of that ingredient will be necessary to prevent recurrence.

Considerations—Generalized pruritus is the most common sign. No other treatment is effective. Corticosteroids usually result in no more than a 50% reduction in signs. Because the offending allergin is usually present in many commercial pet foods, changing brands rarely is effective.

Diets of Choice—Hypoallergenic diet.

Dog or Cat—Prescription Diet Canine d/d or Recipe 6. See appendix Table 1 for other restricted protein source (hypoallergenic) diets that can be used for diagnosis and management of food induced allergy.

ANEMIA

Aim—To supply adequate nutrients to support erythropoiesis. When needed, the blood-building capacity of the body is at least six times the normal replacement rate. Unless supplied in adequate amounts, dietary nutrients become rate-limiting factors in accelerated erythropoiesis.

Management

1. Feed a nutritionally complete growth diet until the hematocrit approaches normal.

2. For a period of at least 2 weeks:
   a. Increase level of B-complex vitamins to 6 times minimum requirements by adding 2 g/kg body weight/day of brewer's yeast to the diet, or giving a B-complex vitamin supplement at a dosage that supplies daily at least 25 μg folic acid, 1 mg niacin, 125 μg pyridoxine, and 4 μg vitamin B-12/kg body weight daily. Do not use supplements that supply more than 500 IU of vitamin A or 50 IU of vitamin D/kg body weight/day.
   b. Increase iron, cobalt, and copper intake by administering sufficient quantity of a trace mineral supplement to supply at least 8 mg iron, 1 mg copper, and 0.35 mg cobalt/kg body weight daily.
   c. Adding 1 oz (30 g) of raw liver/can or 2 cups of food may be beneficial as it provides most nutrients important in erythropoiesis.

Considerations

1. Dietary management only eliminates diet as a limiting factor for correction of the anemia. The determination of the specific cause should be pursued and corrected.
2. If intestinal utilization of iron from the diet is impaired, administer parenterally 10 mg iron/kg body weight/week in divided doses.
3. Kittens fed a high milk diet can develop iron deficiency. In such cases, administer orally 30 mg of ferrous sulfate daily/kitten.

Diets of Choice—High protein and energy diet balanced for growth.

Dog—Prescription Diet Canine p/d, or Recipe 8.

Cat—Prescription Diet Feline p/d or Recipe 8. The canned form is preferred due to its higher protein and energy densities. The dry form should be used only for cats that will not eat canned food.

ANOREXIA & CHANGING THE DIET
(See Chapter 5, Exertion or Stress-page 13-7, and Palatability-page 11-34)

Aim—To provide a balanced nutrient source by appetite stimulation or force, tube, or intravenous feeding.

Management—Administer all nutrients (including fluids and electrolytes) orally whenever possible. If vomiting or severe dehydration exists, administer fluids and electrolytes parenterally.

1. Correct any fluid, electrolyte, and/or acid-base abnormality.

2. Administer daily 70-90 kcal/kg body weight.
3. Administer daily at least 2 g for dogs and 4 g for cats of protein/kg body weight of a biologic value of 80 or greater.
4. Administer vitamins at growth levels.
5. When changing the diet, feeding studies have shown that 95% of hospitalized dogs will eat a new diet in 3 days, or less, if no other food is available. Fasting for several days is normal for non-domesticated dogs and is not harmful unless disease is present which increases nutrient needs. Overweight cats should not be fasted for more than 3 days as hepatic lipidosis may occur. At each regular feeding time, replace any uneaten food with fresh food. Warming the food to body temperature may be helpful. Do not allow the animal access to anything except the new diet. For the few dogs or cats that have not started eating the new diet within 3 days, either of the following procedures are helpful: a) put a very palatable food (such as Prescription Diet Feline c/d) on top of or mixed with the new food, or b) mix a small amount of the new food with the animal's previous food. When the animal is eating this mixture well, which may take anywhere from 1-5 days, increase the amount of new food in the mixture. Continue this procedure until only the new diet is being consumed.
6. Stimulate appetite by giving orally diazepam (Valium, Roche) to cats and puppies at 2 and 14 mg/kg respectively. Most cats will eat immediately following intravenous administration of 0.1-0.5 mg (total dose). Have food available before it is given. Oral administration of 1-2 mg/cat will maintain appetite stimulation.

Considerations–If the animal is anorectic due to a condition which requires dietary alteration, such as renal or heart disease, force feed according to the needs of that condition.

Diets of Choice–Canned food high in energy and protein.

Dogs and Cats—Prescription Diet Feline p/d or c/d or tube feed Recipe 7.

ANTIBIOTIC THERAPY

Aim–To supply vitamins normally produced by intestinal microorganisms which are destroyed by orally administered antimicrobial agents.

Management–When antibiotics are given orally for more than 5 days, provide B-complex vitamins at maintenance or growth levels, whichever is appropriate, with a multivitamin preparation or

add 1 g brewer's yeast/3-5 kg body weight/day to the diet.

CACHEXIA OR STARVATION

Aim–To provide a palatable balanced diet with a high caloric density which supplies high biologic value protein to support tissue repair and immune system stimulation.

Management–Feed a highly palatable diet with a high caloric density.

Considerations

1. Correct any fluid, electrolyte, and/or acid-base abnormalities.
2. Feed small amounts at least 3 and preferably 5-6 times daily.
3. Increase the amount fed gradually over 2-4 days depending on the severity of cachexia present, until the animal is receiving the amount of food needed for growth or all of the food that it will eat. Free choice (ad libitum) feeding may be used after the initial 2-4 day period.
4. Animals on prolonged cancer therapy may develop carbohydrate intolerance and require a high-protein, high-fat diet. Others may develop liver or kidney damage and require a restricted protein diet.

Diets of Choice–High protein and energy diet.

Dogs and Cats—Prescription Diet Canine or Feline p/d, respectively or Feline p/d for either.

COLITIS
(See page 7-49)

Aim–To provide a balanced diet high in fiber (preferably cellulose) which normalizes colonic motility and microflora, decreases clinical signs, and improves healing and nutrient balance.

Management

1. In acute cases withhold food, but not water, for 24-48 hours.
2. Initially feed a diet containing highly-digestible non-fiber ingredients and at least 10% fiber from cellulose in its dry matter.
3. For dogs, the diet dry matter should contain less than 15% fat.
4. Feed small amounts 3-6 times daily.
5. Correct infectious, parasitic, or inflammatory causes.
   a. Sulfasalazine (Azulfidine, Pharmacia Labs) at 25-50 mg/kg 3-4 times daily for dogs and

250 mg/cat once daily for several weeks may be helpful.

b. If whipworms are present, give fenbendazole (Panacur, American Hoechst) at 50 mg/kg once daily for 3 days.

c. If bacterial overgrowth is suspected, give tylosin (Tylan plus Vitamins, Elanco) at 10 mg/kg 2-3 times/day.

d. If eosinophilic colitis is present, give corticosteroids and feed a hypoallergenic diet.

e. Corticosteroid retention enemas (Cortenemas, Rowell) provide prompt relief in patients with tenesmus and dyschezia due to severe colitis.

Consideration–If within 1-2 weeks there is no response to a high fiber diet, switch to a highly digestible diet.

Diets of Choice–Balanced high fiber diet.

1. Dogs or cats at or above optimal body weight, feed a high-fiber reducing diet—Prescription Diets Canine r/d or Feline r/d, or Recipes 4 or 10.

2. Dogs that have difficulty maintaining optimal body weight on the reducing diet, feed a less calorically restricted, moderately high fiber diet—Prescription Diet Canine w/d.

3. Dogs or cats that do not respond to the high fiber diet, feed a highly digestible diet— Prescription Diet Canine i/d or Recipe 1, or Feline c/d or Recipe 8, respectively

CONSTIPATION
(See page 7-50)

Aim–To provide a balanced diet high in fiber to increase intestinal volume and contractions and to retain water in the colon.

Management

1. Feed at least twice daily a diet containing at least 10% fiber in the dry matter to stimulate post-prandial peristalsis.

2. Restrict access to bones, feathers, skin, or foreign material.

3. Thirty to 60 minutes after eating, exercise the dog to encourage defecation and improve abdominal muscle tone. Maintain a clean litter box for cats.

4. Correct any signs of anorectal disease or trauma that may cause pain and reluctance to defecate.

5. To assist in eliminating hair impaction in cats feed a high-fiber diet and periodically administer 1 teaspoon of non-medicated (plain) petroleum jelly orally.

6. Provide free access to fresh water.

Diets of Choice–Low-fat, high-fiber diet.

Dog—Prescription Diet Canine r/d or w/d, or Recipe 4.

Cat—Prescription Diet Feline r/d, or Recipe 10.

COPPER TOXICITY
(See page 7-58)

Aim–To provide a balanced diet that restricts copper intake to an amount that meets nutritional need but eliminates excess.

Management

1. Feed a diet that contains not more than 1.5 mg of copper/100 g of diet dry matter.

2. Do not feed table scraps or vitamin-mineral supplements containing copper.

Considerations–Give D-penicillamine (Cuprimine, Merck) at 10 mg/kg twice daily mixed in the food to increase urinary copper excretion.

Diets of Choice–Low copper diet.

Adults—Prescription Diet Canine u/d or Recipe 3 (without copper in the vitamin-trace mineral supplement).

Puppies

1 cup dry or 1/2 can Prescription Diet Canine u/d

1/2 teaspoon dicalcium phosphate (do not use bone meal or minerals containing copper)

Any **one** of the following:

1 cup cottage cheese

1 cup hamburger

2 hard cooked eggs

Avoid organ tissues (liver, kidney, thymus) and bread.

COPROPHAGY
(See page 7-51)

Aim–To provide a balanced highly digestible diet and alleviate boredom.

Management

1. Promptly remove stools from the environment, and increase the dog's exercise.

2. Feed a good-quality diet which is nutritionally balanced for the particular stage of the life cycle.

Consideration–Since marginal pancreatic insufficiency has been hypothesized as one of the causes of coprophagy, investigate this possibility and manage accordingly.

Diets of Choice–Highly-digestible diet.
Prescription Diet Canine i/d or Recipe 1.

CUSHING'S SYNDROME
(HYPERADRENOCORTICISM)

Aim–To meet the special nutritive needs of the animal suffering from hyperadrenocorticism or undergoing o'p'DDD therapy for Cushing's Syndrome.

Management

1. Feed a low-fiber, low-fat, low-purine, highly-digestible diet.
2. Feed protein of high biologic value at growth levels to minimize the muscle-wasting effects of increased gluconeogenesis.
3. Supply calcium at growth levels. Excessive amounts of calcium above growth levels may contribute to the development of calcinosis cutis.
4. Supply potassium at growth levels.
5. If patient is being treated with o'p'DDD, do not feed a severely restricted sodium diet.
6. Do not limit intake of water.

Diets of Choice–Highly-digestible diet adequate for growth.
Prescription Diet Canine i/d or Recipe 1.

DIABETES MELLITUS

Aim–To maintain a uniform intake of slowly-absorbed carbohydrates and a constant balance between caloric intake and insulin dosage.

Management

1. Feed the same quantity of a diet uniform in ingredients (both in quality and quantity) so that a consistent insulin dosage can be established.
2. Feed a diet containing at least 10% fiber in the diet dry matter and a reduced level of soluble carbohydrates. Such a diet usually allows reduction in insulin dosage and may eliminate need to administer insulin in some cases.

Considerations–Most commercial pet foods are produced from "open" formulas. The resultant ingredient and nutrient fluctuations make it very difficult to establish and maintain a consistent insulin dosage in a diabetic animal. The client may become discouraged and request euthanasia of the diabetic pet.

Diets of Choice–High fiber diet.

1. Dogs or cats at or above optimal body weight with no other disease problem feed a high fiber diet—Prescription Diets Canine r/d or w/d, or Feline r/d respectively.
2. Dogs or cats below optimum body weight or with concomitant pancreatic exocrine insufficiency, feed a highly digestible diet—Prescription Diet Canine i/d, or Prescription Diet Feline c/d, respectively. If necessary, give pancreatic enzymes (Viokase-V, AH Robins) and cimetidine (Tagamet, Smith Kline & French) (see page 7-43).
3. In dogs or cats with other conditions requiring dietary modification, feed the diet indicated for that condition so long as it is uniform and allows insulin standardization.
4. Homemade diet not recommended due to variability.

DIARRHEA
(See Chapter 7)

Aim–To provide foods which are easily digested and absorbed and allow healing of the gastrointestinal tract.

Management

1. Withhold all food, but not water, for 1-4 days (longer the more severe the intestinal disturbance).
2. If the cause of diarrhea is detected from history and initial physical examination, institute specific therapy as indicated.
3. Over the next 3-5 days, gradually return the patient to full feed.
4. Feed small amounts frequently (3-6 times daily) of a highly-digestible diet containing 1% or less fiber in the dry matter except for cases of colitis, (see page 13-4).
5. Feed a diet that provides a moderate amount of highly digestible protein from cottage cheese, chicken, and egg at the rate of 4 g/kg body weight daily. Protein from cereal by-products, commonly present in dry dog foods, and meat by-product and organ tissues, commonly present in canned dog foods, are contraindicated.
6. For the dog, fats in excess of 15% of the diet dry matter should be avoided.
7. Provide easily digested carbohydrates primarily from rice or dextrose. Wheat middlings, bran, and other cereal by-products commonly present in pet foods, are contraindicated.
8. Foods containing more than 10% sucrose (table sugar) or any lactose (milk sugar) should be avoided.

Considerations

1. If dehydration is present, correct it by giving

parenterally Ringer's lactate with 40-70 mEq/L of sodium bicarbonate added.

2. If diarrhea has been a chronic problem, or intestinal parasites or giardiasis are suspected, administer an anthelmenic and metronidazole (Flagyl, Searle) at 25 mg/kg for dogs, or 10 mg/kg for cats, twice daily for 5 days.

Diets of Choice–Highly-digestible diet.

Dog—Prescription Diet Canine i/d or Recipe 1.

Cat—Prescription Diet Feline c/d or Recipe 6.

EXERTION OR STRESS ENVIRONMENTAL, PHYSICAL, OR PSYCHOLOGICAL
(See Chapter 3)

Aim–To provide a palatable balanced diet with a high caloric density to provide the energy need for: 1) physical exertion, 2) cold or hot weather, 3) stress such as dog shows, guard duty, guide, or police work, or 4) when food intake is decreased for any reason.

Management

1. Feed a diet that contains the recommended nutrient levels (see table below).
2. Feed two or more times daily in whatever amount is necessary to maintain optimal body weight.
3. Feed the normal amount 4 hours or more before exertion. From 15 minutes before and every 2-3 hours during exertion feed small amounts of food and water. Feed the majority of the amount of food needed daily within 1-4 hours after exertion.

Considerations–If food intake is inadequate due to psychologically induced stress, feed or add to the dog's ration a highly-palatable, high-energy dense canned cat food (such as Prescription Diet Feline c/d). If dry food is being fed, add warm water prior to feeding to increase food intake.

Diets of Choice–A palatable high-energy diet.

Dog—Science Diet Maximum Stress Diet or

Performance, or other diet that contains the recommended nutrient levels and has been proven to be nutritionally adequate by feeding tests.

Cat—Prescription Diet Feline p/d or c/d.

FELINE UROLOGIC SYNDROME AND UROLITHIASIS
(See Chapter 9)

Aim–To reduce the urinary concentration of minerals found in urinary calculi and crystals, and maintain an acid urine.

Management

1. If cat is obstructed:
   a. Relieve bladder by cystocentesis, if severely distended.
   b. If present, correct dehydration by giving intravenously a mixture of equal parts isotonic saline and isotonic dextrose.
   c. Relieve obstruction by flushing the urolith or plug out of the urethra.
   d. Hospitalize for several days and observe frequently for reobstruction.
2. To all cats showing any signs of FUS feed exclusively for 2-3 months, a severely-restricted magnesium diet that increases urine volume and maintains a urine pH of 5.8-6.2 to allow struvite calculi and crystals to dissolve (Table 5, page 9-10). **Administration of a urine acidifier with a calculolytic diet is contraindicated.**
3. If clinical signs persist beyond 10-14 days, evaluate for other abnormalities and treat accordingly.
4. Identifiable uroliths that enlarge, or do not dissolve within 3 months, should be removed surgically.
5. For prevention, feed exclusively a diet that contains less than 20 mg magnesium/100 kcal ME and maintains a urine pH below 6.4 (Table 5, page 9-10).

Diets of Choice–Restricted-magnesium, high-energy, urine-acidifying diet.

DIET CHARACTERISTICS FOR EXERTION OR STRESS IN ADULTS[a]

	Metabo-lizable kcal/lb	Digesti-ability[c]	% in Food Dry Matter[b]						
			Protein	Fat	Fiber	Ca	P	Sodium	Mag-nesium[e]
Dog	≥ 1900[d]	≥ 82	> 25	> 23	≤ 4	0.8–1.5	0.6–1.2	0.3–0.6	—
Cat	≥ 1900	≥ 82	> 30	> 23	≤ 3	0.8–1.5	0.6–1.2	0.3–0.6	< 0.10

a,b,c,d,e
  See footnotes in Table under Maintenance (page 13-13).

Dissolution—Prescription Diet Feline s/d

Prevention—Prescription Diet Feline c/d or Recipe 8.

FEVER

Aim–To supply sufficient calories to meet the increased metabolic needs attendant with an elevation in temperature.

Management–Increase caloric intake by 7 kcal/kg body weight daily for each degree of fever by increasing amount fed.

Considerations–In prolonged fever with proteinuria, feed a diet designed for growth or add 1/3 cup cottage cheese or 2 hard-cooked eggs to each pound of maintenance-type diet.

Diets of Choice–High protein and energy diet.

Dog and Cat—Prescription Diets Canine p/d and Feline p/d, respectively.

FLATULENCE
(See page 7-51)

Aim–To avoid feeding foods which result in increased fermentation, putrefaction, and gas formation. Feed in a manner that discourages aerophagia by minimizing excitement at feeding.

Management

The influence of foods on gastrointestinal gas formation in dogs is highly variable. A food which results in flatulence in one dog may have little effect when fed to another. The following have been shown to reduce flatulence in some, but not all, dogs:

1. Avoid feeding foods high in soybean products, potatoes, root vegetables, beans, cabbage, cauliflower, onions, etc.
2. Avoid feeding large quantities of milk or milk products to prevent putrefactive fermentation of the lactose.
3. Avoid high protein diets composed of meat or fish by-products.
4. Feed the animal free-choice, or three or more small meals daily, in a flat open pan in a quiet environment to decrease ingestion of air.
5. Avoid vitamin supplementation of prepared diets which may increase microbial activity and intestinal gas formation.

Diets of Choice–Highly-digestible, restricted or moderate protein, low-fiber, soy-free, wheat-free, lactose-free diets.

Dog—Prescription Diets Canine i/d, g/d, d/d,

and k/d meet these criteria (see Appendix Table 1 for additional diets).

Cat—Prescription Diet Feline c/d or Recipe 8.

FRACTURES
(See Chapter 12)

Aim–To supply the nutritive requirements necessary for normal healing of broken bones.

Management–Supply a diet known to be adequate for growth until fixation is removed or healing is complete. If the diet meets the mineral requirements for normal growth, **additional mineral supplementation is of no benefit.** The administration of single nutrient supplements, such as calcium carbonate, may even retard fracture healing and is thus contraindicated.

Diets of Choice–Diet balanced for growth.

Dog and Cat—Prescription Diets Canine and Feline p/d, respectively or other nutritionally complete growth diet (see Growth, page 13-9).

GASTRIC DILATATION OR BLOAT
(See page 7-22)

Aim–To meet nutrient needs with a highly digestible, high-energy diet that allows reduced food intake and prevents gastric distention.

Management

1. Decompress the stomach by passing a tube if possible; if not, by inserting a needle through the abdominal wall into the lumen of the stomach.
2. If poor tissue perfusion is present, give oxygen and administer intravenously large volumes (90 ml/kg in the first hour) of Ringer's lactate containing corticosteroids and antibiotics.
3. If cardiac arrythmia is present, give intravenously a 2-4 mg/kg bolus of lidocaine hydrochloride without epinephrine.
4. If the stomach or pylorus is displaced, correct surgically and do a circumcostal gastropexy to prevent recurrence.
5. Withhold food and water for the first 24 hours, then feed small amounts of water frequently.
6. When vomiting has not occurred for 24 hours, feed one-third of the daily requirement of a highly digestible diet divided into 3-6 small meals. Over the next several days gradually increase the amount fed back to normal.

Prevention

The following have been reported to reduce

the incidence of bloat. None are 100% effective in eliminating bloat in susceptible dogs.

1. Avoid feeding and watering within several hours before, and immediately following, strenuous exercise. Introduce food and water gradually after a rest period to prevent over consumption.

2. Divide daily ration into three or more meals.

3. For working dogs, feed a high-energy, highly-digestible diet 2-3 times daily, so that the quantity eaten at each meal is reduced. Do not allow the patient to gorge on either food or water.

4. To reduce susceptibility to bloat, feed puppies a calorie dense diet in controlled amounts (Chapter 3). This prevents excessive stretching of the suspensory apparatus of the stomach and may help prevent bloat later in life. The diet should contain not more than 1.8% calcium in the dry matter to prevent excessive gastrin secretion which may predispose to bloat.

Diets of Choice–High-energy, highly-digestible diet.

Prescription Diet Canine i/d, Recipe 1, Science Diet Canine Performance or Maximum Stress Diet or other nutritionally adequate high energy food (see Exertion or Stress, page 13-7).

GERIATRICS
(See page 3-22)

Aim–To prolong an enjoyable life by ameliorating existing problems, slowing or preventing the development or progression of disease, and maintaining optimal body weight.

Management

1. Beginning at 7 years of age (5 years for giant breeds of dogs), feed a diet that contains the recommended nutrient levels (see table below).

2. Feed amount necessary to maintain optimal body weight. Many older dogs and cats have a tendency to become less active. If caloric intake is not controlled, obesity will develop.

Considerations

1. Insure adequate physical activity to maintain muscle tone and optimal body weight, enhance circulation, and improve waste elimination.

2. If body weight is above optimal, see obesity (page 13-13). If it is below optimal, see cachexia (page 13-4).

3. If any disease is present, see the management recommended for that particular condition. Early detection and proper nutritional management will delay the onset of clinical signs, and slow the progression of renal and heart failure.

Diets of Choice–Palatable, highly-digestible diet with reduced levels of protein, phosphorus, and sodium.

Dog—Prescription Diet Canine g/d, Recipe 2 or other diet that contains the recommended nutrient levels and has been proven to be nutritionally adequate by feeding tests.

Cat—Prescription Diets Feline c/d (dry) or k/d, Recipe 8, or other diet that contains the recommended nutrient levels and has been proven to be nutritionally adequate by feeding tests.

GROWTH
(See Chapters 3 and 4)

Aim–To feed a diet that provides in a readily available form the increased nutrients needed for maximum disease resistance and optimal musculoskeletal growth, thus preventing malnutrition, stunting, and skeletal diseases.

Management

1. Feed a diet that contains the recommended nutrient levels (see table, page 13-10).

2. Feed kittens (not puppies), free-choice. Feed toy-breed puppies 3 times daily until 6 months of age, and twice daily from 6-12 months of age. Feed other puppies twice daily until 12 months of age (18 months for giant breeds). At each feeding, allow the puppy all it will eat in 20 minutes.

DIET CHARACTERISTICS RECOMMENDED FOR AGED DOGS AND CATS[a]

| | Metabolizable kcal/lb | Digestibility[c] | % in Food Dry Matter[b] | | | | | | |
			Protein	Fat	Fiber	Ca	P	Sodium	Magnesium[e]
Dog	≥ 1700[d]	> 80	14–21	> 10	< 5	0.5–0.8	0.4–0.7	0.2–0.4	——
Cat	≥ 1700	> 80	25–35	> 15	< 5	0.5–0.8	0.4–0.7	0.2–0.4	< 0.10

a,b,c,d,e
   See footnotes in Table under Maintenance (page 13–13).

DIET CHARACTERISTICS RECOMMENDED FOR GROWTH[a]

	Metabo-lizable kcal/lb	Digesti-ability[c]	% in Food Dry Matter[b]					
			Protein	Fat	Fiber	Ca	P	Sodium
Dog	≥ 1750[d]	> 80	> 29	≥ 17	< 5	1.0–1.8	0.8–1.6	0.3–0.7
Cat	≥ 2000	> 80	> 35	≥ 17	< 5	1.0–1.8	0.8–1.6	0.3–0.7

a,b,c,d
    See footnotes in Table under Maintenance (page 13-13).

3. Do not supplement with anything—particularly vitamins or minerals. Supplements are not required if a nutritionally adequate diet is fed. Supplements will not improve a nutritionally adequate diet; they often upset the nutrient balance of a diet.

Considerations

1. If skeletal diseases occur, see page 13-17; or if obesity occurs, see page 13-13. Overfeeding puppies may result in either or both. The development of obesity during growth predisposes to it later in life.
2. A poorly digestible diet may cause diarrhea, increase susceptibility to infectious diseases, predispose to bloat later in life by increasing food intake and stomach distention, and can decrease mature size.

Diets of Choice—High-energy, highly-digestible diet, balanced for growth.

Dog—Prescription Diet Canine p/d, Recipe 1, or other growth diet that contains the recommended nutrient levels and has been proven to be nutritionally adequate by feeding tests.

Cat—Prescription Diet Feline p/d, Recipe 8 substituting 2 tablespoons of dicalcium phosphate for the 1 teaspoon of calcium carbonate and adding 1 teaspoon of table salt, or other feline growth diet that contains the recommended nutrient levels and has been proven to be nutritionally adequate by feeding tests.

HEART FAILURE, CONGESTIVE
(See Chapter 11)

Aim–To meet the animal's nutritive requirements with a diet that restricts sodium intake.

Management

1. Estimate the patient's sodium intake by obtaining a diet history. Restrict sodium intake **as required to control congestion.** The table below provides the approximate average sodium content of various types of foods.
2. During diuresis increase B-complex vitamins to levels comparable to 2 g brewer's yeast/kg body weight daily. B-complex vitamin supplementation is not required if Prescription Diets Canine or Feline k/d or h/d are being fed.
3. For severe congestion, avoid softened water or tap water containing more than 150 ppm sodium. (Contact supplier for sodium content of water). During the period of active diuresis, offer distilled water until congestion is relieved.

Considerations

1. Initiate dietary sodium restriction at the first sign of heart disease to prevent congestion and to accustom the animal to a reduced sodium intake. Use a mild or moderately restricted sodium diet initially. Change to a severely

SODIUM CONTENT OF PET FOODS (mg/100 g of Dry Matter)

Canned dog food	904
Soft-moist dog food	857
Dry dog food	548
Prescription Diet g/d (mild restriction)	300
Prescription Diet k/d (moderate restriction)	230
Prescription Diet h/d (severe restriction) . . . . Canned	90
	Dry 55
Recipe 5	52
Commercial Cat Foods (Avg. of forms range from 560–780)	656
Prescription Diet Feline k/d (mild restriction)	400
Prescription Diet Feline h/d (severe restriction—cats, moderate restriction—dogs)	240
Recipe 8	160

restricted sodium diet when/if required to control clinical signs.

2. Obesity, which may accompany congestive heart failure, increases the severity of heart failure. Compensate by reducing total food intake of a sodium restricted diet. Most reducing diets are contraindicated because of their high sodium content.

3. Edema and ascites, often mistaken for obesity, may conceal emaciation. Following diuresis, if emaciation is present, add 2 Tablespoonfuls of vegetable oil plus 1 oz muscle meat to each lb of sodium-restricted diet fed.

4. For animals with fixed eating habits, mix the new diet with the old diet, gradually increasing the amount of new diet fed, or add **small** quantities of low sodium foods preferred by the individual (see Table below) to encourage eating (also see page 13-3 and 11-34). Finicky dogs may be fed Feline h/d if only moderate sodium restriction is required to alleviate clinical signs.

5. Feeding a sodium-restricted diet may allow a decrease in the dosage of, or cessation of the use of diuretics.

6. If renal failure is also present, restrict protein and phosphorus intakes as well as sodium intake. Diet selection is dictated by the more severe disease.

Diets of Choice–Low-sodium diet.

Dog—Prescription Diets Canine h/d, k/d, g/d, Feline h/d or Recipe 5.

Cat—Prescription Diets Feline h/d, k/d, c/d (dry) or Recipe 8.

HYPERLIPIDEMIA

Aim–To severely reduce fat intake.

Management

1. Feed a diet containing less than 8% fat in the diet dry matter to aid in lowering the serum levels of cholesterol and triglycerides.

2. Increasing dietary fiber may aid in lowering serum lipids in some dogs.

3. Limit foods containing digestible carbohydrates and sugars as they may further increase serum lipids.

Considerations–Inherited defects of lipid metabolism have been reported in Minature Schnauzers and dogs of mixed-breeding. Clinical signs reported were abdominal distress, seizures, and lipid-laden aqueous humor. Control of clinical signs was aided by feeding a restricted fat diet. If the plasma albumin decreases below 2.3% because of intestinal protein loss, add 1 cup of non-creamed cottage cheese or 3-4 oz of fish (fresh, frozen, or canned in water, not oil) to each can of food or 2 cups of dry food.

Diets of Choice–Low-fat diet.

Dog—Prescription Diet Canine r/d, w/d or Recipe 4.

Cat—Prescription Diet Feline r/d or Recipe 10.

HYPERPARATHYROIDISM, NUTRITIONAL SECONDARY
(See page 12-7)

Aim–To provide a balanced diet, especially with respect to the amounts and ratio of calcium to phosphorus.

Management–Feed a diet with a calcium:phosphorus ratio between 1.2:1 and 1.6:1 at a rate to supply at least 500 mg calcium and 400 mg phosphorus/kg body weight daily, supplied by readily available minerals such as dicalcium phosphate or calcium carbonate. Diets that support normal growth are adequate and do not require supplementation with calcium.

TABLE FOODS FOR PATIENTS ON A RESTRICTED SODIUM DIET

Low Sodium Foods	Foods to Avoid
Beef	All processed meats, cheeses, breads, cereals
Domestic rabbit	Carrots
Chicken	Heart
Horsemeat	Kidney
Lamb	Liver
Fresh water fish	Salted fats (butter, margarine)
Egg yolks	Salted snacks and nuts
Oatmeal	Whole egg
Corn	Snack type foods
Rice	
Farina (Cream of Wheat)	

Considerations

1. A change in diet is all that is required. Large quantities of calcium are contraindicated as they not only reduce the digestibility of other nutrients in the diet but alter the calcium:phosphorus ratio in the diet and may produce mineral imbalances and trace mineral deficiencies which retard calcification.

2. Do not administer vitamin D during treatment because vitamin D is rarely deficient and soft tissue calcification due to hypervitaminosis D may result.

Diets of Choice—Balanced growth diet (see 13-9).

Dog or Cat—Prescription Diets Canine p/d or Feline p/d, respectively, or other nutritionally adequate growth diet.

HYPOGLYCEMIA, FUNCTIONAL
(See page 3-25)

Aim—To frequently supply nutrients which are slowly converted by the body to glucose.

Management—Increase frequency of daily feedings to at least 4. Supply calories in the form of protein, fat, and complex carbohydrates. Avoid simple sugars for routine maintenance.

Considerations

1. **During acute attack,** feed dextrose (such as jam and jelly pectins), or if not available, table sugar or corn syrup, at 1 Tablespoon/5 kg body weight/attack, or the equivalent in sugar cubes.

2. Feed additional food to working dogs during periods of exercise. Include a light meal immediately prior (15 minutes or less) to exercise and 100-150 calorie snacks (1/3-1/2 cup of dry food or 1/2 patty of soft-moist food) and water every 4 hours during exercise. Feed the bulk of the diet within 4 hours after exercise, but following a rest period.

3. Train working dogs so that they are physically fit prior to strenuous exercise.

Diets of Choice—High protein and energy diet

Dog—Prescription Diet Canine p/d.

HYPOTHYROIDISM

Aim—To feed a balanced diet uniform in composition and quality to enable evaluation of replacement therapy.

Management—Feed a good quality balanced diet produced from a **fixed** formula. Most commercial pet foods are produced from open formulas; thus, their composition varies making it very difficult to evaluate medical therapy. If obesity exists, reduce weight to optimal (see Obesity, page 13-13).

Diets of Choice—Uniform maintenance diet.

Dog—Prescription Diet Canine c/d, w/d or other appropriate diet.

Homemade diet not recommended due to variability.

LIVER DISEASE
(See page 7-55)

Aim—To (1) reduce the need for liver functions such as gluconeogenesis, fat conversion, deamination, nitrogen and uric acid conversion, and bile secretion, (2) restore liver glycogen, (3) prevent ammonia toxicity (encephalopathy), and (4) prevent sodium retention.

Management

1. Provide readily available energy in the form of dextrose, cornstarch, rice, or other easily digested carbohydrates. Avoid coarse cereal by-products (midlings, bran, etc.) used in many dry pet foods.

2. Feed protein having a biologic value of at least 75 at a rate of 1.75 to 2.5 g/kg body weight daily for dogs and 3 to 3.5 for cats. Diets containing protein primarily from egg or milk (such as cottage cheese or casein) is recommended. Avoid high protein diets and meat by-product proteins of low quality (such as lungs, udders, and viscera) used in many canned pet foods.

3. Restrict purine containing foods and uric acid precursors such as fish meal, shellfish, glandular products such as spleen or thymus, and meat or meat by-products.

4. Feed small amounts of food frequently (4-6 times daily).

5. Ensure sufficient food intake to meet caloric need. If necessary, force-feed or tube-feed (see anorexia, page 13-3).

Considerations

1. If ascites or edema is present, sodium should be restricted to less than 100 mg/100 g of diet dry matter (see page 13-10).

2. If hepatic encephalopathy is present, a low protein diet is essential to lower serum ammonia levels and prevent the development of neurologic signs.

Diets of Choice-Based on clinical signs.

Dog—Initially—Prescription Diet Canine k/d or Recipe 2.

If diarrhea develops—Canine i/d or Recipe 1.

If ascites or edema develop—Canine h/d or Recipe 5.

If encephalopathy develops—Canine u/d or Recipe 3.

Cat—Initially—Prescription Diet Feline k/d or Recipe 9.

If diarrhea develops—Feline c/d.

If ascites or edema develops—Feline h/d or Recipe 9.

MAINTENANCE
(See pages 3-4 and 4-6)

Aim-To feed a diet that provides optimal amounts of all nutrients for maximum health and longevity by preventing the excesses present in many commercial pet foods. Prolonged consumption by adult dogs of diets adequate for growth, or "all purpose" diets containing excessive amounts of protein, calcium, phosphorus, sodium, or magnesium predispose to, and/or promotes the progression of major diseases affecting dogs and cats such as skin, kidney, heart and vascular diseases, bloat, and urolithiasis.

Management

1. Feed a diet that contains the recommended nutrient levels (see table below and 3-5 and 4-6 for dogs and cats, respectively).
2. Feed amount necessary to maintain optimal body weight.

Considerations

1. If body weight is above optimal, see Obesity (page 13-13). If it is below optimal, see Cachexia (page 13-4).
2. If the animal is past 7 years of age (5 years for giant breeds), see Geriatrics (page 13-9).
3. If any disease is present, see the management recommended for that particular condition.

Diets of Choice-High quality maintenance diet—do not use a growth or "all purpose" diet.

Dog—Prescription Diet Canine c/d, Recipe 2 or other maintenance diet that contains the recommended nutrient levels and has been proven to be nutritionally adequate by feeding tests.

Cat—Prescription Diet Feline c/d, Recipe 8 or other maintenance diet that contains the recommended nutrient levels and has been proven to be nutritionally adequate by feeding tests.

OBESITY
(See Chapter 6)

Aim-To produce a caloric deficit in the obese animal and prevent excess caloric intake in the obese-prone animal.

Management

1. During initial weight reduction, reduce the caloric intake to 60-65% of the calculated maintenance needs for dogs or cats at **optimal** (not obese) body weight by feeding a high fiber diet containing not more than 9% fat in the diet dry matter and a reduced level of digestible carbohydrate. This can be accomplished by feeding a diet containing 15-25% indigestible fiber (cellulose).
2. During caloric restriction for weight reduction, maintenance levels of protein, vitamins, and minerals must be provided by the calorie-restricted diet, or deficiencies may result.

DIET CHARACTERISTICS RECOMMENDED FOR MAINTENANCE[a]

	% in Food Dry Matter[b]						
	Digesti-bility[c]	Protein	Fat	Ca	P	Sodium	Mag-nesium[e]
Dog	> 75[d]	15–25	> 8	0.5–0.9	0.4–0.8	0.2–0.5	——
Cat	> 75	> 25	> 10	0.5–0.9	0.4–0.8	0.2–0.5	< 0.10

[a]In addition the label should identify the manufacturer (not just the distributor), that the diet is adequate for maintenance (based on feeding trials, not on meeting NRC recommendations) and an animal source protein is one of the first three ingredients. Dog foods should contain at least one cereal grain.

[b]To determine the amount of the nutrient in the dry matter divide the values given in the Guaranteed Analysis by the food's dry matter content, which is 1 − (% moisture in the food ÷ 100).

[c]% digestibility = [(food dry weight necessary for maintaining body wt − stool dry weight) ÷ (food dry weight necessary for maintaining body wt)] × 100.

[d]> indicates greater than, and < indicates less than.

[e]or not over 5% ash in a dry or soft-moist food if the magnesium content is not known (see FUS, page 13–7).

3. To prevent obesity in obese-prone dogs, feed a moderately calorie-restricted diet containing 10-20% fiber and not more than 12% fat. If necessary to prevent weight gain, an increased amount of the reducing diet can be fed.

4. To prevent recurrence of obesity in cats following weight reduction, restrict intake of a nutritionally adequate maintenance diet or increase the amount of reducing diet fed. This latter method has the additional benefit of helping minimize hair balls, due to the increased volume and movement of fiber and water through the intestinal tract.

Considerations–Obese cats should be reduced slowly (a decrease of not more than 3% body weight weekly). Fasting, or rapid weight loss in obese cats increases hepatic fat deposition, and increases risk of death from hepatic lipidosis. The greater the obesity, the greater the risk. Obese cats should not be allowed to fast for more than a few days.

Diets of Choice–Low-fat, high-fiber diet.

Dog—Weight reduction—Prescription Diet Canine r/d or Recipe 4.

Obesity prevention—Prescription Diet Canine w/d, r/d, Recipe 4 or a nutritionally adequate maintenance diet fed in amounts to maintain optimal weight.

Cat—Prescription Diet Feline r/d, Recipe 10, or a nutritionally adequate maintenance diet fed in amounts to maintain optimal weight.

ORPHANED PUPS AND KITTENS
(See page 3-18)

Aim–To replace the milk and care that would normally be provided by the mother. This requires supplying a balanced nutrient source capable of supporting growth.

Management

1. Provide energy in the following amounts daily:

   1st week . . . . 130 kcal/kg body weight
   2nd week . . . . 150 kcal/kg body weight
   3rd week . . . . 175 kcal/kg body weight
   4th week . . . . 200 kcal/kg body weight

2. Provide protein of a biologic value of 90 or greater from milk and eggs at the rate of at least 6 g/kg body weight until weaning.

3. Provide minerals balanced at growth levels, paying particular attention to a calcium:phosphorus ratio of from 1:1 to 2:1.

4. Provide adequate amounts of vitamins to support growth. Avoid over supplementation.

5. Begin weaning to solid food at 3 weeks of age or as soon as possible. Mix milk replacer with a highly digestible growth diet. Gradually reduce the amount of milk replacer over a 1-2 week period.

Considerations

1. Replacement milk for orphaned puppies and kittens can be administered either by stomach tube, or nursing bottle with a nipple. See Table 5, page 3-19 for feeding rates.

2. Stimulate defecation and urination following feeding by swabbing the perineal area with moist cotton. Control of environmental factors such as maintenance of temperature at 27-30°C (80-86°F), humidity at 40-50%, and the elimination of disturbances, are as important in hand-rearing puppies and kittens as is their diet.

Diets of Choice–See Tables 2 and 3 (pages 3-5 and 3-18).

PANCREATIC INSUFFICIENCY
(See page 7-43)

Aim–To reduce intake of foods which require pancreatic enzymes for their utilization.

Management

1. Feed a highly digestible diet with 1% or less fiber in the diet dry matter.

2. Supply carbohydrates as glucose, sucrose, cornstarch, or rice. Lactose (milk sugar) is contraindicated.

3. Feed the dog a diet containing 10-15% fat in the diet dry matter.

4. Feed proteins from cottage cheese or eggs at restricted levels to avoid excessive intestinal putrefaction.

5. If required, add pancreatic enzymes to the food and give cimetidine at 15 mg/kg twice daily, 5-30 minutes before feeding.

6. Feed the quantity of food required to maintain optimal weight. Required food intake will probably exceed normal maintenance needs.

Diets of Choice–Highly-digestible diet.

Dog—Prescription Diet Canine i/d or Recipe 1.

Cat—Prescription Diet Feline c/d.

PANCREATITIS, ACUTE
(See page 7-22)

Aim–To minimize pancreatic secretion, pain and shock, and meet nutrient needs.

Management

1. Give intravenously large volumes of Ringer's lactate to treat hypotensive shock.
2. Give antibiotics daily.
3. Give meperidine at 5-10 mg/kg 2-3 times daily to relieve pain.
4. Give nothing orally for 2-5 days and only water for the next 3 days. Over the next 3-5 days, gradually return to full feed.
5. Feed small amounts frequently (3-5 times daily) of a highly-digestible, moderately-restricted fat diet.

Considerations—This diet and feeding regimen may be continued thereafter to prevent recurrence and eventual development of either, or both, exocrine or endocrine insufficiency.

Diets of Choice—Highly-digestible diet.

Prescription Diet Canine i/d or Recipe 1.

PANSTEATITIS
(See page 12-13)

Aim—To eliminate the feeding of tuna or cat foods with a high content of unsaturated fatty acids without adequate antioxidants.

Management—Eliminate the feeding of tuna fish containing a high level of unstabilized fat. Feed only balanced commercial rations which have vitamin E and/or ethoxyquin added. Initially, treat by giving vitamin E at 10-20 mg twice daily for 5-7 days, and corticosteroids if needed to control inflammation and pain.

PUERPERAL TETANY (ECLAMPSIA)
(See page 12-11)

Aim—To provide a diet which maintains a normal plasma calcium concentration in the lactating female.

Management

1. During lactation, feed a diet which contains at least 1.4% calcium in the dry matter with a calcium:phosphorus ratio of at least 1:1.
2. Begin feeding the young solid food as early as possible, generally at 3 weeks of age.

Considerations

1. It may be necessary to remove the young from the female and terminate lactation to prevent eclampsia. If the young are not ready for weaning, they should be hand-reared and fed a milk replacer (See Orphaned Pups and Kittens, page 13-14). Withdrawal from the bitch for a 24-hour period is helpful.

2. During gestation, unsupplemented meat-type or other low calcium diets, as well as calcium supplementation are contraindicated.

Diets of Choice—Balanced mineral diet designed for reproduction.

Dog and Cat—Prescription Diet Canine and Feline p/d, respectively.

REGURGITATION
(See page 7-12)

Aim—To manage esophagitis by minimizing gastric acid secretion, increasing gastroesophageal sphincter tone, and providing non-abrasive foods which are easily digested and absorbed.

Management

1. Administer 2-3 times daily for at least 5-7 days:
   a. Cimetidine (Tagamet, Smith Kline & French) at 5 mg/kg orally, or 10 mg/kg intravenously.
   b. Metoclopramide (Reglan, A. H. Robins) at 0.2-0.4 mg/kg orally or subcutaneously into fat pads.
   c. A systemic antibiotic, if warrented.
2. Withhold all food for 3-4 days. Then feed for several days small amounts 3-6 times daily of a highly-digestible, bland canned diet made into a slurry with water. Gradually, over 1-2 days, decrease the amount of water added to the diet.

Considerations

1. Evaluate to determine if surgery or bougienage is warranted.
2. Remove foreign body, if present.
3. If megaesophagus is present:
   a. Feed the animal on stairs or from an elevated platform.
   b. Try different forms of food and feeding regimens to determine what is tolerated best.
   c. Observe closely for aspiration pneumonia and give an antibiotic at first sign.

Diets of Choice—Highly-digestible diet.

Dog—Canned Prescription Diet Canine i/d or Recipe 1 or 6.

Cat—Canned Prescription Diet Feline c/d or Recipe 6.

RENAL FAILURE
(See Chapter 8)

Aim—To reduce the need for, and slow or prevent the loss of, renal function.

Management

1. Initiate dietary management at the first sign of renal failure. Delay in altering the diet will accelerate progression of the disease.

2. Meet energy needs with non-protein calories. Restrict protein and phosphorus intakes as needed to control clinical signs of renal failure, BUN, and hyperphosphatemia. Following diagnosis, the dog should be fed a moderately restricted diet containing in the dry matter:

   a. Not more than 17% protein (14% protein calories) of a biologic value of 80 or greater.

   b. Not more than 0.4% phosphorus.

   c. Between 0.2-0.4% sodium.

Such a diet provides a protein intake of approximately 2.2 g/kg body weight daily .

3. If BUN exceeds 60 mg/dl **when a dog is eating the moderately restricted diet exclusively,** feed a severely restricted protein diet containing in the dry matter:

   a. Not more than 11% protein (8% protein calories) of a biologic value approaching 100.

   b. Not more than 0.2% phosphorus.

   c. Between 0.2-0.4% sodium.

Such a diet provides a protein intake of approximately 1.5 g/kg body weight daily .

4. Provide fresh water free choice.

5. For cats, feed not more than 4.5 g protein/kg body weight daily. The diet should contain not more than 23% protein calories, 0.6% phosphorus, and 0.5% sodium in the dry matter.

Considerations

1. For a discussion of prevention of renal failure see Chapter 8.

2. Phosphate binders are only effective when dietary phosphorus is being restricted.

Diets of Choice–Restricted protein, phosphorus, and sodium diet.

Prevention

Dog—Prescription Diet Canine c/d, w/d, g/d, Recipe 2 or other maintenance diet containing less than 25% protein, 0.8% phosphorus and 0.5% sodium.

Cat—Prescription Diet Feline c/d or other maintenance diet containing less than 0.8% phosphorus and 0.5% sodium.

Management

Dog—Moderate Renal Failure—Prescription Diet Canine k/d or Recipe 2.

Advanced Renal Failure—Prescription Diet Canine u/d or Recipe 3.

Acute Renal Failure—Prescription Diet Canine u/d or Recipe 3.

Cat—Prescription Diet Feline k/d or Recipe 9.

REPRODUCTION
(See pages 3-6 and 4-7)

Aim–To feed a diet that provides in readily utilizable form the increased amounts of nutrients needed for gestation and maximal milk production while maintaining body weight.

Management

1. Prior to breeding:

   a. Perform a thorough physical examination.

   b. Check, and if necessary, treat for internal and external parasites.

   c. Vaccinate so that a good immunity is passed to the young.

   d. Adjust her to optimal body weight.

2. Particularly during the last 3 weeks of gestation and throughout lactation feed a diet that contains the recommended nutrient levels (see table below).

3. Feed the amount necessary so that optimal non-pregnant body weight increases 15-25% during gestation and is maintained during lactation. Frequently this requires limiting food intake during gestation and the feeding of an excellent quality high-energy food free-choice during lactation.

DIET CHARACTERISTICS RECOMMENDED FOR REPRODUCTION[a]

| | Metabolizable kcal/lb | % in Food Dry Matter[b] | | | | | | |
		Digestibility[c]	Protein	Fat	Fiber	Ca	P	Sodium
Dog	≥ 1750[d]	> 80	> 29	≥ 17	< 5	1.0–1.8	0.8–1.6	0.3–0.7
Cat	≥ 2000	> 80	> 35	≥ 17	< 5	1.0–1.8	0.8–1.6	0.3–0.7

a,b,c,d
  See footnotes in Table under Maintenance (page 13-13).

Considerations—If eclampsia has occurred previously, start the puppies eating solid food by 3 weeks of age and, if necessary, supplement them with a milk replacer.

Diets of Choice—Highly-digestible, high-energy diet balanced for reproduction.

Dog—Prescription Diet Canine p/d, Recipe 1, or other diet that contains the recommended nutrient levels and has been proven to be nutritionally adequate by feeding tests.

Cat—Prescription Diet Feline p/d, Recipe 8 substituting 2 tablespoons of dicalcium phosphate for the 1 teaspoon of calcium carbonate and adding 1 teaspoon of table salt, or other diet that contains the recommended nutrient levels and has been proven to be nutritionally adequate by feeding tests.

SKELETAL DISEASES
(See Chapter 12)

Aim—To provide a balanced diet which is nutritionally adequate for the particular stage of the life cycle.

Management—The differential diagnosis of skeletal diseases of nutritional origin from clinical signs is difficult at best. The first consideration is to insure that a diet proven to be nutritionally adequate is being fed in an amount that prevents excessive growth. If a balanced growth diet is being fed (see page 13-10), reduce food intake by 25% rather than adding mineral supplements. The diet should provide calcium and phosphorus at a 1:1 to 2:1 ratio from a readily available source (such as dicalcium phosphate) at the rate of at least 500 mg calcium and 400 mg phosphorus/kg body weight daily. For cats, provide at least one-half this amount. A diet containing more than 2.0% calcium in the dry matter is contraindicated.

Considerations—Do not administer supplemental minerals. Large amounts of calcium, even when balanced with phosphorus, are contraindicated due to their adverse effect on availability of trace minerals and their inducement of hypercalcitoninism and the resulting skeletal problems. Minerals are the least likely nutrients to be deficient if a commercially prepared diet, especially a dry dog food, is being fed, as most contain excessive amounts of minerals, especially calcium and phosphorus.

Diets of Choice—Diet balanced for growth.

Dog—Prescription Diet Canine p/d.

Cat—Prescription Diet Feline p/d.

Homemade diets are not recommended for the dietary management of skeletal diseases due to their susceptibility to nutrient fluctuation at the whim of the pet owner, which can be detrimental to the recovery of the patient.

SOFT TISSUE WOUNDS

Aim—To provide a diet adequate in those nutrients essential to tissue repair, primarily protein and energy.

Management—If the previously fed diet is marginal or questionable, change to a diet designed for growth until healing is complete.

Diets of Choice—High protein and energy diet balanced for growth.

Dog and Cat—Prescription Diet Canine or Feline p/d, respectively or other diet that has been proven to be nutritionally adequate for growth by feeding tests.

SURGERY, GASTROINTESTINAL
(See Chapter 5)

Aim—To provide adequate high quality protein and energy necessary for tissue repair and regeneration in a highly digestible form.

Management

Esophagus

1. Insert a gastrostomy tube at the time of surgery and feed for at least one week a liquid diet that meets all water and nutrient needs. An esophageal incision reaches its maximum strength 6-8 days after surgery.

2. If a gastrostomy tube is not inserted, withhold food and liquid ingestion for 3-4 days postsurgically. Meet fluid needs parenterally. For the next 3-5 days feed small amounts 3-6 times daily of a highly-digestible canned diet made into a slurry with water. Over the next 3-5 days, decrease the amount of water added to the diet so that the animal is eating only the canned diet within 10-14 days postsurgically. Convert gradually to an appropriate diet (growth or maintenance type) 2-3 weeks postsurgically.

Stomach

1. Withhold food, water, and oral medication for 24-48 hours postsurgically.

2. For the next several days, feed small amounts 3-6 times daily of a highly-digestible canned diet made into a slurry with water, or feed a liquid diet such as Recipe 7. Avoid bulky foods.

3. Over several days, decrease the water added to the diet. Convert gradually to an appropriate

diet (growth or maintenance type) 2-3 weeks postsurgically.

Intestine
1. Nothing should be given when ileus is encountered following enterotomy (24-96 hours), unless an enterostomy catheter was inserted at the time of surgery and an elemental diet (Table 11, page 5-30) is being fed (Table 14, page 5-34).
2. Oral alimentation should be started with intestinal peristalsis. Offer small quantities of a highly-digestible diet and water frequently (4-6 times daily).

Diets of Choice—Liquid or highly-digestible diet.

Liquid diet (dogs or cats)—Recipe 7.

Dog—Prescription Diet Canine i/d or Recipe 1.

Cat—Prescription Diet Feline c/d or Recipe 8.

UROLITHIASIS, CANINE
(See Chapter 10)

Aim—To reduce urinary concentration of raw materials available for production of uroliths, maintain proper urine pH, and increase urine volume.

Management
1. If obstructed, manage as described for FUS (page 13-7).
2. Control urinary tract infection, if present, with antibiotics based upon culture and sensitivity (see page 10-19).
3. Determine the type of urolith most likely present (see page 10-13).
4. **Struvite** uroliths
   a. Dissolution—Feed 2-3 times daily a diet which is severely restricted in protein, phosphorus, and magnesium, high in salt, and maintains an acid urine. Continue for 1 month after uroliths are no longer visible radiographically, except to growing dogs, which should be fed the calculolytic diet only until uroliths can no longer be detected. **Urine acidifiers, salt, vitamin-mineral supplements, and any other foods are contraindicated.** If radiographic size or density of the uroliths has not decreased within 60 days:
      1) They are not struvite
      2) Something besides the struvitolytic diet is being consumed
      3) Urinary infection has not been controlled
   b. Prevention—Feed a maintenance diet with

restricted levels of protein, phosphorus, and magnesium, that maintains an acid urine.
5. **Ammonium Urate** uroliths
   a. Dissolution—Feed a diet which is severely restricted in protein, urate precursors (nucleic acids), and phosphorus and maintains an alkaline urine. If urine pH is below 7.0, give 1 g of sodium bicarbonate (1/4 teaspoon)/5 kg body weight every 8 hours. Give 10 mg/kg of allopurinol (Zyloprim, Burroughs Wellcome) 3 times daily. Continue until 4 weeks after the uroliths are no longer visable radiographically. During dissolution observe for obstruction. If it occurs, flush the urolith back into the bladder.
   b. **Prevention—**Feed the same diet recommended for dissolution, but delete allopurinol. If uroliths recur, reduce dosage to 10 mg/kg/day following dissolution.
6. **Calcium oxalate, cystine, or silicate** uroliths
   a. Remove surgically
   b. Prevention—Feed a diet restricted in protein, phosphorus, calcium, sodium, magnesium, oxalate, and silicate.

Diets of Choice—Restricted protein and mineral diet that maintains the proper urine pH.

Struvite uroliths

　Dissolution—Prescription Diet Canine s/d.

　Prevention—Prescription Diet Canine c/d.

Ammonium urate uroliths

　Dissolution—Prescription Diet Canine u/d plus allopurinol.

　Prevention—Prescription Diet Canine u/d.

Calcium oxalate, cystine, or silicate uroliths

　Removal—surgical.

　Prevention—Prescription Diet Canine u/d.

VOMITING
(See page 7-13)

Aim—To manage gastritis and meet nutritional needs with a diet that stimulates minimal gastric secretion, and is easily digested and absorbed.

Management
1. Withhold all food for 24-48 hours and water for 24 hours.
2. If the cause of vomiting is detected from history and physical examination, institute the specific therapy indicated.
3. If vomiting has stopped, over the next 3-5 days gradually return the patient to full feed and water.

4. Feed small amounts of a highly-digestible diet 3-6 times daily. Begin with one-third the amount needed to meet the animal's requirements. Gradually increase amount fed over the next several days.

5. If vomiting persists, do a complete evaluation to determine cause (Figure 3, page 7-14) and appropriate therapy, and give metoclopramide (Reglan, AH Robins) at 0.2-0.4 mg/kg 2-4 times daily.

Considerations—If dehydration is present, correct it by giving parenterally isotonic saline solution with 10-30 mEq/L of potassium chloride.

Diets of Choice—Highly-digestible diet.

Dog—Prescription Diet Canine i/d or Recipe 1 or 6.

Cat—Prescription Diet Feline c/d or Recipe 6.

APPENDIX TABLE 1

DIET TYPES

Occasionally the clinician has need for a specialized type of diet. The purpose of this table is to categorize various diets according to their nutritional characteristics allowing the clinician to rapidly find diets that meet a specific characteristic. Unless specifically stated otherwise, naming of a prepared diet includes both dry and canned forms. All recipes refer to those given in Appendix Table 3.

Low Protein Diets (% protein calories):
Prepared: Canine c/d (19), g/d (17), w/d (17), k/d (13), u/d (8), s/d (6.5)
Feline k/d (22), c/d—dry (27)
Homemade: Recipe 2 (17), Recipe 3 (8), Recipe 9 (21)

High Protein–Low Carbohydrate (% protein calories, % carbohydrate calories)
Prepared: Feline p/d (40, 6.6), many gourmet cat foods (check label for lack of cereal ingredients)
Homemade: To 1 lb of lean cooked ground beef, add 1/2 tsp of calcium carbonate, ground egg shells or 3 Tums Tablets (52, 0)

Low Fat–Low Calorie (% fat, kcal ME/g in dry matter)
Prepared: Canine w/d (7, 3.1), r/d (7, 2.5)
Feline r/d (7, 2.5)
Homemade: Recipe 4 (12, 4.0), Recipe 10 (11, 4.3)

High Fat–High Calorie (% fat, kcal ME/g in dry matter)
Prepared: Canine k/d—can (19.8, 4.7), Science Diet Performance—can (32, 5.3)
Feline p/d—can (32, 5.1), s/d—can (34, 5.2), k/d—can (44, 5.0)
Homemade: Recipe 6 (29, 5.1), Recipe 8 (38, 5.7)

Low Fiber–Highly Digestible (% fiber, % digestibility of dry matter)
Prepared: Canine k/d—can (0.7, 87), k/d—dry (0.9, 90), i/d (0.7, 88)
Feline k/d (0.7, 84)
Homemade: Recipe 1 (0.4, >90)

High Fiber (% fiber in dry matter)
Prepared: Canine w/d (16), r/d—dry (22), r/d—can (25)
Feline r/d—dry (18), r/d—can (28)

Low Sodium (% sodium in dry matter)
Prepared: Canine h/d—dry (0.05), h/d—can (0.09), k/d (0.23), u/d (0.26), w/d (0.23), c/d (0.29)
Feline h/d (0.24)
Homemade: Recipe 5 (0.05), Recipe 8 (0.16)

Low Mineral (% in dry matter)

Prepared—dog	Calcium	Phosphorus	Magnesium
s/d	0.27	0.12	0.02
u/d	0.4	0.13	0.04
k/d	0.78	0.28	0.08
c/d	0.8	0.52	0.10
w/d	0.5	0.48	0.09
Homemade—dog			
Recipe 2	1.0	0.28	0.04
Recipe 3	0.4	0.22	0.03
Prepared—cat			
Feline s/d	0.7	0.6	0.06
Feline c/d	0.8	0.7	0.08
Feline k/d	0.8	0.5	0.07
Homemade—cat			
Recipe 8	0.8	0.5	0.04
Recipe 9	1.2	0.5	0.04

Low Copper (mg/kg dry matter)
Prepared: Canine u/d—can (4.0), dry (4.4)
Homemade: Recipe 1 (4.6) and 3 (1.7)

Low Urate Precursor (low purine–nucleic acids)
Prepared: Canine u/d, s/d, d/d—dry, k/d—dry
Homemade: Recipe 3
Feline 5 eggs, hard-cooked
2 cups cooked rice
1 t calcium carbonate (ground egg shells)

Restricted Protein Source Diets for Food Allergy (Protein Sources)
(Protein Sources)
Dry: Canine d/d (egg, rice), s/d (egg, rice), k/d (corn, rice, egg, casein)
Canned: Canine d/d (mutton, rice), u/d (rice, casein), s/d (egg, liver)
Homemade: Recipe 6 (mutton, rice), Recipe 3 (egg, rice)
Recipe 5 (beef, rice)
Recipe 9 (liver, egg, rice)

Meat Free
Prepared: Canine k/d—dry, u/d—dry, d/d—dry, s/d—dry
Feline—not recommended
Homemade: Recipes 1, 3

Soy Free
Dry: Canine k/d, u/d, i/d, g/d, h/d, d/d, s/d, w/d
Feline—All Prescription Diets
Canned: Canine k/d, u/d, c/d, s/d, h/d, i/d, d/d, g/d, w/d
Feline—All Prescription Diets
Homemade: All Recipes as formulated

Lactose Free
Prepared: Dry—Canine i/d, h/d, r/d, d/d, s/d
Feline c/d, s/d, p/d
Canned—Canine k/d, u/d, i/d, r/d, h/d, d/d, p/d, s/d, c/d
Feline k/d, s/d
Homemade: Recipes, 2, 3, 5, 6, 7, 8, 9, 10

Gluten Free Diets
Prepared: Dry—Canine d/d, s/d
Canned—Canine d/d, u/d, s/d
Homemade: All Recipes as formulated except 1 and 2.

"Additive" Free
Veterinarians are occasionally confronted by a client who wants to feed a diet containing no chemical additives, even though these substances have no adverse effect on the animal. The following dietary foods contain no antioxidants, emulsifiers, colors, flavors or other items frequently referred to as "additives" by the public.
Prepared: Canned—All Prescription Diet products
Homemade: None as formulated

Low Urine pH Producing (urine pH when fed free choice)
Prepared: Canine s/d (5.9–6.2), c/d (6.0–6.3)
Feline s/d (5.9), c/d (6.0–6.3), Science Diet Feline Maintenance (6.0–6.3), Friskies Buffet Beef & Liver Dinner (6.3)

High Urine pH Producing (urine pH when fed free choice)
Prepared: Canine u/d (7.6), Ken-L-Ration (7.3), Purina Dog Chow (7.9)

Liquid or Tube Feeding—See Table 10, page 5–29

Orphan—See Table 3, page 3–18

APPENDIX TABLE 2

PREPARED DIETARY FOODS

PRESCRIPTION DIETS

Prescription Diets are dietary animal foods designed for prevention and/or management of specific physiologic or disease conditions in dogs and cats. Their proper use, like all aspects of clinical management, is dependent upon correct diagnosis and monitoring of alterations, progression, and deviations of the disease process and response to treatment. Therefore, they should be used only under the direction of a veterinarian.

PRESCRIPTION DIET CANINE k/d
Nutritional Characteristics
Protein—moderately restricted, high quality
Fat and Carbohydrate—increased
Calcium, Phosphorus, and Magnesium—restricted
Vitamins—increased
Sodium—moderately restricted

Average Nutrient Contents

	As Fed		Dry Matter	
	Canned	Dry	Canned	Dry
Moisture %	73.3	9.0	0	0
Protein %	4.3	13.5	16.1	14.8
Fat %	7.3	18.0	27.3	19.8
Carbohydrate %	14.1	56.0	52.8	61.5
Fiber %	0.2	0.8	0.7	0.9
Ash %	0.8	2.7	3.0	3.0
Calcium %	0.12	0.36	0.45	0.4
Phosphorus %	0.07	0.26	0.26	0.28
Sodium %	0.06	0.21	0.22	0.23

ME (kcal)	1.4/g	4.3/g	5.1/g	4.7/g
	612/can	350/cup		
% Protein Calories	13.2	12.7		

Discussion
Animal proteins from chicken, egg, and liver, and plant protein from corn and rice form a protein blend which is utilized by the dog's body in excess of 90%. Protein of this quality allows reduction of amino acids consumed in excess of requirements, thereby reducing the load on the liver for deamination and on the kidneys for the excretion of nitrogenous wastes. Readily available sources of glucose to aid liver function, combined with readily digestible animal fat from chicken, provide sufficient calories from non-protein sources to meet the energy requirements and prevent the excessive utilization of protein for energy. Unsaturated fatty acids from vegetable oil and egg are important for healthy skin and hair coat. A phosphorus level, which meets adult maintenance needs but limits excesses, reduces urinary phosphorus excretion and aids in reducing phosphate retention that occurs with reduced renal function. A moderately-restricted sodium level is beneficial in preventing hypertension associated with renal failure, in providing moderate dietary sodium restriction for the early phases of heart failure, and in controlling ascites and/or edema that may occur with hepatic dysfunction. In addition to its use in dogs with renal, cardiac, and hepatic diseases not requiring a low fat diet, it also can be used successfully to manage other conditions requiring a uniform diet with moderately restricted protein balanced to a moderate calorie density. It is nutritionally adequate for adult dogs, but should not be fed to puppies or reproducing bitches due to the restricted protein and mineral levels. Due to its high energy content, food intake should be controlled to maintain optimal body weight..

PRESCRIPTION DIET CANINE u/d
Nutritional Characteristics
Protein—restricted, high quality
Urate precursors—severely restricted
Fat and Carbohydrate—increased
Calcium, Phosphorus, Magnesium, and Oxalate—
    severely restricted
Vitamins—increased
Sodium—moderately restricted
Urine pH—alkaline

Average Nutrient Contents

	As Fed		Dry Matter	
	Canned	Dry	Canned	Dry
Moisture %	72.1	9.0	0	0
Protein %	2.9	8.6	10.4	9.5
Fat %	7.6	19.1	27.2	21.0
Carbohydrate %	16.3	58.8	58.4	64.6

Fiber %	0.4	2.0	1.4	2.2
Ash %	0.7	2.5	2.5	2.7
Calcium %	0.11	0.37	0.39	0.4
Phosphorus %	0.04	0.12	0.14	0.13
Potassium %	0.1	0.40	0.36	0.44
Sodium %	0.07	0.24	0.24	0.26
Magnesium %	0.009	0.04	0.03	0.04
Copper mg/kg	1.1	4.0	4.0	4.4
ME (kcal)	1.5/g	4.5/g	5.3/g	5.0/g
	662/can	291/cup		
% Protein Calories	7.9	8.0		

Discussion

Dogs with advanced renal failure have difficulty in excreting even small amounts of protein catabolic wastes and phosphorus. This diet contains restricted levels of protein and phosphorus and a moderate level of sodium. The protein is derived from casein and methionine, which contain no nucleic acids (urate precursors), and has a biological value of 100, which means it is completely utilized by the dog, resulting in very little excess nitrogen to be excreted by the impaired kidneys. Although this diet is low in protein, due to the high digestibility and biological value of the protein, healthy dogs still obtain 30% more protein than required for maintenance. The extra dietary protein for dogs with renal failure is required because, while these dogs have a decreased ability to tolerate excess protein, their minimum protein requirement is higher than healthy dogs. This necessitates a higher dietary protein level than would be required in a diet consumed by dogs with normal renal function. To accomplish this low protein level, energy is supplied from animal fat, vegetable oil and highly-digestible carbohydrates from starch, sugar, and rice.

Prescription Diet u/d contains high amounts of B-vitamins to compensate for their loss with polyuria. As a result, supplementation with vitamins or minerals is not necessary in most cases of renal failure. The diet is designed to combat the metabolic acidosis that may occur with advanced renal failure. Its metabolism results in an alkaline urine.

A diet such as u/d, with restriction of protein, calcium, phosphorus, and nucleic acids, and moderate restriction of sodium, should be fed to dogs with advanced renal failure which develop uremia when eating Prescription Diet k/d exclusively, or dogs with acute renal failure.

Consumption of u/d results in an alkaline urine and reduced urinary concentrations of urea, ammonium, urate, cystine, phosphorus, calcium, and oxalate. As a result, it is beneficial in the dietary management of ammonium urate, cystine, and calcium oxalate uroliths. It should not be fed to dogs with struvite urolithiasis, which require a diet whose metabolism results in an acid urine, or puppies or reproducing bitches. Supplementation with other foods, vitamins, or minerals is contraindicated.

PRESCRIPTION DIET CANINE s/d
Nutritional Characteristics

Protein—severely restricted, high quality
Fat and Carbohydrate—increased
Magnesium, Phosphorus, and Calcium—severely restricted
Sodium—moderately elevated
Urine pH—acid

Average Nutrient Contents

	As Fed		Dry Matter	
	Canned	Dry	Canned	Dry
Moisture %	71.0	9.0	0	0
Protein %	2.2	8.5	7.6	9.4
Fat %	7.6	20.3	26.2	22.3
Carbohydrate %	17.2	55.4	59.3	60.9
Fiber %	0.7	2.2	2.4	2.4
Ash %	1.3	4.6	4.5	5.0
Calcium %	0.08	0.31	0.27	0.34
Phosphorus %	0.036	0.13	0.12	0.14
Magnesium %	0.005	0.03	0.017	0.032
Sodium %	0.35	1.1	1.2	1.2
ME (kcal)	1.5/g	4.4/g	5.1/g	4.9/g
	670/can	336/cup		
% Protein Calories	6.5	8.1		

Discussion

Calories are supplied by carbohydrates, animal fats, and vegetable oil. Protein is derived from egg and liver— a protein blend of high biologic value. This makes possible a severely restricted level, which is adequate for maintenance of most mature dogs. Minimizing protein intake reduces urinary urea available for ammonia production by urease positive bacteria. Along with magnesium and phosphorus restriction, and the elevated salt content, which induces diuresis, these dietary characteristics reduce urine concentrations of the "building blocks" for magnesium-ammonium-phosphate (struvite) calculi. The metabolism of the diet results in the production of an acid urine. The hypoconcentrated and acid urine allows struvite calculi to dissolve. Supplements of **any** type, including human or prepared pet foods and urine acidifiers, will delay or prevent urolith dissolution. An untreated urinary tract infection will also delay urolith dissolution. Because of its severely restricted protein and mineral contents and elevated sodium content, it is not recommended if edema, ascites, or congestion are present, or during growth, reproduction, following surgery, or for prevention of recurrence of struvite urolithiasis following dissolution or surgical removal. Prescription Diet Canine c/d should be fed for prevention of struvite urolithiasis.

PRESCRIPTION DIET CANINE c/d
Nutritional Characteristics

Protein—restricted
Fat and carbohydrate—increased
Calcium, Phosphorus, and Magnesium—restricted
Sodium—moderately restricted
Urine pH—acid

Average Nutrient Contents

	As Fed		Dry Matter	
	Canned	Dry	Canned	Dry
Moisture %	72.8	9.0	0	0

Protein %	6.2	20.2	22.8	22.2
Fat %	6.5	19.5	24.0	21.4
Carbohydrate %	13.3	44.8	48.9	49.3
Fiber %	0.1	2.2	0.3	2.4
Ash %	1.1	4.2	4.0	4.7
Calcium %	0.16	0.74	0.60	0.81
Phosphorus %	0.12	0.47	0.44	0.52
Sodium %	0.07	0.26	0.25	0.29
Magnesium %	0.02	0.09	0.07	0.10
ME (kcal)	1.4/g	4.3/g	4.9/g	4.7/g
	602/can	364/cup		
% Protein Calories	19.5	19.0		

Discussion

This diet combines low ash animal proteins from liver, meat by-products, chicken, and egg with plant proteins from rice, corn, and soy, resulting in an amino acid blend that allows reduction in dietary protein content. The cooked carbohydrates from rice and corn, with animal fats, and vegetable oil produce a highly-digestible, restricted-mineral diet. Since adult dogs have very low mineral requirements and consumption of excessive minerals over extended periods of time have been shown to accelerate the development of renal and cardiac failure and urolithiasis, such a diet is beneficial in preventing or delaying their development.

Maintenance of an acid urine and reduction of urine concentrations of phosphorus, magnesium, ammonia, and urea are important in allowing struvite uroliths to dissolve, and in preventing their recurrence. This diet accomplishes these goals due to its restricted content of protein and minerals. In addition to its use in dogs to prevent recurrence of struvite uroliths following dissolution with Prescription Diet Canine s/d or surgical removal, it is also beneficial for maintenance of active adult dogs as a part of a preventive medicine program to delay or reduce the incidence of renal or cardiac diseases.

PRESCRIPTION DIET CANINE p/d
Nutritional Characteristics

Protein—increased
Fat—increased
Carbohydrate—decreased
Minerals and Vitamins—increased

Average Nutrient Contents

	As Fed		Dry Matter	
	Canned	Dry	Canned	Dry
Moisture %	70.1	9.0	0	0
Protein %	9.4	29.4	31.4	32.3
Fat %	7.8	21.0	26.1	23.1
Carbohydrate %	10.3	31.1	34.4	34.2
Fiber %	0.3	3.0	1.0	3.3
Ash %	2.1	7.5	7.0	8.2
Calcium %	0.38	1.6	1.24	1.75
Phosphorus %	0.32	1.1	1.14	1.32
Sodium %	0.17	0.31	0.57	0.34
Potassium %	0.24	0.75	0.80	0.82
ME (kcal)	1.5/g	4.2/g	4.9/g	4.6/g
	663/can	395/cup		

Discussion

Adequate amounts of digestible protein and energy are imperative for optimal growth, lactation, and recovery from debilitation. By combining large quantities of animal protein from chicken, liver, egg, soy, and meat by-products, a highly usable protein blend is formed. The energy derived when the carbohydrate from cooked cereal is combined with animal and vegetable fats supplies both the immediate and long-term needs of the growing dog.

Because of the rapid development of bone during the growth period, minerals, particularly calcium and phosphorus, are supplied in a form highly available to dogs. Dicalcium phosphate, calcium carbonate, finely ground bone, and phosphorus contained in meat are readily digested forms of these minerals. While supplying adequate amounts of these important minerals, it avoids the excessive amounts of calcium present in many dog foods, which cause hypercalcitoninism and skeletal problems during growth. The availability of minerals has added significance in the pregnant and lactating bitch. If poorly available, as is the case with phytin phosphorus in high-cereal dry dog foods, the bitch will mobilize these minerals from her own bones to maintain levels in her milk.

Although rarely a problem in non-reproducing adult dogs, the most common deficiency in a lactating bitch's diet is energy. By providing an increased level of dietary fat, it is possible to provide adequate calories to maintain the lactating bitch at a constant weight, and still furnish her with sufficient energy to produce the milk needed for a large litter of rapidly growing pups.

A high-protein, high-energy diet has several applications in clinical medicine. It can be used for dietary management of debilitation, anemias, hypoproteinemia, prior to and during immunization, and for pre- and postoperative care, as well as optimal growth of puppies and reproducing bitches. It should not be fed long-term to adult dogs, especially those which are overweight or those suffering from renal or hepatic failure.

PRESCRIPTION DIET CANINE r/d
Nutritional Characteristics

Fat—severely restricted
Carbohydrate (digestible)—restricted
Fiber—greatly increased

Average Nutrient Contents

	As Fed		Dry Matter	
	Canned	Dry	Canned	Dry
Moisture %	75.8	9.0	0	0
Protein %	6.2	22.7	25.6	25.0
Fat %	1.7	6.4	7.0	7.0
Carbohydrate %	8.7	35.2	36.0	38.7
Fiber %	6.1	19.8	25.2	21.8
Ash %	1.5	6.9	6.2	7.6
Calcium %	0.13	0.9	0.5	1.0
Phosphorus %	0.09	0.6	0.36	0.66
Sodium %	0.07	0.3	0.3	0.3
ME (kcal)	0.6/g	2.3/g	2.4/g	2.5/g
	260/can	200/cup		

Discussion

By using low-calorie ingredients such as lean meat by-products, liver, meat meal and soy as protein sources and soybean hulls and cellulose flour as carbohydrate sources, the digestibility of the calories in the diet is reduced and the fiber content (bulk) increased. The amount of fat in the diet is restricted to a small amount of vegetable oil to supply unsaturated fatty acids. The resulting low-calorie, high-fiber diet is effective in reducing or controlling body weight.

Consumption of a high fiber diet tends to satisfy hunger, whereas simply reducing food intake creates a food beggar. This type of diet can be used in any case where restriction of energy or fat intake is desirable, such as obesity, weight control, hypothyroidism with obesity, and hyperlipidemia. It is also useful in conditions where increased fiber intake is desirable, such as constipation, diabetes mellitus, lymphangietasia, and colitis. A high-fiber diet helps prevent constipation as it increases intestinal volume and contractions and holds more water in the colon. In the management of diabetes mellitis, fiber minimizes fluctuation of blood glucose and allows reduction and stabilization of insulin dosage. Its sodium content is mildly restricted to allow its use in obesity complicated with congestive heart failure. It should not be used in pancreatic exocrine insufficiency due to the large amount of bulky indigestible carbohydrates. It is also contraindicated in dogs requiring a high energy intake, such as during growth, reproduction, stress, or physical exertion.

PRESCRIPTION DIET CANINE w/d
Nutritional Characteristics

Protein—restricted
Fat and Carbohydrate (digestible)—moderately restricted
Fiber—increased
Calcium, Phosphorus, and Magnesium—restricted
Sodium—moderately restricted

Average Nutrient Contents

	As Fed		Dry Matter	
	Canned	Dry	Canned	Dry
Moisture %	73.5	9.0	0	0
Protein %	4.3	15.4	16.2	16.9
Fat %	3.2	6.7	12.1	7.4
Carbohydrate %	14.7	49.1	55.5	53.9
Fiber %	3.5	14.5	13.2	15.9
Ash %	0.8	5.3	3.0	5.8
Calcium %	0.12	0.5	0.45	0.55
Phosphorus %	0.10	0.44	0.38	0.48
Sodium %	0.06	0.21	0.22	0.23
Magnesium %	0.025	0.08	0.09	0.09
ME (kcal)	1.0/g	2.9/g	3.6/g	3.1/g
	432/can	220/cup		
% Protein Calories	16.2	18.6		

Discussion

This diet combines cellulose, rice, chicken, liver, egg, and milk, which results in a diet that contains high quality protein, low fat, increased fiber, and low contents of minerals. Such a diet is effective for the dietary management of several common canine clinical diseases, obesity being the most common (see Chapter 6). The optimal management of obesity requires consumption of a very low calorie diet that will result in weight loss, and a moderately low calorie maintenance diet that prevents recurrence of obesity after the patient reaches its optimum body weight. In theory, it should be possible for the owner to control the dog's food intake to maintain optimum body weight once it has been reached. The reality is that the owner cannot or will not control the dog's food intake. The solution is to feed a diet moderately restricted in calories.

In addition to its use in dogs to prevent obesity, a diet containing increased fiber has been shown to be beneficial in the clinical management of diabetes mellitus, due to the reduced and delayed absorption of glucose from the intestine following eating. This effect reduces the fluctuations in blood glucose that occur when diets containing more digestible carbohydrates are fed, and allows reduction and stabilization of insulin dosage. The clinical management of both constipation and colitis also are benefited by feeding a diet with an increased fiber content.

Any effective canine preventive medicine program includes prevention of obesity and renal and cardiac diseases. This diet can be beneficially used for maintenance of inactive adult dogs to prevent these extremely common canine diseases.

PRESCRIPTION DIET CANINE i/d
Nutritional Characteristics

Protein—high quality and digestible
Fat—moderately restricted and highly digestible
Carbohydrate—highly digestible
Fiber—restricted
Electrolytes and Vitamins—increased

Average Nutrient Contents

	As Fed		Dry Matter	
	Canned	Dry	Canned	Dry
Moisture %	70.1	9.0	0	0
Protein %	7.6	24.8	25.4	27.3
Fat %	4.4	13.2	14.7	14.5
Carbohydrate %	15.3	45.0	51.2	49.4
Fiber %	0.2	0.8	0.7	0.9
Ash %	2.4	7.2	8.0	7.9
Calcium %	0.36	1.3	1.2	1.4
Phosphorus %	0.27	1.0	0.9	1.1
Sodium %	0.15	0.48	0.5	0.5
ME (kcal)	1.3/g	3.9/g	4.3/g	4.3/g
	580/can	332/cup		

Discussion

Eggs, chicken, and liver are some of the most easily digested, low-residue sources of high-quality protein for dogs. Dextrose, and properly cooked rice and cornstarch are highly-digestible carbohydrate sources having a low-fiber content, essential factors in a low-residue diet. A highly-digestible diet that leaves little

residue is a versatile tool for the veterinary clinician. The most obvious use is in gastrointestinal disturbances. It also can be used for early weaning of pups (3-5 weeks of age) and for pre- and postoperative nutritional support, especially for patients recovering from gastrointestinal surgery.

Some patients with disorders of the liver are able to tolerate increased dietary fat, while others cannot tolerate a high fat intake due to reduced bile secretion. For these patients, energy must be supplied by easily utilized, digestible carbohydrates which help restore liver glycogen. The protein content of a diet for hepatic disease patients should be mildly restricted, adequate to allow tissue regeneration, but not excessive to prevent hepatic encephalopathy. For liver disease patients which are able to tolerate fat, Prescription Diet Canine k/d is the diet of choice. For those with steatorrhea or diarrhea requiring a fat restricted diet, Prescription Diet Canine i/d is preferred. For those with ascites or edema requiring sodium restriction, Prescription Diet Canine h/d is preferred, and if hepatic encephalopathy develops, Prescription Diet u/d is the proper diet.

Many cases of pancreatic insufficiency can be managed by feeding a highly-digestible diet without added pancreatic enzymes. For severe pancreatic disease, both dietary management and pancreatic enzyme therapy are necessary to maximize digestion of orally consumed food.

PRESCRIPTION DIET CANINE g/d
Nutritional Characteristics
Protein—mildly restricted
Fat and Carbohydrate—mildly restricted
Fiber—increased
Vitamins—increased
Minerals—mildly restricted
Unsaturated fatty acids—increased
Salt—mildly restricted

Average Nutrient Contents

	As Fed		Dry Matter	
	Canned	Dry	Canned	Dry
Moisture %	73.3	9.0	0	0
Protein %	5.0	16.8	18.7	18.5
Fat %	4.0	9.7	15.0	10.7
Carbohydrate %	15.9	58.3	59.5	64.0
Fiber %	0.8	3.1	3.7	3.4
Ash %	0.8	3.1	3.0	3.4
Calcium %	0.16	0.61	0.6	0.67
Phosphorus %	0.12	0.45	0.45	0.61
Sodium %	0.08	0.26	0.30	0.28
Potassium %	0.1	0.32	0.37	0.35
ME (kcal)	1.2/g 540/can	3.7/g 282/cup	4.5/g	4.0/g
% Protein Calories	16.9	17.7		

Discussion
The incidence of a number of diseases requiring dietary management increases significantly with age. The geriatric dog has a low protein requirement compared to the growing pup. Prescription Diet Canine g/d

contains high quality protein at a mildly restricted level. This reduces the excess which must be metabolized for energy and the waste nitrogen excreted, thereby delaying the onset of the clinical signs of renal failure common in older dogs.

Vitamins of specific interest in canine geriatrics are the B-complex vitamins, thiamine, choline, folic acid, and B-12. Vitamin E and niacin are recommended to improve circulation. A decreased intake of vitamin D is appropriate, due to its role in enhancing calcium deposition in arthritic joints. Prescription Diet Canine g/d contains increased amounts of all B-complex vitamins and vitamin E, a reduced level of vitamin D, and fresh liver and whole egg to supply choline, inositol, and lipotropic vitamins.

Mild phosphorus restriction is indicated in a diet for all adult dogs, especially geriatric dogs, to prevent parathyroid hormone and phosphorus retention, which occur as renal function declines. Sodium is present at a mildly restricted level compared to regular dog foods. This aids in delaying the onset of the clinical signs of congestive heart disease which is common in older dogs.

PRESCRIPTION DIET CANINE h/d
Nutritional Characteristics
Sodium—severely restricted
Potassium—increased
Protein—mildly restricted
Fat and Carbohydrate—increased
Vitamins—increased

Average Nutrient Contents

	As Fed		Dry Matter	
	Canned	Dry	Canned	Dry
Moisture %	72.2	9.0	0	0
Protein %	4.8	15.9	17.3	17.5
Fat %	8.0	19.3	28.8	21.2
Carbohydrate %	13.6	49.8	48.9	54.7
Fiber %	0.2	1.0	0.7	1.1
Ash %	1.2	5.0	4.3	5.5
Calcium %	0.15	0.7	0.54	0.77
Phosphorus %	0.12	0.5	0.43	0.55
Sodium %	0.026	0.05	0.09	0.055
Potassium %	0.33	0.94	1.18	1.03
ME (kcal)	1.4/g 648/can	4.2/g 336/cup	5.2/g	4.6/g
% Protein Calories	13.9	15.0		

Discussion
A balanced, low sodium diet must be composed of ingredients supplying adequate amounts of other nutrients yet a reduced amount of sodium. Sodium salts of trace minerals and vitamins are avoided. The fat level should be increased to supply needed calories in a smaller amount of food, thus reducing sodium intake even further. The potassium level should be adequate to replace losses from increased excretion caused by digitalis and diuretics, commonly used in treating congestive heart failure.

In addition to congestive heart failure, a diet low in

sodium also is valuable in the management of sodium retention from liver disease or corticosteroids. A low-sodium diet should not be fed to pregnant or rapidly growing dogs or those suffering from electrolyte imbalance, debilitation, or diarrhea.

PRESCRIPTION DIET CANINE d/d

Nutritional Characteristics

Protein and Fat—derived solely from rice and mutton tissues (canned), or rice and egg (dry)
Carbohydrate—derived solely from rice
Unsaturated fatty acids—increased

Average Nutrient Contents

	As Fed		Dry Matter	
	Canned	Dry	Canned	Dry
Moisture %	70.4	9.0	0	0
Protein %	7.9	14.8	26.7	16.3
Fat %	6.4	10.9	21.6	12.0
Carbohydrate %	12.9	60.6	43.6	66.6
Fiber %	1.0	1.4	3.4	1.5
Ash %	1.4	3.3	4.7	3.6
Calcium %	0.16	0.46	0.54	0.51
Phosphorus %	0.12	0.33	0.41	0.36
Sodium %	0.15	0.27	0.51	0.3
ME (kcal)	1.4/g	3.9/g	4.6/g	4.3/g
	617/can	295/cup		
% Protein Calories	22.9	16.1		

Discussion

The accurate diagnosis of the individual items responsible for food-induced allergy requires that the patient be fed a food containing ingredients either to which the patient has not been exposed or which have a tendency to be hypoallergenic. Because mutton, egg, and rice are suitable nutrient sources for dogs and cats and are not commonly present in prepared pet foods, mutton and rice are used to form the base of the canned hypoallergenic diet, and egg and rice the dry hypoallergenic diet. No preservatives are added to the canned diet, and only antioxidant ethoxyquin, to prevent fatty acid oxidation, is added to the dry diet. In addition to its use as a diagnostic tool, diets containing such infrequently consumed ingredients also can be used as a maintenance diet for dogs or cats which have been diagnosed as being allergic to ingredients commonly used in commercially prepared pet foods.

PRESCRIPTION DIET FELINE c/d

Nutritional Characteristics

Magnesium, Phosphorus, and Calcium—restricted
Fat—increased
Urine pH—acid

Average Nutrient Contents

	As Fed		Dry Matter	
	Canned	Dry	Canned	Dry
Moisture %	71.5	9.0	0	0
Protein %	12.5	31.0	43.9	34.0
Fat %	8.5	23.7	29.8	26.0
Carbohydrate %	5.7	30.6	20.0	33.7
Fiber %	0.4	1.6	1.4	1.8
Ash %	1.4	4.1	4.9	4.5
Calcium %	0.21	0.7	0.8	0.8
Phosphorus %	0.19	0.62	0.7	0.7
Magnesium %	0.02	0.07	0.07	0.08
Sodium %	0.15	0.42	0.52	0.46
ME (kcal)	1.4/g	4.3/g	5.0/g	4.7/g
	604/can	519/cup		
% Protein Calories	33.7	26.2		

Discussion

In contrast to protein and vitamins, cats do not require higher dietary levels of minerals than dogs. Minerals assimilated in excess of body needs are excreted in the urine and are available as building blocks for the formation of struvite crystals. If an individual cat is prone to develop feline urological syndrome (FUS), a high urinary magnesium concentration aids in the formation of struvite crystals leading to cystitis, hematuria, and obstruction. A restricted magnesium diet, whose metabolism results in an acid urine, is beneficial in the prevention and control of FUS (see Chapter 9).

The ingredients for this diet have been selected so the level of magnesium is restricted, yet adequate for normal maintenance, and urine remains acid even following eating, when the alkaline tide normally occurs. As a result, **urine acidifiers should not be given when it is being fed.**

PRESCRIPTION DIET FELINE s/d

Nutritional Characteristics

Fat—increased
Magnesium, Phosphorus, and Calcium—severely restricted
Sodium—increased
Urine pH—consistently acid

Average Nutrient Contents

	As Fed		Dry Matter	
	Canned	Dry	Canned	Dry
Moisture %	71.0	9.0	0	0
Protein %	12.0	31.9	41.4	35.0
Fat %	9.9	25.9	34.1	28.5
Carbohydrate %	5.2	26.3	17.9	28.9
Fiber %	0.4	1.0	1.4	1.1
Ash %	1.5	5.9	5.2	6.5
Calcium %	0.20	0.64	0.62	0.70
Phosphorus %	0.16	0.53	0.55	0.58
Magnesium %	0.017	0.05	0.058	0.055
Sodium %	0.23	0.7	0.79	0.76
ME (kcal)	1.5/g	4.4/g	5.2/g	4.8/g
	645/can	530/cup		

Discussion

The high fat content and digestibility of the diet increases its caloric density, which reduces the amount of the food and minerals consumed and minerals ex-

creted in the urine. The combination of magnesium and phosphorus restriction and increased sodium content, which increases urine volume, reduces urine concentrations of the "building blocks" for magnesium-ammonium-phosphate (struvite) calculi formation. The diet also results in the maintenance of a urine pH of 5.9 in the absence of urinary tract infection. The hypoconcentrated acid urine allows struvite calculi and crystals to dissolve. These calculi and crystals are responsible for the clinical signs of FUS, which include hematuria and pollakiuria and, in some cases, obstruction. Most supplements will delay or prevent calculi dissolution as they increase urine mineral concentrations and raise urine pH. Because of its increased sodium content, it should not be fed if edema, ascites, or congestion are present. It should not be fed if liver disease or metabolic acidosis are present and it is not recommended during growth, reproduction or for routine adult maintenance. Prescription Diet Feline c/d should be fed for prevention of FUS.

Urine acidifiers are contraindicated when Prescription Diet Feline s/d is being fed. The diet results in the proper urine pH for dissolutin of struvite calculi. Additional acidification can result in metabolic acidosis.

PRESCRIPTION DIET FELINE k/d
Nutritional Characteristics

Protein—moderately restricted
Fat and Carbohydrate—increased
Magnesium, Phosphorus, and Calcium—restricted
Vitamins—increased
Sodium—moderately restricted

Average Nutrient Contents

	As Fed		Dry Matter	
	Canned	Dry	Canned	Dry
Moisture %	72.0	9.0	0	0
Protein %	8.5	26.0	30.4	28.6
Fat %	12.0	25.3	42.9	27.8
Carbohydrate %	6.0	34.7	21.4	38.2
Fiber %	0.2	1.5	0.7	1.6
Ash %	1.3	3.5	4.6	3.8
Calcium %	0.17	0.7	0.6	0.8
Phosphorus %	0.13	0.4	0.46	0.5
Magnesium %	0.02	0.06	0.07	0.07
Sodium %	0.11	0.25	0.40	0.27
ME (kcal)	1.6/g	4.4/g	5.7/g	4.9/g
	680/can	537/cup		
% Protein Calories	21.0	22.1		

Discussion

The combination of animal proteins from liver, meat by-products, and egg form a protein blend with a high biological value. This allows the restriction of the quantity of amino acids consumed in excess of requirements, which reduces the load on the liver for deamination, and on the kidneys for the excretion of nitrogenous wastes. Because of the detrimental effect of excessive phosphorus intake in renal failure, phosphorus is restricted. Animal fat and carbohydrates provide

sufficient calories to meet energy requirements and reduce the utilization of protein for energy. The diet is designed to reduce the metabolic acidosis which commonly occurs with renal failure.

PRESCRIPTION DIET FELINE p/d
Nutritional Characteristics

Protein—increased
Fat—increased
Carbohydrate—reduced
Vitamins—increased
Magnesium—restricted

Average Nutrient Contents

	As Fed		Dry Matter	
	Canned	Dry	Canned	Dry
Moisture %	68.6	9.0	0	0
Protein %	15.7	36.4	50.0	40.0
Fat %	10.0	25.3	31.8	27.8
Carbohydrate %	3.3	22.2	10.5	24.4
Fiber %	0.4	1.2	1.3	1.3
Ash %	2.0	5.9	6.4	6.5
Calcium %	0.33	1.2	1.1	1.3
Phosphorus $	0.28	0.9	0.9	1.0
Magnesium %	0.039	0.09	0.12	0.10
Sodium %	0.15	0.45	0.48	0.49
ME (kcal)	1.6/g	4.4/g	5.1/g	4.9/g
	675/can	535/cup		
% Protein Calories	39.0	30.9		

Discussion

A cat requires twice as much protein as a dog. By using liver, meat by-products, and eggs, a high-quality protein blend results, which furnishes the cat's increased protein need. The energy requirement of the cat during lactation, growth, and recovery from debilitation also is high. Even with the energy supplied by these fresh ingredients, additional fat is added to meet the demand. Cats have high requirements for B-complex vitamins. By using brewer's yeast and vitamins at high levels in the diet, the necessary increases can be met.

Cats have low requirements for minerals, and an excessive amount of magnesium plays a role in the development of feline urological syndrome. Therefore, mineral levels in the diet are adequate to meet needs for reproduction and growth, but below the excessive levels present in many cat foods.

The concentrated nature of a diet suitable for cats also makes it useful in meeting the increased energy needs of small breeds of dogs. It is especially useful during periods of stress such as pregnancy, lactation, and disease when nutrient needs increase, but food intake may be reduced.

PRESCRIPTION DIET FELINE r/d
Nutritional Characteristics

Fat—restricted
Carbohydrate (digestible)—restricted
Fiber—increased
Minerals—restricted

Average Nutrient Contents

	As Fed		Dry Matter	
	Canned	Dry	Canned	Dry
Moisture %	76.6	9.0	0	0
Protein %	8.1	34.6	34.6	38.0
Fat %	2.0	7.5	8.5	8.2
Carbohydrate %	6.8	29.6	29.0	32.5
Fiber %	5.2	16.1	22.2	17.7
Ash %	1.3	3.2	5.6	3.5
Calcium %	0.22	0.61	0.94	0.67
Phosphorus %	0.11	0.50	0.47	0.55
Magnesium %	0.014	0.06	0.06	0.066
Sodium %	0.14	0.2	0.6	0.22
ME (kcal)	0.8/g	2.7/g	3.5/g	3.0/g
	350/can	268/cup		

Discussion

By using low fat meat by-products, liver, and cellulose flour the digestibility of the calories in the diet is reduced and the fiber is increased. Consumption of a high fiber diet tends to satisfy hunger, whereas simply reducing food intake creates a hungry pest. The higher fiber content helps to retain water in the colon, and the bulk stimulates bowel activity, which is helpful in constipation and colitis. The diet is especially designed for obesity and weight control. It is also indicated for the dietary management of diabetes mellitus, where the less digestible carbohydrates minimize fluctuation in blood glucose, and allow reduction and stabilization of insulin dosage. Because of its restricted magnesium content, it can be fed to obese cats with a history of FUS.

PRESCRIPTION DIET FELINE h/d

Nutritional Characteristics

Sodium—restricted
Potassium—increased
Vitamins—increased
Minerals—restricted

Average Nutrient Contents

	Canned	
	As Fed	Dry Matter
Moisture %	70.7	0
Protein %	12.6	43.0
Fat %	7.8	26.6
Carbohydrate %	6.7	22.9
Fiber %	0.5	1.7
Ash %	1.7	5.8
Calcium %	0.24	0.82
Phosphorus %	0.23	0.78
Sodium %	0.07	0.24
Potassium %	0.22	0.75
Magnesium %	0.02	0.07
ME (kcal)	1.4/g	4.7/g
	594/can	

Discussion

Cats suffering from feline cardiomyopathy are quite ill and usually have a depressed appetite. Thus, a so-dium restricted diet must be extremely palatable. The combination of liver and meat by-products is used as a palatable, low sodium protein source. Sodium salts of trace minerals and vitamins are avoided, and no salt is added. Additional potassium is added to compensate for losses caused by cardiac drugs and diuretics. With the sodium restriction supplied by this diet, it is possible to decrease the dosage or eliminate diuretics in many cases.

Other congestive states in the cat, and finicky small dogs, may be managed with this palatable restricted sodium diet.

CONTROL DIETS

Control diets are medicated foods designed to provide optimum nutrition along with specific drug therapy. This allows for the proper nutritional management of the pathologic condition for which the drug is indicated.

HRH

Control Diet HRH is a highly-palatable soft-dry food originally developed for the Armed Forces for the nutritional management of highly stressed and parasitized military working dogs.

Average Drug Contents

Styrylpyridinium Chloride % .... 0.035 (160 mg/lb)
Diethylcarbamazine (as the base) % .... 0.021 (96 mg/lb)

Average Nutrient Contents

	As Fed	Dry Matter
Moisture %	9.0	0
Protein %	28.0	30.8
Fat %	26.5	29.1
Carbohydrate %	26.8	29.4
Fiber %	3.6	4.0
Ash %	6.1	6.7
Calcium %	1.0	1.1
Phosphorus %	0.85	0.9
Sodium %	0.27	0.3
ME (kcal)	4.7/g	5.2/g
	586/cup	

Discussion

HRH is a nutritionally complete, high-calorie medicated diet to provide optimal nutrition for reproduction, exertion, or stress while controlling hookworms and roundworms and preventing heartworms in dogs. The drugs included in the diet have been shown to have no adverse effect on reproduction or physical performance. When fed to adult dogs, food intake should be adjusted to maintain optimal body weight. HRH is designed to be fed continuously during periods of exposure to hookworms, roundworms, and heartworms. The drug diethylcarbamazine prevents the maturation of immature heartworms (third stage infective larvae) into adults. Dogs with heartworms should be converted to a microfilaria-free status before being fed HRH.

APPENDIX TABLE 3

RECIPES FOR HOMEMADE DIETARY FOODS

RECIPE 1
Highly Digestible Diet for Dogs

½ cup farina (113 ml) (Cream of Wheat®) cooked to
   make 2 cups (490 g)
1½ cups (340 g) creamed cottage cheese
  1 large egg (50 g), hard-cooked
  2 T (25 g) brewer's yeast
  3 T (45 g) sugar
  1 T (15 g) vegetable oil
  1 t (5 g) potassium chloride
  1 t (4.5 g) dicalcium phosphate
  1 t (5 g) calcium carbonate

Balanced supplement which fulfills the canine MDR for
  all vitamins and trace minerals.

Cook farina according to package directions including
salt. Cool. Add remaining ingredients to farina and mix
well. Yield: 2.2 lb (980 g).

NUTRIENT CONTENTS		
	As Fed	Dry Matter
Moisture %	75.8	0
Protein %	7.1	29.3
Fat %	3.7	15.3
Carbohydrate %	11.2	46.3
Fiber %	0.1	0.4
Ash %	2.1	8.7
Calcium %	0.33	1.4
Phosphorus %	0.19	0.8
Sodium %	0.16	0.7
Potassium %	0.36	1.5
Copper-mg/kg	1.1	4.6
Copper-mg/kg excluding yeast	0.3	1.1
ME (kcal/lb)	485	2008

RECIPE 2
Restricted Protein/Phosphorus Diet for Dogs

¼ lb (115 g) ground beef (regular)*
1 large egg (50 g), hard-cooked
2 cups (350 g) cooked rice without salt
3 slices (75 g) white bread, crumbled
1 t (5 g) calcium carbonate

Balanced supplement which fulfills the canine MDR for
  all vitamins and trace minerals.

*Do not use lean ground round or chuck.

Braise the meat, retaining fat. Combine all ingredients
and mix well. This mixture is somewhat dry. The palatability can be improved by adding some water (not milk).
Yield: 1¼ lb (595 g).

NUTRIENT CONTENTS		
	As Fed	Dry Matter
Moisture %	65.5	0
Protein %	6.9	20.0
Fat %	5.5	15.9
Carbohydrate %	21.1	61.1
Fiber %	0.01	0.04
Ash %	1.0	2.9
Calcium %	0.36	1.03
Phosphorus %	0.1	0.29
Sodium %	0.1	0.26
Potassium %	0.1	0.27
Magnesium %	0.01	0.04
**ME (kcal/lb)	750	2175

**This diet supplies 17% protein calories, 30% fat calories, and 53%
carbohydrate calories.

RECIPE 3
Restricted Purine/Phosphorus Ultra Low Protein
Diet for Dogs

2½ cups (440 g) cooked rice
  2 T (1 oz/28 g) vegetable oil
  1 large egg (50 g), hard-cooked
  ¼ t (1.25 g) calcium carbonate
  ¼ t (1.25 g) potassium chloride

Balanced supplement which fulfills the canine MDR for
  all vitamins and trace minerals.

Cook rice as per package instructions, except use only
¼ t salt. Add other ingredients and mix well. Yield:
1.1 lb (520 g).

NUTRIENT CONTENTS		
	As Fed	Dry Matter
Moisture %	69.2	0
Protein %	3.0	9.7
Fat %	6.7	21.7
Carbohydrate %	20.5	66.6
Fiber %	0.01	0.03
Ash %	0.6	2.1
Calcium %	0.12	0.39
Phosphorus %	0.07	0.22
Sodium %	0.10	0.32
Potassium %	0.17	0.55
Magnesium %	0.01	0.03
Copper-mg/kg	0.5	1.7
**ME (kcal/lb)	690	2240

**This diet supplies 8% protein calories, 39% fat calories, and 53%
carbohydrate calories.

RECIPE 4
Low Fat Reducing Diet for Dogs

¼ lb (115 g) lean ground beef
½ cup (75 g) cottage cheese, **uncreamed**
2 cups (310 g) carrots, canned solids
2 cups (270 g) green beans, canned solids
1½ t (7 g) dicalcium phosphate

Balanced supplement which fulfills the canine MDR for
  all vitamins and trace minerals.

Cook beef, drain fat, and cool. Add the remaining
ingredients and mix. Yield: 1¾ lb (775 g).

NUTRIENT CONTENTS

	As Fed	Dry Matter
Moisture %	86.4	0
Protein %	5.5	40.4
Fat %	1.7	12.5
Carbohydrate %	4.1	30.1
Fiber %	0.7	5.1
Ash %	1.6	11.8
Calcium %	0.17	1.3
Phosphorus %	0.17	1.3
Sodium %	0.23	1.7
Potassium %	0.14	1.0
ME (kcal/lb)	220	1614

RECIPE 5
Low Sodium Diet for Dogs

¼ lb (115 g) lean ground beef
2 cups (350 g) cooked rice without salt
1 T (15 g) vegetable oil
2 t (9 g) dicalcium phosphate

Balanced supplement which fulfills the canine MDR for
  all vitamins and trace minerals.

Braise meat, retaining fat. Add the remaining ingredients
and mix. Yield: 1.1 lb (490 g).

NUTRIENT CONTENTS

	As Fed	Dry Matter
Moisture %	68.5	0
Protein %	6.3	20.0
Fat %	5.5	17.4
Carbohydrate %	17.6	55.8
Fiber %	0.07	0.22
Ash %	2.0	6.3
Calcium %	0.44	1.4
Phosphorus %	0.44	1.4
Sodium %	0.016	0.052
Sodium, mg/100 kcal ME	11	11
Potassium %	0.44	1.4
ME (kcal/lb)	660	2100

RECIPE 6
Hypoallergenic Diet for Dogs or Cats

¼ lb (115 g) lamb
1 cup (175 g) cooked rice
1 t (5 g) vegetable oil
1½ t (7 g) dicalcium phosphate
⅛ t (0.6 g) potassium chloride

Balanced supplement which fulfills the canine or feline
  MDR for all vitamins and trace minerals.

Combine all ingredients and mix well. Yield: 2/3 lb
(300 g).

NUTRIENT CONTENTS

	As Fed	Dry Matter
Moisture %	66.0	0
Protein %	7.0	20.6
Fat %	10.0	29.4
Carbohydrate %	14.0	41.2
Fiber %	0.06	0.2
Ash %	2.9	8.5
Calcium %	0.53	1.6
Phosphorus %	0.51	1.5
Sodium %	0.24	0.7
Potassium %	0.24	0.70
ME (kcal/lb)	795	2340

RECIPE 7
Liquid Diet for Dogs and Cats

½ can (224 g) Prescription Diet Feline p/d canned
¾ cup (170 ml) water

Blend to smooth consistency in a blender. Strain through
a kitchen strainer (1 mm mesh). Yield: 390 ml.

NUTRIENT CONTENTS

	As Fed	Dry Matter
Moisture %	83.0	0
Protein %	7.4	44.2
Fat %	5.0	29.6
Carbohydrate %	2.8	17.0
Calcium %	0.19	1.1
Phosphorus %	0.13	0.8
Sodium %	0.10	0.6
**ME (kcal)	0.8/ml	4.76/g

**This diet supplies 33% protein calories, 55% fat calories, and 12%
  carbohydrate calories.

Daily dose (dog or cat)—1 oz/lb (60 ml/kg) body weight. Fulfills all
normal fluid and nutrient needs. Excessive fluid losses must be
replaced by additional water or parenteral fluids.

RECIPE 8
Restricted Mineral and Sodium Diet for Cats

1 lb (450 g) regular ground beef, cooked
¼ lb (115 g) liver
1 cup (175 g) cooked rice without added salt
1 t (5 g) vegetable oil
1 t (5 g) calcium carbonate

Balanced supplement which fulfills the feline MDR for all vitamins and trace minerals.

Combine all ingredients. Yield: 1¾ lb (750 g).

NUTRIENT CONTENTS	As Fed	Dry Matter
Moisture %	64.0	0
Protein %	14.3	39.7
Fat %	13.9	38.6
Carbohydrate %	6.3	17.5
Fiber %	0.02	0.06
Ash %	1.4	3.9
Calcium %	0.27	0.75
Phosphorus %	0.16	0.44
Sodium %	0.06	0.16
Potassium %	0.20	0.56
Magnesium %	0.014	0.04
Magnesium, mg/100 kcal ME	7	7
ME (kcal/lb)	940	2610
Taurine %	0.07	0.20

RECIPE 9
Restricted Protein/Phosphorus Diet for Cats

¼ lb (115 g) liver
2 large eggs (100 g), hard-cooked
2 cups (350 g) cooked rice without added salt
1 T (15 g) vegetable oil
1 t (5 g) calcium carbonate
¼ t (1 g) potassium chloride (salt substitute)

Balanced supplement which fulfills the feline MDR for all vitamins and trace minerals.

Dice and braise the liver, retaining fat. Combine all ingredients and mix well. This mixture is somewhat dry and the palatability may be improved by adding some water (not milk). Yield: 1¼ lb (585 g).

NUTRIENT CONTENTS	As Fed	Dry Matter
Moisture %	70.0	0
Protein %	7.3	24.3
Fat %	5.3	17.7
Carbohydrate %	15.8	52.7
Fiber %	0.06	0.2
Ash %	1.5	5.0
Calcium %	0.36	1.20
Phosphorus %	0.14	0.47
Phosphorus, mg/100 kcal ME	100	100
Sodium %	0.05	0.17
Potassium %	0.21	0.70
Magnesium %	0.01	0.04
Magnesium, mg/100 kcal ME	7	7
**ME (kcal/lb)	635	2140
Taurine %	0.03	0.09

**This diet supplies 21% protein calories, 35% fat calories, and 44% carbohydrate calories.

RECIPE 10
Low Fat Reducing Diet for Cats

1¼ lb (565 g) liver, cooked and ground
1 cup (175 g) cooked rice
1 t (5 g) vegetable oil
1 t (5 g) calcium carbonate

Balanced supplement which fulfills the feline MDR for all vitamins and trace minerals.

Combine all ingredients. Yield: 1¾ lbs (750 g).

NUTRIENT CONTENTS	As Fed	Dry Matter
Moisture %	70.0	0
Protein %	15.5	51.7
Fat %	3.4	11.3
Carbohydrate %	9.2	30.7
Fiber %	0.02	0.07
Ash %	1.9	6.3
Calcium %	0.28	0.9
Phosphorus %	0.28	0.9
Sodium %	0.19	0.6
Potassium %	0.22	0.7
Magnesium %	0.012	0.04
Magnesium, mg/100 kcal ME	9	9
ME (kcal/lb)	585	1950
Taurine %	0.03	0.10

APPENDIX TABLE 4

NUTRIENT CONTENTS OF HUMAN FOODS*
(Grams per 100 grams as fed)

Foods	Calories	Moisture	Protein	Fat	Calcium	Phos-phorus	Sodium	Measures**
Meats								
Chicken								
Meat, raw (fryers)	107	77.2	19.3	2.7	0.01	0.20	0.06	
(hens)	155	70.5	21.6	7.0	0.01	0.20	0.06	
Skin, raw	223	66.3	16.1	17.1	0.01	0.17	—	
Giblets, raw	103	78.4	17.5	3.1	0.01	0.22	—	
Necks (ground with bone)	233	64.4	13.2	18.6	0.80	0.50	0.10	
Fish								
Cod, raw	78	81.2	17.6	0.3	0.01	0.19	0.07	
Halibut, raw	100	76.5	20.9	1.2	0.01	0.21	0.05	
Shrimp, raw	91	78.2	18.1	0.8	0.06	0.17	0.14	
Tuna, canned, in oil	288	52.6	24.2	20.5	0.01	0.29	0.80	
in water	127	70.0	28.0	0.8	0.02	0.19	0.04	
Ground Beef, raw, lean	179	68.3	20.7	10.0	0.01	0.19	0.06	
raw, regular	268	60.2	17.9	21.2	0.01	0.16	0.06	
Heart, beef, raw	108	77.5	17.1	3.6	—	0.18	0.09	
Kidney, beef, raw	130	75.9	15.4	6.7	0.01	0.22	0.18	
Lamb, shoulder, raw	265	61.2	15.5	22.0	0.01	0.14	0.08	
Liver, beef, raw	140	69.7	19.9	3.8	0.01	0.35	0.14	
Milk and Egg Products								
Cheese, cottage, creamed	106	78.3	13.6	4.2	0.10	0.15	0.23	1 c = 225g
non-creamed	86	79.0	17.0	0.3	0.09	0.18	0.29	1 c = 145g
cheddar	398	37.0	25.0	32.2	0.75	0.48	0.70	1 in³ = 17g
Egg, whole	163	73.7	12.9	11.5	0.05	0.20	0.12	1 large = 50g
white	51	87.6	10.9	—	0.01	0.15	0.15	from 1 = 33g
yolk	348	51.1	16.0	30.6	0.14	0.57	0.05	from 1 = 17g
Milk, whole	65	87.4	3.5	3.5	0.12	0.09	0.05	1 c = 244g
skimmed	59	90.5	3.6	0.1	0.12	0.10	0.06	1 c = 246g
dried, non-fat	363	3.0	35.9	0.8	1.31	1.02	0.53	1 c = 68 g
Vegetables								
Carrots, canned								
solids and liquid	28	91.8	0.6	0.2	0.02	0.02	0.24	
drained solids	30	91.2	0.8	0.3	0.03	0.02	0.24	1 c = 155g
Green Beans, canned								
solids and liquid	18	93.5	1.0	0.1	0.03	0.02	0.24	
drained solids	24	91.9	1.4	0.2	0.04	0.02	0.24	1 c = 135g
Soybean Flour								
high fat	380	8.0	41.2	12.1	0.24	0.65	tr	
low fat	356	8.0	43.4	6.7	0.26	0.63	tr	
Cereals and Bread								
Bread, white	270	35.6	8.7	3.2	0.08	0.01	0.51	1 slice = 25g
whole wheat	243	36.4	10.5	3.0	0.10	0.23	0.53	1 slice = 28g
Corn, flour	368	12.0	7.8	2.6	0.01	0.16	tr	
meal (whole ground)	362	12.0	9.0	3.4	0.02	0.22	tr	1 c = 122g
flakes (breakfast cereal)	386	3.8	7.9	0.4	0.02	0.04	1.00	1 c = 28g
Macaroni, dry	369	10.4	12.5	1.2	0.03	0.16	tr	
cooked (8-10 min.)	148	63.6	5.0	0.5	0.01	0.06	tr	1 c = 130g
Oatmeal, dry	390	8.3	14.2	7.4	0.05	0.40	tr	
cooked	55	86.5	2.0	1.0	0.01	0.06	0.22	1 c = 240g

APPENDIX TABLE 4—Continued

NUTRIENT CONTENTS OF HUMAN FOODS*
(Grams per 100 grams as fed)

Foods	Calories	Moisture	Protein	Fat	Calcium	Phos-phorus	Sodium	Measures**
Rice, long grain parboiled								
dry	369	10.3	7.4	0.3	0.06	0.2	0.01	1 c = 185g
Rice, cooked with salt	106	73.4	2.1	0.1	0.02	0.06	0.36	1 c = 175g
without salt							0.003	
Wheat, cream of or farina								
dry	371	10.3	11.4	0.9	0.02	0.11	tr	
cooked	42	89.5	1.3	0.1	tr	0.01	0.14	1 c = 245g
flour (whole)	335	12.0	13.3	2.0	0.04	0.37	tr	1 c = 125g
Fats and Oils								
Fat, trimmed from beef	736	15.2	5.2	78.8	tr	0.05	0.06	
Lard	902	0	0	100	0	0	0	1 T = 15g
Margarine	720	15.5	0.6	81	0.02	0.02	0.99	1 T = 15g
Oils—salad or cooking	884	0	0	100	0	0	0	1 T = 15g

Linoleic Acid Content (%)—Beef Fat 1, Lard 10, Margarine 25, Corn Oil 53, Cottonseed Oil 50, Safflower Seed Oil 72, Soybean Oil 52

Foods	Calories	Moisture	Protein	Fat	Calcium	Phos-phorus	Sodium	Measures**
Minerals								
Bone Meal					30	17	0.5	1 t = 4g
Calcium Carbonate,								
ground limestone								
ground eggshell or					39	0.04	0.02	1 t = 5g
Tums® (1 Tab = 0.5g CaCO₃)								
Dicalcium Phosphate					23	19	2.7	1 t = 4g
Salt					0	0	39.3	1 t = 5g
Lite Salt = ½ sodium chloride and ½ potassium								
chloride (29.3% K, 53.4% Cl & 17.3% Na)					0	0	17.3	1 t = 5g
Salt Substitute = potassium chloride (52.3% K & 47.7% Cl)					0	0	0	1 t = 5g

*From Agriculture Handbook No. 8, Composition of Foods, Agriculture Research Service, U.S.D.A. and Home and Garden Bulletin Number 72, Nutritive Value of Foods, Agriculture Research Service, U.S.D.A.

**c = 8 oz volume cup, T = level tablespoon and t = level teaspoon.

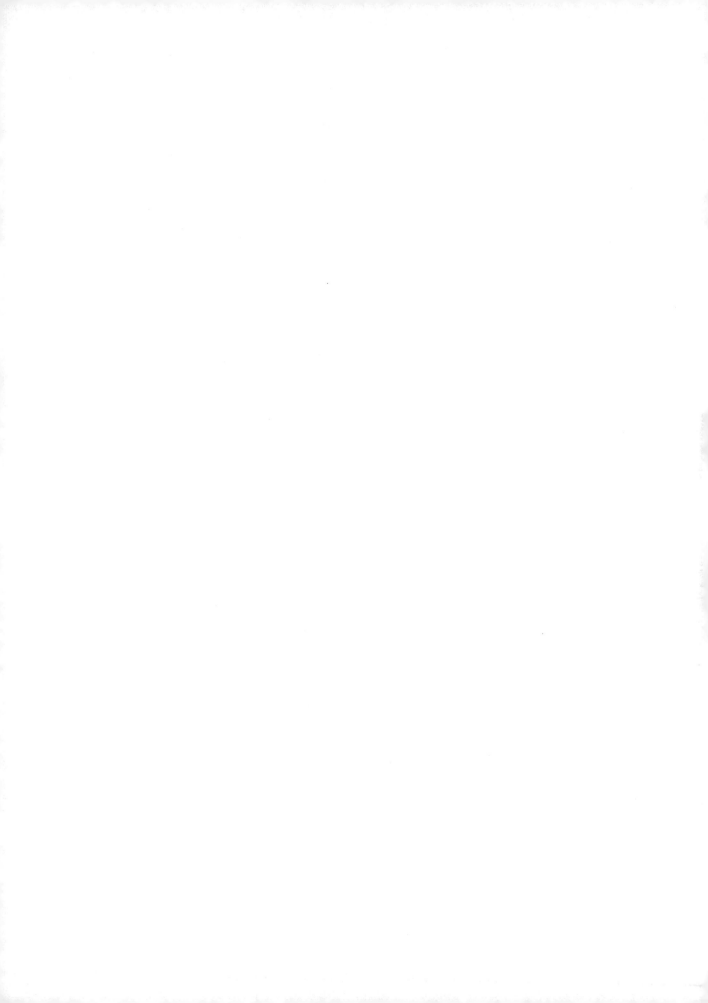

INDEX